CLINICAL ANATOMY

Dr. Ankush Chandra

ALLIED HEALTH PRESS

AF794562

Clinical Anatomy

Author: **Dr. Ankush Chandra**

Allied Health Press
4164 Lakeshore Road
Burlington ON L7L 1A4
Canada
www.alliedhealthpress.com
Email: orders@arclereducation.com

ISBN: 978-1-77956-238-8

ABOUT THE AUTHOR

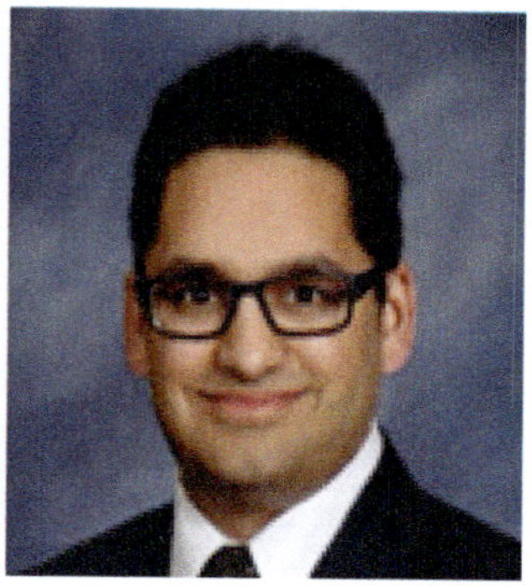

Dr Ankush Chandra, M.D., M.S. born in New York on 19th August 1989, grew up in Boston, Massachusetts, a distinguished neurological surgeon. He has made significant contributions to the field of neuroscience and neurosurgery. Ankush received his Doctor of Medicine (M.D.) degree in Neurological Surgery from Wayne State University School of Medicine, Detroit, Michigan and graduated with honors in Biomedical Research. This accolade was conferred upon him during a special convocation.

Dr Chandra also holds a Master of Science (MS) degree in Medical Sciences from Boston University School of Medicine, Boston, MA, and a Bachelor's degree (BA) in Neuroscience and Biology from Boston University. His academic journey is marked by excellence and dedication, reflected in numerous awards and honors. Ankush's research career began as a Research Fellow at Massachusetts General Hospital (MGH) Harvard University School of Medicine, Boston where he made significant contributions to neuroscience research. He also served as a Research Fellow at Merrimack Pharmaceuticals, Inc. in Cambridge, MA. One of the most notable achievements of Dr Chandra is being awarded the prestigious Howard Hughes Medical Institute (HHMI) Medical Research Fellowship in Neurosurgery at the University of California, San Francisco (UCSF) School of Medicine, spanning from 2016 to 2023. This fellowship is one of the highest honors for a young investigator in the United States. Dr Chandra has received numerous accolades throughout his career, including the Comprehensive Academic Honors, Howard Hughes Medical Institute Medical Research Fellowship (HHMI), AOA Carolyn Kuckein Research Award, AANS Medical Student Research Fellowship, BCBS Michigan Research Award, Ralph Wadley MD Scholarship, BMA Endowed Scholarship, Wayne State Board of Governors Scholarship, Sarah and John Tait Endowed Scholarship for Cancer Research, Robert F. Troxley Award in Biochemistry, Boston University Scarlet Key Award, Commitment to Residence Life Award, Distinction in Neuroscience, and the Summer Undergraduate Research Grant. He is also a member of the prestigious Alpha Omega Alpha (AOA) Medical Honor Society.

He has published more than 100 original research papers in prestigious journals, such as- JAMA Oncology, Lancet Neurology, Proceedings of the National Academy of Sciences (PNAS), Cancer Research, Journal of Neuro-Oncology, Journal of Clinical Investigation (JCI), Journal of Neuroscience, and Journal of Neurosurgery. Additionally, he has edited two volumes of the book titled "Makers of Indian History".

Dr Chandra's early interest in medicine and research was evident during his summer internship in 2007 at the New York-Presbyterian Hospital of Weill Cornell Medical College, where he was trained under the guidance of Prof. Brij B. Saxena in the laboratory of Reproductive Endocrinology, Department of Obstetrics & Gynecology. This experience provided him with a solid foundation in understanding the immunological and molecular mechanisms involved in hypothalamic-pituitary-gonadal regulation and function, after completing his High School with distinction from Springdale's School, New Delhi, India in 2007.

Currently, Dr Ankush Chandra is pursuing a challenging career in Neurological Surgery at McGovern Medical School, University of Texas Health Sciences Center, Houston, Texas. He specializes in glioblastoma and brain surgery, continuing his dedication to advancing medical science and improving patient outcomes.

Dr Ankush Chandra has also served as the President and Captain of the Boston University Cricket Club, Chief Curriculum Officer-Innoworks United Academy at Boston University

Word Roots, Prefixes, and Suffixes by Chapter

Chapter 1 The Structure of the Body – The Systems and Organs

Acous/o-: Hearing

Aden/o-: Gland

-ac: Pertaining to

-ium: a body structure or tissue

cardi-: heart muscle

Chapter 2 The Thoracic Wall, Diaphragm, and Cavity

diaphragmat/o: diaphragm

epiglott/o: epiglottis

nas/o: nose

thorac/o: thorax, chest cavity

Pneumo-: Pneumothorax(air in the thoracic cavity causing lung collapse)

Mediastin-: Mediastinum (the central compartment of the thoracic cavity).

-ectomy: Lobectomy (surgical removal of a lobe of the lung)

Chapter 3 The Mediastinal Structures, Pleura, and Lungs

Phlebo/veno: veins, phlebitis, phlebotomy

pect-: chest

hepat-: hepatocytes (main functional cells of the liver)

-pnea: breathing

-cele: hernia, protrusion

Chapter 4 The Abdomen

laryng/o: larynx

radi/o: x-rays, ionizing radiation

abdom-: the abdomen

adip-: fat/fatty tissue adipocyte (fat cell)

bronch(i)-: the lungs bronchitis (inflammation in the lungs)

-emia: in the blood

-tomy: cut into, incision

Chapter 5 The Pelvis and Perineum

Sacr-: Pertains to the sacrum (bone at the base of the spine).

arthr-, articul-: joints arthritis (inflammation of a joint), articulation (joint between two parts, typically bones)

gastr-: gastroenterology, gastropod

pelv(o)-: Pelvis

-ectomy: Surgical removal.

-rrhaphy: Surgical suturing.

Chapter 6 The Back

Kyph/o: Humpback (posterior curvature of thoracic spine)

Lumb/o: Lower back, lumbar region

myel-: spinal cord

occipit-: back of the head external occipital protuberance

plant-, sole-, tars-: sole of foot plantar flexion, soleus muscle, tarsal bones

-algia: pain, such as neuralgia, meaning nerve pain.

Chapter 7 The Upper Limb

Fibul/o: Lower leg bone

Humer/o: Upper arm bone

Lumb/o: Lumbar region

Cervi: (neck) cervical, cervix

Carp-: Refers to the wrist

Scapul-: Refers to the shoulder blade

Chapter 8 The Lower Limb

Arthr-: Joint

Burs-: Bursa (fluid-filled sac near joints)

Femor-: Femur (thigh bone)

Gon-: Knee

Patell-: Patella (kneecap)

Chapter 9 The Head and Neck

Cephal-: Head Example: Cephalalgia (headache)

Cranio-: Skull Example: Craniotomy (surgical opening of the skull)

Cervic-: Neck Example: Cervical (pertaining to the neck)

Encephal-: Brain Example: Encephalitis (inflammation of the brain)

Faci-: Face Example: Facial (pertaining to the face)

Mandibul-: Mandible (lower jaw)

Chapter 10 The Central Nervous System

cephal/o: Head

Encephal-: Brain Example: Encephalopathy (disease of the brain)

Gli-: Glial cells (supportive cells in the CNS) Example: Glioma (tumor of glial cells)

Mening-: Meninges (membranes covering the brain and spinal cord)

Psych-: Mind Example: Psychiatry (medical specialty dealing with mental disorders)

Hemi-: Half Example: Hemiplegia (paralysis of one side of the body)

Table of Contents

LIST OF FIGURES

LIST OF TABLES

PREFACE

Throughout history, anatomy has consistently been a cornerstone of surgical procedures, providing the fundamental understanding necessary for successful interventions. However, in recent decades, the field of musculoskeletal surgery has witnessed remarkable progress, particularly in minimally invasive techniques. These advancements have revolutionized surgical practices, enabling procedures such as arthroscopy across multiple joints, spinal surgery, and more physiological approaches to major joint arthroplasties, foot and ankle surgery, hand surgery, and beyond.

Minimally invasive surgery, including arthroscopy, has become a preferred method for many orthopedic procedures due to its reduced tissue trauma, faster recovery times, and overall improved patient outcomes. Arthroscopic procedures allow surgeons to visualize, diagnose, and treat joint problems through small incisions, using specialized tools and a tiny camera called an arthroscope. This technique has greatly expanded the scope of what can be accomplished with less invasive means, offering patients less pain, shorter hospital stays, and quicker return to normal activities compared to traditional open surgeries.

In spinal surgery, advancements have led to more precise and less invasive procedures, often performed with the assistance of specialized tools and navigation systems. These innovations have significantly reduced the risk of complications and improved outcomes for patients undergoing spinal interventions.

Similarly, major joint arthroplasties, such as hip and knee replacements, have benefited from more physiological approaches that aim to preserve as much healthy tissue as possible while restoring joint function. This approach has led to improved longevity and functionality of joint replacements, enhancing the quality of life for many patients.

Foot and ankle surgery, as well as hand surgery, have also seen significant advancements in techniques and technologies, allowing for more precise and effective treatments with reduced morbidity and faster recovery times.

The field of musculoskeletal surgery continues to evolve rapidly, driven by innovations in technology, surgical techniques, and a deeper understanding of anatomy and biomechanics. These advancements have not only improved surgical outcomes but also have the potential to further enhance patient care and quality of life in the years to come.

"Clinical Anatomy" serves as a guide laying a robust groundwork for collaborative clinical endeavors, and fostering innovative approaches among researchers, scientists, educators, and healthcare practitioners. It bridges the gap between anatomical advancements and modern

technologies, leveraging tools such as cloud computing, artificial intelligence (AI), the internet of things (IoT), and digital twins to revolutionize medical education, particularly in the era of the COVID-19 pandemic, where traditional methods face constraints.

Augmented reality (AR) emerges as a promising, albeit costly, solution offering personalized instruction and virtual preparation for medical procedures, enhancing spatial understanding and facilitating deeper anatomical insights. It represents a new frontier in medical education, enriching learning experiences and expanding diagnostic capabilities. Furthermore, advancements in technology enable enhanced visualization and diagnosis of normal and pathological conditions, significantly impacting clinical practice by integrating morphological and clinical perspectives, thereby revolutionizing patient care and health outcomes. The book provides a comprehensive and authoritative resource for healthcare professionals looking to enhance their knowledge and clinical skills in this field.

Chapter

1

THE STRUCTURE OF THE BODY – THE SYSTEMS AND ORGANS

Contents

Introduction

The foundation of medical education is clinical anatomy, which gives medical professionals a comprehensive understanding of the composition and operation of the human body. Fundamentally, clinical anatomy explores how the body is organized, including all of its systems and organs. The human body is a complex organism made up of various systems that cooperate to support life. The musculoskeletal system, respiratory system, digestive system, urinary system, reproductive system, nervous system, and endocrine system are some of these systems. Specialized organs, tissues, and cells, each with distinct roles and functions, make up each system. When diagnosing and treating medical conditions, healthcare professionals must have a thorough understanding of the anatomy and physiology of these systems and organs. A thorough analysis of the connections between anatomical structures and their applicability to clinical practice can be found in clinical anatomy. It helps medical practitioners to precisely navigate the human body, spot anomalies, decipher test results, and create efficient treatment regimens. Clinical anatomy lays the groundwork for excellence in medical practice by thoroughly examining the body's structure as well as its complex systems and organs. This ensures that medical professionals have the knowledge and abilities needed to give patients the best care possible. The body's organs and systems are made up of neural, muscular, connective, and epithelial tissues.

Orientation and Directional Terms

Term	Definition	Illustration
Human Body	Human body is a complex, highly organized structure made up of unique cells that work together to accomplish the specific functions necessary for sustaining life.	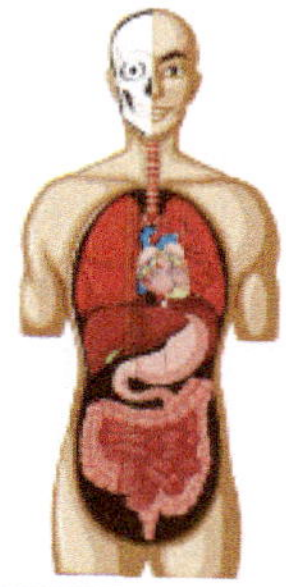
Epithelial Tissue	Epithelial tissues are widespread throughout the body. They form the covering of all body surfaces, line body cavities and hollow organs, and are the major tissue in glands. They perform a variety of functions that include protection, secretion, absorption, excretion, filtration, diffusion, and sensory reception.	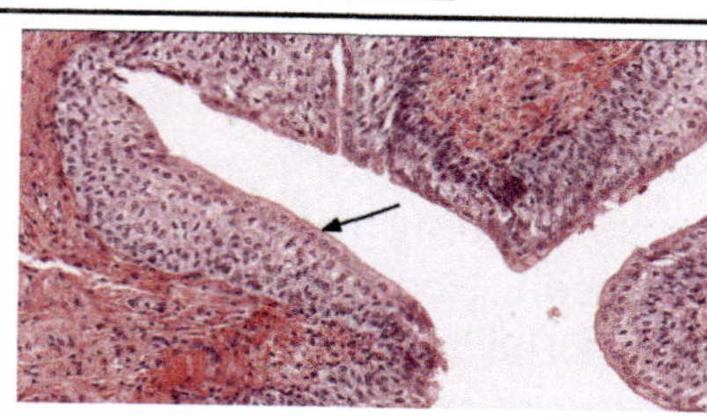
Reproductive System	Reproductive system of an organism, also known as the genital system, is the biological system made up of all the anatomical organs involved in sexual reproduction. Many non-living substances such as fluids, hormones, and pheromones are also important accessories to the reproductive system.	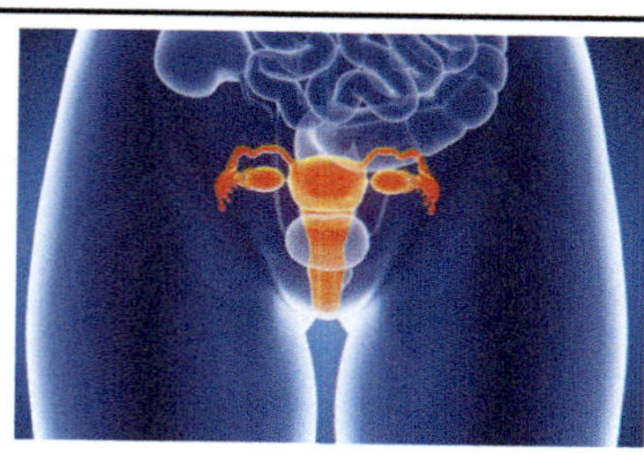
Areolar Tissue	Areolar Tissue is a type of loose connective tissue that consists of a meshwork of collagen, elastic tissue, and reticular fibres - with many connective tissue cells in between the meshwork of fibers.	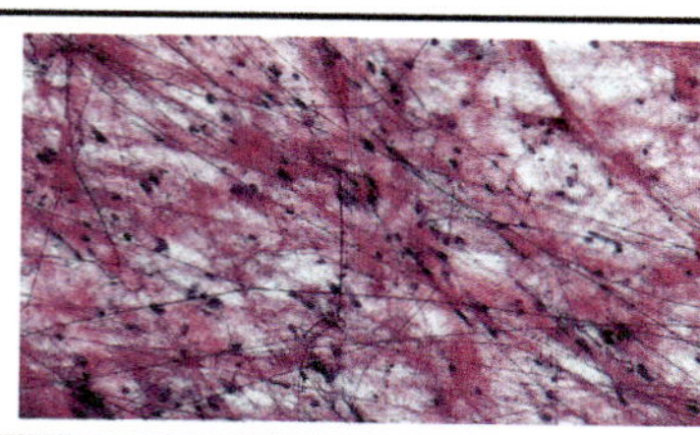
Hyaline Cartilage	Hyaline cartilage is the glass-like (hyaline) and translucent cartilage found on many joint surfaces. It is also most commonly found in the ribs, nose, larynx, and trachea.	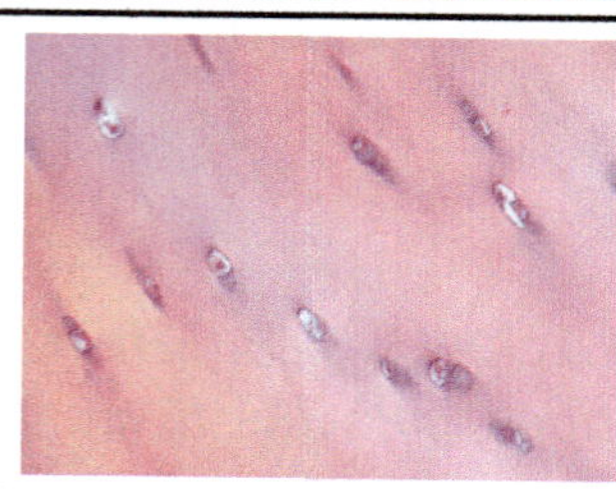

1.1. Epithelial Tissue

The epithelium covers the body's external and internal surfaces to provide protection. It originates from each of the three early embryonic layers. The skin is formed by the ectoderm, the gut and blood vessel endothelium by the mesoderm, and the pleura, pericardium, and peritoneum by the endoderm. Since they arise from the invagination of an epithelial surface, the majority of glands have an epithelial origin. Epithelium is impervious to dehydration's effects as well as physical and chemical harm. It can function as a barrier that is selective and resistant to chemicals, bacteria, and hazardous metabolites. It is distinguished by having very little intercellular material and a propensity to form sheets of cells with one or more layers that can be continuously replaced. It could be stratified, simple, or transitional.

1.1.1. Simple Epithelium

A single layer of cells on top of a basement membrane makes up this structure. Its cell shape determines whether it is referred to as columnar, cuboidal, or squamous (paving). Squamous cells can be seen lining the blood vessels (endothelium), the serous cavities (mesothelium), and the lungs' alveoli. Numerous glands have ducts lined with cuboidal cells. Columnar cells line a large portion of the respiratory, alimentary, and reproductive tracts. They are frequently ciliated and can be altered to become mucus-forming goblet cells. A glycoprotein called mucus builds up inside the cell and is released from its free (luminal) surface (Figure 1.1).

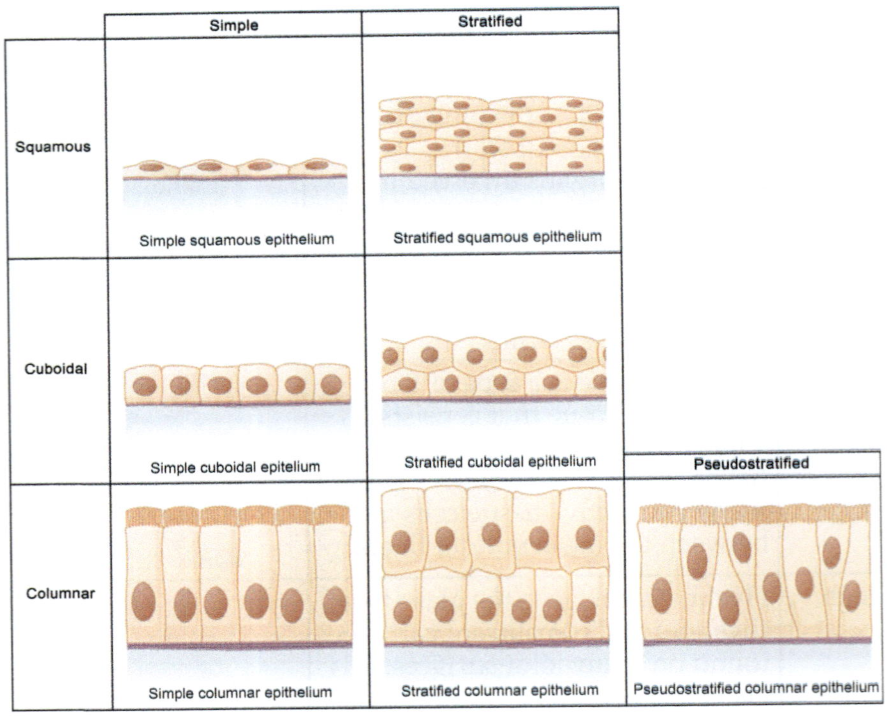

Figure 1.1. *Cells of Epithelial Tissue. Simple epithelial tissue is organized as a single layer of cells and stratified epithelial tissue is formed by several layers of cells.*

Source: https://courses.lumenlearning.com/suny-ap1/chapter/epithelial-tissue/.

1.1.2. Transitional Epithelium

This is made up of two or three layers of nucleated cells, the majority of which are adhered to the basement membrane. It is flexible, does not desquamate, and lines the majority of the urinary tract. Its gland count is small.

1.1.3. Stratified Squamous Epithelium

This likewise has two or more cell layers. Columnar cells are those in which the basement membrane comes into contact. The surface cells lack nuclei (enucleate) and are constantly being rubbed away, while the more superficial cells are flattened (desquamated). The skin, both ends of the gastrointestinal tract, and areas of the body subjected to abrasion are covered by this type of epithelium. The upper respiratory tract's pseudostratified columnar epithelium, which is made up of a large number of mucous cells, appears as a double layer due to the varying lengths of the columnar cells.

1.1.4. Skin

There are two layers to this: the inner dermis (corium) and the outer epidermis. Squamous epithelium that is stratified and keratinized makes up the epidermis. The epidermis is modified by sweat and sebaceous glands, hair follicles, and nails. Melanocytes, the pigment-producing cells found in the basal layer of the epidermis, and blood flow both affect skin color. The primary component of the skin's surface scales is keratin, a fibrous protein rich in sulfur that is primarily in charge of the skin's barrier and protective qualities. The dermis is a layer of vascular connective tissue that is firmly molded to the epidermis and eventually blends into the subcutaneous tissues at a deeper level. The coiled tubular sweat glands that open onto the skin's surface and hair follicles are located in the dermis. The arrector pili muscle is attached to each of these follicles. The subcutaneous tissue is home to the sweat gland and hair roots.

1.1.5. Mucous and Serous Membranes

These are made up of two layers: an epithelium and a corium, and they border the body's moist interior surfaces. The mucous membrane epithelium is typically of a simple type with a large number of mucous or serous cells; however, transitional epithelium lines the urinary tract, while pseudostratified columnar ciliated epithelium with mucous cells lines the respiratory tract. The majority of the closed body cavities are lined with serous membranes. The connective tissue-based corium sits beneath the epithelium. The muscularis mucosa, a thin layer of smooth muscle, lines the digestive tract (Figure 1.2).

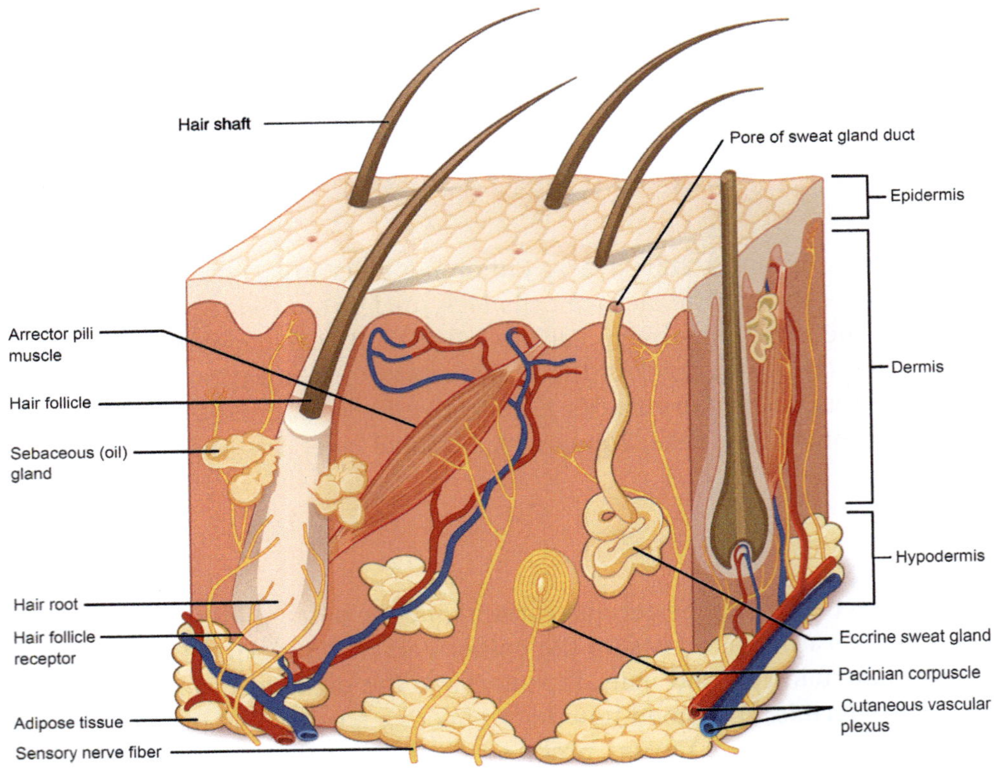

Figure 1.2. *Diagram of a cross-section through the skin.*

Source: https://commons.wikimedia.org/wiki/File:501_Structure_of_the_skin.jpg.

1.1.6. Glands

These are modified epithelial ingrowths with secretory functions. These secretions can enter the bloodstream through endocrine glands or travel to the epithelial surface through exocrine glands. Exocrine glands can have multiple cells or just one (a goblet). The latter can be either simple, with just one duct, or complex, with many smaller ducts opening up into one main duct. The gland's secretory portion can be intermediate, such as tubuloalveolar, globular (acinar), oval (alveolar), or long and thin (tubular). Exocrine gland secretions can be produced by the disintegration of the entire cell (holocrine, such as sebaceous glands), the disintegration of the cell's free end (apocrine, e.g., mammary glands), or in the case of most other glands (merocrine or eccrine, for example) without causing cellular damage. The majority of glands in the body are endocrine. When an exocrine gland's duct gets clogged and the gland keeps secreting, the fluid builds up and forms a cyst. The term "adenopathy" refers to a widespread enlargement of the glands (Moore, Dalley & Agur, 2014; Agur & Lee, 2017; Drake, Vogl, & Mitchell, 2019).

1.2. Connective Tissue

This is distinguished by having a high content of material between cells. It creates blood, cartilage, bone, and areolar tissue, which serve as the body's packing material. Mesenchyme refers to the connective tissue found in embryos.

1.2.1. Areolar Tissue

The semisolid intercellular material consists of proteins and mucopolysaccharides. There are three different types of fibers: reticular fibers, which form a very fine network of silver-staining throughout the tissues; elastic fibers, which are yellowish in bulk, less frequent, and arranged in bundles; and coarse collagen fibers, which are white in bulk, flexible, inelastic, and arranged in bundles (Figure 1.3).

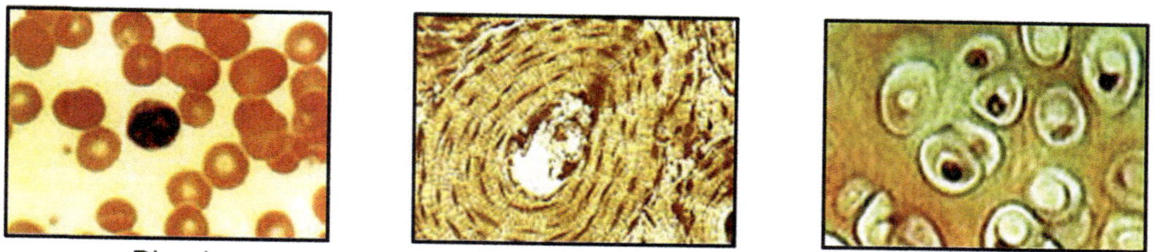

Figure 1.3. *Connective tissue.*

Source: Public Domain; https://commons.wikimedia.org/w/index.php?curid=1394212.

The cells can be classified into five main types: oval plasma cells with their cartwheel-shaped staining nucleus, which are involved in the production of antibodies; granular basophilic mast cells, which are involved in the production of histamine and heparin; large, slender, poorly staining fibroblasts, which are closely concerned with the production of the three types of tissue fiber; and tissue macrophages, which are phagocytic and can engulf particulate matter. The body is composed of different proportions of intercellular and cellular material. Loose fibrous tissue and varying amounts of fat are found in subcutaneous tissue. Fat typically predominates on the surface, but deeper down, fibrous tissue connects to the deep fascia that invests the limbs and trunk to form a distinct superficial fascial sheet. Ligaments, tendons, aponeuroses, and retinacula are formed in different locations by condensations of non-elastic fibrous tissue. Aponeuroses are thin, flattened tendinous sheets through which muscles gain wider attachments. Ligaments are typically attached to the bones on either side of a joint, maintaining its stability. Tendons connect the muscles to the bones by blending with the periosteum. Retinacula are typically thickenings of the joint-related deep fascia (Moore, Dalley & Agur, 2014; Agur & Lee, 2017; Drake, Vogl, & Mitchell, 2019).

1.3. Supporting Tissue

1.3.1. Cartilage

This is a firm, avascular tissue made up of cells called chondrocytes surrounded by a copious amount of intercellular matrix. It is composed of the perichondrium, an underlying fibrous layer, and is divided into hyaline cartilage, fibrocartilage, and yellow elastic cartilage based on the predominant fibers in each (Figure 1.4).

- Hyaline cartilage contains many cells, a few fine collagen-like fibers, and is found in the rib cartilages and over most articular surfaces. It also forms the precursor in cartilaginous ossification.

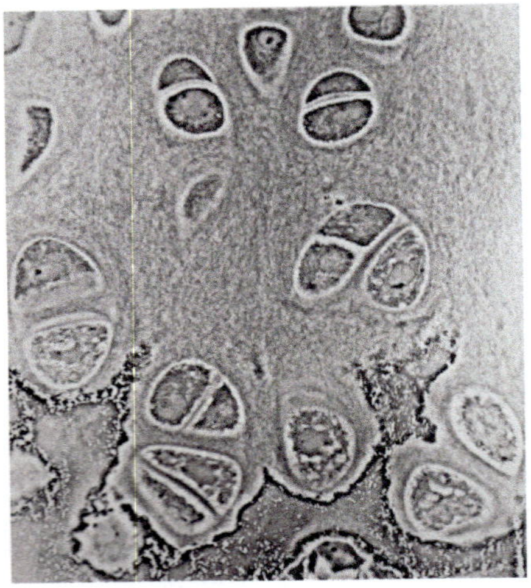

Figure 1.4. *Hyaline cartilage.*

Source: By Robert M. Hunt – Own work, Public Domain; https://commons.wikimedia.org/w/index.php?curid=9543639.

- Fibrocartilage is found in intra-articular cartilages such as the menisci of the knee and over the articular surface of bones that ossify in membranes, such as the mandible, as well as intervertebral discs. It is composed of many dense fibrous bundles and fewer cells.
- Elastic fibers are present in yellow elastic cartilage, which is located in the head's auricular, epiglottic, and arytenoid cartilage apices.

1.3.2. Bone

This is a strong supporting tissue made mostly of an impregnated network of collagen fibers by inorganic calcium salts. A Haversian system is the fundamental component, consisting of concentric layers encircling a central vessel. Osteocytes, or bone cells, are found in the gaps (lacunae) between the layers, and the processes of these cells enter the canaliculi of the bone. The outermost portion of most bones is made of compact bone, which is robust and dense. The osteocytes are located within lacunae in the network of thin partitions, or trabeculae, that surround intercommunicating spaces that make up the cancellous (spongy) bone. A thick layer of fibrous tissue called the periosteum covers the outside of a bone. Many of the cells in this layer are the granular osteoblasts that form new bone. These cells develop into osteocytes when they are encased in the hard intercellular substance. The periosteum, muscle vessels, and, in the case of long bones, one or two nutrient arteries that enter the shaft provide blood to the bone.

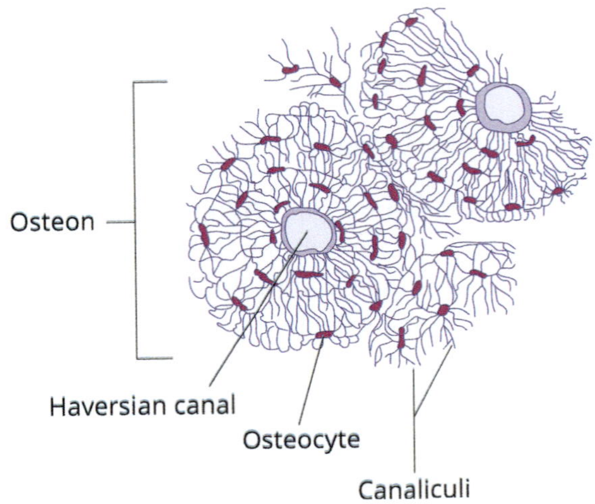

Figure 1.5. *Haversian bony systems with osteoblasts in circular layers with central canals carrying nutrient vessels.*

Source: By Source digital bitmap graphics: BDB recreated in vector format: Nyq – Original analog graphics: Gray's anatomy of the human body from the classic 1918 publication available online at Bartleby.com. Digital bitmap graphics: Transverse section of Bone.png recreated in vector format: Own work, CC BY-SA 4.0; https://commons.wikimedia.org/w/index.php?curid=50064939.

The architecture of the trabeculae, the ratio of compact to cancellous tissue, and the shape of the body's bones are all designed to provide maximum strength and material economy. A bone's size and form are influenced by both local and genetic factors. The bone is somewhat shaped by the muscles or organs that are nearby, such as the brain. With the use of X-rays, many of these factors can be examined in a living individual. There are several types of bones: sesamoid, long, short, flat, and irregular. Long bones are present in the limbs. The body (shaft) is a cylinder of compact bone surrounding a medullary cavity which is filled with some cancellous bone and a large amount of yellow fatty marrow (Figure 1.5).

Spongy bone makes up the two ends, which have a thin layer of compact bone covering them. The lines of force determine how the trabeculae in the cancellous bone are arranged. A child's growing long bone contains blood-forming tissue, which is not typically present in an adult's bone marrow. The tarsus and carpus contain the short bones. They are made of porous bone that is lightly coated in compact bone (Figure 1.6).

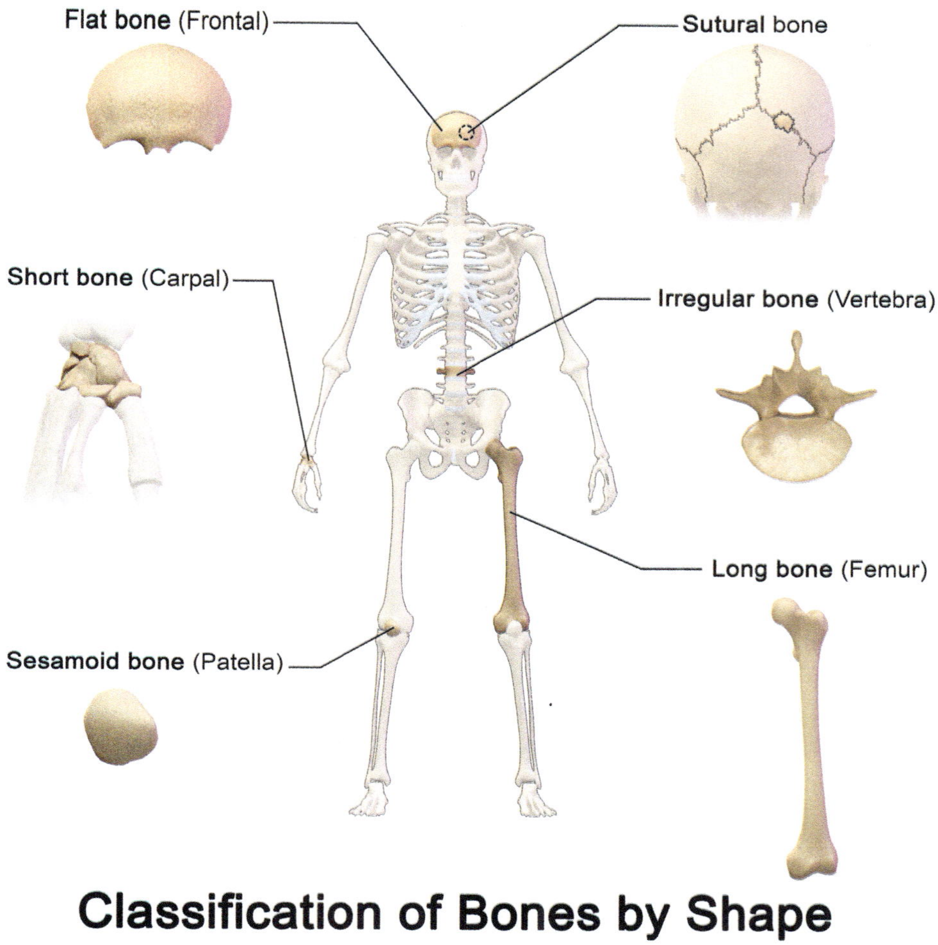

Figure 1.6. *Bone types by shape.*

Source: By BruceBlaus - Own work, CC BY 3.0; https://commons.wikimedia.org/w/index.php?curid=29849179.

The flat bones, such as the scapula, serve as a protective covering and point of attachment for muscles (the skull vault's bones). They are made up of two compact bone layers separated by a thin layer of spongy tissue (the dipole in the skull). Sesamoid bones, which are produced inside tendons, help to reduce friction and change a muscle's pull direction. The patella is the largest sesamoid bone. The remaining atypical bones might have air spaces (sinuses) or red, blood-forming marrow (the vertebrae) (Figure 1.7).

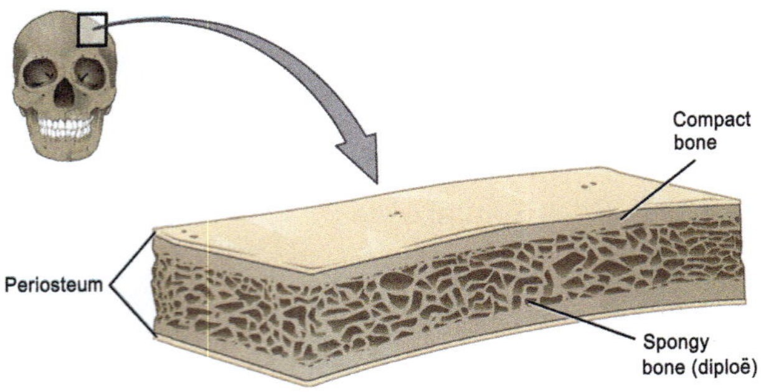

Figure 1.7. *Pneumatized bone, for example, the skull sinuses around the nasal cavity.*

Source: By OpenStax College - Anatomy and Physiology, Connexions Web site. http://cnx.org/content/col11496/1.6/, CC BY 3.0; https://commons.wikimedia.org/w/index.php?curid=30131423.

A bone may break (fracture) as a result of excessive force applied to it; in such cases, the force and the broken ends of the bone may injure the surrounding soft tissues. Understanding the anatomical relationships between the bone and injury allows the clinician to anticipate the likelihood that a fracture will result from damage to the nerve, artery, and muscle. Since it allows pathogenic organisms to enter, a break in the skin covering a fracture site is a serious consequence. The fracture is considered compound under these conditions. A bone may fracture if an excessive amount of force is applied to it; in these cases, the force and the broken ends of the bone may injure the surrounding soft tissues (Figure 1.8).

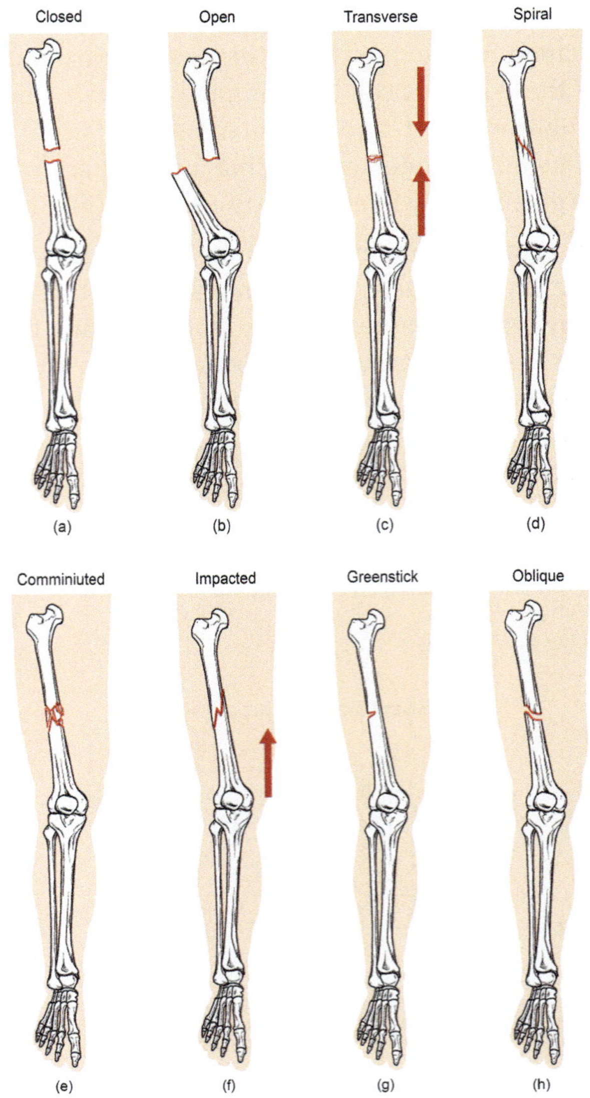

Figure 1.8. *Types of Fracture.*

Source: By OpenStax College - Anatomy and Physiology, Connexions Web site. http://cnx.org/content/col11496/1.6/, CC BY 4.0; https://commons.wikimedia.org/w/index.php?curid=30127535.

1.3.3. Ossification

In a condensed fibrous tissue model, the process of bone formation is known as membranous (mesenchymal) ossification; in a cartilage model, where the mesenchyme has been replaced, the process is known as cartilaginous (endochondral) ossification. Mesenchymal ossification, which is present in the bones of the face, clavicle, and skull vault, typically begins in the fifth or sixth week of intrauterine life. With the exception of the clavicle, all long bones experience cartilaginous ossification. About the eighth week of intrauterine life is when the primary center for the body of a long bone appears, and between birth and puberty, secondary centers for each end appear. For males, the fusion of the body and these centers happens around the age of 18. In females, secondary centers can form and fuse up to a year earlier. During puberty, additional ossification centers may form in major muscle attachment sites, such as the crests of the scapula and hip, as well as the processes of the vertebrae. About the 25th year, they fuse with the rest of the bone.

1.3.4. Development of a Long Bone

A cartilaginous model with an outer perichondrium and an irregular cartilaginous matrix gives rise to a long bone; the deep layers of the perichondrium can form new bone (Figure 1.9).

The middle of the body's cartilage cells (the diaphysis) undergo the initial alterations. Their enlargement results in a corresponding reduction and calcification of the matrix. The spaces left by the dying and shrinking cells are referred to as primary alveoli. The periosteum is the term for the deeper layer of perichondrium that forms bone around the midline of the body. From the periosteum to the calcified zone, blood vessels and bone cells—the osteoblasts that form bone and the osteoclasts that remove it—pass inward.

Instead of being changed into bone, the cartilage is replaced with it when the osteoclasts remove it. Larger spaces known as secondary alveoli are created when the calcified material is absorbed by the multinucleated osteoclasts. Layers of bone are deposited and osteoblasts line the secondary alveoli.

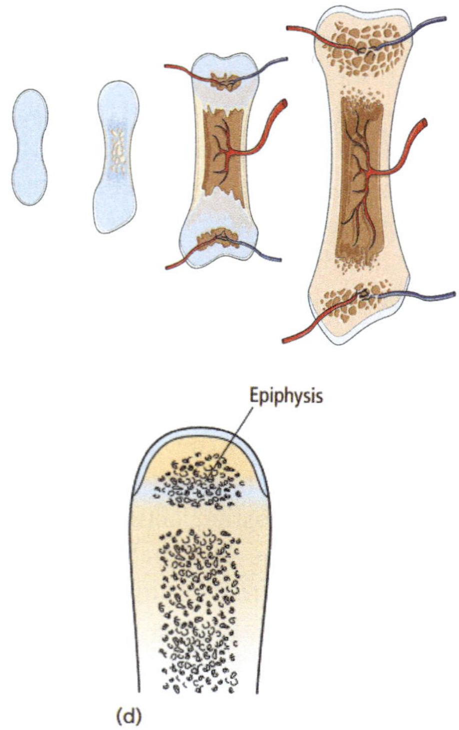

Figure 1.9. *Ossification of a long bone. The ossification starts in the shaft of the bone usually within uterine life. Secondary centers start in the epiphysis, one end often preceding the other, and appear after puberty.*

Source: By Laboratoires Servier – Smart Servier website: Images related to bone growth, skeleton and bones, and bones – Download in PowerPoint format. Flickr: Images related to bone growth, skeleton and bones, and bones (in French), CC BY-SA 3.0; https://commons.wikimedia.org/w/index.php?curid=82681289.

A portion of osteoblasts integrates into the bone to form osteocytes or bone cells. Ossification radiates from this main center throughout the body. After aligning themselves into parallel longitudinal rows, the neighboring cartilage cells are replaced in the previously mentioned way. This form of ossification is known as endochondral (cartilaginous) (Moore, Dalley & Agur, 2014; Agur & Lee, 2017; Drake, Vogl, & Mitchell, 2019).

The epiphyses, which are secondary centers of ossification, develop later in life. After the cells have experienced hypertrophy, death, and shrinkage, osteogenic cells infiltrate the calcified cartilage. The epiphyseal plate is the layer of cartilage that remains between the diaphysis and the epiphysis. The cartilage next to the metaphysis is continuously ossifying; the metaphysis is the portion of the diaphysis that borders the plate. The epiphyseal plate is where new cartilage cells are created. The diaphysis and epiphysis fuse after the cartilage cells cease to proliferate, at which point the bone continues to grow longer. Both osteoclastic and osteoblastic activity remodel the internal architecture of the bone. Subperiosteal ossification, a kind of mesenchymal ossification, is the simultaneous laying down of bone layers by the periosteum around the body. This process increases the girth of the bone. Up until adulthood, the bone continues to grow and change as a result of osteoclasts' constant destruction and osteoblasts' constant replacement.

Three types of epiphyses can be distinguished: "atavistic" epiphyses, which are defunct skeletal remnants that may appear on an X-ray and be misinterpreted for illness or damage; pressure epiphyses, which are found at the ends of weight-bearing bones; and traction epiphyses, which are found at the site of muscle attachments. Before puberty, the majority of epiphyseal centers and most primary ossification centers of long bones typically emerge by the end of the second month of intrauterine life. The knee joint epiphyses, which show the age of the fetus, develop shortly before birth. For the most part, long bones stop growing in length between the ages of 18 and 20 in men and around 1 year earlier in women.

1.3.5. The Skeleton

An axial portion (the bones of the head and trunk) and an appendicular part (the bones of the limbs) make up the skeleton. The mobile muscular pectoral girdle connects the upper limb to the trunk, while the stable bony pelvic girdle connects the lower limb to the trunk (Moore, Dalley & Agur, 2014; Agur & Lee, 2017; Drake, Vogl, & Mitchell, 2019).

1.4. Joints

These are unions between two or more bones and may be of four types: bony, fibrous, cartilaginous, or synovial.

1.4.1. Bony

The three elements of the hip bone are joined by bony union, as are the occipital and the sphenoid in the skull after the completion of the second dentition (Figure 1.10).

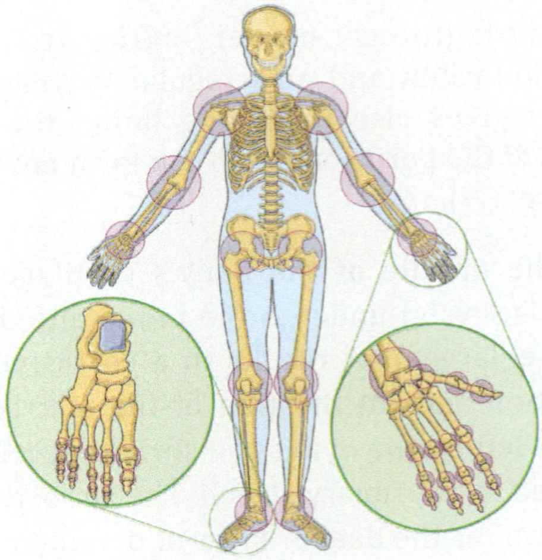

Figure 1.10. *Bony joints.*

Source: By Laboratoires Servier – Smart Servier website: Images related to joints, skeleton and bones, and bones – Download in PowerPoint format. Flickr: Images related to joints, skeleton and bones, and bones (in French), CC BY-SA 3.0; https://commons.wikimedia.org/w/index.php?curid=82641187.

1.4.2. Fibrous

Fibrous tissue connects the bony surfaces. These include the inferior tibiofibular joint, the articulations of the tooth roots, and the sutures in the skull (Table 1.1).

Table 1.1. *Comparison Among Different Published Sensor Technologies for Monitoring Joints*

Types of Sensor/ Technology	Monitored Joint Parameters *	Measure	Method of Analysis	Advantages	Limitations	References
Optical fiber sensors	Angle	Attenuation of the transmitted optical signal power.	Using the relation between the attenuation and the bending angle of the fiber.	• High resolution. • Flexibility. • Light-weight. • Long term reliability. • Immunity to electromagnetic interference.	• Limited measurement range (angle). • Nonlinearity. • Sensitive to temperature and humidity.	[Pinet, É.; et al. 2007, Bilro, L.; et al. 2011, Stupar, D.Z.; et al. 2012, Babchenko, A.; et al. 2007]
Optical-based goniometer.	Angle	Planar motion of an optical navigation sensor.	Detecting navigation of the sensor using a miniature camera to calculate the bending of the joint.	• Compact and light-weight. • Flexibility. • High accuracy. • High speed of reaction.	• Sensitive to placement location. • May hinder natural joint movement during operation. • 3D sensing may not be possible.	[Donno, M.; et al. 2008, Lim, C.K.; et al. 2010, Vimal, A.K.; et al. 2015]
Imaging and video-based tracking system.	Angle, motion, skeletal tracking.	Visual data of several human actions.	Skeletal tracking using anthropometric constraints and known joint locations in reference videos **	• High accuracy and sensitivity. • Able to capture movements of multiple joints at a time. • No body-worn sensors are needed.	• Complex procedure with expensive infrastructure and sophisticated analyses. • Limited coverage area. • Requires body markers and adequate lighting condition for accurate measurements. • Unreliable to differentiate between near and far parts of human body, and for postures having self-occlusions ***	[Mobini, A.; et al. 2014, Wang, Z.; et al. 2017, Gritai, A.; et al. 2006, Islam, M.U.; et al. 2017, Jalal, A.; et al. 2017, Abiddin, W.Z.; et al. 2016]

Textile-based conductive wire sensors.	Angle	Changes of resistance	Changes of resistance are directly proportional to joint angles.	• Comfortable and suitable for long-term monitoring. • Simple mechanism. • One-time calibration. • Low-cost.	• Low resolution. • Low accuracy. • Nonlinearity. • Material uncertainties and hysteresis.	[Gibbs, P.T.; et al. 2005]
Textile-based flex sensors	Angle	Changes of resistance	Changes of resistance are directly proportional to joint angles.	• Flexibility and stretchability. • Easily attachable with comfortable garments. • Low-cost.	• Fragile and lower lifetime (prone to be damaged due to numerous bending). • Low accuracy with noisy signal. • Nonlinearity. • Sensors are wide and affixing multiple sensors on the supportive garments is not feasible.	[Bergmann, J.H.M.; et al. 2013, Bakhshi, S.; et al. 2011, Gioberto, G. 2014, Totaro, M.; et al. 2017, Zhang, H.; et al. 2018]
Textile-based strain sensors	Angle, motion, and rotation	Changes of resistance	Changes of resistance are directly proportional to joint angles and motion.	• Flexibility and stretchability. • High sensitivity. • Low-cost.	• Performance degradation due to large mechanical strains and rigorous deformations. • Signal drift due to the viscoelasticity of materials. • Limited to sense movements in the sagittal plane.	[Jeong, S.-M.; et al. 2018, Park, S.; et al. 2019, Wang, C.; et al. 2017, Zheng, Y.; et al. 2018, Ryu, S.; et al. 2015]
Piezoresistive sensors – chopped carbon fiber (CCF)/ polydimethylsiloxane (PDMS) yarns.	Motion	Changes of resistance	Variation of relative resistance under mechanical deformation due to joint movements.	• Flexibility. • High sensitivity. • Easy integration into textile structures.	• Nonlinearity. • Material uncertainties and hysteresis. • Applying higher strain may cause piezoresistive performance (i.e., sensitivity) decay and delays the piezo resistivity transition.	[Montazerian, H.;et al. 2019]

Smartphone sensors – accelerometer, gyroscope, magnetometer, and camera.	Angle, motion	Acceleration, inclination, and camera measurements.	Using smartphone applications to gather inbuilt sensors and camera data for measuring the range of motion.	• No external sensors are needed. • No external communication and data processing module are needed. • Applications are easy to implement.	• Lower accuracy comparing to other external sensors-based applications. • Difficult to place smartphones around different body joints. • Unable to monitor complex joint movements. • No standardized testing procedures are reported for clinical application.	[Støve, M.P.; et al. 2018, Jenny, J.-Y.; et al. 2016, Vohralik, S.L.; et al. 2015, Milanese, S.; et al. 2014, Johnson, L.B.; et al. 2015, Majumder, S.; et al. 2019]
Acoustic emission (AE) sensors – piezoelectric-films/ MEMS-based microphones.	Angle, motion	High-frequency sound signal occurring during joint motion.	Changes of surface resistance due to acoustic emission.	• Low-cost. • Light-weight. • Easy to attach around different body joints.	• High background and interface noise. • Nonlinearity. • Low accuracy.	[Feng, G.-H.; et al. 2016, Browne, M.; et al. 2016, Toreyin, H.; et al. 2016, Teague, C.N.; et al. 2016 Teague, C.N.; et al. 2017]
Gyroscope	Angle	Three axes angular rate	Joint angle is calculated by comparing the angular rate between two calibrated gyroscopes (below and above the joint).	• Small size. • Low-cost. • Light-weight. • High resolution. • Easy to attach around different body joints.	• Produces some large drift over time. • Complex algorithms are needed to reduce noise and drift error. • At least two sensors are needed to measure accurate angle.	[Sudin, S.B. et al. 2012]
Magnetometer	Angle, motion	Change of magnetic field.	Change of magnetic field is directly proportional to joint motion.	• Feasible to measure complex joint angles. • Easy to control with digital circuits.	• Interference in the magnetic field by ferromagnetic and EMF-producing objects in the environment may decrease the accuracy of measurement.	[Friedman, N.; et al. 2014]

					• Unreliable for detecting the orientations of joints in a 3D environment.	
Inertial measurement unit (IMU) sensors – accelerometer, gyroscope, and magnetometer.	Angle, motion, skeletal tracking.	Three-dimensional acceleration, angular rate and the magnetic field vector.	Three-dimensional angular velocities and linear accelerations are used to detect the position and orientation. Relative data from two calibrated IMUs are compared for tracking the joint angle and gait analysis.	• A combination of three sensors (accelerometer, gyroscope, and magnetometer). • Compact and light-weight. • Small size. • Low-cost. • High resolution. • High accuracy. • Easy to attach around different body joints. • Built-in wireless module. • Built-in algorithms in new generation IMU sensors for calibration and to fix the sensors' orientation with respect to a global fixed coordinate system. • Reliable for detecting the position and orientations of joints in a 3D environment.	• Sensor's alignment is required in a multiple IMUs-based joint monitoring system. • Drift error from gyroscope (possible to compensate by fusing data from accelerometer and gyroscope).	[Seel, T.; et al. 2014, Bakhshi, S.; et al. 2011, Favre, J.; et al. 2008, Crews, D.J. et al. 2017, Castañeda, J.J.; et al. 2017, Vargas-Valencia, L.; et al. 2016, Favre, J.; et al. 2009, Seel, T.; et al. 2013, El-Gohary, M.; et al. 2008, Salehi, S.; et al. 2015, Bonnet, V.; et al. 2016, Ribeiro, N.F.; et al. 2017, Yost Labs 2013, Masdar, A.; et al. 2013, Pathirana, P.N.; et al. 2018, Karatsidis, A.; et al. 2018, Ahmadi, A.; et al. 2016, Wang, X.; et al. 2016, Kim, J.N.J.; et al. 2018, Hung, L.-P.; et al. 2018, Matula, T. 2016]

Source: Faisal, A. I., Majumder, S., Mondal, T., Cowan, D., Naseh, S., & Deen, M. J., (2019). Monitoring methods of human body joints: State-of-the-art and research challenges. Sensors, 19(11), 2629. https://doi.org/10.3390/s19112629.

*Joint angle: The angle between the two segments on either side of the joint; joint motion: the combination of the angle and the orientation of the joint; and skeletal tracking: a technique to build a skeletal model of a human body by detecting the joint positions.

** Anthropometric constraints: Size, shape, and composition of the human body.

*** Self-occlusion: One part of an object is occluded by another part from a certain viewpoint.

1.4.3. Cartilaginous

They could be intermediate or main. As in the union of the body and ends in a growing long bone, hyaline cartilage unites the bony surfaces in the primary cartilaginous joints.

A fibrocartilaginous disc connects the bony surfaces of the symphyses, secondary cartilaginous joints, which are covered in hyaline cartilage. The symphysis pubis, the manubriosternal and xiphisternal junctions, and the intervertebral discs are among these midline joints.

1.4.4. Synovial

Hyaline cartilage covers the bony articular surfaces (facets) of the joints (except the temporomandibular and sternoclavicular joints, which are covered in fibrocartilage). A fibrous capsule is connected close to the bone's articular margins. The delicate vascular synovial membrane that lines the interior surfaces of the joint, with the exception of those covered by cartilage, secretes a lubricating synovial fluid into the joint cavity (Figure 1.11).

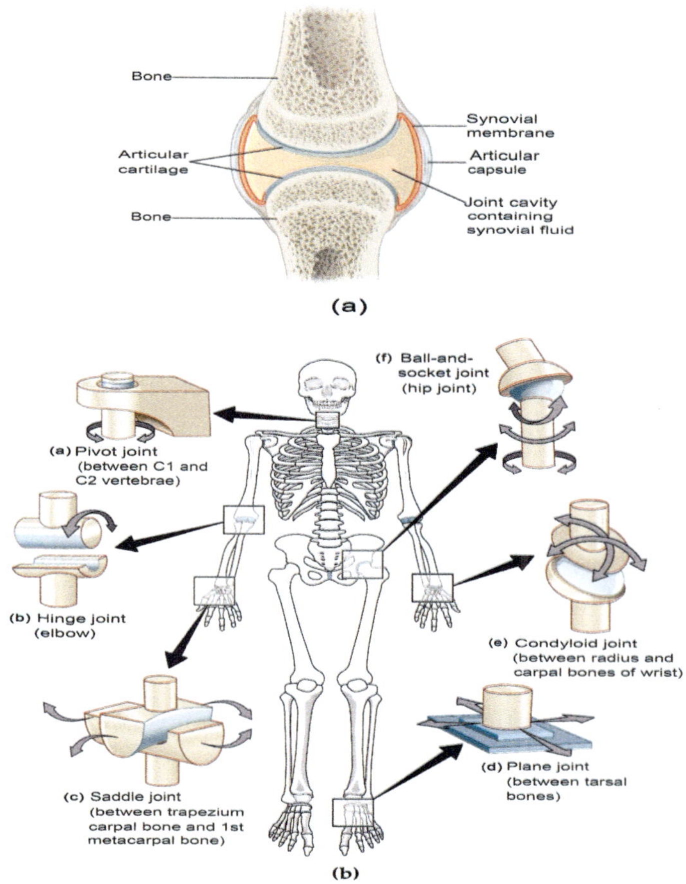

Figure 1.11. *Synovial joints.*

Source: Faisal, A. I., Majumder, S., Mondal, T., Cowan, D., Naseh, S., & Deen, M. J., (2019). Monitoring methods of human body joints: State-of-the-art and research challenges. Sensors, 19(11), 2629. https://doi.org/10.3390/s19112629.

Ligamentous thickenings may be present in the capsule, and there is a possibility that extracapsular and intracapsular auxiliary ligaments will cross the joint. Certain joints have fibrous intra-articular discs that can occasionally split the joint's cavity in half (temporomandibular joint, for example). Sometimes a tendon pierces the capsule (biceps brachii) to enter the joint cavity, and there may be fat pads between the capsule and the synovial lining (knee joint). Synovial sheaths or sacs, whose fluid reduces friction, may shield muscles or tendons that cross the joint superficially. Bursae are the name for the sacs, and there may be communication between the cavity and the joint.

1.4.5. Functional Aspects of Joints

1.4.5.1. Movement

While synovial joints move freely, bone, fibrous, and primary cartilaginous joints are immobile, and secondary cartilaginous joints are only slightly mobile. The different types of synovial joints are classified based on the range of motions that are possible at the joint. The best way to understand these varieties—which are listed below—is to look at the examples provided (Figures 1.12 and 1.13; Table 1.2):

- **Hinge** – elbow, ankle and interphalangeal joints, the knee and temporomandibular joints are modified hinge joints.
- **Pivot** – the proximal radioulnar joint and the dens articulation of the atlantoaxial joint.
- **Condyloid** – metacarpophalangeal joint.
- **Ellipsoid** – radiocarpal (wrist) joint.
- **Saddle** – carpometacarpal joint of the thumb.
- **Ball and Socket** – hip and shoulder joints.
- **Plane** – intercarpal joints and joints between the articular processes of adjacent vertebrae.

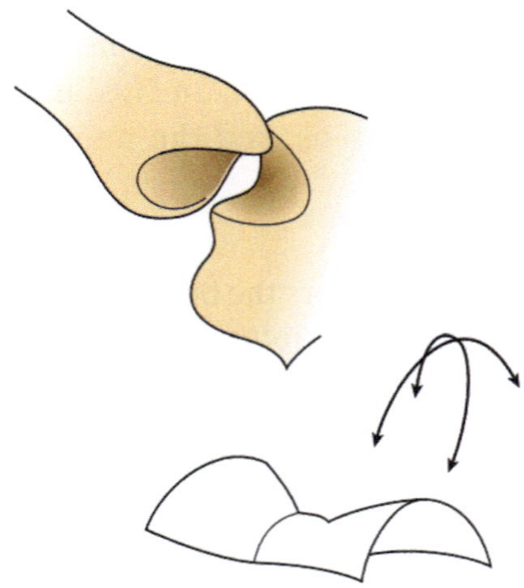

Figure 1.12. *Saddle joint. The carpometacarpal joint of the thumb is shaped like the saddle of a horse where the rider can slide off from side to side as well as move backwards and forwards.*

Source: http://repository.stikesrspadgs.ac.id/62/1/Illustrated%20Clinical%20Anatomy-402hlm.pdf.

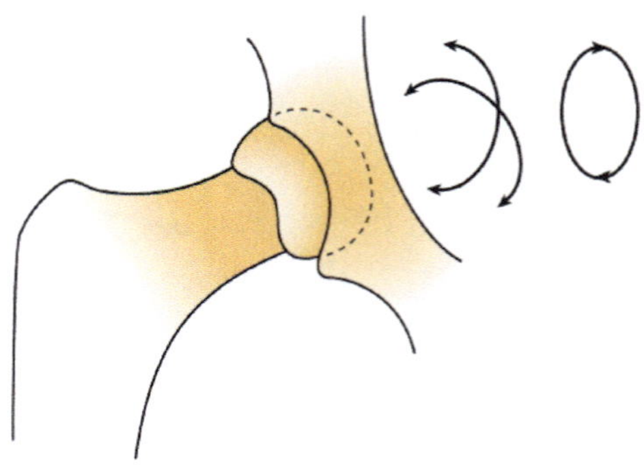

Figure 1.13. *Ball and socket joint, for example, the hip. The hip joint has all the movements of the condyloid joint and in addition the head can rotate within the socket, i.e., additional medial and lateral rotation.*

Source: http://repository.stikesrspadgs.ac.id/62/1/Illustrated%20Clinical%20Anatomy-402hlm.pdf.

Table 1.2. *Joint Movements: Active Range of Motion (ROM) (°) for Human Joints by Gender and Age*

Age		2-8 Years		9-19 Years		20-44 Years		45-69 Years	
		Females (39)	**Males (55)**	**Females (56)**	**Males (48)**	**Females (143)**	**Males (114)**	**Females (123)**	**Males (96)**
Joint motion	Hip extension	26.2 (23.9–28.5)	28.3 (27.2–29.4)	20.5 (18.6–22.4)	18.2 (16.6–19.8)	18.1 (17.0–19.2)	17.4 (16.3–18.5)	16.7 (15.5–17.9)	13.5 (12.5–14.5)
	Hip flexion	140.8 (139.2–142.4)	131.1 (129.4–132.8)	134.9 (133.0–136.8)	135.2 (133.0–137.4)	133.8 (132.5–135.1)	130.4 (129.0–131.8)	130.8 (129.2–132.4)	127.2 (125.7–128.7)
	Knee flexion	152.6 (151.2–154.0)	147.8 (146.6–149.0)	142.3 (140.8–143.8)	142.2 (140.4–144.0)	141.9 (140.9–142.9)	137.7 (136.5–138.9)	137.8 (136.5–139.1)	132.9 (131.6–134.2)
	Knee extension	5.4 (3.9–6.9)	1.6 (0.9–2.3)	2.4 (1.5–3.3)	1.8 (0.9–2.7)	1.6 (1.1–2.1)	1.0 (0.6–1.4)	1.2 (0.7–1.7)	0.5 (0.1–0.9)
	Ankle dorsiflexion	24.8 (22.5–27.1)	22.8 (21.3–24.3)	17.3 (15.6–19.0)	16.3 (14.9–17.7)	13.8 (12.9–14.7)	12.7 (11.6–13.8)	11.6 (10.6–12.6)	11.9 (10.9–12.9)
	Ankle plantar flexion	67.1 (64.8–69.4)	55.8 (54.4–57.2)	57.3 (54.8–59.8)	52.8 (50.8–54.8)	62.1 (60.6–63.6)	54.6 (53.2–56.0)	56.5 (55.0–58.0)	49.4 (47.7–51.1)
	Shoulder flexion	178.6 (176.9–180.3)	177.8 (176.7–178.9)	171.8 (169.8–173.8)	170.9 (169.1–172.7)	172.0 (170.9–173.1)	168.8 (167.3–170.3)	168.1 (166.7–169.5)	164.0 (162.3–165.7)
	Elbow flexion	152.9 (151.5–154.3)	151.4 (150.8–152.0)	149.7 (148.5–150.9)	148.3 (146.8–149.8)	150.0 (149.1–150.9)	144.6 (143.6–145.6)	148.3 (147.3–149.3)	143.5 (142.3–144.7)
	Elbow extension	6.8 (5.2–8.4)	2.2 (0.9–3.5)	6.4 (4.7–8.1)	5.3 (3.6–7.0)	4.7 (3.9–5.5)	0.8 (0.1–1.5)	3.6 (2.6–4.6)	-0.7 (-1.5-0.1)
	Elbow pronation	84.6 (82.8–86.4)	79.6 (78.8–80.4)	81.2 (79.6–82.8)	79.8 (77.8–81.8)	82.0 (81.0–83.0)	76.9 (75.6–78.2)	80.8 (79.7–81.9)	77.7 (76.5–78.9)
	Elbow supination	93.7 (91.4–96.0)	86.4 (85.3–87.5)	90.0 (88.0–92.0)	87.8 (85.7–89.9)	90.6 (89.2–92.0)	85.0 (83.8–86.2)	87.2 (86.0–88.4)	82.4 (80.9–83.9)

Source: Faisal, A. I., Majumder, S., Mondal, T., Cowan, D., Naseh, S., & Deen, M. J., (2019). Monitoring methods of human body joints: State-of-the-art and research challenges. Sensors, 19(11), 2629. https://doi.org/10.3390/s19112629.

1.4.5.2. Stability

Muscular, ligamentous, and bony components all contribute to stability. They typically have an inverse relationship with the joint's mobility. Radiology can evaluate many of these functional aspects of joints. Dislocation is the displacement of a joint's articulating surfaces. Subluxation is the term for a partial displacement of the articulating surfaces. A severe injury may be followed by a dislocation, which is always accompanied by damage to the accessory and capsular ligaments.

In addition, fractures of the joint's osseous components and sporadic injury to nearby nerves and blood vessels are possible. Chronic inflammatory processes can damage the synovial membrane (rheumatoid arthritis) and the ends of bones (osteoarthritis). As a result, affected joints may be painful, deformed, and have a significant range of motion.

1.4.5.3. Nerve Supply

Pain, proprioceptive, and stretch fibers are found in the capsule and ligaments of a joint; these fibers provide information about the joint's position and any abnormal forces. A joint receives its nerve supply from the nerves that supply the muscles that use the joint (Moore, Dalley & Agur, 2014; Agur & Lee, 2017; Drake, Vogl, & Mitchell, 2019).

1.5. Muscular Tissue

This is a contractile tissue. There are skeletal, smooth and cardiac varieties.

1.5.1. Skeletal (Striated, Voluntary) Muscle

This forms certain sphincters and primarily acts as a diaphragm or on the bony skeleton. It is also present in the vicinity of the larynx and pharynx. It is made up of numerous nuclei and unbranched sarcoplasmic fibers that are confined by the sarcolemma membrane. Every fiber has a motor endplate and numerous myofibrils, which are contractile units with alternating bands of light (I) and dark (A). The Z disc, a dark line, passes through the center of the I band. The striated appearance of the muscle fiber is caused by the coincidence of bands between neighboring myofibrils. Fibrous endomysium envelops each fiber and attaches it to its neighbor; fibrous perimysium encloses bundles of fibers. A muscle with numerous bundles is encircled by an epimysium (Figure 1.14).

The motor nuclei of the brain stem and the anterior horn cells of the spinal cord supply the motor nerves that power the muscles. In addition to the more basic touch and pain endings, the sensory supply also originates in the more specialized spindles and tendon organs. Sensory endings send impulses into the spinal cord's posterior horn. Voluntary fibers form the structure of skeletal muscles. The periosteum, either directly or through tendons and aponeuroses, attaches the muscles to the bone at each end. The muscles then cross one or more joints. Sometimes two muscles come together at a common, stretchable union called a raphe, such as the mylohyoid muscles. A very rich blood supply nourishes muscles. Pennate muscles are made up of muscle fibers that are arranged either obliquely to the direction of the action or parallel to it (sartorius). Oblique fibers are inserted into one side of a tendon (extensor digitorum longus) in unipennate muscles. Oblique fibers are inserted into the rectus femoris tendon on both sides of bipennate muscles. A multipennate muscle is either circular with a central tendon (tibialis anterior) or has several parallel bipennate tendons (deltoid). An oblique arrangement of fibers produces more power but less movement in muscles with equal volumes than a parallel arrangement. A muscle's origin is often referred to as its least mobile attachment, and its insertion as its most mobile attachment. However, since this is a subjective differentiation, the text refers to muscle attachments rather than origin or insertion. An aponeurosis, which is observed in the muscles of the abdominal wall, is a thin, flat tendinous expansion that offers a wide attachment (Figure 1.15).

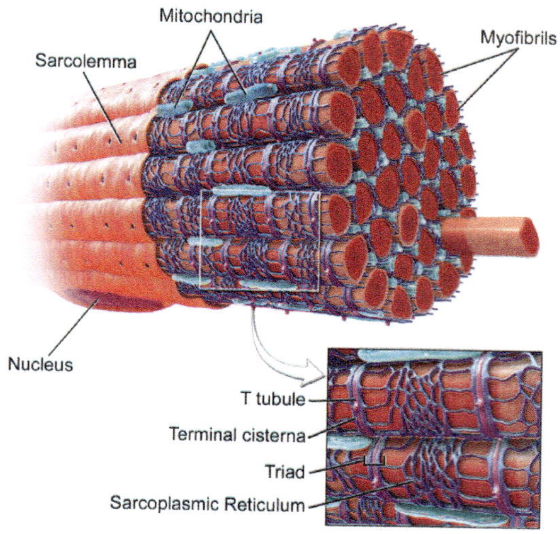

Figure 1.14. *Muscle fibers of striated muscle. The strands of myosin and actin interlock during muscle contraction in a similar fashion to Velcro.*

Source: By BruceBlaus. When using this image in external sources it can be cited as: Blausen.com staff (2014). "Medical gallery of Blausen Medical (2014)." Wiki Journal of Medicine, 1(2). doi: 10.15347/wjm/2014.010. ISSN: 2002-4436. Own work, CC BY 3.0; https://commons.wikimedia.org/w/index.php?curid=29452230.

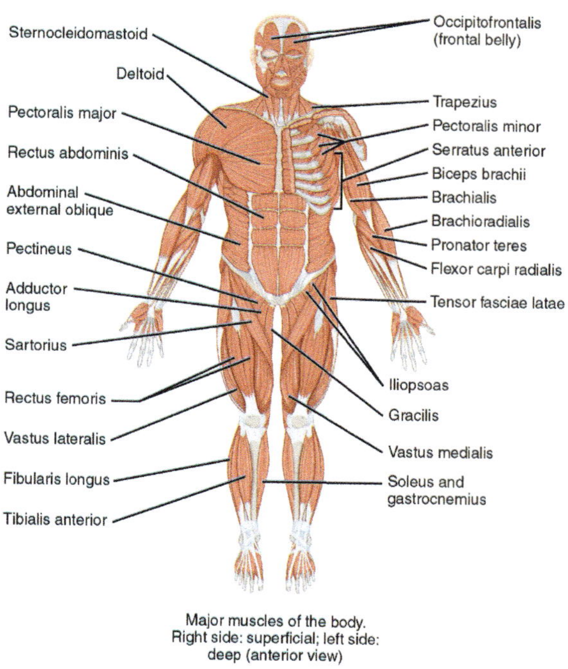

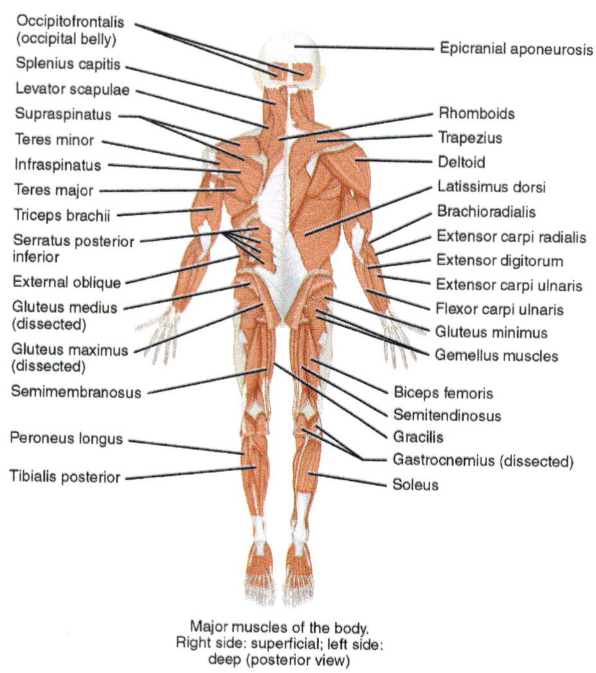

Figure 1.15. *Muscles.*

Source: https://courses.lumenlearning.com/suny-dutchess-ap1/chapter/the-muscular-system/.

The muscles involved in generating a movement at a joint are referred to as the prime movers, or agonists, and the muscles opposing the movement, or antagonists. Synergists are muscles that contract to stabilize the joint that is being moved across. Another kind of movement is called a paradoxical action, where a muscle progressively relaxes against the force of gravity. An example of this would be bending forward, which is caused by relaxing the back muscles.

1.5.2. Smooth (Unstriated, Involuntary) Muscle

This is found in the walls of the majority of the body's hollow organs and vessels. It has many unstriated myofibrils and is made up of unbranched, spindle-shaped cells with a single central nucleus. The autonomic nervous system supplies the fibers, which are arranged in interlocking bundles (Figure 1.16).

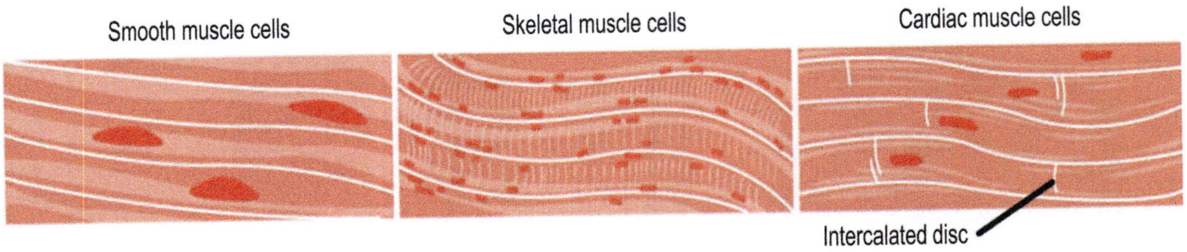

Figure 1.16. *Smooth muscle fibers contained within a loose muscle bundle; cardiac muscle showing the striations of striated muscle and branching, producing a continuous network of muscle.*

Source: https://courses.lumenlearning.com/suny-dutchess-ap1/chapter/the-muscular-system/.

1.5.3. Cardiac Muscle

The heart contains this. It is made up of short, cylindrical fibers that are joined end to end and branched. Dark intercalated discs are created by the adherent ends of neighboring fibers. Each fiber has striated myofibrils that resemble voluntary muscle fibers and a single central nucleus. The autonomic nervous system supplies it, but the heart muscle also possesses the ability to contract spontaneously and rhythmically. Modified cardiac muscle cells make up the heart's conducting system (Moore, Dalley & Agur, 2014; Agur & Lee, 2017; Drake, Vogl, & Mitchell, 2019).

1.6. Nervous Tissue

Both conductivity and excitability are possible with this. It is made up of excitable cells (neurons) and supporting cells, known as Schwann cells in the peripheral nervous system and neuroglial cells in the central nervous system (Figure 1.17).

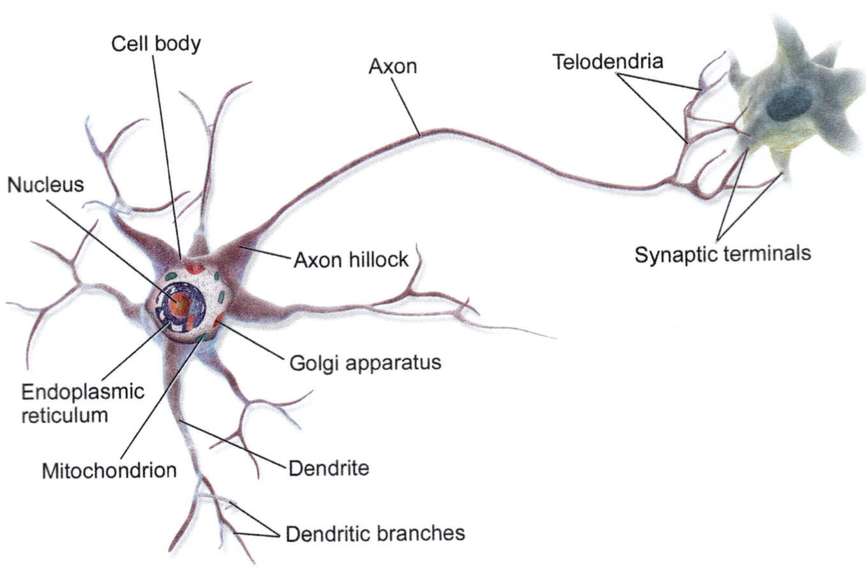

Figure 1.17. *Neuron.*

Source: By BruceBlaus – Own work, CC BY 3.0; https://commons.wikimedia.org/w/index.php?curid=28761830.

The neuron, which is the nervous system's functional unit, is made up of an axon and one or more dendrites as well as a cell body. The cell bodies are located in the peripheral ganglia or the central nervous system. They have distinct cellular inclusions and a sizable nucleus. The impulses are carried away from the cell body by the axon (fiber), which starts at a tiny axon hillock on the cell body. This frequently lengthy, thin process terminates by splitting into numerous branches, each of which has a small bouton—a terminal knob connected to the cell body or branch of another neuron. A synapse is a relationship that can be either facilitatory or inhibitory, depending on the original neuron and possibly the second neuron's receptor area. When a nerve terminates at a motor endplate on a muscle fiber, a highly specialized synapse is created.

Short collateral branches can emerge from axons in one or more instances. They can either be myelinated or not. Known as the node of Ranvier, these constrictions sever the myelin approximately every millimeter. All internodal segments of the sheath in the peripheral nervous system are produced by Schwann cells, the surface of which contains the nucleus. In peripheral nerve regeneration, these cells are crucial. An additional thin fibrous membrane covering peripheral nervous system fibers is called a neurilemma. Schwann cells are replaced in the central nervous system by oligodendroglia. Usually, dendrites are brief, unsynapsed processes that transport depolarizations of the membrane to the cell body. The term dendritic field refers to the area that a single cell's dendrites stretch.

Instructions are carried out by efferent neurons away from the central nervous system, and information is carried by afferent neurons towards it. Many intercalated (also known as intermediate or internuncial) neurons frequently connect afferent and efferent neurons within the central nervous system. The central and peripheral nervous systems are made up of the arrangement of neurons. The cranial nerves, spinal nerves, and autonomic nervous system are included in the latter, while the brain and spinal cord are included in the former. A collection of neurons is referred to as a ganglion outside the central nervous system (CNS) and as a nucleus inside the CNS. Neuroglial cells, also referred to as astrocytes, oligodendroglia, and microglia, comprise nearly half of the brain's mass and are found within the central nervous system.

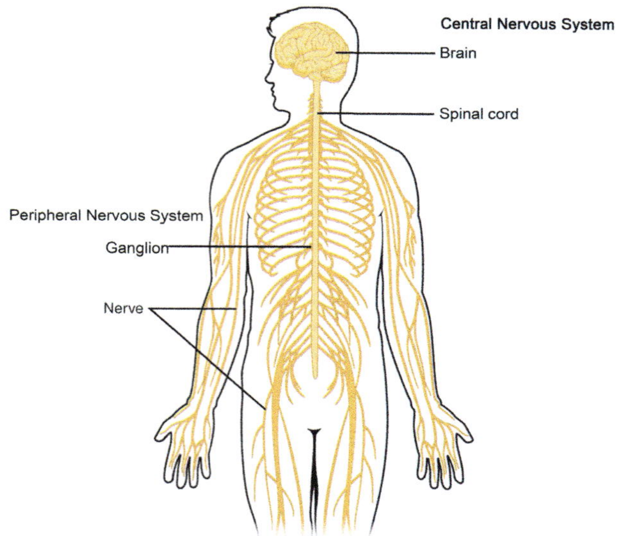

Figure 1.18. *Brain and spinal cord.*

Source: By OpenStax – https://cnx.org/contents/FPtK1zmh@8.25:fEI3C8Ot@10/Preface, CC BY 4.0; https://commons.wikimedia.org/w/index.php?curid=30147907.

Astrocytes are stellate cells with large nuclei and multiple processes. They can be either thin fibrous type, which is primarily found in the white matter, or thick protoplasmic type, which is primarily found in the gray matter. It is believed that the astrocytes are involved in the nutrition of the neurons and the fluid balance in the central nervous system. Some of the processes terminate in blood vessels. Oval cells that stain darkly and have few processes are called oligodendroglia. They are the ones who make the central nervous system's myelin. A component of the macrophage system, microglia are tiny, mobile phagocytic cells (Figure 1.18).

The cavities of the brain and spinal cord are lined with columnar-shaped ependymal cells. Cerebrospinal fluid is produced by the brain's choroid plexuses, which are formed by modifications to the ependyma in specific regions.

1.6.1. Cranial Nerves

Around 12 pairs of nerves are attached to the brain. Some are mainly sensory, some are mainly motor, and others are mixed sensory and motor.

1.6.2. Spinal Nerves

Within the vertebral canal, each of the 31 paired spinal nerves—eight cervical, 12 thoracic, five lumbar, five sacral, and one coccygeal—is formed by the union of a ventral and a dorsal root. The anterolateral and posterolateral spinal cord sulci give rise to several rootlets, which eventually form the roots. Afferent (sensory) fibers are carried to the cord by the dorsal root, and efferent (motor) fibers are carried out of the cord by the ventral root. Located in a ganglion on the dorsal root are the cell bodies of the sensory fibers. As a result, the spinal nerves are a combination of sensory and motor fibers. An intervertebral foramen allows each nerve to exit the vertebral canal. From there, it quickly splits into a larger ventral and a smaller dorsal ramus (branch).

While the adjacent ventral rami of the thoracic region become the intercostal and subcostal nerves, those of the majority of regions communicate to form plexuses (cervical, brachial, and lumbosacral). The dorsal rami split into medial and lateral branches after passing backward into the postvertebral muscles. These rami do not provide branches to the limbs, but they do supply the muscles and skin over the posterior aspect of the body (Figure 1.19).

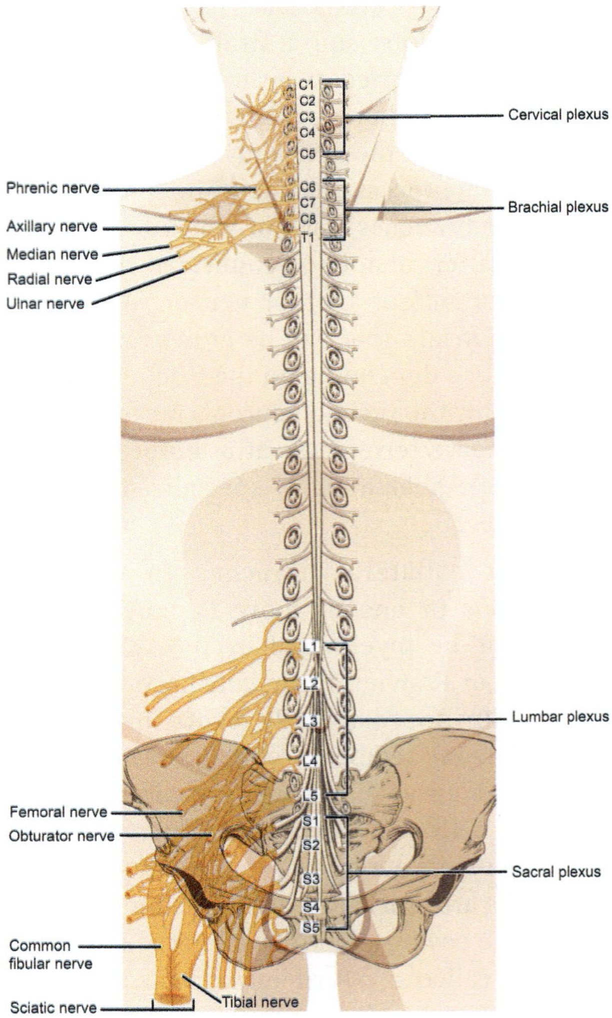

Figure 1.19. *Nerve plexuses of the body: There are four main nerve plexuses in the human body. The cervical plexus supplies nerves to the posterior head and neck, as well as to the diaphragm. The brachial plexus supplies nerves to the arm. The lumbar plexus supplies nerves to the anterior leg. The sacral plexus supplies nerves to the posterior leg.*

Source: https://open.oregonstate.education/aandp/chapter/13-3-spinal-and-cranial-nerves/.

1.6.3. Autonomic Nervous System

This system's motor component innervates smooth and cardiac muscle as well as glands. Its fibers in the blood vessels and nerves form a delicate network. Before reaching the organs they supply, all of its fibers synapse with peripheral ganglion cells, where they are derived from neurons found in the brain and spinal cord's visceral columns. The sympathetic and parasympathetic branches of this intricate network split off at different locations from the central nervous system and work in tandem. Their effects on the structure they supply through endings are typically antagonistic, primarily adrenergic or cholinergic.

1.6.3.1. Sympathetic System

The sympathetic chain or trunk receives a bundle of myelinated (preganglionic) fibers from each ventral ramus, which extends from the first thoracic to the second lumbar nerve. The bundles, known as white rami communicantes, form the sympathetic outflow of the central nervous system and arise close to the formation of a ramus. A gray ramus communicans, or bundle of unmyelinated (postganglionic) fibers, is subsequently transferred from the sympathetic trunk to each ventral ramus. (The terms "white" and "gray" rami communicantes, respectively, also refer to the myelinated and unmyelinated fibers.)

The two sympathetic trunks that run parallel to the spinal column contain the system's peripheral ganglia. There are three cervical, 12 thoracic, four lumbar, and five sacral ganglia in the trunks, which run from the base of the skull to the coccyx. The thoracolumbar outflow's preganglionic fibers can synapse – (i) in the ganglion next to it; (ii) in ganglia further up or down the chain; or (iii) in the collateral ganglia located in the plexuses surrounding the aorta (e.g., celiac). Widespread activity can result from the synapse of each preganglionic fiber with at least 15 ganglionic cells. The suprarenal gland's medulla is the destination of several preganglionic fibers.

Postganglionic (unmyelinated) fibers may – (a) return to a spinal nerve in a gray ramus communicans to be distributed to peripheral smooth muscle, e.g., arterial walls; (b) pass along the major arteries and their branches to be distributed to the organs these supply; or (c) form named nerves, e.g., cardiac, running to the viscus concerned.

The cell bodies of the sympathetic fibers supplying the upper and lower limbs are situated in ganglia in the cervicothoracic and lumbosacral regions, respectively. The visceral branches supply the smooth circular muscle, including the sphincters of the viscera.

1.6.3.2. Parasympathetic System

This system receives preganglionic fibers from four cranial nerves (oculomotor, facial, glossopharyngeal, and vagus) as well as the second, third, and fourth sacral spinal nerves (craniosacral outflow). The peripheral ganglia of this system are located close to the organs they innervate, typically within the organ walls. There are also four distinct parasympathetic ganglia associated with the cranial nerves. The postganglionic fibers are typically short and unmyelinated. The visceral branches primarily supply the smooth muscle responsible for organ emptying and also cause dilation of blood vessels. There is limited evidence of parasympathetic supply to the limbs. Afferent (e.g., pain) fibers from the viscera are present in both sympathetic and parasympathetic systems and pass to the central nervous system without synapsing. Their subsequent paths are similar to those of somatic pain. Afferent (reflex) fibers, e.g., from the lungs, heart, bladder, and visceral sensations of nausea, hunger, rectal distension, also reach the central nervous system, probably along parasympathetic pathways. Most transmitter chemicals can be classified as adrenergic (for the sympathetic system) or cholinergic (for the parasympathetic system) (Moore, Dalley & Agur, 2014; Agur & Lee, 2017; Drake, Vogl, & Mitchell, 2019).

1.7. The Cardiovascular System

The heart, blood vessels, arteries, veins, capillaries, and sinusoids make up the cardiovascular system. Nerves typically accompany the arteries and veins that supply muscles and organs, forming a compact neurovascular bundle. Three coats cover the artery walls: the intima, which is primarily made up of smooth muscle in small and medium-sized arteries and endothelial lining and a small amount of connective tissue; the media in larger arteries, which is mostly made up of elastic tissue; and the outer fibrous adventitia. The artery and vein coats are similar, but there is less smooth muscle and elastic fiber in the media. The adventitia is thicker than the media in the larger veins. The majority of veins have valves. They aid in determining the direction of flow and are made up of paired endothelial folds. The venae comitantes, or companion veins, frequently accompany medium- and smaller-sized arteries instead of just one. Venules are the tiniest postcapillary veins. A single endothelial layer made up of large, angular, flattened cells forms the walls of the capillaries, which connect the arteries and veins.

Anastomosis is the term used to describe the direct union of two vessels. Arteriovenous anastomoses, which are found around nail beds, are a crucial component of the blood flow regulation system in digital devices. Sinusoids are dilated, thin-walled channels that connect veins and arteries. They are present in the liver, spleen, bone marrow, and suprarenal glands. A portal circulation occurs when blood travels through two capillary beds before returning to the heart. One example of such a system is the blood that passes through the liver from the stomach, intestine, pancreas, and spleen. Emissary veins are small blood vessels that join veins outside and venous channels (sinuses) inside the skull through foramina in the skull (Figure 1.20).

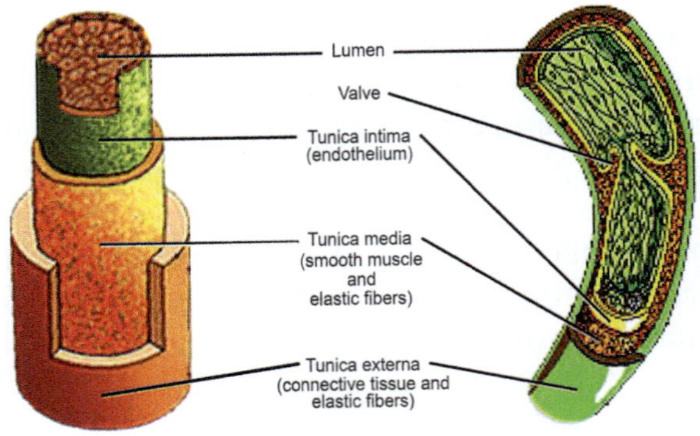

Figure 1.20. *Structure of: (a) artery; and (b) vein.*

Source: By CNX OpenStax – http://cnx.org/contents/GFy_h8cu@10.53:rZudN6XP@2/Introduction see also: https://www.training.seer.cancer.gov/anatomy/cardiovascular/blood/classification.html, CC BY 4.0; https://commons.wikimedia.org/w/index.php?curid=49935655.

1.8. The Lymphatic System

Plasma and cells, primarily lymphocytes, make up lymph. Tissue fluid is gathered by the lymphatic system and delivered to the bloodstream. It is made up of the lymph nodes, lymph capillaries, and aggregations of lymph tissue in the spleen, thymus, and surrounding digestive tract. The body's fine vessels are difficult to distinguish, but the system nonetheless forms a vast network throughout. The lymph capillaries consist of a single layer of endothelial cells and are bigger than blood capillaries. The lymph vessels have numerous pairs of valves and resemble veins. The larger collecting vessels emerge close to the brachiocephalic vein formation and open into the venous system.

An accumulation of lymph tissue along a lymph vessel's path is called a lymph node. It has a bean-like shape, with an efferent vessel exiting its hilus (opening) and several afferent vessels entering its convex surface, which carry lymph away from the node. Fibrous trabeculae pass inward from a fibrous capsule that encloses it. The cells inside it are either fixed macrophages or primitive lymphocyte precursors, and it is filled with a reticular network of fine collagen fibers. There is a subcapsular lymph space because few monocytes and many lymphocytes are absent from the periphery and lie freely within the meshwork. The tightly packed cells that make up the cortex, or outer layer of the node, are referred to as germinal centers. Lymphocytes are loosely packed in the hilar (medullary) regions of the node and in the center of the follicle. A mixture of follicles and loosely packed lymphocytes make up lymph aggregations in other parts of the body (Figure 1.21).

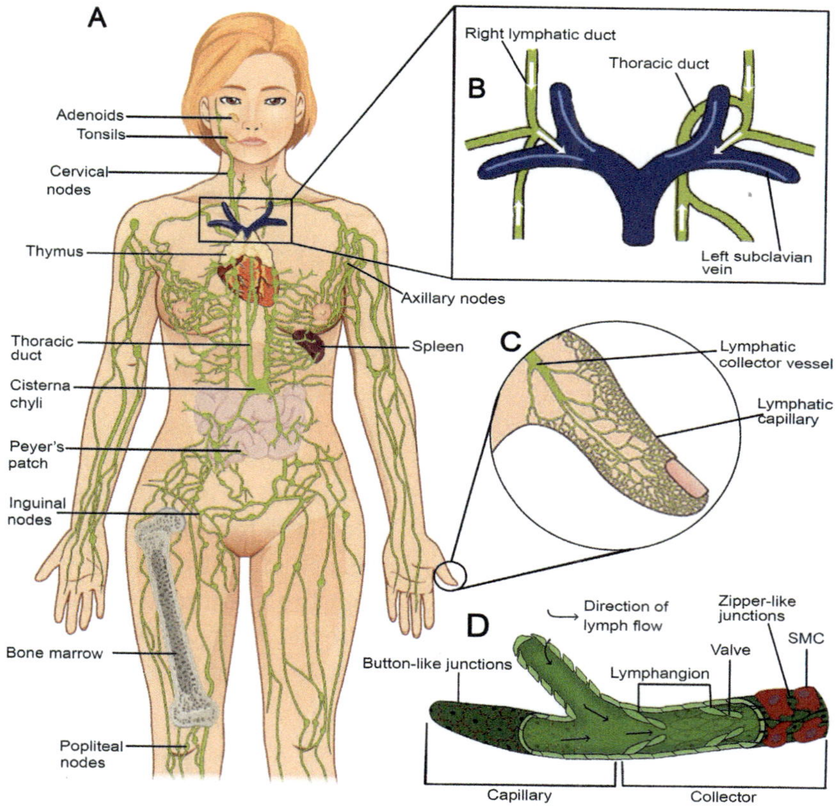

Figure 1.21. *Lymphatic system.*

Source: By SGUL lymres – Own work, CC BY-SA 4.0; https://commons.wikimedia.org/w/index.php?curid=99532989.

1.9. Orientation

Every anatomical description refers to the anatomical position. It's the kind where the person stands straight, feet together, arms straight down the side of the body, palms facing forward, and eyes forward. Structures behind are referred to as posterior (dorsal) and those in front as anterior (ventral). The terms "palmar" and "dorsal" refer to the surfaces of the hands and feet, respectively.

Superior structures are cranial and rostral, while inferior structures are caudal. Structures in the midline are referred to as median, while those that are farther from the midline are referred to as lateral. Paramedian refers to being next to and in line with the midline. The terms "superficial" and "deep" describe how structures relate to the body's surface. Within the body, a coronal plane intersects a sagittal plane at a right angle and travels vertically Antero posteriorly. The body is traversed horizontally by transverse planes. Referring to a structure's distance from the body's center, terms like proximal and distal are employed. Shoulder and elbow joints are proximal and distal, respectively. The veins carry blood proximally (centrally) and distally (peripherally) through their lumen (Figure 1.22).

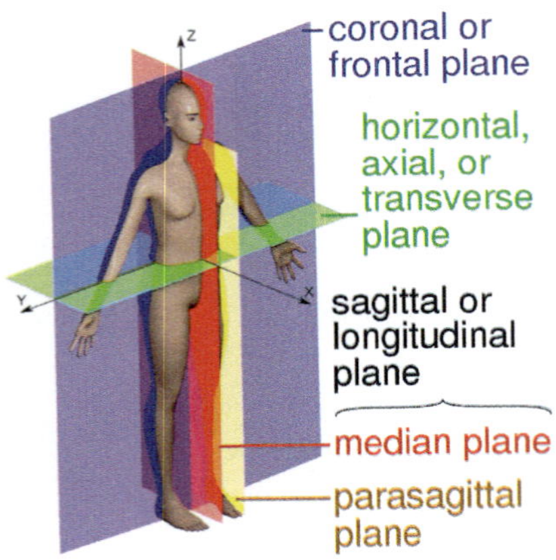

Figure 1.22. *Anatomical position.*

Source: By David Richfield and Mikael Häggström, M. D. and Cmglee – Human anatomy planes, labeled.jpg, CC BY-SA 4.0; https://commons.wikimedia.org/w/index.php?curid=91212408.

1.9.1. Movements

Extension is the term used to describe movement backward and flexion in a sagittal plane, respectively. Backward leg movement extends the hip and flexes the knee due to lower limb rotation during development; downward movement of the toes is flexion. At the ankle joint, dorsiflexion (extension) refers to movement upward and plantar flexion (flexion) to movement downward. In the coronal plane, movement in the direction of the midline is called adduction and movement away from it is called abduction. In reference to the middle finger and second toe, abduction and adduction of the fingers and toes are measured. As the thumb develops, its axis rotates with respect to the fingers; as a result, movement is explained in terms of the thumbnail's plane. Lateral flexion is the term for the side-to-side movement of the neck and trunk. When a bone's distal end describes the base of a cone with its apex at the proximal end, the movement is known as circumduction. In the limbs, rotation can be medial, or toward the midline, or lateral, or away from it. Rotation happens along a bone's long axis. Pronation and supination are the terms for the medial and lateral rotation of the forearm, which is achieved through the axis drawn through the heads of the ulna and radius, respectively. Opposition of the two digits is the movement of the thumb and little finger to bring their pulps together. The thumb exhibits this movement more than the other digits. When the sole of the forefoot is turned toward the midline, it is called eversion, and when it is turned away from the midline, it is called inversion (Moore, Dalley & Agur, 2014; Agur & Lee, 2017; Drake, Vogl, & Mitchell, 2019).

1.10. Imaging – The Essentials

One of the medical disciplines that is growing the fastest is the study of the healthy and ill human body. This is thanks to the development of X-rays more than a century ago. Ultrasound (US), computed tomography (CT), contrast studies, radionuclide scans, and, in the last 30 years, significant advancements in magnetic resonance imaging and angiography (MRI and MRA, respectively) and, more recently, electron beam computed tomography (EBCT) are among the diagnostic tools available to us in the 21st century.

1.10.1. X-Rays

The majority of X-rays are absorbed by materials like bone, calcium stones, or heavy metals (radio-opaque), but they are easily absorbed by air or fatty tissues (radiotransparent). When X-rays collide with molecules inside the body, they release energy that damages those molecules and do not travel through to the X-ray plate. This is the mechanism through which X-rays cause harm; the effect is especially noticeable on rapidly dividing cells, such as gonadal and fetal cells. Therefore, when X-raying pregnant women or people who are of reproductive age, care is taken to protect the fetus. The name of the view depends on which way the beam travels through the subject. For example, a postero-anterior chest X-ray is taken with the subject facing the beam and the chest on the "cold" X-ray plate. While the antero-posterior chest X-ray is superior for seeing the vertebral bodies, this view is perfect for determining lung and heart size.

1.10.2. Contrast Media

It is possible to outline body cavities, the lumen of vessels (such as arteries and veins), ureters, or hollow viscera (such as the bowel) using heavy metal or halogen suspensions. There are several methods to introduce these contrast media: intravenous urogram for outlining the kidneys and urinary tract; direct introduction (barium enema); injection (arteriograms, venograms); or injection into the bloodstream followed by concentration by particular organs. These days, soft tissue background images can be "removed" and the system being studied can be seen more easily thanks to the use of digital, computerized images (digital subtraction angiography, or DSA). The development of non-invasive angiography techniques, like magnetic resonance angiography (MRA), in recent times has contributed to a decrease in the need for numerous invasive procedures.

1.10.3. Nuclear Medicine

Nuclear medicine uses radioactive isotopes, mainly for diagnosis but occasionally for therapeutic uses such as in hyperthyroid disease. In the diagnostic field, myocardial perfusion imaging, lung scans to detect pulmonary embolism and bone scans to find widespread metastases are now routine procedures.

1.10.4. Ultrasound

The use of high-frequency sound waves and their interaction with biological tissues to create "echograms" through ultrasound techniques, on the other hand, is far easier to perform. The Doppler principle has led to duplex scanning, which measures movement and blood flow in real-time and has the added benefit of producing easily understood color images. Modern ultrasound hardware now permits real-time tomographic images. The ability to use ultrasound at the bedside and its multi-planar nature make it an extremely valuable tool. These advantages now mean that many interventional procedures (e.g., biopsy and drainage of cysts or abscesses) can be done under ultrasound guidance. Usage of a variety of different transducers has improved the range of ultrasound imaging, but this technique is still totally operator-dependent and as it is a real-time interactive process, it is not best seen with hardcopy images.

1.10.5. Computed Tomography

Through the use of a computer to process a series of various angular X-ray projections, computed tomography (CT) produces X-ray views of a section or slice with a predetermined thickness. The X-ray tube is positioned across from a set of detectors in a stiff metal frame that makes up the CT machine. For the tube and detectors to revolve around the patient, every view for each slice is gathered at the same time. It takes 15–30 seconds for one slice. Examinations of the brain, spine, musculoskeletal system, and chest do not require any special preparation. It is frequently necessary to opacify the gastrointestinal tract for studies on the abdomen and pelvis by using a diluted contrast medium solution (either a water-soluble or a barium compound). CT is particularly helpful for analyzing bony structures, and the most recent 64-slice machines offer incredibly detailed 3D reconstructions that surgeons value for their precise pre-operative evaluation.

1.10.6. Magnetic Resonance Imaging

A strong magnetic field and radiofrequency energy are combined in magnetic resonance imaging (MRI) to examine the distribution and behavior of hydrogen protons in water and fat. The magnetic field strength that MRI systems generate is used to rank them. Systems that can generate a magnetic field strength of 1–2 Tesla are classified as high-field systems. Although there are no known biological hazards associated with MRIs, individuals who have an implanted electro inductive device or pacemaker should not have their scans performed due to potential harm to these devices. Ferromagnetic intracranial aneurysm clips, specific cardiac valve replacement procedures, and metallic foreign bodies inserted into the eyes are among the other items that are forbidden. Extracranial vascular clips and orthopedic prostheses are generally safe to examine, but they may produce local artifacts. You must keep loose metal objects out of the examination room, and you should expect your credit cards to be canceled.

Magnetic resonance imaging offers much better visualization of the soft tissues than computed tomography (CT). This is the true benefit of magnetization. Additionally, soft tissues like the brain, muscles, fascial planes, and intervertebral discs can be imaged in exceptionally detailed detail. To emphasize vascular, inflammatory, and tumor abnormalities, an intravenous injection of gadolinium complex contrast medium may be administered. A rise in MR angiography (MRA)—a non-invasive technique that detects blood flow in vessels without the need for contrast material—will occur over the course of the next 10 years.

1.10.7. New Techniques and Future Developments

Since patients dislike invasive procedures like contrast injections, it makes sense that non-invasive procedures would be approved more quickly. But it's not just this feature that has expanded the possibilities; new imaging modalities have also allowed us to see images in three dimensions and reconstruct the body in real-time. Contemporary medical equipment is becoming more and more rapid in its investigations. For example, 3D chest reconstructions can be completed in a matter of minutes using an electron-beam CT scanner that has high-speed cardiac cycle sequencing. A full torso scan on a 64-slice CT can be completed in less than 15 seconds. This is especially helpful in trauma cases where multiple systems may be damaged. The ability to reconstruct images in three dimensions is constantly improving with increased computer power, and resolution has now improved as computer-generated slices become thinner, down to 0.35 mm resolution (Moore, Dalley & Agur, 2014; Agur & Lee, 2017; Drake, Vogl, & Mitchell, 2019).

A Closer Look

Epithelium

Epithelium, in anatomy, is a layer of cells closely bound to one another to form continuous sheets covering surfaces that may come into contact with foreign substances.

Outgrowths or ingrowths from these surfaces form structures consisting largely or entirely of cells derived from the surface epithelium. In this way, the central nervous system, the sensitive surfaces of special sense organs, glands, hair, nails, and other structures all originate. The epithelial cells possess typical microscopic characteristics: the cell outline is clearly marked, and the nucleus is large and spherical or ellipsoidal. The cytoplasm of the cell is usually large in amount and often contains large numbers of granules.

Epithelium may be protective, absorptive, or secretory. It may produce special outgrowths and manufacture chemical material (e.g., keratin), in which case the whole cell becomes modified. In other instances, it contains fat droplets, granules of various kinds, protein, mucin, watery granules, or glycogen. In a typical absorbing cell, granules of material are absorbed. A secreting cell forming specific substances stores them until they are utilized—e.g., fat in sebaceous and mammary glands; enzymes in salivary and gastric glands; and various excretory substances in the renal epithelium of the kidney.

The cells forming an epithelial membrane are of various types: columnar, cuboidal, squamous (flattened), irregular, or ciliated (i.e., with hairlike projections). The membranes formed by these cells may be only one cell thick, as in the major part of the gastrointestinal tract, or consist of several layers, as in the epidermis of the skin. Columnar epithelium covers the intestinal tract from the end of the esophagus to the beginning of the rectum. It also lines the ducts of many glands. A typical form covers the villi (nipple-like projections) of the small intestine. Cuboidal epithelium is found in many glands and ducts (e.g., the kidney), the middle ear, and the brain. Squamous, or flattened, epithelial cells, very thin and irregular in outline, occur as the covering epithelium of the alveoli of the lung and of the glomeruli and capsule of the kidney. Ciliated epithelium lines the trachea, bronchi of the lungs, parts of the nasal cavities, the uterus and oviduct of the female, and the vas deferens and epididymis of the male. A single projection from the exposed surface of a cell, usually large and long, is called a flagellum.

When the cells of an epithelial surface are several layers deep, various epithelial types can be distinguished: stratified, stratified ciliated, and transitional epithelium. In stratified epithelium, which is found in the epithelium of the skin and of many mucous membranes (e.g., mouth, esophagus, rectum, conjunctiva, vagina), the surface cells are flattened, those of the middle layer are polyhedral, and those of the lowest layer are cubical or columnar. This type of epithelium covers surfaces exposed to friction. The surface cells are constantly being rubbed off and are replaced by new cells growing up from below. Hence, the deepest layer is formative, and successive stages upward reveal a gradual transformation into scaly cells that no longer show any sign of being alive. In stratified ciliated epithelium, the superficial cells are ciliated and columnar. This epithelium lines parts of the respiratory passages, the vas deferens, and the epididymis. Transitional epithelium lines the urinary bladder; its appearance depends on whether the bladder is contracted or distended (Moore, Dalley & Agur, 2014; Agur & Lee, 2017; Drake, Vogl, & Mitchell, 2019).

Summary

- Epithelium forms a protective covering over the internal and external surfaces of the body. It is derived from all three primitive embryonic layers.
- Hyaline cartilage contains many cells, a few fine collagen-like fibers, and is found in the rib cartilages and over most articular surfaces. It also forms the precursor in cartilaginous ossification.
- Sesamoid bones are formed within tendons and serve to relieve friction and to alter the line of pull of a muscle.
- Excessive force applied to a bone may cause it to break (fracture), and in such injuries, the adjacent soft tissues may be damaged both by the force and by the broken ends of the bone.
- The bony surfaces are united by fibrous tissue. These comprise the skull sutures, the articulations of the roots of the teeth and the inferior tibiofibular joint.
- The bony articular surfaces (facets) are covered with hyaline cartilage (except for the temporomandibular and sternoclavicular joints, where they are covered with fibrocartilage).
- The motor nerve supply of the muscle comes from the anterior horn cells of the spinal cord and the motor nuclei of the brain stem.
- The neuron is the functional unit of the nervous system and consists of a cell body and processes, usually an axon and one or more dendrites.
- The cardiovascular system comprises the heart and blood vessels, arteries, veins, capillaries, and sinusoids.
- Lymph consists of cells, mainly lymphocytes, and plasma. The lymphatic system collects tissue fluid and conveys it to the bloodstream (Moore, Dalley & Agur, 2014; Agur & Lee, 2017; Drake, Vogl, & Mitchell, 2019).

References

1. Agur, A. M. R., & Lee, M. J. (2017). *Grant's Atlas of Anatomy*. Wolters Kluwer.
2. Drake, R. L., Vogl, W., & Mitchell, A. W. M. (2019). *Gray's Atlas of Anatomy*. Elsevier.
3. Ellis, H., Logan, B. M., & Dixon, A. K. (2019). *Human Sectional Anatomy: Pocket Atlas of Body Sections, CT and MRI Images*. CRC Press.
4. Haines, D. E., & Mihailoff, G. A. (2018). *Fundamental Neuroscience for Basic and Clinical Applications*. Philadelphia, PA: Elsevier.
5. Moore, K. L., & Persaud, T. V. N. (2015). *Before We are Born: Essentials of Embryology and Birth Defects*. Elsevier.
6. Moore, K. L., Dalley, A. F., & Agur, A. M. R. (2014). *Clinically Oriented Anatomy* (7th ed.). Philadelphia, PA: Lippincott Williams & Wilkins.
7. Moore, K. L., Dalley, A. F., & Agur, A. M. R. (2018). *Clinically Oriented Anatomy*. Wolters Kluwer.
8. Netter, F. (2019). *Atlas of Human Anatomy* (7th ed.). Philadelphia, PA: Saunders.

9. Netter, F. H. (2019). *Atlas of Human Anatomy*. Elsevier.
10. Rohen, J. W., Yokochi, C., & Lütjen-Drecoll, E. (2018). *Color Atlas of Anatomy*. Thieme.
11. Snell, R. S., & Lemp, M. A. (2019). *Clinical Anatomy by Regions*. Wolters Kluwer.
12. Standring, S. (2016). *Gray's Anatomy* (41st ed.). Edinburgh: Elsevier Churchill Livingstone.
13. Standring, S. (Ed.). (2016). *Gray's Anatomy: The anatomical basis of clinical practice*. Elsevier.
14. Tamura, R., Yoshida, K., & Toda, M. (2019). Current understanding of lymphatic vessels in the central nervous system. *Neurosurgical Review, 43*(4), 1055–1064. https://doi.org/10.1007/s10143-019-01144-3.
15. Tortora, G. J., & Derrickson, B. (2017). *Principles of Anatomy and Physiology*. John Wiley & Sons.
16. Gray, H. Anatomy of the Human Body. *Am. J. Med. Sci.* 1919, *157*, 704.
17. Mow, V.C.; Lai, W.M. Recent Developments in Synovial Joint Biomechanics. *SIAM Rev.* 1980, *22*, 275–317.
18. Hui, A.Y.; McCarty, W.J.; Masuda, K.; Firestein, G.S.; Sah, R.L. A systems biology approach to synovial joint lubrication in health, injury, and disease. *Wiley Interdiscip. Rev. Syst. Biol. Med.* 2012, *4*, 15–37.
19. OpenStax. Anatomy and Physiology: Chapter 9.4 Synovial Joints. OpenStax CNX. 26 February 2016. Available online: http://cnx.org/contents/14fb4ad7-39a1-4eee-ab6e-3ef2482e3e22@8.24 (accessed on 06 June 2019).
20. Aging & Health A to Z. Health in Aging. 2017. Available online: http://www.healthinaging.org/aging-and-health-a-to-z/topic:joint-problems/ (accessed on 30 August 2018).
21. Schofield, D.; Kelly, S.; Shrestha, R.; Callander, E.; Passey, M.; Percival, R. The impact of back problems on retirement wealth. *Pain* 2012, *153*, 203–210.
22. Schofield, D.J.; Shrestha, R.N.; Cunich, M.; Tanton, R.; Kelly, S.; Passey, M.E.; Veerman, L.J. Lost productive life years caused by chronic conditions in Australians aged 45–64 years, 2010–2030. *Med. J. Aust.* 2015, *203*, 260.
23. Briggs, A.M.; Cross, M.J.; Hoy, D.G.; Sanchez-Riera, L.; Blyth, F.M.; Woolf, A.D.; March, L. Musculoskeletal Health Conditions Represent a Global Threat to Healthy Aging: A Report for the 2015 World Health Organization World Report on Ageing and Health. *Gerontologist* 2016, *56*, S243–S255.
24. Dadoun, S.; Zeboulon-Ktorza, N.; Combescure, C.; Elhai, M.; Rozenberg, S.; Gossec, L.; Fautrel, B. Mortality in rheumatoid arthritis over the last fifty years: Systematic review and meta-analysis. *Jt. Bone Spine* 2013, *80*, 29–33.
25. Murray, C.J.; Vos, T.; Lozano, R.; Naghavi, M.; Flaxman, A.D.; Michaud, C.; Ezzati, M.; Shibuya, K.; Salomon, J.A.; Abdalla, S.; et al. Disability-adjusted life years (DALYs) for 291 diseases and injuries in 21 regions, 1990–2010: A systematic analysis for the Global Burden of Disease Study 2010. *Lancet* 2012, *380*, 2197–2223.
26. Arthritis Foundation. Arthritis by the Numbers. *Arthritis Found.* 2017, *15*, 1–70.
27. Papi, E.; Belsi, A.; McGregor, A.H. A knee monitoring device and the preferences of patients living with osteoarthritis: A qualitative study. *BMJ Open* 2015, *5*, e007980.
28. Brennan-Olsen, S.L.; Cook, S.; Leech, M.T.; Bowe, S.J.; Kowal, P.; Naidoo, N.; Ackerman, I.N.; Page, R.S.; Hosking, S.M.; Pasco, J.A.; et al. Prevalence of arthritis according to age, sex and

socioeconomic status in six low and middle income countries: Analysis of data from the World Health Organization study on global AGEing and adult health (SAGE) Wave 1. *BMC Musculoskelet. Disord.* 2017, *18*, 271.

29. Arthritis and Osteoporosis Victoria. *A Problem Worth Solving—The Rising Cost of Musculoskeletal Conditions in Australia*; Arthritis and Osteoporosis Victoria: Elsternwick, Australia, 2013.
30. Nisar, K.; Ibrahim, A.A.A.; Wu, L.; Adamov, A.; Deen, M.J. Smart home for elderly living using Wireless Sensor Networks and an Android application. In Proceedings of the 2016 IEEE 10th International Conference on Application of Information and Communication Technologies (AICT), Baku, Azerbaijan, 12–14 October 2016.
31. Tognetti, A.; Lorussi, F.; Carbonaro, N.; de Rossi, D. Wearable Goniometer and Accelerometer Sensory Fusion for Knee Joint Angle Measurement in Daily Life. *Sensors* 2015, *15*, 28435–28455.
32. Donno, M.; Palange, E.; di Nicola, F.; Bucci, G.; Ciancetta, F. A new flexible optical fiber goniometer for dynamic angular, measurements: Application to human joint movement monitoring. *IEEE Trans. Instrum. Meas.* 2008, *57*, 1614–1620.
33. Harada, T.; Uchino, H.; Mori, T.; Sato, T. Portable absolute orientation estimation device with wireless network under accelerated situation. In Proceedings of the 2004 IEEE International Conference on Robotics and Automation, New Orleans, LA, USA, 26 April–1 May 2004.
34. Edwards, J.Z.; Greene, K.A.; Davis, R.S.; Kovacik, M.W.; Noe, D.A.; Askew, M.J. Measuring flexion in knee arthroplasty patients. *J. Arthroplast.* 2004, *19*, 369–372.
35. Majumder, S.; Mondal, T.; Deen, M. Wearable Sensors for Remote Health Monitoring. *Sensors* 2017, *17*, 130.
36. Majumder, S.; Chen, L.; Marinov, O.; Chen, C.-H.; Mondal, T.; Deen, M.J. Noncontact Wearable Wireless ECG Systems for Long-Term Monitoring. *IEEE Rev. Biomed. Eng.* 2018, *11*, 306–321.
37. Nemati, E.; Deen, M.J.; Mondal, T. A wireless wearable ECG sensor for long-term applications. *IEEE Commun. Mag.* 2012, *50*, 36–43.
38. Deen, M.J. Information and communications technologies for elderly ubiquitous healthcare in a smart home. *Pers. Ubiquitous Comput.* 2015, *19*, 573–599.
39. Mukhopadhyay, S.C. Wearable Sensors for Human Activity Monitoring: A Review. *IEEE Sens. J.* 2015, *15*, 1321–1330.
40. Pinet, É.; Hamel, C.; Glišić, B.; Inaudi, D.; Miron, N. Health monitoring with optical fiber sensors: From human body to civil structures. *Proc. SPIE* 2007, *6532*, 653219.
41. Bilro, L.; Oliveira, J.G.; Pinto, J.L.; Nogueira, R.N. A reliable low-cost wireless and wearable gait monitoring system based on a plastic optical fibre sensor. *Meas. Sci. Technol.* 2011, *22*, 045801.
42. Stupar, D.Z.; Bajic, J.S.; Manojlovic, L.M.; Slankamenac, M.P.; Joza, A.V.; Zivanov, M.B. Wearable Low-Cost System for Human Joint Movements Monitoring Based on Fiber-Optic Curvature Sensor. *IEEE Sens. J.* 2012, *12*, 3424–3431.
43. Babchenko, A.; Maryles, J. A sensing element based on 3D imperfected polymer optical fibre. *J. Opt. A Pure Appl. Opt.* 2007, *9*, 1–5.
44. Lim, C.K.; Luo, Z.; Chen, I.-M.; Yeo, S.H. A low cost wearable optical-based goniometer for human joint monitoring. *Front. Mech. Eng. China* 2010, *6*, 13–22.

45. Vimal, A.K.; Bhasin, S.; Sharma, S.; Anand, S.; Swami, P. Brace design for knee-angle measurement in human gait using infrared sensor. In Proceedings of the 2015 International Conference on Signal Processing and Communication (ICSC), Noida, India, 16–18 March 2015; pp. 201–203.

46. Mobini, A.; Behzadipour, S.; Foumani, M.S. Accuracy of Kinect's skeleton tracking for upper body rehabilitation applications. *Disabil. Rehabil. Assist. Technol.* 2014, *9*, 344–352.

47. Wang, Z.; Liu, G.; Tian, G. Human skeleton tracking using information weighted consensus filter in distributed camera networks. In Proceedings of the 2017 Chinese Automation Congress (CAC), Jinan, China, 20–22 October 2017; pp. 4640–4644.

48. Gritai, A.; Shah, M. Tracking of Human Body Joints using Anthropometry. In Proceedings of the 2006 IEEE International Conference on Multimedia and Expo, Toronto, ON, Canada, 9–12 July 2006; pp. 1037–1040.

49. Islam, M.U.; Mahmud, H.; Ashraf, F.B.; Hossain, I.; Hasan, M.K. Yoga posture recognition by detecting human joint points in real time using microsoft kinect. In Proceedings of the 2017 IEEE Region 10 Humanitarian Technology Conference (R10-HTC), Dhaka, Bangladesh, 21–23 December 2017; pp. 668–673.

50. Jalal, A.; Kamal, S.; Kim, D. A Depth Video-based Human Detection and Activity Recognition using Multi-features and Embedded Hidden Markov Models for Health Care Monitoring Systems. *Int. J. Interact. Multimed. Artif. Intell.* 2017, *4*, 54.

51. Abiddin, W.Z.; Jailani, R.; Omar, A.R.; Yassin, I.M. Development of MATLAB Kinect Skeletal Tracking System (MKSTS) for gait analysis. In Proceedings of the 2016 IEEE Symposium on Computer Applications & Industrial Electronics (ISCAIE), Batu Feringghi, Malaysia, 30–31 May 2016; pp. 216–220.

52. Gibbs, P.T.; Asada, H.H. Wearable conductive fiber sensors for multi-axis human joint angle measurements. *J. Neuroeng. Rehabil.* 2005, *2*, 7.

53. Bergmann, J.H.M.; Anastasova-Ivanova, S.; Spulber, I.; Gulati, V.; Georgiou, P.; McGregor, A. An Attachable Clothing Sensor System for Measuring Knee Joint Angles. *IEEE Sens. J.* 2013, *13*, 4090–4097.

54. Bakhshi, S.; Mahoor, M.H. Development of a Wearable Sensor System for Measuring Body Joint Flexion. In Proceedings of the 2011 International Conference on Body Sensor Networks, Dallas, TX, USA, 23–25 May 2011; pp. 35–40.

55. Gioberto, G. Garment-integrated wearable sensing for knee joint monitoring. In Proceedings of the 2014 ACM Int. Symposium on Wearable Computers Adjunct Program, Seattle, WA, USA, 13–17 September 2014; pp. 113–118.

56. Totaro, M.; Poliero, T.; Mondini, A.; Lucarotti, C.; Cairoli, G.; Ortiz, J.; Beccai, L. Soft Smart Garments for Lower Limb Joint Position Analysis. *Sensors* 2017, *17*, 2314.

57. Zhang, H.; Niu, W.; Zhang, S. Extremely Stretchable, Stable, and Durable Strain Sensors Based on Double-Network Organogels. *ACS Appl. Mater. Interfaces* 2018, *10*, 32640–32648.

58. Jeong, S.-M.; Kang, Y.; Lim, T.; Ju, S. Hydrophobic Microfiber Strain Sensor Operating Stably in Sweat and Water Environment. *Adv. Mater. Interfaces* 2018, *5*, 1801376.

59. Park, S.; Ahn, S.; Sun, J.; Bhatia, D.; Choi, D.; Yang, K.S.; Bae, J.; Park, J.J. Highly Bendable and Rotational Textile Structure with Prestrained Conductive Sewing Pattern for Human Joint Monitoring. *Adv. Funct. Mater.* 2019, *29*, 1808369.

60. Wang, C.; Xia, K.; Jian, M.; Wang, H.; Zhang, M.; Zhang, Y. Carbonized silk georgette as an ultrasensitive wearable strain sensor for full-range human activity monitoring. *J. Mater. Chem. C* 2017, *5*, 7604–7611.

61. Zheng, Y.; Li, Y.; Dai, K.; Wang, Y.; Zheng, G.; Liu, C.; Shen, C. A highly stretchable and stable strain sensor based on hybrid carbon nanofillers/polydimethylsiloxane conductive composites for large human motions monitoring. *Compos. Sci. Technol.* 2018, *156*, 276–286.

62. Ryu, S.; Lee, P.; Chou, J.B.; Xu, R.; Zhao, R.; Hart, A.J.; Kim, S.G. Extremely Elastic Wearable Carbon Nanotube Fiber Strain Sensor for Monitoring of Human Motion. *ACS Nano* 2015, *9*, 5929–5936.

63. Montazerian, H.; Dalili, A.; Milani, A.S.; Hoorfar, M. Piezoresistive sensing in chopped carbon fiber embedded PDMS yarns. *Compos. Part B Eng.* 2019, *164*, 648–658.

64. Støve, M.P.; Palsson, T.S.; Hirata, R.P. Smartphone-based accelerometry is a valid tool for measuring dynamic changes in knee extension range of motion. *Knee* 2018, *25*, 66–72.

65. Jenny, J.-Y.; Bureggah, A.; Diesinger, Y. Measurement of the knee flexion angle with smartphone applications: Which technology is better? *Knee Surg. Sport Traumatol. Arthrosc.* 2016, *24*, 2874–2877.

66. Vohralik, S.L.; Bowen, A.R.; Burns, J.; Hiller, C.E.; Nightingale, J.E. Reliability and Validity of a Smartphone App to Measure Joint Range. *Am. J. Phys. Med. Rehabil.* 2015, *94*, 325–330.

67. Milanese, S.; Gordon, S.; Buettner, P.; Flavell, C.; Ruston, S.; Coe, D.; O'Sullivan, W.; McCormack, S. Reliability and concurrent validity of knee angle measurement: Smart phone app versus universal goniometer used by experienced and novice clinicians. *Man. Ther.* 2014, *19*, 569–574.

68. Johnson, L.B.; Sumner, S.; Duong, T.; Yan, P.; Bajcsy, R.; Abresch, R.T.; de Bie, E.; Han, J.J. Validity and reliability of smartphone magnetometer-based goniometer evaluation of shoulder abduction—A pilot study. *Man. Ther.* 2015, *20*, 777–782.

69. Majumder, S.; Deen, M.J. Smartphone Sensors for Health Monitoring and Diagnosis. *Sensors* 2019, *19*, 2164.

70. Feng, G.-H.; Chen, W.-M. Piezoelectric-film-based acoustic emission sensor array with thermoactuator for monitoring knee joint conditions. *Sens. Actuators A Phys.* 2016, *246*, 180–191.

71. Browne, M.; Barrett, D.; Balabanis, A.; Rowland, C. Passive Monitoring of Knee Joint Condition Using Acoustic Emission. *Orthop. Proc.* 2016, *98*, 54.

72. Toreyin, H.; Hersek, S.; Teague, C.N.; Inan, O.T. A Proof-of-Concept System to Analyze Joint Sounds in Real Time for Knee Health Assessment in Uncontrolled Settings. *IEEE Sens. J.* 2016, *16*, 2892–2893.

73. Teague, C.N.; Hersek, S.; Töreyin, H.; Millard-Stafford, M.L.; Jones, M.L.; Kogler, G.F.; Sawka, M.N.; Inan, O.T. Novel Methods for Sensing Acoustical Emissions From the Knee for Wearable Joint Health Assessment. *IEEE Trans. Biomed. Eng.* 2016, *63*, 1581–1590.

74. Teague, C.N.; Hersek, S.; Conant, J.L.; Gilliland, S.M.; Inan, O.T. Wearable knee health rehabilitation assessment using acoustical emissions. *AIP Conf. Proc.* 2017, *1806*, 070008.

75. Sudin, S.B. Wireless Knee Joint Angle Measurement System Using Gyroscope. Ph.D. Thesis, University Tun Hussein Onn Malaysia, Parit Raja, Malaysia, 2012.

76. Friedman, N.; Rowe, J.B.; Reinkensmeyer, D.J.; Bachman, M. The Manumeter: A Wearable Device for Monitoring Daily Use of the Wrist and Fingers. *IEEE J. Biomed. Health Inform.* 2014, *18*, 1804–1812.

77. Seel, T.; Raisch, J.; Schauer, T. IMU-Based Joint Angle Measurement for Gait Analysis. *Sensors* 2014, *14*, 6891–6909.

78. Bakhshi, S.; Mahoor, M.H.; Davidson, B.S. Development of a body joint angle measurement system using IMU sensors. In Proceedings of the 2011 Annual International Conference of the IEEE Engineering in Medicine and Biology Society, Boston, MA, USA, 30 August–3 September 2011; pp. 6923–6926.

79. Favre, J.; Jolles, B.M.M.; Aissaoui, R.; Aminian, K. Ambulatory measurement of 3D knee joint angle. *J. Biomech.* 2008, *41*, 1029–1035.

80. Crews, D.J. *Real-Time Estimation of Knee Angle, Heel-Strike, and Toe-Off Events for Gait Rehabilitation Devices*; California State University: Long Beach, CA, USA, 2017.

81. Castañeda, J.J.; Roldán, F.Z. Knee Joint Angle Monitoring System Based on Inertial Measurement Units for Human Gait Analysis. *IFMBE Proc.* 2017, *60*, 690–693.

82. Vargas-Valencia, L.; Elias, A.; Rocon, E.; Bastos-Filho, T.; Frizera, A. An IMU-to-Body Alignment Method Applied to Human Gait Analysis. *Sensors* 2016, *16*, 2090.

83. Favre, J.; Aissaoui, R.; Jolles, B.M.; de Guise, J.A.; Aminian, K. Functional calibration procedure for 3D knee joint angle description using inertial sensors. *J. Biomech.* 2009, *42*, 2330–2335.

84. Seel, T.; Schauer, T. IMU-based joint angle measurement made practical. In Proceedings of the 4th European Conference on Technically Assisted Rehabilitation, Berlin, Germany, 14–15 March 2013; p. 6.

85. El-Gohary, M.; Pearson, S.; McNames, J. Joint Angle Tracking with Inertial Sensors. In Proceedings of the 2008 30th Annual International Conference of the IEEE Engineering in Medicine and Biology Society, Vancouver, BC, Canada, 21–24 August 2008; pp. 1068–1071.

86. Salehi, S.; Bleser, G.; Reiss, A.; Stricker, D. Body-IMU autocalibration for inertial hip and knee joint tracking. In Proceedings of the 10th EAI International Conference on Body Area Networks, Sydney, Australia, 28–30 September 2015.

87. Bonnet, V.; Joukov, V.; Kulic, D.; Fraisse, P.; Ramdani, N.; Venture, G. Monitoring of Hip and Knee Joint Angles Using a Single Inertial Measurement Unit During Lower Limb Rehabilitation. *IEEE Sens. J.* 2016, *16*, 1557–1564.

88. Ribeiro, N.F.; Ferreira, C.; Reis, L.P.; Silva, H.; Macedo, P.; Rocha, L.; Santos, C.P. Validation Of A Knee Angle Measurement System Based On IMUs, Human-Centric Robotics. In Proceedings of the 20th International Conference on CLAWAR, Porto, Portugal, 11–13 September 2017; pp. 645–652.

89. Yost Labs. *Calculating Angles between Two Yost Labs 3-Space Sensor™ Devices on a Human Body*; Yost Labs: Portsmouth, OH, USA, 2013.

90. Masdar, A.; Ibrahim, B.S.; Hanafi, D.; Jamil, M.M.; Rahman, K.A. Knee Joint Angle Measurement System using Gyroscop and Flex-Sensors for Rehabilitation. In Proceedings of the 6th 2013 Biomedical Engineering International Conference, Amphur Muang, Thailand, 23–25 October 2013; pp. 5–8.

91. Pathirana, P.N.; Karunarathne, M.S.; Williams, G.L.; Nam, P.T.; Durrant-Whyte, H. Robust and Accurate Capture of Human Joint Pose Using an Inertial Sensor. *IEEE J. Transl. Eng. Health Med.* 2018, *6*, 1–11.

92. Karatsidis, A.; Jung, M.; Schepers, H.M.; Bellusci, G.; de Zee, M.; Veltink, P.H.; Andersen, M.S. Predicting kinetics using musculoskeletal modeling and inertial motion capture. *arXiv* 2018, arXiv:1801.01668.

93. Ahmadi, A.; Destelle, F.; Unzueta, L.; Monaghan, D.S.; Linaza, M.T.; Moran, K.; O'Connor, N.E. 3D Human Gait Reconstruction and Monitoring Using Body-Worn Inertial Sensors and Kinematic Modeling. *IEEE Sens. J.* 2016, *16*, 8823–8831.

94. Wang, X.; Kyrarini, M.; Ristic-Durrant, D.; Spranger, M.; Graser, A. Monitoring of gait performance using dynamic time warping on IMU-sensor data. In Proceedings of the 2016 IEEE International Symposium on Medical Measurements and Applications (MeMeA), Benevento, Italy, 15–18 May 2016; pp. 1–6.

95. Kim, J.N.J.; Kim, J.N.J.; Jo, J.H.; Kim, K.; Kim, S.H.; Chong, W.S. Development of real-time knee joint angle measurement technology for posture analysis monitoring. In Proceedings of the 2018 Global Medical Engineering Physics Exchanges/Pan American Health Care Exchanges (GMEPE/PAHCE), Porto, Portugal, 19–24 March 2018.

96. Hung, L.-P.; Chao, Y.-H.; Tseng, Y.-L.; Chung, Y.-L. Constructing a Home-Based Knee Replacement Exercise Monitoring System with G Sensor. *Lect. Notes Electr. Eng.* 2018, *422*, 627–636.

97. Matula, T. Estimating Human Movement Using Accelerometers. Ph.D. Thesis, Brno University of Technology, Brno, Czechia, 2016.

98. Majumder, S.; Aghayi, E.; Noferesti, M.; Memarzadeh-Tehran, H.; Mondal, T.; Pang, Z.; Deen, M. Smart Homes for Elderly Healthcare—Recent Advances and Research Challenges. *Sensors* 2017, *17*, 2496.

99. Agoulmine, N.; Deen, M.; Lee, J.-S.; Meyyappan, M. U-Health Smart Home. *IEEE Nanotechnol. Mag.* 2011, *5*, 6–11.

100. Kim, J.; Choi, H.; Wang, H.; Agoulmine, N.; Deerv, M.J.; Hong, J.W.-K. POSTECH's U-Health Smart Home for elderly monitoring and support. In Proceedings of the 2010 IEEE International Symposium on "A World of Wireless, Mobile and Multimedia Networks" (WoWMoM), Montrreal, QC, Canada, 14–17 June 2010.

101. Bergmann, T.; Peterson, D. Chiropractic Technique: Chapter 2 Joint Anatomy and Basic Biomechanics. In *Chiropractic Technique*; Elsevier/Mosby: Amsterdam, The Netherlands, 2010; pp. 11–34.

102. Ha, M.; Han, D. The relationship between knee joint angle and knee flexor and extensor muscle strength. *J. Phys. Ther. Sci.* 2017, *29*, 662–664.

103. Baltzopoulos, V.; Brodie, D.A. Isokinetic Dynamometry. *Sport. Med.* 1989, *8*, 101–116.

104. Anthropometry and Biomechanics. NASA. Available online: https://msis.jsc.nasa.gov/sections/section03.htm (accessed on 7 November 2018).

105. Greene, W.B.; Heckman, J.D. *The Clinical Measurement of Joint Motion*; American Academy of Orthopaedic Surgeons: Rosemont, IL, USA, 1994.

106. Slightam, J.E. Modeling and Simulation of Biologically Inspired 3D-Printed Fluid Power

Robotic System Architectures. Ph.D. Thesis, Milwaukee School of Engineering, Milwaukee, WI, USA, 2016.

107. Moromizato, K.; Kimura, R.; Fukase, H.; Yamaguchi, K.; Ishida, H. Whole-body patterns of the range of joint motion in young adults: Masculine type and feminine type. *J. Physiol. Anthropol.* 2016, *35*, 23.

108. Soucie, J.M.; Wang, C.; Forsyth, A.; Funk, S.; Denny, M.; Roach, K.E.; Boone, D.; Hemophilia Treatment Center Network. Range of motion measurements: Reference values and a database for comparison studies. *Haemophilia* 2011, *17*, 500–507.

109. Khayani, S.B. Development of Wearable Sensors for Body Joint Angle Measurement. Master's Thesis, University of Denver, Denver, CO, USA, 2011.

110. Rakheja, P.; Vats, A. Knee Deformity Recognition and Deform Angle Measurement. *Int. J. Appl. Inf. Syst.* 2012, *3*, 47–51.

111. Rome, K.; Cowieson, F. A Reliability Study of the Universal Goniometer, Fluid Goniometer, and Electrogoniometer for the Measurement of Ankle Dorsiflexion. *Foot Ankle Int.* 1996, *17*, 28–32.

112. Tesio, L.; Monzani, M.; Gatti, R.; Franchignoni, F. Flexible electrogoniometers: Kinesiological advantages with respect to potentiometric goniometers. *Clin. Biomech.* 1995, *10*, 275–277.

113. Zhang, W.; Tomizuka, M.; Byl, N. A Wireless Human Motion Monitoring System for Smart Rehabilitation. *J. Dyn. Syst. Meas. Control* 2016, *138*, 111004.

114. Chiang, C.-Y.; Chen, K.-H.; Liu, K.-C.; Hsu, S.; Chan, C.-T. Data Collection and Analysis Using Wearable Sensors for Monitoring Knee Range of Motion after Total Knee Arthroplasty. *Sensors* 2017, *17*, 418.

115. Webb, J.; Ashley, J. Skeleton Tracking. In *Beginning Kinect Programming with the Microsoft Kinect SDK*; Apress: Berkeley, CA, USA, 2012; pp. 85–120.

116. Pedersoli, F.; Benini, S.; Adami, N.; Leonardi, R. XKin: An open source framework for hand pose and gesture recognition using kinect. *Vis. Comput.* 2014, *30*, 1107–1122.

117. Charles, J.; Everingham, M. Learning shape models for monocular human pose estimation from the Microsoft Xbox Kinect. In Proceedings of the 2011 IEEE International Conference on Computer Vision, Barcelona, Spain, 6–13 November 2011; pp. 1202–1208.

118. Zhang, Z.; Liu, Y.; Li, A.; Wang, M. A novel method for user-defined human posture recognition using Kinect. In Proceedings of the 2014 7th International Congress on Image and Signal Processing, Dalian, China, 14–16 October 2014; pp. 736–740.

119. Le, T.L.; Nguyen, M.Q.; Nguyen, T.T.M. Human posture recognition using human skeleton provided by Kinect. In Proceedings of the 2013 International Conference on Computing, Management and Telecommunications, Ho Chi Minh City, Vietnam, 21–24 January 2013; pp. 340–345.

120. Rector, K.; Bennett, C.L.; Kientz, J.A. Eyes-Free Yoga: An Exergame using Depth Cameras for Blind & Low Vision Exercise. In Proceedings of the 15th International ACM SIGACCESS Conference on Computers and Accessibility, Bellevue, WA, USA, 21–23 October 2013.

121. Obdržálek, Š.; Kurillo, G.; Han, J.; Abresch, T.; Bajcsy, R. Real-time human pose detection and tracking for tele-rehabilitation in virtual reality. *Stud. Health Technol. Inform.* 2012, *173*, 320–324.

122. Patsadu, O.; Nukoolkit, C.; Watanapa, B. Human gesture recognition using Kinect camera. In Proceedings of the 2012 Ninth International Conference on Computer Science and Software Engineering (JCSSE), Bangkok, Thailand, 30 May–1 June 2012; pp. 28–32.

123. Yuan, Q.; Chen, I.-M.; Sin, A.W. Method to calibrate the skeleton model using orientation sensors. In Proceedings of the 2013 IEEE International Conference on Robotics and Automation, Karlsruhe, Germany, 6–10 May 2013; pp. 5297–5302.

124. Saul, K.R.; Hu, X.; Goehler, C.M.; Vidt, M.E.; Daly, M.; Velisar, A.; Murray, W.M. Benchmarking of dynamic simulation predictions in two software platforms using an upper limb musculoskeletal model. *Comput. Methods Biomech. Biomed. Eng.* 2015, *18*, 1445–1458.

125. Lee, K.; Kwon, D.S. Wearable master device using optical fiber curvature sensors for the disabled. In Proceedings of the 2001 ICRA. IEEE International Conference on Robotics and Automation (Cat. No. 01CH37164), Seoul, Korea, 21–26 May 2001; pp. 892–896.

126. Rantala, J.; Hännikäinen, J.; Vanhala, J. Fiber optic sensors for wearable applications. *Pers. Ubiquitous Comput.* 2011, *15*, 85–96.

127. Udd, E.; Spillman, W.B. *Fiber Optic Sensors: An Introduction for Engineers and Scientists*, 2nd ed.; John Wiley & Sons: Hoboken, NJ, USA, 2011; p. 512.

128. Wood, K.; Brown, T.; Rogowski, R.; Jensen, B. Fiber optic sensors for health monitoring of morphing airframes: II. Chemical sensing using optical fibers with Bragg gratings. *Smart Mater. Struct.* 2000, *9*, 170–174.

129. Yin, S.S.; Ruffin, P. Fiber Optic Sensors. In *Wiley Encyclopedia of Biomedical Engineering*; John Wiley & Sons, Inc.: Hoboken, NJ, USA, 2006.

130. Kuang, K.S.C.; Cantwell, W.J.; Scully, P.J. An evaluation of a novel plastic optical fibre sensor for axial strain and bend measurements. *Meas. Sci. Technol.* 2002, *13*, 1523–1534.

131. Dunne, L.; Walsh, P.; Smyth, B.; Caulfield, B. Design and Evaluation of a Wearable Optical Sensor for Monitoring Seated Spinal Posture. In Proceedings of the 2006 10th IEEE International Symposium on Wearable Computers, Montreux, Switzerland, 11–14 October 2006; pp. 65–68.

132. Fu, Y.; Di, H. Fiber-optic curvature sensor with optimized sensitive zone. *Opt. Laser Technol.* 2011, *43*, 586–591.

133. Behrad, A.; Roodsarabi, N. 3D Human Motion Tracking and Reconstruction Using DCT Matrix Descriptor. *ISRN Mach. Vis.* 2012, *2012*, 1–11.

134. MTw Awinda—Products—Xsens 3D Motion Tracking. Available online: https://www.xsens.com/products/mtw-awinda/ (accessed on 28 November 2018).

135. Muro-de-la-Herran, A.; Garcia-Zapirain, B.; Mendez-Zorrilla, A. Gait Analysis Methods: An Overview of Wearable and Non-Wearable Systems, Highlighting Clinical Applications. *Sensors* 2014, *14*, 3362–3394.

136. Majumder, S.; Mondal, T.; Deen, M.J. A Simple, Low-cost and Efficient Gait Analyzer for Wearable Healthcare Applications. *IEEE Sens. J.* 2018, *19*, 2320–2329.

137. Jin, B.; Thu, T.H.; Baek, E.; Sakong, S.H.; Xiao, J.; Mondal, T.; Deen, M.J. Walking-Age Analyzer for Healthcare Applications. *IEEE J. Biomed. Health Inform.* 2014, *18*, 1034–1042.

138. Mandal, P.; Tank, K.; Mondal, T.; Chen, C.-H.; Deen, M.J. Predictive Walking-Age Health Analyzer. *IEEE J. Biomed. Health Inform.* 2018, *22*, 363–374.

139. Ji, X.S.; Wang, S.; Xu, Y.; Shi, Q.; Xia, D. Application of the digital signal procession in the MEMS gyroscope de-drift. In Proceedings of the 1st IEEE International Conference on Nano Micro Engineered and Molecular Systems, 1st IEEE-NEMS, Zhuhai, China, 18–21 January 2006; pp. 218–221.

140. Fahn, C.-S.; Sun, H. Development of a Fingertip Glove Equipped with Magnetic Tracking Sensors. *Sensors* 2010, *10*, 1119–1140.

141. Micera, S.; Cavallaro, E.; Belli, R.; Zaccone, F.; Gulielmelli, E.; Dario, P.; Collarini, D.; Martinelli, B.; Santin, C.; Marcovich, R. Functional assessment of hand orthopedic disorders using a sensorised glove: Preliminary results. In Proceedings of the 2003 IEEE International Conference on Robotics and Automation (Cat. No. 03CH37422), Taipei, Taiwan, 14–19 September 2003; pp. 2212–2217.

142. Elmenreich, W. *An Introduction to Sensor Fusion*; Vienna University of Technology: Vienna, Austria, 2002; pp. 1–28.

143. Li, Y.; Zhang, X.; Gong, Y.; Cheng, Y.; Gao, X.; Chen, X. Motor Function Evaluation of Hemiplegic Upper-Extremities Using Data Fusion from Wearable. *Sensors* 2017, *17*, 582.

144. Kröning, O.; Rothe, H. Gait motion analysis using optical and inertial sensor fusion to design human kinetic energy harvesting systems. In *Novel Optical Systems Design and Optimization XX*; International Society for Optics and Photonics: Bellingham, WA, USA, 2017; p. 16.

145. Menard, H.A.; Paquette, D. Skin temperature of the knee: An unrecognized physical sign of inflammatory disease of the knee. *Can. Med. Assoc. J.* 1980, *122*, 439–440.

146. Dhaher, Y.Y.; Kahn, L.E. The effect of vastus medialis forces on patello-femoral contact: A model-based study. *J. Biomech. Eng.* 2002, *124*, 758–767.

147. Besier, T.F.; Lloyd, D.G.; Ackland, T.R. Muscle Activation Strategies at the Knee during Running and Cutting Maneuvers. *Med. Sci. Sport Exerc.* 2003, *35*, 119–127.

148. Besier, T.F.; Fredericson, M.; Gold, G.E.; Beaupré, G.S.; Delp, S.L. Knee muscle forces during walking and running in patellofemoral pain patients and pain-free controls. *J. Biomech.* 2009, *42*, 898–905.

149. Kim, J.; Kwon, S.; Seo, S.; Park, K. Highly wearable galvanic skin response sensor using flexible and conductive polymer foam. In Proceedings of the 2014 36th Annual International Conference of the IEEE Engineering in Medicine and Biology Society, Chicago, IL, USA, 26–30 August 2014; pp. 6631–6634.

150. Sim, J.K.; Yoon, S.; Cho, Y.-H. Wearable Sweat Rate Sensors for Human Thermal Comfort Monitoring. *Sci. Rep.* 2018, *8*, 1181.

151. Banaee, H.; Ahmed, M.; Loutfi, A. Data Mining for Wearable Sensors in Health Monitoring Systems: A Review of Recent Trends and Challenges. *Sensors* 2013, *13*, 17472–17500.

152. Liu, Y.; Zhang, L.; Yang, Y.; Zhou, L.; Ren, L.; Wang, F.; Liu, R.; Pang, Z.; Deen, M.J. A Novel Cloud-Based Framework for the Elderly Healthcare Services Using Digital Twin. *IEEE Access* 2019, *7*, 49088–49101.

153. Sow, D.; Turaga, D.S.; Schmidt, M. Mining of Sensor Data in Healthcare: A Survey. In *Managing and Mining Sensor Data*; Springer: Boston, MA, USA, 2013; pp. 459–504.

154. Rashidi, P.; Mihailidis, A. A Survey on Ambient-Assisted Living Tools for Older Adults. *IEEE J. Biomed. Health Inform.* 2013, *17*, 579–590.

155. Giri, D.; Acharya, U.R.; Martis, R.J.; Sree, S.V.; Lim, T.C.; VI, T.A.; Suri, J.S. Automated diagnosis of Coronary Artery Disease affected patients using LDA, PCA, ICA and Discrete Wavelet Transform. *Knowl. Based Syst.* 2013, *37*, 274–282.
156. Guyon, I.; Elisseeff, A. Feature Extraction, Foundations and Applications: An introduction to feature extraction. In *Feature Extraction*; Springer: Berlin/Heidelberg, Germany, 2006; pp. 1–28.
157. Bellos, C.C.; Papadopoulos, A.; Rosso, R.; Fotiadis, D.I. Extraction and Analysis of features acquired by wearable sensors network. In Proceedings of the 10th IEEE International Conference on Information Technology and Applications in Biomedicine, Corfu, Greece, 3–5 November 2010.
158. Avci, A.; Bosch, S.; Marin-Perianu, M.; Marin-Perianu, R.; Havinga, P. Activity Recognition Using Inertial Sensing for Healthcare, Wellbeing and Sports Applications: A Survey. In Proceedings of the 2010 23th International Conference on Architecture of Computing Systems, Hannover, Germany, 22–23 February 2010.
159. Singh, R.R.; Conjeti, S.; Banerjee, R. An approach for real-time stress-trend detection using physiological signals in wearable computing systems for automotive drivers. In Proceedings of the 2011 14th International IEEE Conference on Intelligent Transportation Systems (ITSC), Washington, DC, USA, 5–7 October 2011; pp. 1477–1482.
160. Apiletti, D.; Baralis, E.; Bruno, G.; Cerquitelli, T. Real-Time Analysis of Physiological Data to Support Medical Applications. *IEEE Trans. Inf. Technol. Biomed.* 2009, *13*, 313–321.
161. Charbonnier, S.; Gentil, S. On-line adaptive trend extraction of multiple physiological signals for alarm filtering in intensive care units. *Int. J. Adapt. Control Signal Process.* 2010, *24*, 382–408.
162. Gialelis, J.; Chondros, P.; Karadimas, D.; Dima, S.; Serpanos, D. Identifying Chronic Disease Complications Utilizing State of the Art Data Fusion Methodologies and Signal Processing Algorithms. *Lect. Notes Inst. Comput. Sci. Soc. Inform. Telecommun. Eng.* 2012, *83*, 256–263.
163. Roffo, G. Feature Selection Library (MATLAB Toolbox). Ranking to Learn and Learning to Rank: On the Role of Ranking in Pattern Recognition Applications. 5 July 2018. Available online: https://arxiv.org/pdf/1607.01327.pdf (accessed on 12 February 2019).
164. Gu, Q.; Li, Z.; Han, J. Generalized Fisher Score for Feature Selection. *arXiv* 2012, arXiv:1202.3725.
165. Roffo, G.; Melzi, S.; Castellani, U.; Vinciarelli, A. Infinite Latent Feature Selection: A Probabilistic Latent Graph-Based Ranking Approach. In Proceedings of the 2017 IEEE International Conference on Computer Vision (ICCV), Venice, Italy, 22–29 October 2017; pp. 1407–1415.
166. Roffo, G.; Melzi, S. Ranking to Learn: Feature Ranking and Selection via Eigenvector Centrality. *Lect. Notes Comput. Sci. (Incl. Subser. Lect. Notes Artif. Intell. Lect. Notes Bioinform.)* 2017, *10312*, 19–35.
167. Guo, J.; Zhu, W. Dependence Guided Unsupervised Feature Selection. In Proceedings of the 2018 Thirty-Second AAAI Conference on Artificial Intelligence, New Orleans, LA, USA, 2–7 February 2018; pp. 2232–2239.
168. Du, L.; Shen, Y.-D. Unsupervised Feature Selection with Adaptive Structure Learning. In Proceedings of the 21th ACM SIGKDD International Conference on Knowledge Discovery and Data Mining, Sydney, Australia, 10–13 August 2015; pp. 209–218.
169. Guo, J.; Quo, Y.; Kong, X.; He, R. Unsupervised feature selection with ordinal locality. In

Proceedings of the 2017 IEEE International Conference on Multimedia and Expo (ICME), Hong Kong, China, 10–14 July 2017; pp. 1213–1218.

170. Liu, H.; Motoda, H. *Computational Methods of Feature Selection*; CRC Press: Chapman and Hall, FA, USA, 2007.

171. Bradley, P.S.; Mangasarian, O.L. Feature Selection via Concave Minimization and Support Vector Machines. In Proceedings of the 15th International Conference on Machine Learning (ICML 1998), Madison, WI, USA, 24–27 July 1998; pp. 82–90.

172. Widodo, A.; Yang, B.-S. Application of nonlinear feature extraction and support vector machines for fault diagnosis of induction motors. *Expert Syst. Appl.* 2007, *33*, 241–250.

173. Yousefpour, A.; Ibrahim, R.; Hamed, H.N.A.; Hajmohammadi, M.S. A comparative study on sentiment analysis. *Adv. Environ. Biol.* 2014, *8*, 53–64.

174. Kubat, M. *An Introduction to Machine Learning*; Springer International Publishing: Cham, Switzerland, 2017.

175. Iqbal, Z.; Ilyas, R.; Shahzad, W.; Inayat, I. A comparative study of machine learning techniques used in non-clinical systems for continuous healthcare of independent livings. In Proceedings of the 2018 IEEE Symposium on Computer Applications & Industrial Electronics (ISCAIE), Penang, Malaysia, 28–29 April 2018; pp. 406–411.

Chapter

THE THORACIC WALL, DIAPHRAGM, AND CAVITY

2

Contents

Introduction

The area between the inferior root of the neck and the inferior abdomen is known as the thorax. The thoracic wall, the thoracic cavity, and its superficial structures—the skin, muscles, and breast—combine to form the thorax. A complicated and crucial system that is necessary for breathing, thoracic organ protection, and structural support is made up of the thoracic wall, diaphragm, and thoracic cavity. The tissues, muscles, and bones that enclose the thoracic cavity make up the thoracic wall, commonly referred to as the chest wall. The thoracic vertebrae, ribs, sternum, and related muscles like the intercostal muscles are all included. The thoracic wall serves a vital role in breathing mechanics and serves as a barrier against physical harm to the heart, lungs, and major blood vessels. The diaphragm is a musculotendinous structure with a dome shape that divides the thoracic and abdominal cavities. This is the main breathing muscle. The diaphragm flattens and contracts during inhalation, expanding the thoracic cavity's volume and producing negative pressure that draws air into the lungs. It relaxes and returns to its dome shape during exhalation, reducing the volume of the thoracic cavity and releasing air from the lungs. Additionally, by raising intra-abdominal pressure, the diaphragm facilitates functions like coughing, vomiting, and defecation. The space bounded by the diaphragm and thoracic wall is known as the thoracic cavity. It is separated into three main compartments: the mediastinum, which houses the heart, esophagus, trachea, thymus, and major blood vessels like the vena cava and aorta, and the left and right pleural cavities, which house the lungs. A pleural membrane enclosing each lung is made up of two layers: the parietal layer lining the thoracic wall and the visceral layer adhered to the lung surface. Pleural fluid, which is found in the narrow space between these layers called the pleural cavity, lessens friction when breathing. For effective breathing and the defense of important organs, the thoracic wall, diaphragm, and thoracic cavity must interact. The diaphragm helps breathing by adjusting the pressure inside the thoracic cavity, the thoracic cavity houses and protects the heart and lungs, and the thoracic wall offers structural integrity and protection. It is essential to comprehend these structures' anatomy and physiology to diagnose and treat respiratory and cardiovascular diseases.

Orientation and Directional Terms

Term	Definition	Illustration
Thorax	The area of the body between the neck and the abdomen. The thorax contains vital organs, including the heart, major blood vessels, and lungs.	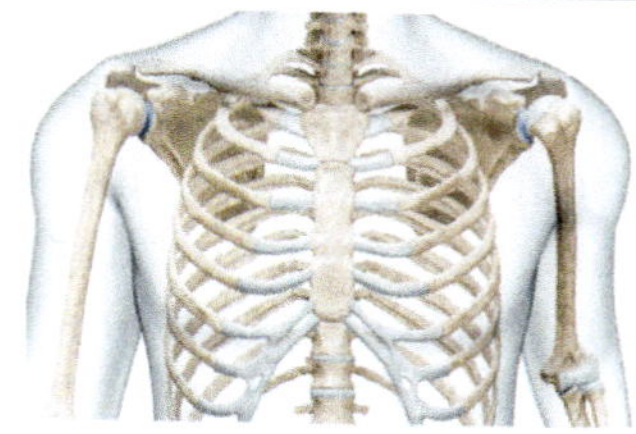
Thoracic Cavity	Thoracic cavity (chest cavity) is a space inside your thorax (chest) that contains your heart, lungs and other organs and tissues. It's the second biggest hollow space in your body, with only your abdominal cavity being larger.	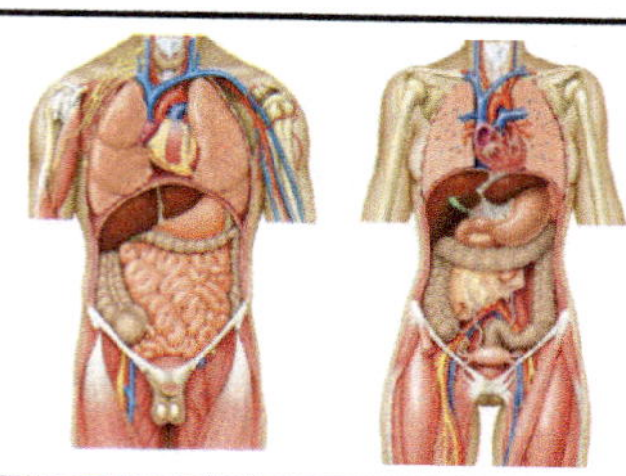
Tension pneumothorax	Tension pneumothorax is a life-threatening condition caused by the continuous entrance and entrapment of air into the pleural space, thereby compressing the lungs, heart, blood vessels, and other structures in the chest.	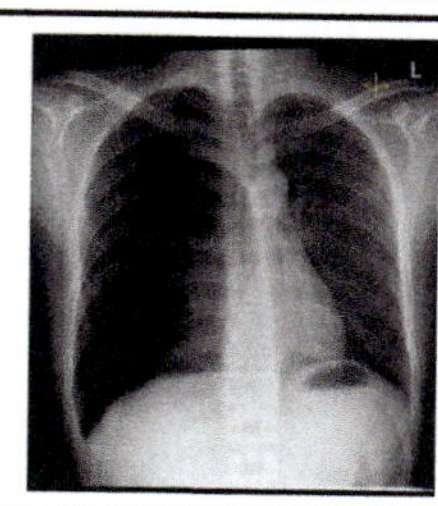
Lymphatic drainage	Lymphatic drainage massage, also known as manual lymphatic drainage, relieves swelling that happens when medical treatment or illness blocks your lymphatic system. Lymphatic drainage massage involves gently manipulating specific areas of your body to help lymph move to an area with working lymph vessels.	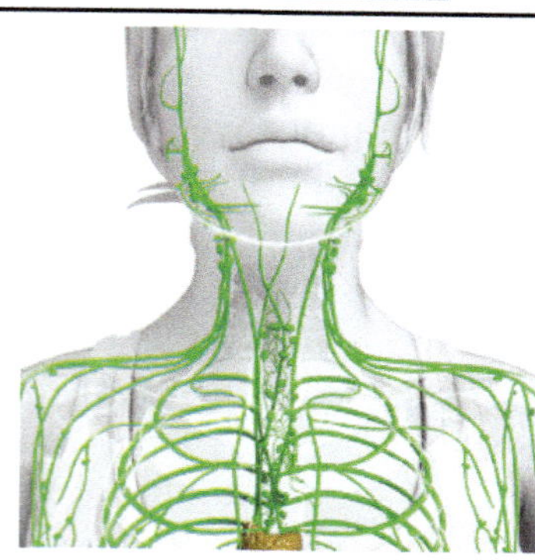
Subareolar lymphatic plexus	Subareolar lymphatic plexus, also known as Sappey's plexus is the lympatic drainage of the areola of the breast. It is a dense network of lympatics located in the dermis. The subareolar plexus of Sappey communicated with the plexus of lymph nodes located in the deep fascia of pectoralis major muscle.	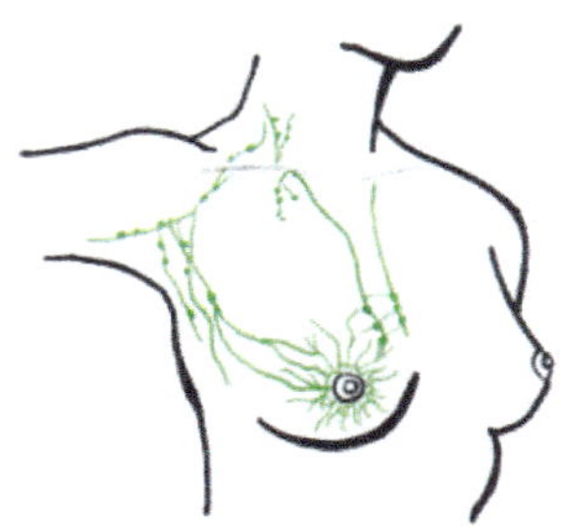

2.1. Structure and Function

2.1.1. Thoracic Wall

The thoracic wall consists of 12 ribs, 12 thoracic vertebrae, cartilage, sternum, and five muscles. Its main functions include movement, respiration, and protection of the thoracic cavity. The posterior thoracic wall is made up of thoracic vertebral bodies and intervertebral discs. Each rib articulates with two vertebral bodies, curving laterally, anteriorly, and inferiorly. The first seven true ribs connect to the sternum, while the false ribs 8 to 10 have cartilaginous extensions to reach the sternum, and floating ribs 11 and 12 do not connect to the sternum. These ribs create the structural support for the thoracic wall along with parts of the vertebral column. The muscles of the thoracic wall, from superficial to deep, are the external intercostal, internal intercostal, innermost intercostal, subcostal (posteriorly), and the transversus thoracic muscle (anteriorly). These muscles aid in respiration by moving the ribs and changing the volume of the thoracic cavity. Some muscles also attach to or are located superficially to the thorax, helping with the movement of the shoulder girdle, spine, thorax, and pelvis. Breast tissue covers the anterior portion of the thoracic wall above the pectoralis major muscle. It is made up of mammary glands, fibrous tissue, fat, the areolar complex, and the nipple.

2.1.2. Thoracic Cavity

The thoracic cavity is situated below the thoracic aperture, the root of the neck, and deep within the thoracic wall, above the diaphragm. The thoracic cavity is home to organs and tissues involved in the immune system (the thymus), nervous system (the vagus nerve, sympathetic chain, phrenic nerve, recurrent laryngeal nerve), cardiovascular system (the heart, pericardium, great vessels, lymphatics), and digestive system (the esophagus). There are usually distinct compartments within the thoracic cavity. The mediastinum and the pleural cavities are the main components. The lungs and pleura are located in the left and right pleural cavities, respectively. Located in the space between the two bilateral pleural cavities, the mediastinum is central. The mediastinum reaches the entire vertical length of the thoracic cavity and the inner border of the sternum anteriorly and the thoracic vertebral bodies posteriorly. The angle formed by the sternum's body and manubrium joining together is traversed by the transverse thoracic plane. The superior and inferior mediastinum are separated by the transverse thoracic plane, which passes over the T4–T5 vertebral junction (Nordström et al., 2023). Because of the anterior and posterior surfaces of the pericardium, the inferior mediastinum is further divided into anterior, middle, and posterior compartments. The heart and pericardium are located in the middle mediastinum, which is behind the pericardial sac; the anterior mediastinum is ahead of the sac. The posterior mediastinum is behind the sac.

The gross contents of each mediastinal compartment are as follows:

- **Pleural Cavities –** lungs and pleura.
- **Superior Mediastinum –** great vessels, trachea, esophagus, vagus nerve, phrenic nerve, sympathetic nerves, thoracic lymphatic duct, thymus.
- **Anterior Mediastinum –** connective tissue, thymus, and lymph nodes.
- **Middle Mediastinum –** heart, roots of great vessels, phrenic nerve, and pericardium.
- **Posterior Mediastinum –** descending aorta, azygos veins, esophagus, vagus nerve, sympathetic nerves, bronchi, and thoracic lymphatic duct.

2.2. Embryology

Three separate layers form during the development of the embryo (the trilaminar disc). The outer ectoderm, middle mesoderm, and inner endoderm are these layers. The mesoderm's neural tube, which is formed by the differentiation of neural cells along the midline, continues to grow. All of the thoracic structures originate from a three-layered tubular structure that is created when the endoderm is folded in a way that causes it to become internalized.

2.2.1. Thoracic Wall

Paraxial mesodermal somites form on opposing sides of the neural tube during development. Bone, cartilage, muscle, and dermis are formed by somite differentiation. The thoracic wall and the enclosure of the thoracic cavity will also develop as a result of elongation and folding.

2.2.2. Thoracic Cavity

The cardiogenic field, a collection of cardiac myoblasts, is where the cardiovascular system begins in the mesoderm layer. This field has a horseshoe-like initial shape before rotating to resemble a crude heart tube. Blood travels from the venous system to the primitive aorta (from caudal to cephalic direction) via a tube formed by the differentiation of endothelial, myocardial, and pericardial cells. The cardiac loop is formed at three weeks when the tube elongates and bends. The heart's ventricles, septum, valves, and trabeculae are formed by cell division and proliferation. Perfusion of the lungs is the result of several physiological changes that occur at birth, most notably the closure of the ductus arteriosus and the alteration in flow through the foramen ovale.

At three to six weeks, the respiratory system emerges as a diverticulum from the ventral wall of the primitive foregut endoderm. In front of the foregut, this diverticulum elongates caudally to form a parallel tube known as the primitive trachea (primitive esophagus). The future lungs' two left and three right lobes are formed by the trachea's formation of bronchial buds caudally. The surrounding mesoderm that engulfs the bronchial buds forms the pleura. The bronchial tree, bronchioles, alveoli, and lung vasculature develop as a result of the morphogenesis and differentiation of the bronchial buds. At 24 weeks, pulmonary surfactant production starts, and by 32 weeks, it can stop atelectasis. Even after giving birth, alveoli continue to develop for eight years.

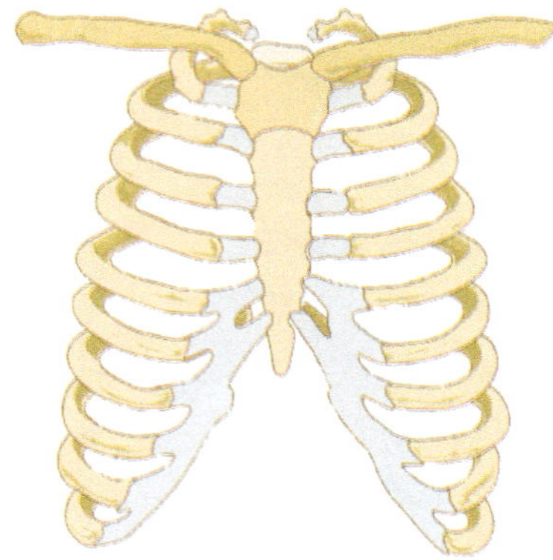

Figure 2.1. *Thoracic cage.*

Source: By Mikael Häggström – Image: Human_skeleton_front.svg (Public domain license), Public Domain; https://commons.wikimedia.org/w/index.php?curid=6111860.

Developing in the thoracic cavity, the thymus has its origins in the ventral third pharyngeal pouch. The thymus shrinks as an adult, despite being large at birth. The thoracic bony–cartilaginous skeleton shields the heart, lungs, and major blood vessels. It is made up of 12 pairs of ribs with costal cartilages medially, the sternum anteriorly, and 12 thoracic vertebrae posteriorly. It has a conical shape with a narrow inlet superiorly and a wide outlet inferiorly. The first thoracic vertebra posteriorly, the upper border of the manubrium anteriorly, the first rib and costal cartilage anteriorly, and the thoracic inlet, which is 10 cm wide and 5 cm Antero posteriorly, are the boundaries of this downward-sloping inlet (Remien, 2023) (Figure 2.1).

The esophagus, trachea, and large vessels of the head and neck pass through it, and the pleura's dome is located on either side. The 12th thoracic vertebra posteriorly, the 11th and 12th ribs posteriorly, and the costal cartilages of the 7th, 8th, 9th, and 10th ribs, which ascend to meet the sternum anteriorly, are the boundaries of the thoracic outlet, which is also the widest from side to side. The diaphragm divides the abdomen from the thorax. The sternum consists of three parts: the manubrium, the body, and the xiphoid process. It is a flat bone that can be felt all the way around. The thickest portion, the manubrium, has the jugular notch for articulation with the clavicles between the two lateral facets on its upper border. The palpable sternal angle, also known as the Louis angle, is where its inferior border articulates with the body (Figure 2.2).

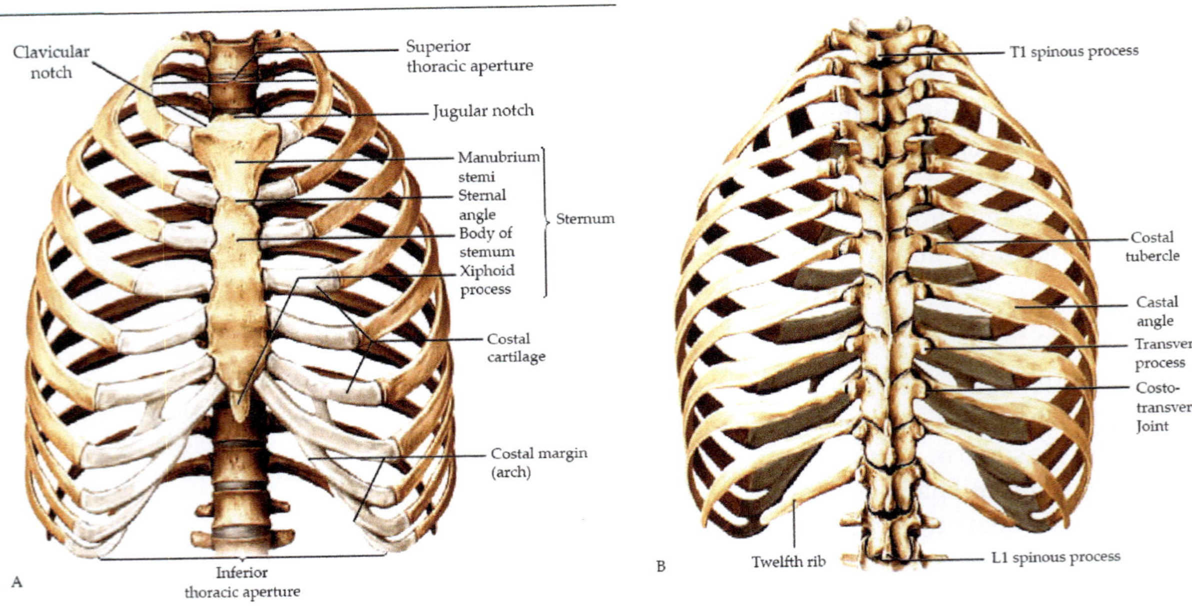

Figure 2.2. *Anterior chest wall.*

Source: Source: THIEME Atlas of Anatomy, General Anatomy and Musculoskeletal System, Thieme 2005, Illustration by Karl Wesker

This easily felt protuberance is a significant landmark because it marks the location of the bifurcation of the trachea, the beginning and end of the aortic arch, and the second costal cartilage's articulation on the same plane as the fourth thoracic vertebra. The sternum's body, which is about 10 centimeters long, articulates with the second through seventh costal cartilages on its lateral borders. The heart valves are located behind the body in the following order: pulmonary, aortic, mitral, and tricuspid. The xiphoid cartilage, which is cartilaginous in infancy and provides attachment to the diaphragm and rectus abdominis, articulates with the narrow lower end.

As the xiphoid calcifies in later life, an inexperienced clinician may mistake it for a stomach tumor. Since it is less common for drivers to forcefully strike the steering column with their chest in auto accidents when wearing seatbelts, sternal fractures have become more common. There may then be damage to the aorta, heart, or pericardium. Multiple rib fractures can also cause a flail chest, in which the entire chest wall moves paradoxically when breathing. The likelihood of this injury is decreased by safety belts and airbags. Even though sternum aspiration is less common these days, it is still a viable option for adult bone marrow aspiration if iliac crest aspiration fails (Figure 2.3).

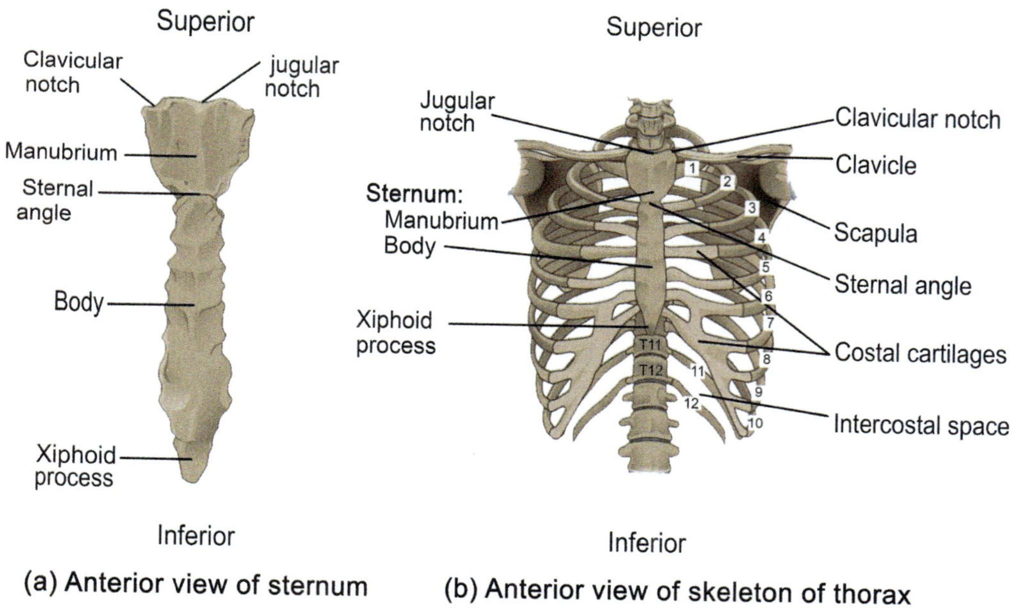

Figure 2.3. *The thoracic cage is formed by the (a) sternum; and (b) 12 pairs of ribs with their costal cartilages. The ribs are anchored posteriorly to the 12 thoracic vertebrae. The sternum consists of the manubrium, body, and xiphoid process. The ribs are classified as true ribs (1–7) and false ribs (8–12). The last two pairs of false ribs are also known as floating ribs (11–12).*

Source: http://repository.stikesrspadgs.ac.id/62/1/Illustrated%20Clinical%20Anatomy-402hlm.pdf.

The ribs, which typically number 12 on each side, all articulate posteriorly with the thoracic vertebrae; the upper seven, referred to as the true ribs, articulate with the sternum through their costal cartilages; the eighth through tenth ribs, referred to as the "false ribs," articulate with the cartilage above; and the 11th and twelfth ribs, referred to as the "floating ribs," have free anterior ends. The synovial joints known as the costochondral and costosternal joints are small and strengthened by fibrous bands. Tietze's syndrome, which is characterized by painful inflammation of these joints, is often mistakenly identified as heart disease. The "clicking rib" syndrome, a unique type of costochondritis, is caused by a rib causing subluxation that irritates the underlying intercostal nerve. The pain this causes can be mistaken for abdominal pathology.

There is a head, neck, tubercle, and body on a typical rib. The head is joined to the intervertebral disc and articulates with nearby vertebrae. The tubercle articulates with the transverse process, and the neck provides attachment for the costotransverse ligaments. The flattened, curved body has a lower border that is sharper and a rounded upper border. The intercostal nerve and vessels are located inside the costal groove on the inside of the upper border.

The 1st, 10th, 11th, and 12th ribs are not typical. All articulate with only one vertebra. The 1st rib is short, wide, and has superior and inferior surfaces. The lower smooth surface lies on the pleura; the upper surface has two grooves separated by the scalene tubercle, to which scalenus anterior is attached; the anterior groove is for the subclavian vein and the posterior for the subclavian artery and the lower trunk of the brachial plexus. The 11th and 12th ribs are short and have neither necks nor tubercles. Their costal cartilages lie free within the abdominal wall musculature (Tables 2.1–2.4).

Table 2.1. *Cervical Ribs Classification Proposed by Gruber [Gruber W.1869]*

Type	CR Type Description
I	CR extends to the transverse process of the 7th cervical vertebrae.
II	CR extends beyond TPs with no connection to FR.
III	CR extends beyond TP with partial fusion to FR by fibrous bands or cartilage.
IV	CR is fully fused to FR.

Abbreviations: CR: Cervical rib; TP: transverse process; and FR: first rib.

Source: Maślanka, K., Zielinska, N., Karauda, P., Balcerzak, A., Georgiev, G., Borowski, A., Drobniewski, M., & Olewnik, Ł., (2023). Congenital, acquired, and trauma-related risk factors for thoracic outlet syndrome – Review of the literature. Journal of Clinical Medicine, 12(21), 6811. https://doi.org/10.3390/jcm12216811.

Table 2.2. *Types of Bands and Ligaments in the Thorax Distinguished by Roos*

- **Type 1:** A band from the anterior apex of an incomplete CR to the middle of the upper surface (posterior to scalene tubercle) of the FR.
- **Type 2:** A strip originated at elongated C7 that attached to the FR in the same place as a type 1.
- **Type 3:** A band that had origin near the neck of FR and insertion behind the scalene tubercle.
- **Type 4:** A band lies along the anterior edge of SM, which has an origin on the transverse process and is inserted into the FR with SM.
- **Type 5:** The scalene minimus muscle (SMM)—described in more detail later in this chapter.
- **Type 6:** SMM inserts into Sibson's fascia (not to the FR) above the cupola of the pleura.
- **Type 7:** A fibrous strand running in front of AS, down to FR, and inserts to the sternum or costochondral junction (CJ). Due to the close relation to the subclavian vein (right behind it), it may cause her obstruction.
- **Type 8:** A strip arising from MS passes below the subclavian vessels (vein and artery) to insert into CJ.
- **Type 9:** The network filling the inner, posterior arch of the FR, consisting of muscles and their fascia's.

- **Type 10:** AS-derived muscle fibers attaching to the brachial bundle (perinerium).
- **Type 11:** Muscle fibers that form bands that connect the AS and AM and run between the cords of BP.
- **Type 12:** An anomalous AS (inferior part) runs posterior to the C5 and C6 roots.
- **Type 13:** n-band consisting of fused scalene muscles.
- **Type 14:** Fibrous bands run vertically, behind the AS, and anteriorly to the roots of BP.

Source: *Maślanka, K., Zielinska, N., Karauda, P., Balcerzak, A., Georgiev, G., Borowski, A., Drobniewski, M., & Olewnik, Ł., (2023). Congenital, acquired, and trauma-related risk factors for thoracic outlet syndrome – Review of the literature. Journal of Clinical Medicine, 12(21), 6811. https://doi.org/10.3390/jcm12216811.*

Table 2.3. *Crucial Anatomical Spaces for the Pathogenesis of Thoracic Outlet Syndrome or TOS*

Space	Borders	Contents
Scalene triangle	Anterior: Scalenus anterior Posterior: Scalenus middle Inferior: 1st rib	Brachial plexus (trunks) Subclavian artery
Costoclavicular space	Anterior: Clavicle (or sub-clavicular muscle) Posterolateral: Upper board of the scapula Posteromedial: 1st rib	Brachial plexus (division) Subclavian vessels
Sub-coracoid space	Anterior: Pectoralis minor muscle Superior: Coracoid process of the scapula Posterior: 2nd–4th ribs	Brachial plexus (cords) Axillary vessels

Source: *Maślanka, K., Zielinska, N., Karauda, P., Balcerzak, A., Georgiev, G., Borowski, A., Drobniewski, M., & Olewnik, Ł., (2023). Congenital, acquired, and trauma-related risk factors for thoracic outlet syndrome – Review of the literature. Journal of Clinical Medicine, 12(21), 6811. https://doi.org/10.3390/jcm12216811.*

Table 2.4. *Risk Factors for Thoracic Outlet Syndrome or TOS*

Congenital Risk Factors	Acquired Risk Factors	Trauma-Related Risk Factors
• Cervical rib [Sanders R.J., et al. 2002]. • Pseudoarthrosis of the clavicle [Lozano P., et al. 2002]. • First rib variation (increased width, congenital malformation) [Chang C.S., et al. 2011]. • Ectopic insertion of pectoralis minor [Le Double A.F. 1897]. • Morphological variations of scalene muscles (AS, MS, SMM) [Collins R.M., et al. 2014, Thomas G.I., et al. 1983]. • Subclavius posticous muscle presence [Akita K., et al. 2000]. • Brachial plexus variation (piercing AS and/or MS) [Leonhard V., et al. 2016]. • Superior pleural sinus presence [Hardy A., et al. 2019]. • Congenital ligaments and bands [Roos D.B. 1976]. • Elongated transverse process of C7 [White R., et al. 2008].	• Hypertrophy of the AS, MS, and subclavius muscle [1, Baltopoulos P., et al. 2008, Telford E.D., et al. 1948]. • Repetitive overhead shoulder movements [Garraud T., et al. 2022]. • Sports associated with risk of TOS (baseball, swimming, water polo, judo, climbing) [Garraud T., et al. 2022, Chandra V., et al. 2014]. • Lower position of the shoulder girdle [Cho Y.J., et al. 2012]. • Hypermobility of the shoulder joint [Hudson N., et al. 1995]. • Occupations with overhead movements or sedentary work patterns (e.g., computer users or musicians) [Franklin G.M. et al. 2015, Pascarelli E.F., et al. 2001, Sällström J., 1984].	• Whiplash injury car/motorcycle accident [Schwartzman R.J. 2022]. • Arthritis of the first costovertebral joint and hydrocortisone injection into the costovertebral joint [Weinberg H., et al. 1972]. • Neuritis of the brachial plexus [Feinberg J.H., et al. 2017].

Source: Maślanka, K., Zielinska, N., Karauda, P., Balcerzak, A., Georgiev, G., Borowski, A., Drobniewski, M., & Olewnik, Ł., (2023). Congenital, acquired, and trauma-related risk factors for thoracic outlet syndrome – Review of the literature. Journal of Clinical Medicine, 12(21), 6811. https://doi.org/10.3390/jcm12216811.

The body anterior to the angle is the weakest part of the rib and is where most fractures from blunt trauma occur. Any part of the ribs can fracture as a result of direct trauma. The adjacent structures, such as the pleura, lung, spleen, or intercostal vessels, may sustain damage from the fracture fragments in either scenario. Air in the pleural cavity, or pneumothorax, is a common consequence of severe rib fractures that rupture the lung beneath. There are situations where the valvular nature of the lung tissue tear results in air building up in the pleural cavity with each inspiration, which causes the mediastinum to move to the other side (tension pneumothorax).

2.3. The Thoracic Cage

- The cavity is kidney-shaped in cross-section because the vertebral column intrudes into the cage posteriorly.
- The ribs increase in length from the 1st to the 7th and thereafter become shorter.
- The ribs lie at an angle of about 45° to the vertebral column, the maximum obliquity being reached by the 9th rib.
- The costal cartilages increase in length from above downwards – from ribs 1–10.
- The cage gives attachment to the muscles of the upper limb, the abdominal wall muscles, the extensor muscles of the back, the diaphragm and the intercostal muscles.

The intercostal vessels and nerves are located in the intercostal spaces, which are defined by the ribs and costal cartilages. Adjacent to them, the pleura is present. The external, internal, and innermost intercostal muscles are the three layers of muscles that make up the spaces, arranged from outer to inner. They move the ribs and are supplied by the intercostal nerves. When the intercostal muscles bring the ribs together and the scalene muscles contract to stabilize the first rib, the sternum rises and air is drawn into the lungs. The sternum descends and air is expelled from the lungs when the lower ribs come together and are supported by the abdominal muscles (Boron & Boulpaep, 2016; West, 2016; Berne & Levy, 2018).

2.3.1. Intercostal Vessels and Nerves

The neurovascular bundle made up of the intercostal vessels and nerves travels deep into the subcostal groove and forward to the internal intercostal muscle, which is the only muscle that separates the pleura from the interior of the intercostal space. Anastomosing in each intercostal space, the posterior and anterior intercostal arteries supply the space. All of the other arteries originate directly from the descending aorta, except for the first and second posterior arteries, which are branches of the subclavian artery; the anterior arteries are branches of the internal thoracic artery, which is also a subclavian branch. Draining into the internal thoracic and azygos veins, the intercostal veins are located in the costal groove above their arteries.

The ventral rami of the upper 11 thoracic spinal nerves give rise to the intercostal nerves. Dorsal and ventral roots connect each to the spinal cord. A sensory ganglion is located in the intervertebral foramen of the dorsal root. The nerve splits into dorsal and ventral rami after the roots unite. Every dorsal ramus provides blood to the back's cutaneous branches, which in turn supply the skin and extensor muscles. The intercostal nerve, which supplies the intercostal muscles and the skin of the lateral and anterior chest wall, is formed by the ventral ramus and travels forward in the costal groove beneath the artery. It is safest to insert a needle into the lower intercostal space, away from the intercostal neurovascular bundle located in the subcostal groove, in order to remove fluid or blood from the pleural cavity (Figure 2.4).

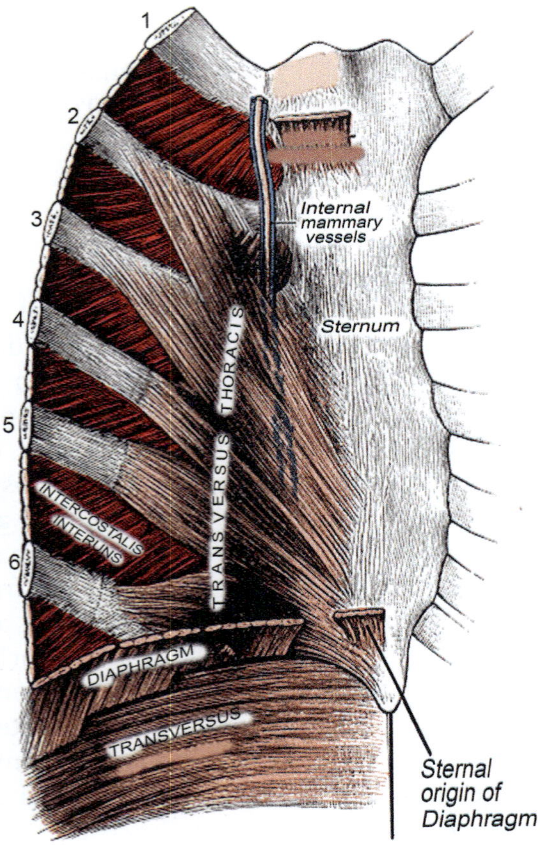

Figure 2.4. *Intercostal space.*

Source: By Henry Gray; modified by user: Gautehuus – Gray's Anatomy, Public Domain; https://commons.wikimedia.org/w/index.php?curid=36324969.

2.4. Dermatomes

A dermatome is a skin strip that lies between the anterior and posterior midlines. It is supplied by the cutaneous branches of the ventral and dorsal rami of each spinal nerve. Due to the fact that these originate from spinal cord segments, they are arranged in a segmental fashion. The dermatomes of adjacent tissues overlap. To determine whether a specific spinal cord segment functions normally or not, clinicians must have a working understanding of the dermatomal innervation of the skin (Figure 2.5 and Table 2.5).

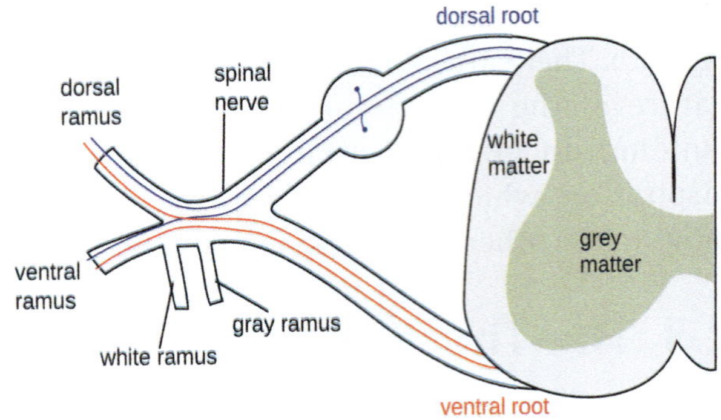

Figure 2.5. *Typical spinal nerve.*

Source: By Mysid (original by Tristanb) – Vectorized in CorelDraw by Mysid on an existing image at en-wiki by Tristanb, CC BY-SA 3.0; https://commons.wikimedia.org/w/index.php?curid=1420508.

Table 2.5. *Molecular Therapies for Spinal Cord Injury*

Therapeutic Agent	Molecular Target	Mechanisms of Action
Diazoxide	K-ATP channels	Aids spinal cord ischemia-reperfusion injury by decreasing apoptosis and preserving neuronal viability and motor function. The synergistic effect with erythropoietin contributes to higher therapeutic effects.

Glibenclamide	NCCa-ATP	Acts as an NCCa-ATP antagonist, improving behavioral outcomes, decreasing lesion volume, and significantly preserving white matter.
Levetiracetam	SV2A	Reduces glutamate excitotoxicity, lipid peroxidation, and apoptosis, and improves astrocitic function. Significant functional and histological improvements were observed.
Riluzole	Na^+ channels	Reduces glutamate excitotoxicity and inflammatory cytokines and induces a less active state in microglia and macrophages. Decreases cavity size and neuropathic pain and improves motor function recovery.
Progesterone	PR	Increases TGFβ1 positive astrocytes and microglia cells. Attenuates axonal dieback, neuronal death, and pro-inflammatory cytokines. Contradictory results were observed.
Estrogen	ER-α and ER-β receptors	Attenuates the expression of several inflammasome components, apoptosis, and ROS production. Reduces glial scar formation and demyelination and improves axonal regeneration.
Atorvastatin	HMG-CoA reductase inhibitor	Reduces oxidative stress markers, pro-inflammatory cytokines, and apoptosis. Improve motor functions and increase spare axons. Synergic treatment with and L-carnitine enhances therapeutic outcomes. No improvements were observed when tested in humans aside from a decrease in neuropathic pain.
Resveratrol	Pleiotropic interactions	Activates autophagy and inhibits apoptosis and pro-inflammatory cytokines. Reduces astrocyte activation and glial scar formation. Improves motor function and survival of motor neurons.
Omega-3 fatty acids	Pleiotropic interactions	Reduces oxidative stress, apoptosis, and inflammatory markers, and increases autophagy. Inhibits microgliosis and demyelination and increases oligodendrocytes. Locomotor recovery was observed.
Minocycline	Pleiotropic interactions	Improves behavior outcomes. Reduction in free radicals, lipid peroxidation, glial fibrillary, and acidic protein expression, as well as an increase in brain-derived neurotrophic factor were observed. Synergic effects with olfactory ensheathing cells graft were observed.

IL-10	IL-10R1 and IL-10R 2	Improves motor function, reduces lesion volume, decreases TNF-α levels and modulation of macrophages.
IL-4	IL-4Rα	Reduction in tissue damage and inflammatory markers were observed. Favors macrophage and microglia phenotype to a pro-regenerative phenotype. Improves locomotor recovery.
Maresin	RORα/LGR6	Reduces pro-inflammatory cytokines, induces pro-regenerative macrophages phenotype, improves neutrophil clearance, and reduces macrophages in the lesion site. Improves locomotor recovery.
Hypothermia	–	Reduces inflammatory cell infiltration, cell death, MPO activity, and vasogenic edema, and increases BSCB stabilization.
Anti-Nogo A	Nogo-A receptor	Promotes axonal regrowth and sprouting. Improves functional recovery and reduces urodynamic abnormalities.
ChABC	CSPGs	Promotes functional recovery, neural plasticity, and regeneration. Synergic treatment with cell therapies.

Source: *Lima, R., Monteiro, A., Salgado, A. J., Monteiro, S., & Silva, N. A., (2022). Pathophysiology and therapeutic approaches for spinal cord injury. International Journal of Molecular Sciences, 23(22), 13833. https://doi.org/10.3390/ijms232213833.*

A viral infection of the dorsal root ganglia causes herpes zoster, also known as shingles. The dermatome supplied by the infected segment experiences a sharp burning pain due to infection. A few days later, vesicular eruptions and a reddening of the affected dermatome are visible.

2.5. The Mediastinum

For description, the mediastinum is divided into:

- The superior mediastinum extending from the thoracic inlet to the transverse plane, T4.
- The posterior mediastinum below the plane and behind the heart.
- The anterior mediastinum below the plane and anterior to the heart.
- The middle mediastinum containing the pericardium, heart and main bronchi (Boron & Boulpaep, 2016; West, 2016; Berne & Levy, 2018).

2.6. The Diaphragm

This musculotendinous septum separates the thoracic and abdominal cavities; it has a central tendinous part and a peripheral muscular part. It has peripheral attachments around the outlet of the thoracic cavity (Figure 2.6):

- **Sternal** – from the back of the xiphoid process.
- **Costal** – from the inner surfaces of the lower six costal cartilages.
- **Vertebral** – from the sides of the upper lumbar vertebrae by two crura and from medial and lateral arcuate ligaments.

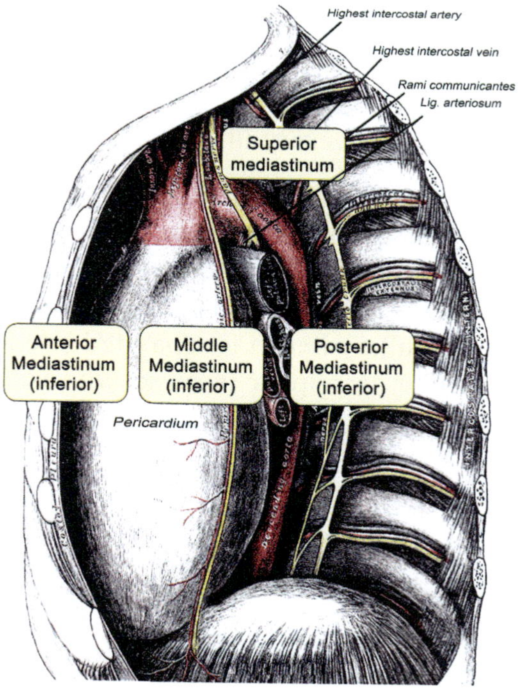

Figure 2.6. *The mediastinum.*

Source: By No machine-readable author provided. Arcadian assumed (based on copyright claims). No machine-readable source provided. Own work assumed (based on copyright claims). Public Domain; https://commons.wikimedia.org/w/index.php?curid=1224440.

The bodies of the top three vertebrae give rise to the right crus, while the first two vertebrae give rise to the left crus. The lateral arcuate ligament is anterior to the quadratus lumborum and extends between the transverse process of the 12th rib and the tip of the rib. The medial arcuate ligament, which is the thickened upper edge of the psoas fascia, passes between the body of the first lumbar vertebra and its transverse process. Its central attachment is made to a trefoil central tendon's periphery. The main breathing muscle is the diaphragm. The diaphragm's dome flattens and descends during contraction, increasing the chest's vertical diameter and drawing air into the lungs. Expiration causes the diaphragm to relax.

On both sides, the diaphragm curves upward, ending at the fifth intercostal space on the left and marginally higher on the right.

2.6.1. Nerve Supply

The two halves of the diaphragm are each supplied by a phrenic nerve and its periphery receives sensory branches from the lower intercostal nerves.

2.6.2. Openings

There are three large openings in the diaphragm:

- **The Caval Opening** – at the level of the 8th thoracic vertebra. This transmits the inferior vena cava and the right phrenic nerve.
- **The Esophageal Opening** – in the right crus, to the left of the midline at the level of the 10th thoracic vertebra. It transmits the esophagus, the gastric branches of the vagus nerves and gastric vessels.
- **The Aortic Opening** – between the diaphragmatic crura in front of the 12th thoracic vertebra. It conveys the aorta, the thoracic duct and the azygos vein.

The left diaphragm's dome is punctured by the left phrenic nerve. On its upper surface are the pericardium and pleural sacs, which house the heart and lungs, respectively. Its upper surface is securely attached to the fibrous pericardium. The liver, kidney, and suprarenal gland are inferiorly located on the right side, while the stomach fundus, spleen, left kidney, and suprarenal gland are inferiorly located on the left.

2.6.3. Respiration

The thoracic cavity's volume increases and decreases during inspiration and expiration.

The weight of the liver, which is attached to the underside of the diaphragm, helps with inspiration during quiet respiration, which only involves the diaphragm:

1. **Inspiration:** The diaphragm contracts, descends, and the height of the thoracic cavity thus increases. The upper ribs are fixed by the scalenes and contraction of the intercostals thus raises the ribs, thereby increasing the anteroposterior and transverse diameters of the chest.
2. **Expiration:** It is largely produced by relaxation of the diaphragm and elastic recoil of the lungs and the costal cartilages. Simultaneous contraction of the abdominal muscles forces the diaphragm upwards in forced expiration, such as in coughing and sneezing. Moreover, the diaphragm facilitates defecation. Straining entails closing the glottis to stop expiration as well as deep inspiration and fixation of the contracted diaphragm. Additionally, this action helps with lifting large objects off the ground (Boron & Boulpaep, 2016; West, 2016; Berne & Levy, 2018).

2.7. The Breast

A hemispherical, soft structure makes up the adult female breast. Located in the superficial fascia of the upper anterior thoracic wall, it is made up of glandular tissue, varying amounts of fat, and fibrous tissue. It is invested by the fascia, which also forms radial septae, or suspensory ligaments (Cooper). These ligaments pass through the gland from the underlying fascia to the skin above it. The gland is divided into 15–20 lobules by them. The ducts join to form a lactiferous duct from each lobule's alveoli. The pectoralis major fascia, on which the breast rests, is separated from it by loose connective tissue. Male breasts are simple organs with tiny ducts but no alveoli. On the other hand, they are prone to every illness that affects the female breast.

The female breast primarily rests on the pectoralis major muscle and spans the second to sixth ribs, slightly lateral to the sternum, up to the midaxillary line. It is separated into four quadrants for descriptive purposes; the axillary tail, or upper outer quadrant, extends laterally into the axilla.

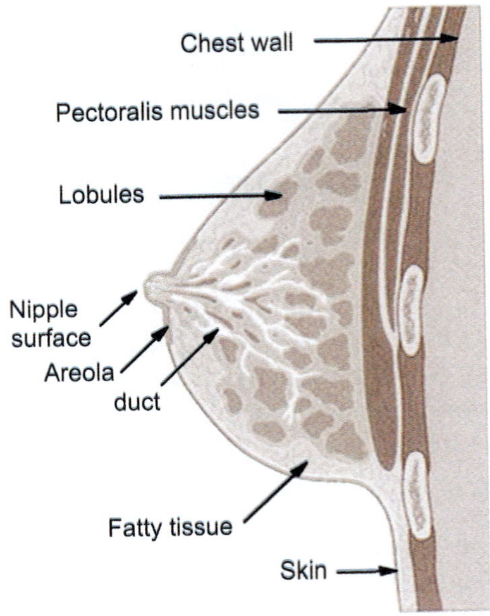

Figure 2.7. *The female breast.*

Source: https://upload.wikimedia.org/wikipedia/commons/6/64/Illu_breast_anatomy.jpg.

The lactiferous duct that connects each of the approximately 15 breast lobules empties into the nipple, which is encircled by a thin layer of pigmented skin called the areola that contains smooth muscle and modified sebaceous glands. Blood supply is via branches of the internal thoracic, intercostal and lateral thoracic arteries (Figure 2.7 and Table 2.6).

Table 2.6. *The Thermal and Physiological Properties of Human Fatty Breast Tissue*

Reference	Tissue	Status	*nsns*	*Ts*	*ρ*	**c**	**k**	q_m	ω_t
				(°C)	(kg/m³)	(J/kg/K)	(W/m/K)	(W/m³)	(kg/s/m³)
Johnson (1976) *	Normal Breast	*In vivo*	1	19	–	–	–	–	0.014
Hammerstein (1979) *	adipose Tissue	*In vitro*	8	–	930	–	–	–	–
Gautherie (1980) *	Fatty breast	*In vivo*	–	–	–	–	0.171 ± 0.012	–	–
		In vitro	–	–	–	–	0.120 ± 0.008	–	–
Beaney (1984) *	Normal breast	*In vivo*	10	–	–	–	–	–	0.700 ± 0.157
Johns (1987) [37] *	Fat (breast)	*In vitro*	14	–	928	–	–	–	–
Robinson (1991) [57] *	Fat (breast)	*In vitro*	1	–	934	–	–	–	–
		In vitro	2	37–43	–	2,220			
Wilson (1992) [56] *	Normal breast	*In vivo*	17	–	–	–	–	–	0.980 ± 0.245
Hamilton (1998) [60] *	Breast fat	*In vitro*	22	25	–	–	0.209 ± 0.022	–	–
Mankoff (2002) [59] *	Breast	*In vivo*	37	–	–	–	–	–	0.978
Ng (2001) [39]	Subcutaneous fat [a]	–	–	–	1,080	–	0.210	400	0.190
Ekstrand (2005) [54]	Fat (breast)	–	–	–	920	3,000	0.120	–	–
He (2006) [43]	Subcutaneous fat	–	–	–	930	2,770	0.220 [b]	–	–
Converse (2006) [36]	Breast [c]	–	–	–	1,069	2,279	0.306	350	0.615
Bakker (2009) [46]	Fat (breast)	–	–	–	950	2,493	0.240	–	0.416
Jiang (2011) [34]	Subcutaneous fat 1 [d]	–	–	–	–	–	0.246	1,180	0.190
	Subcutaneous fat 2 [d]	–	–	–			0.385		
Chanmugam (2012) [41]	Subcutaneous fat	–	–	–	930	2,770	0.210	400	0.210
Singh (2021) [61]	Highly perfused fat	–	–	–	920	3,000	0.210	400	4.240
	Moderately perfused fat	–	–	–	920	3,000	0.210	400	8.798

Source: *Said, C. J., Farrugia, L., Curto, S., Rodrigues, D. B., Farina, L., Caruana, D. G., Bonello, J., Farhat, I., & Sammut, C. V., (2022). Review of thermal and physiological properties of human breast tissue. Sensors, 22(10), 3894. https://doi.org/10.3390/s22103894.*

* *Measured values.*

[a] *Values obtained from generic fat tissue from [Werner J.,et al. 1988], but they are not exact.*

[b] *k given in units of (W/m).*

[c] *Referenced as "breast tissue," no distinction between fatty and glandular tissue. However, the properties are cited in other papers as fatty breast tissue.*

[d] *k was assumed to vary with orientation, so two values of k were used in the modeling study.*

The subcutaneous subareolar plexus and the sub-mammary plexus on the pectoralis major are the two lymphatic plexuses that carry lymph out of the gland along vascular branches. Although these plexuses' lymphatics communicate with one another, they primarily drain laterally to the axillary nodes, superiorly to the lower deep cervical and infraclavicular nodes, inferiorly to the lymphatics in the anterior abdominal wall, and medially to the nodes surrounding the internal thoracic artery. From the medial side of the breast into the opposing breast, a tiny quantity of lymph flows. Anywhere along the "milk line," which runs from the axilla to the groin, can result in the formation of extra breasts or nipples. Increased blood supply, increased pigmentation of the areola and nipple, and marked glandular proliferation are all facilitated by pregnancy and lactation.

An infected breast can occur during lactation. To protect the duct system, abscess drainage should be accomplished through a radial incision. Breast cancer that has infiltrated and spread may invade, attaching itself to the pectoralis major muscle underneath it as well as the fascia. The nipple may retract if the suspensory ligaments contract as a result of an invasion. Skin edema, or peau d'orange, will develop if the spread has infected and obstructed the breast's lymphatics. Arm edema (lymphedema) may result from cancerous infiltration of the axillary lymph nodes (Table 2.7).

Table 2.7. *Summary of the Studies Addressing Nutritional Status and Epigenetic Modifications in Breast Cancer*

Authors	Study Design	Model	Sample Size	Intervention	Key Findings
Li et al. (2020)	*In vivo*	Her 2/neu female mice that develop ER (–) tumors.	N = 42 broods	Mothers treated with BSps from 3 weeks of age until the weaning of their offspring.	↓ The development of mammary tumors in offspring. Methylated histone H3K9 was enriched in the promoter regions of tumor suppressor genes.
Arora et al. (2022)	*In vivo*	SV40 female mice that develop ER (–) tumors.	N = 40 broods	Mothers treated with BSps from 4 weeks of age until the weaning of their offspring.	Preventive effects of breast cancer in offspring. Histone acetylation and global DNA methylation were affected. SFN downregulated HDAC expression, leading to an increase in histone acetylation.

Abbas et al. (2021)	*In vivo*	BALB/c female mice	N = 200 broods	Mothers treated with canola oil during gestation and lactation of their offspring.	Epigenetic modifications that contributed to the activation of pathways that suppressed cell proliferation in tumorigenesis, with ↑ survival, ↓ tumor size, and ↓ mortality.
Chen et al. (2022)	*In vivo*	SV40 female mice that develop mammary tumors spontaneously.	N = 30 broods	Mothers treated with GE from 4 weeks of age until the weaning of their offspring.	Tumor demethylation in the progeny.
Chen et al. (2022)	*In vivo*	Her 2/neu and SV40 female mice that develop ER (−) mammary tumors spontaneously.	N = 75 broods	Mothers treated with GE from 4 weeks of age until weaning of their calves (Ma-LT-GE), GE from gestation to weaning of their offspring (Ma-ST-GE), and offspring treated with GE postnatally (from 4 weeks of age to the end of the experiment) (Post-GE).	Ma-ST-GE: ↓ protection against breast cancer compared with Ma-LT-GE. Ma-LT-GE: ↑ expression of *Trp63*, ↓ than that of *Myc*. Results of chemoprevention similar to Post-GE.
Bowers et al. (2022)	*In vivo*	C57BL/5 female mice	N = 100 broods	Mothers subjected to weight loss regimes 5 days a week for 10 weeks.	Caloric restriction: ↓ predominance to hypermethylation of DNA. Four of six genes that were differentially methylated and differentially expressed were also differentially expressed without being methylated.

Abbreviations: BSps: Broccoli sprouts; ER (−): estrogen receptor negative; GE: genistein; HDACs: histone deacetylases; Ma-ST-GE: short-term maternal treatment with genistein; Ma-LT-GE: long-term maternal treatment with genistein; N: number; Post-GE: postnatal dietary exposure of offspring to genistein; SFN: sulforaphane; ↑: increase; and ↓: decrease.

Source: Soldado-Gordillo, A., & Álvarez-Mercado, A. I., (2024). Epigenetics, microbiota, and breast cancer: A systematic review. Life, 14(6), 705. https://doi.org/10.3390/life14060705.

It is now understood that the previous approach to treating breast cancer, which involved attempting to surgically remove the entire breast, including the cancer-containing portion, the pectoralis major, and any potentially affected lymph nodes, was predicated on the false belief that most breast cancers could be surgically removed along with the local lymphatic spread. It is now acknowledged that the majority of the time the disease has spread too far for any surgical field to contain, so the surgical approach is restricted to removing the breast and the axillary nodes (or, in the case of small cancers, the tumor and surrounding tissue). Chemotherapy and/or radiation therapy are used to treat the cancer's increased spread (Table 2.8).

Table 2.8. *Summary of Various Imaging Modalities for Screening of Breast Cancer*

Imaging Modality	Principle	Diagnostic Accuracy	Advantages	Limitations
Mammography (first-line tool for breast screening).	Low-dose ionizing X-ray creates detailed images of the breast.	Sensitivity: 75–90% Specificity: 90–95% Spatial resolution: 50 μm	Most cost-effective. Good response with high specificity and sensitivity. Portable device.	Uses ionizing radiation. Sensitivity decreases with increasing breast density. Accuracy is low in young women. High false-positive results in young women due to dense breasts. Poor contrast compared to MRI.
Magnetic resonance imaging	Uses low-energy radio waves and strong magnets to obtain detailed images of structures within the breast.	Sensitivity: 75–100% Specificity: 83–98.4% Spatial resolution: 25–100 μm	Ability to detect breast malignancies that often escape from clinical, mammograms, and ultrasound detection.	Expensive, inability to standardize the test. Unnecessary breast biopsies due to inability to distinguish between malignant and benign lesions.
Magnetic resonance spectroscopy	Employs magnetic field on body fluids and tissue samples to obtain chemical information of that region.	Sensitivity: 93% Specificity: 70% Spatial resolution: up to 0.25 cm^3	Overcomes limitations of mammography. Radiation-free imaging technology. Excellent Sensitivity. Excellent spatial resolution. All imaging planes possible.	Expensive and time-consuming. Low specificity. Not portable. False-positive results in some benign tumors.
Dynamic contrast enhanced MRI (DCE-MRI)	Multiple MRI scans taken post i.v. injection of contrast agent.	Sensitivity: 89–99% Specificity: 37–86% Spatial resolution: 25–100 μm	Exhibits good performance in monitoring response post therapy.	False-negative results observed due to artifacts based on bleeding and tumor structure.

Diffusion-weighted imaging	Employs diffusion of water molecules to generate contrast.	Sensitivity: 83% Specificity: 84% Spatial resolution: 25–100 μm	Non-radioactive imaging technique	Failure to detect high water content malignant lesions due to high apparent diffusion coefficients.
MR elastography (MRE)	Dynamic elasticity imaging technique that combines MRI imaging with low frequency. Employs mechanical waves to create an elastogram to assess tissue stiffness.	Sensitivity: 90–100% Specificity: 37–80% Spatial resolution: 25–100 μm	Non-invasive, non-ionizing, and cross-sectional imaging modality.	Lacking in spatial resolution and detection of small focal lesions.
Positron emission tomography conjugated with computed tomography (PET-CT)	Combines nuclear medicine technique and computed tomography resulting in high detailed images.	Sensitivity: 90–100% Specificity: 75–90% Spatial resolution: 2–10 mm	Non-invasive. Provides twice the diagnostic benefits (elevated activity within the body detected by PET scan and intricate images of tissues and organs by CT scan).	High-cost. Unable to detect tumors less than 8 mm.
Sentinel lymph node biopsy (SLNB)	Surgical procedure to detect spreading of cancer in lymphatic system.	Sensitivity: 90.5% Specificity: 85.7% Spatial resolution: Not applicable	Significantly reduces post-operative complications.	Not useful for patients with locally advanced cancers and inflammatory breast cancer.
Breast specific gamma imaging	Employs use of a radiotracer. Image captured using a special camera.	Sensitivity: 90–96% Specificity: 71–80% Spatial resolution: ≥7 mm	Able to identify smaller lesions (<1 cm)	High radiation dose. Not suited for routine tumor screening.
Ultrasound	Employs sound waves to image breast tissues.	Sensitivity: 80–89% Specificity: 34–88% Spatial resolution: 50–500 μm	Accessible, real-time lesion visualization, cost-effective, patient compliant.	Failure to detect microcalcifications, possibility of false-positives.

Source: Bhushan, A., Gonsalves, A., & Menon, J. U., (2021). Current state of breast cancer diagnosis, treatment, and theranostics. Pharmaceutics, 13(5), 723. https://doi.org/10.3390/pharmaceutics13050723.

2.8. The Thoracic Cavity

The central mediastinum separates the right and left pleural cavities from the thoracic cavity. The mediastinum extends from the diaphragm below to become continuous above the structures in the root of the neck. It is bounded in front by the sternum and behind by the vertebral column. It includes the trachea, lymphatics, esophagus, great vessels, and heart.

2.8.1. The Heart

The pulmonary and systemic circulations are powered by the heart, a muscular pump. It consists of two ventricles and two atria, or four chambers. Unidirectional valves between the ventricles and the emerging aorta and pulmonary trunk, as well as between the ventricles and the atria, regulate the direction of blood flow. The heart is about 300 g in weight, shaped like a flattened cone with a base and an apex, and it is about the size of a closed fist. It is suspended by the pericardial sac and lies obliquely across the lower mediastinum behind the sternum, away from the great vessels (Figure 2.8).

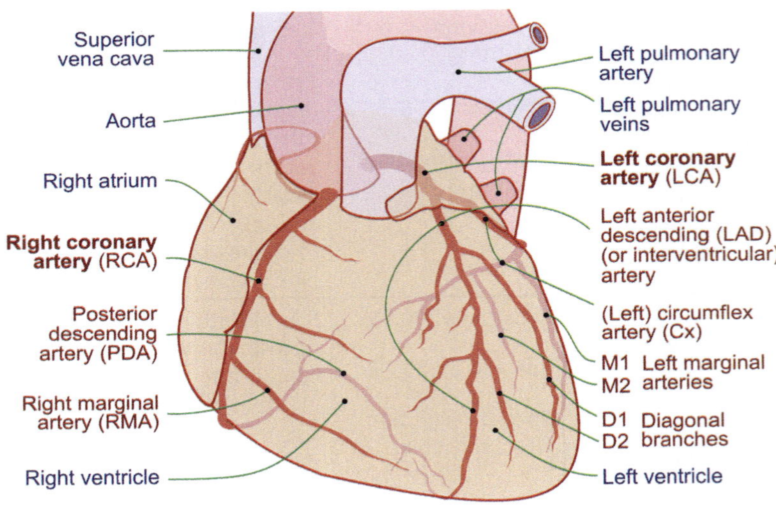

Figure 2.8. *Surface anatomy of the heart.*

Source: *By Coronary.pdf: Patrick J. Lynch, medical illustrator derivative work: Fred the Oyster adaption and further labeling: Mikael Häggström, M. D. Author info – Reusing images – Conflicts of interest: NoneMikael Häggström, M. D. – Coronary.pdf, CC BY-SA 3.0; https://commons.wikimedia.org/w/index.php?curid=9967381.*

Shaped by the left atrium and the four pulmonary veins, its square base faces posteriorly. The lower left extremity of the heart is home to the tip of the left ventricle, which forms the apex. The right atrium and the ventricles, which are divided by the anterior interventricular grooves, make up the anterior surface. The inferior surface is made up of both ventricles, primarily the left one, and is situated on the diaphragm's central tendon. The posterior interventricular groove divides them. The left ventricle and a tiny portion of the left atrium form the left surface, which is in contact with the left lung. The superior and inferior vena cavae enter the right atrium, which forms the right surface in contact with the right lung.

2.8.1.1. Surface Markings

The right sternal border is slightly beyond the right border of the heart, which lies between the 3rd and 6th right costal cartilages. Its inferior border extends from the apex, which is located in the 5th intercostal space of the midclavicular line, to the right 6th cartilage. The left border starts at the apex and ends approximately 2 centimeters from the sternal edge at the left second costal cartilage.

2.8.2. The Chambers of the Heart

Blood is pumped by the right chamber through the lungs and the left through the circulatory system. The coronary sinus, superior and inferior venae cavae, and the right atrium are the blood vessels that supply this thin-walled chamber. The right auricle, a small projection, crosses the aortic root superomedially. A vertical ridge known as the crista terminalis runs between the cavae on the right side. The smooth atrial wall with a shallow central depression known as the fossa ovalis separates the right atrium from the left atrium behind the caval openings (Figure 2.9).

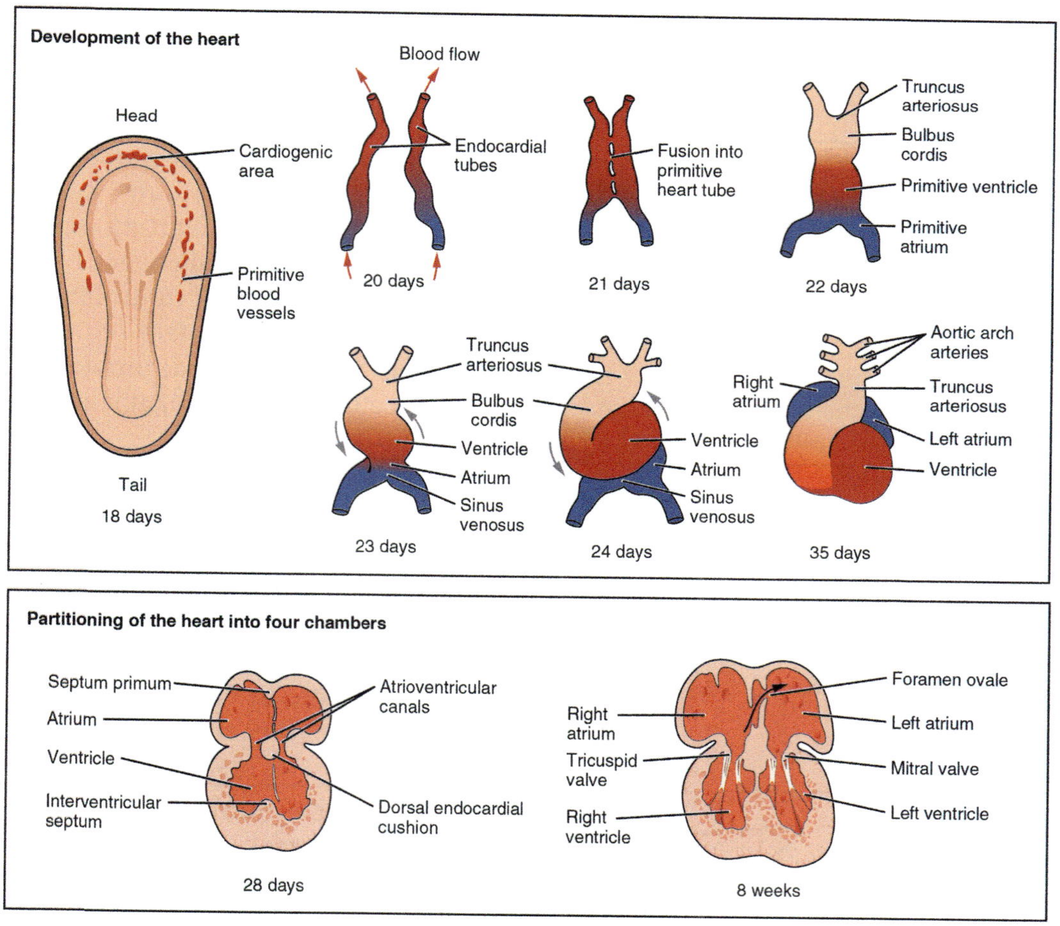

Figure 2.9. *Development.*

Source: By OpenStax College – Anatomy and Physiology, Connexions Web site. http://cnx.org/content/col11496/1.6/, CC BY 3.0; https://commons.wikimedia.org/w/index.php?curid=30148240.

Table 2.9. *Interaction of the Circulatory System with Other Body Systems*

System	Diagram	Roles of Circulatory System
Digestive	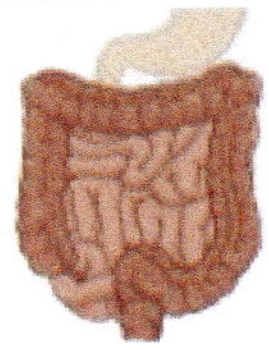	Absorbs nutrients and water; delivers nutrients (except most lipids) to liver for processing by hepactic portal vein; provides nutrients essential for hematopoiesis and building hemoglobin.
Endocrine	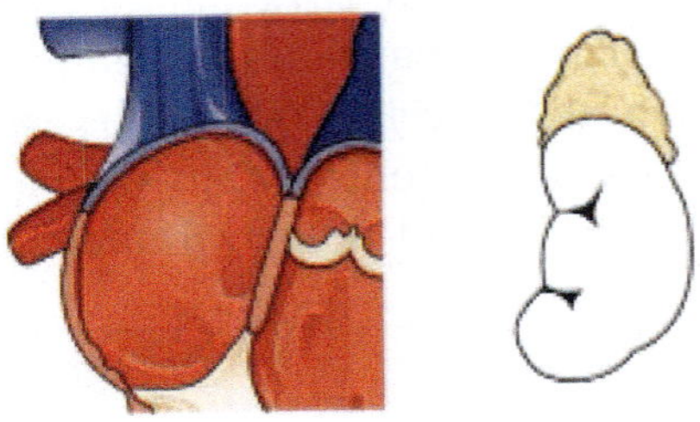	Delivers hormones: atrial natriuretic hormone (peptide) secreted by the heart atrial cells to help regulate blood volumes and pressures; epinephrine, ANH, angiotensin II, ADH, and thyroxine to help regulate blood pressure; estrogen to promote vascular health in women and men.
Integumentary	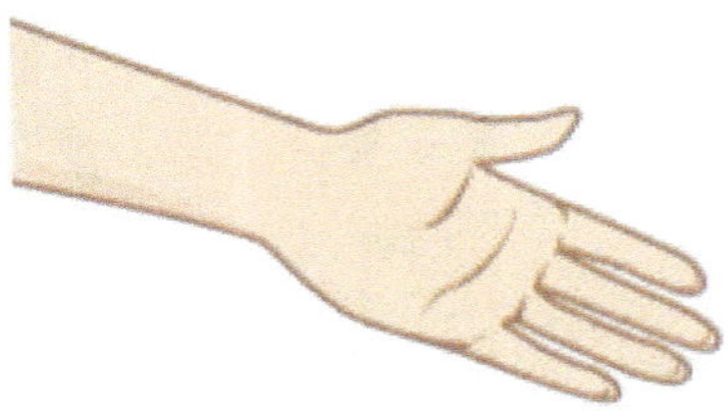	Carries clotting factors, platelets, and white blood cells for homeostasis, fighting infection, and repairing damage; regulates temperature by controlling blood flow to the surface, where heat can be dissipated; provides some coloration of integument; acts as a blood reservoir.
Lymphatic	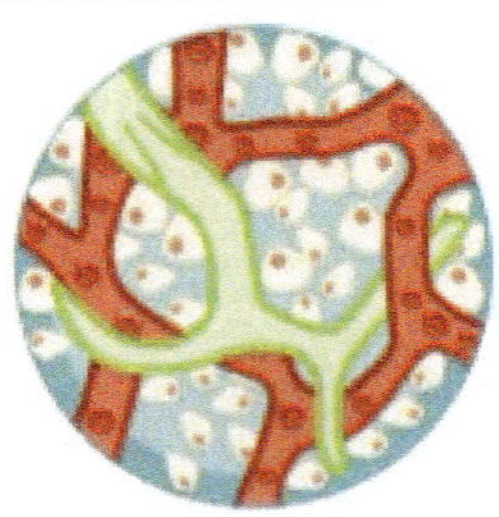	Transports various white blood cells, including those produced by lymphatic tissue, and immunoglobulins (antibodies) throughout the body to maintain health; carries excess tissue fluid not able to be reabsorbed by the vascular capillaries back to the lymphatic system for processing.
Muscular	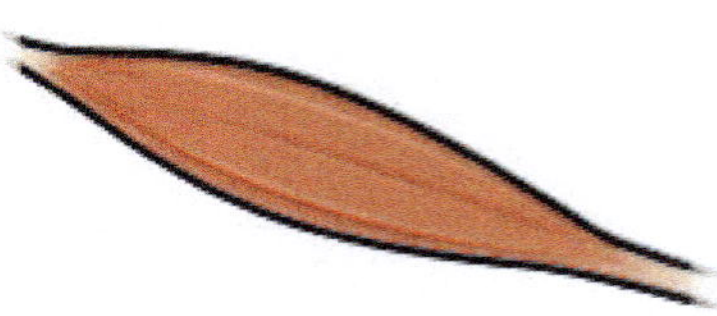	Provides nutrients and oxygen for contraction; removes lactic acid and distributes heat generated by contraction; muscular pumps aid in venous return; exercise contributes to cardiovascular health and helps to prevent atherosclerosis.

Nervous	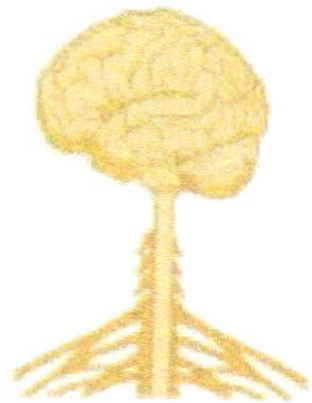	Produces cerebrospinal fluid (CSF) within choroid plexuses; contributes to blood–brain barrier; cardiac and vasomotor centers regulate cardiac output and blood flow through vessels via autonomic system.
Reproductive	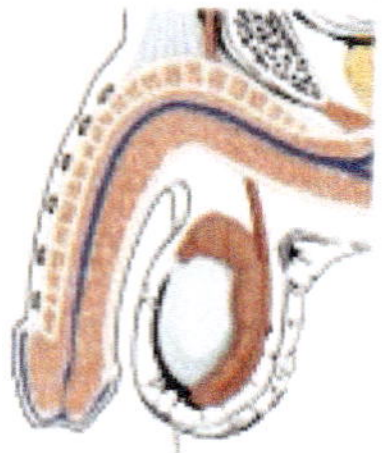	Aids in erection of genetalia in both sexes during sexual arousal; transports gonadotropic hormones that regulate reproductive functions.
Respiratory	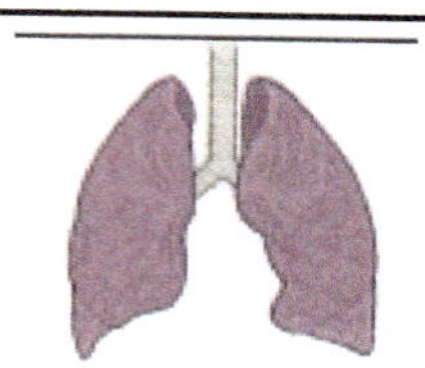	Provides blood for critical exchange of gases to carry oxygen needed for metabolic reactions and carbon dioxide generated as byproducts of these processes.
Skeletal	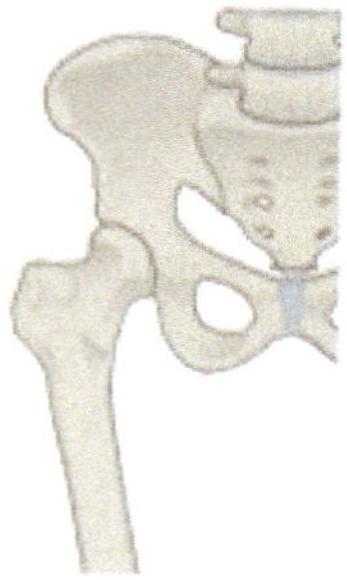	Provides calcium, phosphate, and other minerals critical for bone matrix; transports hormones regulating buildup and absorption of matrix including growth hormone (somatotropin), thyroid hormone, calcitonin's, and parathyroid hormone; erythropoietin stimulates myeloid cell hematopoiesis; some level of protection for select vessels by bony structures.
Urinary	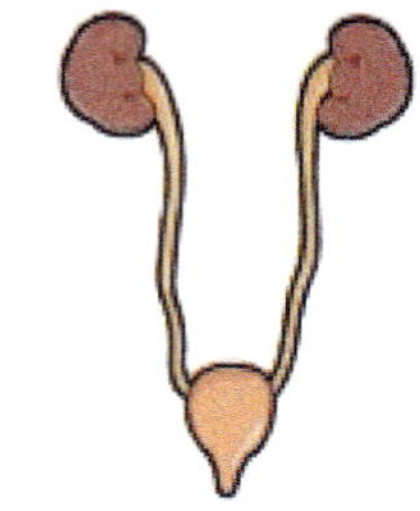	Delivers 20% of resting circulation to kidneys for filtering, reabsorption of useful products, and secretion of excesses; regulates blood volume and pressure by regulating fluid loss in the form of urine and by releasing the enzyme renin that is essential in the renin-angiotensin-aldosterone mechanism.

Source: https://courses.lumenlearning.com/suny-ap2/chapter/circulatory-pathways/.

The wall is composed of parallel muscular ridges that cross transversely to form the crista terminalis, a vertical ridge. The wall is thicker anteriorly. The inferior vena cava orifice has a primitive valve anteriorly, and the smaller coronary sinus opening is located posteriorly between them. The superior caval orifice is valveless. The right atrium projects forward and to the left of the right ventricle, a chamber with thick walls. It protrudes into the right cavity and is divided from the left ventricle by an interventricular septum. Except for the superior region, where the smooth-walled infundibulum leads to the pulmonary orifice, the ventricular walls are identified by interlacing muscular bands. The tricuspid valve, which has three cusps, protects the posteroinferior atrioventricular orifice. Their conical papillary muscles, which originate from the anterior and inferior ventricular walls, or the ventricular septum, provide the fine tendinous cords that anchor their rough ventricular surfaces to the ventricular walls. Blood regurgitation into the atrium is prevented by these cords and papillary muscles, which also stop the eversion of the valve cusps into the atrial cavity during ventricular contraction. Three semilunar cusps, which are concave when viewed from above, make up the pulmonary valve, which is located at the upper end of the infundibulum (Boron & Boulpaep, 2016; West, 2016; Berne & Levy, 2018).

Behind the right atrium is the rectangular chamber that is the left atrium. Overlying the left side of the pulmonary trunk is its appendix, the left auricular projection. Its posterior surface is entered by four pulmonary veins, two on each side; these orifices are valveless. The anterior atrial wall contains the left atrioventricular orifice. The descending thoracic aorta, left bronchus, and esophagus are all located anterior to the posterior wall. The left ventricle is primarily located behind the right ventricle and extends forward and to the left of the left atrium. Except for the vestibule, a smooth area located beneath the aortic orifice, its extremely thick walls are covered in muscular ridges on the inside. It has two openings: the aortic superiorly and the left atrioventricular posteriorly. The mitral valve, which has two cusps attached to papillary muscles by tendinous cords, protects the left atrioventricular orifice. The aortic valve consists of three cusps, and the aortic sinuses are tiny dilations located above them (Table 2.9).

2.8.3. Blood Supply

The left and right coronary arteries are the source of this. The right coronary artery originates in the anterior aortic sinus and travels down to the anterior surface of the heart, where it supplies the ventricular and atrial branches of the heart's atrioventricular groove. It gains the posterior surface, from which it arises a posterior and a marginal interventricular artery, which may form an anastomosis with the left coronary arteries anterior interventricular branch. The left posterior aortic sinus gives rise to the larger left coronary artery. It supplies the ventricular and atrial branches by moving forward. The anterior interventricular artery, also referred to as the left anterior descending artery or LAD in clinical terminology, is its most significant branch. It descends in the anterior interventricular groove to the apex and lower border before anastomosing with the right coronary arteries posterior interventricular branch (Table 2.10).

Table 2.10. *A Select List of Blood Vessels*

Vessel	Description
Pulmonary trunk	Single large vessel exiting the right ventricle that divides to form the right and left pulmonary arteries.
Pulmonary arteries	Left and right vessels that form from the pulmonary trunk and lead to smaller arterioles and eventually to the pulmonary capillaries.
Pulmonary veins	Two sets of paired vessels—one pair on each side—that are formed from the small venules, leading away from the pulmonary capillaries to flow into the left atrium.
Aorta	Largest artery in the body, originating from the left ventricle and descending to the abdominal region, where it bifurcates into the common iliac arteries at the level of the fourth lumbar vertebra; arteries originating from the aorta distribute blood to virtually all tissues of the body.
Ascending aorta	Initial portion of the aorta, rising superiorly from the left ventricle for a distance of approximately 5 cm.
Aortic arch	Graceful arc to the left that connects the ascending aorta to the descending aorta; ends at the intervertebral disk between the fourth and fifth thoracic vertebrae.
Descending aorta	Portion of the aorta that continues inferiorly past the end of the aortic arch; subdivided into the thoracic aorta and the abdominal aorta.
Thoracic aorta	Portion of the descending aorta superior to the aortic hiatus.
Abdominal aorta	Portion of the aorta inferior to the aortic hiatus and superior to the common iliac arteries.
Brachiocephalic artery	Single vessel located on the right side of the body; the first vessel branching from the aortic arch; gives rise to the right subclavian artery and the right common carotid artery; supplies blood to the head, neck, upper limb, and wall of the thoracic region.
Subclavian artery	The right subclavian artery arises from the brachiocephalic artery while the left subclavian artery arises from the aortic arch; gives rise to the internal thoracic, vertebral, and thyrocervical arteries; supplies blood to the arms, chest, shoulders, back, and central nervous system.
Internal thoracic artery	Also called the mammary artery; arises from the subclavian artery; supplies blood to the thymus, pericardium of the heart, and anterior chest wall.
Vertebral artery	Arises from the subclavian artery and passes through the vertebral foramen through the foramen magnum to the brain; joins with the internal carotid artery to form the arterial circle; supplies blood to the brain and spinal cord.

Thyrocervical artery	Arises from the subclavian artery; supplies blood to the thyroid, the cervical region, the upper back, and shoulder.
Common carotid artery	The right common carotid artery arises from the brachiocephalic artery and the left common carotid artery arises from the aortic arch; each gives rise to the external and internal carotid arteries; supplies the respective sides of the head and neck.
External carotid artery	Arises from the common carotid artery; supplies blood to numerous structures within the face, lower jaw, neck, esophagus, and larynx.
Internal carotid artery	Arises from the common carotid artery and begins with the carotid sinus; goes through the carotid canal of the temporal bone to the base of the brain; combines with the branches of the vertebral artery, forming the arterial circle; supplies blood to the brain.
Arterial circle or circle of Willis	An anastomosis located at the base of the brain that ensures continual blood supply; formed from the branches of the internal carotid and vertebral arteries; supplies blood to the brain.
Anterior cerebral artery	Arises from the internal carotid artery; supplies blood to the frontal lobe of the cerebrum.
Middle cerebral artery	Another branch of the internal carotid artery; supplies blood to the temporal and parietal lobes of the cerebrum.
Ophthalmic artery	Branch of the internal carotid artery; supplies blood to the eyes.
Anterior communicating artery	An anastomosis of the right and left internal carotid arteries; supplies blood to the brain.
Posterior communicating artery	Branches of the posterior cerebral artery that form part of the posterior portion of the arterial circle; supplies blood to the brain.
Posterior cerebral artery	Branch of the basilar artery that forms a portion of the posterior segment of the arterial circle of Willis; supplies blood to the posterior portion of the cerebrum and brain stem.
Basilar artery	Formed from the fusion of the two vertebral arteries; sends branches to the cerebellum, brain stem, and the posterior cerebral arteries; the main blood supply to the brain stem.
Visceral branches	A group of arterial branches of the thoracic aorta; supplies blood to the viscera (i.e., organs) of the thorax.
Bronchial artery	Systemic branch from the aorta that provides oxygenated blood to the lungs; this blood supply is in addition to the pulmonary circuit that brings blood for oxygenation.
Pericardial artery	Branch of the thoracic aorta; supplies blood to the pericardium.
Esophageal artery	Branch of the thoracic aorta; supplies blood to the esophagus.
Mediastinal artery	Branch of the thoracic aorta; supplies blood to the mediastinum.

Parietal branches	Also called somatic branches, a group of arterial branches of the thoracic aorta; include those that supply blood to the thoracic wall, vertebral column, and the superior surface of the diaphragm.
Intercostal artery	Branch of the thoracic aorta; supplies blood to the muscles of the thoracic cavity and vertebral column.
Superior phrenic artery	Branch of the thoracic aorta; supplies blood to the superior surface of the diaphragm.
Celiac trunk	Also called the celiac artery; a major branch of the abdominal aorta; gives rise to the left gastric artery, the splenic artery, and the common hepatic artery that forms the hepatic artery to the liver, the right gastric artery to the stomach, and the cystic artery to the gall bladder.
Left gastric artery	Branch of the celiac trunk; supplies blood to the stomach.
Splenic artery	Branch of the celiac trunk; supplies blood to the spleen.
Common hepatic artery	Branch of the celiac trunk that forms the hepatic artery, the right gastric artery, and the cystic artery.
Hepatic artery proper	Branch of the common hepatic artery; supplies systemic blood to the liver.
Right gastric artery	Branch of the common hepatic artery; supplies blood to the stomach.
Cystic artery	Branch of the common hepatic artery; supplies blood to the gall bladder.
Superior mesenteric artery	Branch of the abdominal aorta; supplies blood to the small intestine (duodenum, jejunum, and ileum), the pancreas, and a majority of the large intestine.
Inferior mesenteric artery	Branch of the abdominal aorta; supplies blood to the distal segment of the large intestine and rectum.
Inferior phrenic arteries	Branches of the abdominal aorta; supply blood to the inferior surface of the diaphragm.
Adrenal artery	Branch of the abdominal aorta; supplies blood to the adrenal (suprarenal) glands.
Renal artery	Branch of the abdominal aorta; supplies each kidney.
Gonadal artery	Branch of the abdominal aorta; supplies blood to the gonads or reproductive organs; also described as ovarian arteries or testicular arteries, depending upon the sex of the individual.
Ovarian artery	Branch of the abdominal aorta; supplies blood to ovary, uterine (Fallopian) tube, and uterus.
Testicular artery	Branch of the abdominal aorta; ultimately travels outside the body cavity to the testes and forms one component of the spermatic cord.
Lumbar arteries	Branches of the abdominal aorta; supply blood to the lumbar region, the abdominal wall, and spinal cord.

Common iliac artery	Branch of the aorta that leads to the internal and external iliac arteries.
Median sacral artery	Continuation of the aorta into the sacrum.
Internal iliac artery	Branch from the common iliac arteries; supplies blood to the urinary bladder, walls of the pelvis, external genitalia, and the medial portion of the femoral region; in females, also provides blood to the uterus and vagina.
External iliac artery	Branch of the common iliac artery that leaves the body cavity and becomes a femoral artery; supplies blood to the lower limbs.
Axillary artery	Continuation of the subclavian artery as it penetrates the body wall and enters the axillary region; supplies blood to the region near the head of the humerus (humeral circumflex arteries); the majority of the vessel continues into the brachium and becomes the brachial artery.
Brachial artery	Continuation of the axillary artery in the brachium; supplies blood to much of the brachial region; gives off several smaller branches that provide blood to the posterior surface of the arm in the region of the elbow; bifurcates into the radial and ulnar arteries at the coronoid fossa.
Radial artery	Formed at the bifurcation of the brachial artery; parallels the radius; gives off smaller branches until it reaches the carpal region where it fuses with the ulnar artery to form the superficial and deep palmar arches; supplies blood to the lower arm and carpal region.
Ulnar artery	Formed at the bifurcation of the brachial artery; parallels the ulna; gives off smaller branches until it reaches the carpal region where it fuses with the radial artery to form the superficial and deep palmar arches; supplies blood to the lower arm and carpal region.
Palmar arches (superficial and deep)	Formed from anastomosis of the radial and ulnar arteries; supply blood to the hand and digital arteries.
Digital arteries	Formed from the superficial and deep palmar arches; supply blood to the digits.
Femoral artery	Continuation of the external iliac artery after it passes through the body cavity; divides into several smaller branches, the lateral deep femoral artery, and the genicular artery; becomes the popliteal artery as it passes posterior to the knee.
Deep femoral artery	Branch of the femoral artery; gives rise to the lateral circumflex arteries.
Lateral circumflex artery	Branch of the deep femoral artery; supplies blood to the deep muscles of the thigh and the ventral and lateral regions of the integument.
Genicular artery	Branch of the femoral artery; supplies blood to the region of the knee.

Popliteal artery	Continuation of the femoral artery posterior to the knee; branches into the anterior and posterior tibial arteries.
Anterior tibial artery	Branches from the popliteal artery; supplies blood to the anterior tibial region; becomes the dorsalis pedis artery.
Dorsalis pedis artery	Forms from the anterior tibial artery; branches repeatedly to supply blood to the tarsal and dorsal regions of the foot.
Posterior tibial artery	Branches from the popliteal artery and gives rise to the fibular or peroneal artery; supplies blood to the posterior tibial region.
Medial plantar artery	Arises from the bifurcation of the posterior tibial arteries; supplies blood to the medial plantar surfaces of the foot.
Lateral plantar artery	Arises from the bifurcation of the posterior tibial arteries; supplies blood to the lateral plantar surfaces of the foot.
Dorsal or arcuate arch	Formed from the anastomosis of the dorsalis pedis artery and the medial and plantar arteries; branches supply the distal portions of the foot and digits.
Plantar arch	Formed from the anastomosis of the dorsalis pedis artery and the medial and plantar arteries; branches supply the distal portions of the foot and digits.

Source: https://courses.lumenlearning.com/suny-ap2/chapter/circulatory-pathways/.

To supply a large portion of the left ventricle, the circumflex branch passes posteriorly. The right coronary artery typically supplies the right ventricle, the left by the left, both the left and the right supply the interventricular septum, and the atria variably supply the left. Typically, the right coronary artery supplies both the atrioventricular node and the sinoatrial node.

The most commonly afflicted heart valve is the mitral valve; fibrosis shortens the cusps, resulting in valve incompetence and/or stenosis. It is possible to have congenital stenosis of the aortic and pulmonary valves, which can lead to cardiac decompensation and right and left ventricle hypertrophy, respectively. Even though there are anastomoses between the two coronary arteries, a sudden blockage of a major branch can cause ischemia and myocardial infarction, which is the death of part of the heart muscle. If the affected area is large or includes the conducting system, the patient may not survive. Less severe ischemic damage reduces the heart's ability to pump blood, and angina (pain) may appear with effort. By reducing the blood supply to the heart muscle, coronary artery narrowing may also result in angina, a pain that is typically felt in the substernal area.

The myocardium's ischemia stimulates its nerve endings. The sympathetic branches transport sensory impulses to the thoracic segments T1–4, mostly on the left side. Although heart-related pain is felt substernally, it is frequently reported to be in the left arm and neck. Sometimes balloon dilatation, stenting, or surgical bypass of the blockage can be used to treat this coronary narrowing (CABG – coronary artery bypass graft). The mitral or tricuspid valve may become inoperable as a result of a ruptured papillary muscle, such as that which occurs after ischemic damage. Incompetence or valvular stenosis may necessitate surgical valve replacement.

2.8.3.1. Venous Drainage

The coronary sinus, which empties into the right atrium close to the inferior vena cava opening, is primarily responsible for this. The great cardiac vein ascends the anterior interventricular groove, the middle cardiac vein runs in the posterior interventricular groove, and a small cardiac vein reaches it in the coronary sulcus, branching from the posterior of the left ventricle and atrium. The cardiac vein is approximately 3 cm long. Numerous anterior cardiac veins empty the anterior right ventricle and empty into the right atrium. Much of the heart wall is drained by the Venae Cordii Minimae. They are tiny and lead straight into the chambers of the heart.

2.8.4. Nerve Supply

This originates from the sympathetic (cardio excitatory) and vagus (cardioinhibitory) nerves via the cardiac plexus. The fibers travel alongside the coronary artery branches. Within the heart wall are the parasympathetic ganglia. Pain fibers travel with sympathetic nerves, passing through the cervical and upper thoracic sympathetic ganglia before entering the spinal nerves T1–4. The vagus nerve carries sensory fibers. Ischemic heart tissue is the source of cardiac pain. The somatic structures with the same nerve supply—the left upper limb, the precordium, and the left neck—are often associated with the visceral pain caused by ischemia because the afferent sensory fibers travel through the cervical and upper thoracic ganglia before entering the upper thoracic spinal cord segments.

The heart's conducting system, which is made up of specialized cardiac muscle cells, starts, plans, and controls the intricate contraction pattern that makes up the cardiac cycle. The AV bundle of His, its right and left branches, the terminal subendocardial plexus of Purkinje fibers, the atrioventricular (AV) node, and the sinoatrial (SA) node make up this structure. A tiny patch of conducting tissue located in the right atrial wall anterior to the superior vena cava opening is called the SA node, sometimes referred to as the pacemaker. The atrial wall muscle conducts impulses from it to the AV node, a nodule that is similar and located near the coronary sinus entrance on the right side of the atrial septum. From there, the AV bundle descends the interventricular septum and splits into the right and left branches, which supply the corresponding ventricle primarily. These branches then branch out to form the subendocardial plexus, which supplies the papillary muscles and ventricular walls.

2.8.5. The Pericardium

The pericardium is a protective membrane that surrounds the heart and the nearby large blood vessels. It is made up of an outer layer of fibrous tissue and an inner layer of serous tissue, which is further divided into visceral and parietal layers. These layers enclose the pericardial sac, creating a closed sac that contains a thin pericardial cavity around the heart. The visceral pericardium covers the outer surface of the heart and is connected to the parietal pericardium lining the inside of the fibrous pericardium.

2.8.5.1. Electrocardiogram (ECG)

The ECG is a record of the electrical potential detected at the body surface. Around 10 electrodes are placed as shown in Figure 2.10–four limb leads on the muscular parts of each forearm and lower leg and six precordial leads, named V_1–V_6, are placed:

- **V_1** – right side of sternum, 4th intercostal space.
- **V_2** – left side of sternum, 4th intercostal space.
- **V_3** – midway between V_2 and V_4.

- **V_4** – midclavicular line, 5th intercostal space.
- **V_5** – anterior axillary line horizontal to V_4.
- **V_6** – mid-axillary line horizontal to V_4.

The ECG traces detect the electrical potential produced by the heart muscle contracting. Each trace represents a distinct area of the heart muscle, allowing for the identification and localization of any abnormalities. This method is crucial for measuring and diagnosing irregular heart rhythms resulting from issues with the conducting tissue or electrolyte imbalances. Additionally, in cases of myocardial infarction, it can pinpoint the specific region of the heart muscle that has been damaged.

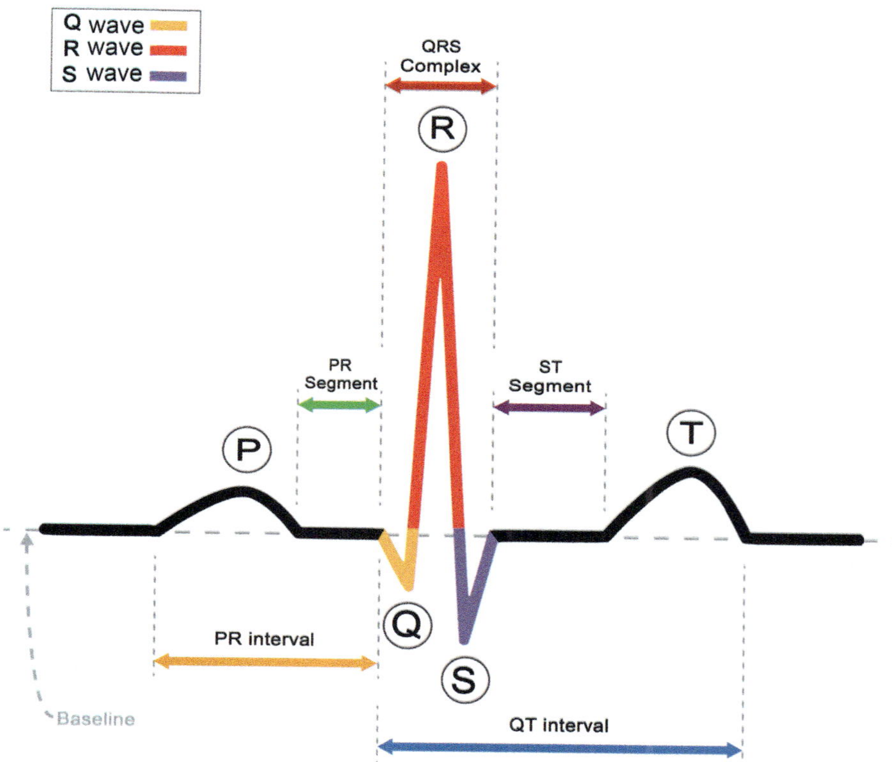

Figure 2.10. *The electrocardiogram (ECG) records the electrical activity of the heart. Leads, attached by adhesive pads, are placed on the shoulders, left leg and around the chest (V_1–V_6). Leads I, II, and III record voltage between two limb leads; AVR, AVL, and AVF, between one limb and the other two; and V_1–V_6 between a point on the chest and an average of the three limb leads. AVR and V1 are oriented towards the cavity of the heart; II, III, and AVF face the inferior surface; I, AVL, and V_6 face the lateral wall of the left ventricle; V_1 and V_2 are directed at the right ventricle; V_3 and V_4 at the interventricular septum; and V_5 and V_6 at the left ventricle.*

Source: By Created by Agateller (Anthony Atkielski), converted to svg by atom. SinusRhythmLabels.png, Public Domain; https://commons.wikimedia.org/w/index.php?curid=1560893; http://repository.stikesrspadgs.ac.id/62/1/Illustrated%20Clinical%20Anatomy-402hlm.pdf.

An electrocardiogram (ECG) can record the generation and passage of the impulses from the SA node, and this diagnostic tool is very useful in identifying cardiac irregularities and the location of cardiac ischemia. The ventricles beat slowly at their own rate independent of the atria, which continue to contract at the rate set by the SA node if the AV bundle is damaged, as might happen after a coronary artery thrombosis. This condition is known as total heart block. Atheroma can damage the AV node, which delays the propagation of impulses and can result in ischemia or myocardial infarction (heart block). A cardiac pacemaker with an electrode positioned in the right ventricle is inserted to treat this (Figure 2.10).

Cardiac tamponade is the limitation of the heart's filling and output due to fluid in the pericardium caused by trauma or infection. Congestion develops in the veins of the face and neck as a result, and eventually, the cardiac output falls as the fluid pressure in the inextensible pericardial sac rises. Aspirating the fluid is required in these situations. A needle inserted between the xiphoid process and the left costal margin and directed headwards, backwards, and medially through the central tendon of the diaphragm is the most convenient way to enter the pericardial sac (Figure 2.11).

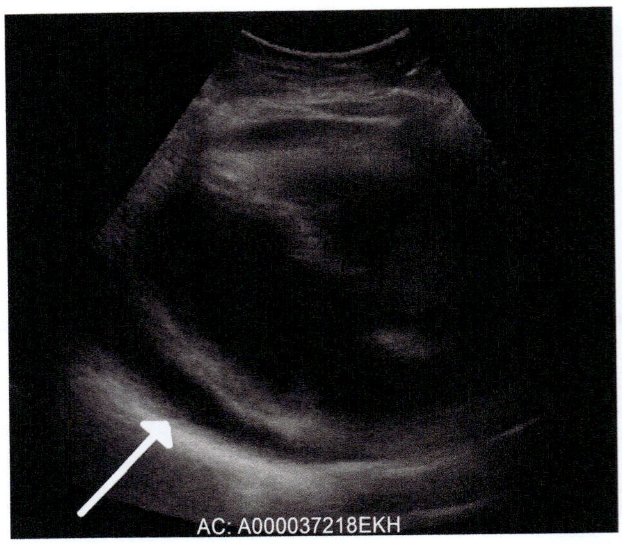

Figure 2.11. *Pericardial effusion.*

Source: By James Heilman, M. D. – Own work, CC BY-SA 3.0; https://commons.wikimedia.org/w/index.php?curid=19364446.

The fibrous pericardium encircles the heart and serous pericardium in a robust, flask-shaped sac that merges with the pulmonary veins behind, the adventitia of the aorta, pulmonary trunk, and inferior vena cava above, and the central tendon of the diaphragm in Figure 2.11.

2.8.6. Development of the Heart

A vascular tube that hangs from the dorsal wall of the pericardial portion of the coelomic sac gives rise to the heart. There are two primary processes at play: division into the left and right sides and bending with differential growth.

2.8.6.1. Bending and Differential Growth

The dorsal mesocardium, a mesentery, suspends the heart from the embryo's dorsal wall. The vessels that become the pulmonary veins and the superior and inferior venae cavae are received at the caudal (venous) end of the heart tube. These vessels are encased in a common pericardial sheath. The aorta and pulmonary artery, which are also contained within a single pericardial tube, are formed by the division of the cephalic (arterial) end. The cephalic end becomes S-shaped as it elongates and descends in front of the veins. The oblique and transverse sinuses are spaces left in the pericardial sac by the heart's twisting development. In the primitive heart, the sinus venosus, atrium, ventricle, and bulbus cordis develop into four dilatations. A small atrioventricular canal connects the ventricle and atrium.

2.8.6.2. Division into Right and Left Sides

The right and left atria, the right and left ventricles, and the pulmonary and aortic trunks are separated, respectively, by longitudinal partitions in the atrium, ventricle, and bulbus cordis. The atrioventricular canal is divided into the right and left sides by the union of two tiny endocardial cushions.

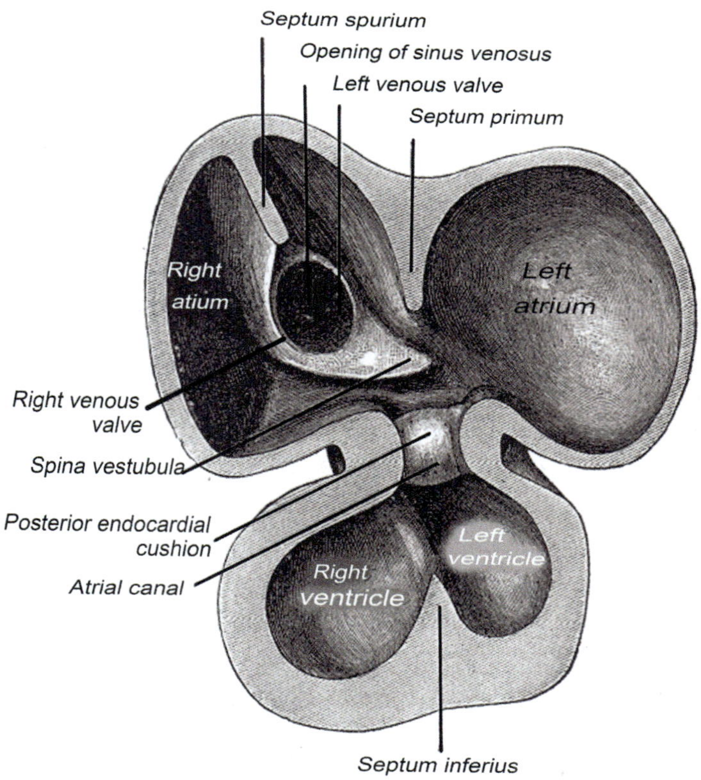

Figure 2.12. *The development of the cardiovascular system.*

Source: By Henry Vandyke Carter – Henry Gray, (1918). Anatomy of the human body (see "Book" section below) Bartleby.com: Gray's Anatomy, Plate 465, Public Domain; https://commons.wikimedia.org/w/index.php?curid=567229.

A septum (septum primum) penetrates the atrial cavity and becomes perforated in its upper part as it descends to fuse with the endocardial cushions. By virtue of its construction, the foramen ovale acts in the fetus like a valve, allowing blood to flow from the right to the left atria but not the other way. A septum secundum descends on the right of the septum primum to partially overlap the perforation, leaving an oblique communication between the atria (Figure 2.12).

The bulbus cordis cavity is divided by a spiral septum to form the pulmonary and aortic trunks, while the ventricular cavity is divided by a septum that fuses with the endocardial cushions above. The right ventricle leads to the pulmonary trunk, while the left ventricle leads to the aorta due to the union of the ventricles and the bulbar septa. The pulmonary veins are included in the left atrium, and the sinus venosus is included in the right atrium.

2.8.6.3. Fetal Circulation

The ductus venosus transports oxygenated blood from the placenta to the liver, where it is subsequently transported to the right atrium and inferior vena cava. The angle formed by the inferior and superior vena cava then directs the placental blood into the left atrium via the foramen ovale, the left ventricle, and finally the aorta. A significant portion of this blood is directed toward the head and growing brain. It goes back to the heart via the pulmonary artery and the right ventricle after exiting through the superior vena cava.

The ductus arteriosus then directs it into the aorta, avoiding the lungs in the process. While some of it travels through the placenta through the umbilical arteries, the majority flows to the rest of the body. The inferior vena cava receives blood from the placenta in the umbilical vein and the ductus venosus, as well as the venous return from the rest of the body. As soon as breathing starts, there is a rise in both the amount of blood going to the lungs and the amount of venous return in the pulmonary veins. As a result, the left atrial pressure increases, closing the foramen ovale. At this point, the ductus venosus and ductus arteriosus also shut, establishing the adult pattern of circulation.

Many people are born with congenital cardiac defects, some of which are not compatible with long-term survival. Although they are frequently symptomless, bicuspid aortic valves are among the most prevalent. Surgical correction is typically necessary for a patent ductus arteriosus, ventricular defects, and atrial septal defects (caused by a persistent foramen ovale). Heart failure typically ensues from pulmonary hypertension, which is caused by higher-pressure systemic blood being diverted into the pulmonary circulation if the ductus is unable to close. It needs to be corrected surgically. Congenital narrowing of the aorta near the ductus is known as aortic coarctation. Anastomoses between the scapular and intercostal vessels, as well as the internal thoracic and inferior epigastric vessels, are typically responsible for maintaining circulation in the lower body and limbs when the coarctation is short.

Atrioventricular septal defect (ASD) is a defect in which the septa overlap but the fusion of the septum primum and septum secundum is incomplete in 10% of the population. This defect usually has no functional significance. A surgical repair is necessary in a small number of patients because the defect permits blood to be shunted from the left to the right atrium. The membranous portion of the interventricular septum, a region with a complex developmental origin, is where ventricular septal defects (VSDs) are typically located. The larger ones result in a blood shunt from the left ventricle to the right, which raises pulmonary blood flow, pulmonary hypertension, and cardiac failure. They differ in size and clinical significance. If congenital pulmonary stenosis is linked to a VSD, it can lead to some syndromes, including Fallot's tetralogy. This includes right ventricular hypertrophy, pulmonary stenosis, an overriding aorta, and a ventricular septal defect (Boron & Boulpaep, 2016; West, 2016; Berne & Levy, 2018).

A Closer Look

Breast Tissue

Breast tissue, a vital component of the female anatomy, is a complex structure composed of glandular, fibrous, and adipose tissues, each playing a crucial role in the breast's function and overall health. The glandular tissue, which includes lobules and ducts, is responsible for the production and transportation of milk during lactation. Lobules are small, milk-producing glands, and ducts are the channels that carry milk from the lobules to the nipple. Surrounding these glandular structures is fibrous tissue, which provides support and maintains the shape of the breast. Adipose tissue, or fat, fills the spaces between the lobules and ducts, contributing to the size and shape of the breast and serving as a protective cushion. The proportion of these tissues varies among individuals and can change over time due to factors such as age, hormonal fluctuations, and body weight. Hormones, particularly estrogen and progesterone, play a significant role in the development and function of breast tissue. During puberty, these hormones stimulate the growth of ductal tissue and the accumulation of adipose tissue, leading to the development of mature breasts. Throughout the menstrual cycle, hormonal changes cause fluctuations in breast tissue, often resulting in temporary swelling and tenderness. During pregnancy, increased levels of estrogen, progesterone, and prolactin prepare the breasts for lactation by promoting the growth of lobules and ducts. After childbirth, prolactin continues to stimulate milk production, while oxytocin triggers the milk ejection reflex during breastfeeding. Breast tissue is also subject to various pathological conditions, such as benign breast lumps, cysts, fibroadenomas, and malignant tumors like breast cancer. Regular self-examinations and screenings, such as mammograms, are essential for early detection and treatment of breast abnormalities. Lifestyle factors, including diet, exercise, and avoiding harmful substances like tobacco and excessive alcohol, can influence breast health. Additionally, genetic factors, such as mutations in the BRCA1 and BRCA2 genes, significantly increase the risk of developing breast cancer. Understanding the anatomy and function of breast tissue is crucial for recognizing changes and maintaining breast health. Awareness and education about breast health can empower individuals to take proactive steps in monitoring their breasts and seeking medical advice when necessary. Advances in medical research continue to improve our understanding of breast tissue, leading to better prevention, diagnosis, and treatment options for breast-related conditions. Ultimately, a comprehensive approach to breast health involves a combination of regular medical check-ups, a healthy lifestyle, and being informed about the risks and signs of breast diseases. This approach helps in maintaining the overall health and well-being of individuals, ensuring that any issues with breast tissue are addressed promptly and effectively (Boron & Boulpaep, 2016; West, 2016; Berne & Levy, 2018).

Summary

- The thorax is the region between the abdomen inferiorly and the root of the neck superiorly. The thorax forms from the thoracic wall, its superficial structures (breast, muscles, and skin), and the thoracic cavity.
- The thoracic wall is formed by 12 ribs, 12 thoracic vertebrae, cartilage, sternum, and five muscles. The thoracic wall functions in movement, respiration, and protection of the thoracic cavity.
- The thoracic cavity can typically be divided into well-established compartments. The pleural cavities and the mediastinum are the primary constituents. There are two pleural cavities which respectively contain the left and right lungs and the pleura.
- The embryo's development undergoes the formation of three distinct layers (the trilaminar disc). These layers are the outer ectoderm, middle mesoderm, and inner endoderm.
- The cardiovascular system originates from the mesoderm layer as a coalescence of cardiac myoblasts known as the cardiogenic field. This field is initially horseshoe-shaped but rotates to form a primitive heart tube.
- The intercostal vessels and nerves form a neurovascular bundle that passes forward in the subcostal groove deep into the internal intercostal muscle, separated from the pleura only by the innermost intercostal muscle.
- The adult female breast is a soft, hemispherical structure. It is composed of glandular, and a variable amount of fat and fibrous tissue and lies in the superficial fascia of the upper anterior thoracic wall.
- The wall is thicker anteriorly and formed of parallel muscular ridges which pass transversely to a vertical ridge, the crista terminalis. The superior caval orifice has no valves; that of the inferior vena cava has a rudimentary valve anteriorly, and between them, posteriorly, is the smaller opening of the coronary sinus.
- The pericardium is a fibro serous membrane that surrounds the heart and the adjacent parts of the large vessels entering and leaving it. It consists of an outer fibrous and an inner serous layer, and the latter is divided into two layers, the visceral and parietal, between which is the pericardial sac.
- The heart is suspended from the dorsal wall of the embryo by a mesentery, the dorsal mesocardium. The caudal (venous) end of the heart tube receives vessels, enclosed in a common sheath of pericardium, which become the superior and inferior venae cavae and the pulmonary veins (Boron & Boulpaep, 2016; West, 2016; Berne & Levy, 2018).

References

1. Allen, E., Minutello, K., & Murcek, B. W. (2023). Anatomy, head and neck, larynx recurrent laryngeal nerve. In *StatPearls*. StatPearls Publishing. Retrieved from: https://www.ncbi.nlm.nih.gov/books/NBK499964/ (accessed on 3 July 2024).
2. Alshak, M. N., & Das, J. M. (2023). Neuroanatomy, sympathetic nervous system. In *StatPearls*. StatPearls Publishing. Retrieved from: https://www.ncbi.nlm.nih.gov/books/NBK482476/ (accessed on 3 July 2024).

3. Aroor, A. R., Prakasha, S. R., Seshadri, S., S, T., & Raghuraj, U. (2014). A study of clinical characteristics of mediastinal mass. *Journal of Clinical and Diagnostic Research, 8*(2), 77–80.
4. Banning, A. P., Baumbach, A., Blackman, D., Curzen, N., Devadathan, S., Fraser, D., & British Cardiovascular Intervention Society. (2015). Percutaneous coronary intervention in the UK: Recommendations for good practice 2015. *Heart, 101*(Suppl 3), 1–13.
5. Berne, R. M., & Levy, M. N. (2018). *Cardiovascular Physiology* (10th ed.). Elsevier.
6. Boron, W. F., & Boulpaep, E. L. (2016). *Medical Physiology* (3rd ed.). Elsevier.
7. Brochhausen, C., Turial, S., Müller, F. K., Schmitt, V. H., Coerdt, W., Wihlm, J. M., & Kirkpatrick, C. J. (2012). Pectus excavatum: History, hypotheses and treatment options. *Interactive CardioVascular and Thoracic Surgery, 14*(6), 801–806.
8. Brown, K. N., Devarapally, S. R., Lee, L. S., & Gupta, N. (2023). Catheter-directed thrombolysis of pulmonary embolism. In *StatPearls*. StatPearls Publishing. Retrieved from: https://www.ncbi.nlm.nih.gov/books/NBK507860/ (accessed on 3 July 2024).
9. Choi, W. I. (2014). Pneumothorax. *Tuberculosis and Respiratory Diseases (Seoul), 76*(3), 99–104.
10. Clemens, M. W., Evans, K. K., Mardini, S., & Arnold, P. G. (2011). Introduction to chest wall reconstruction: Anatomy and physiology of the chest and indications for chest wall reconstruction. *Seminars in Plastic Surgery, 25*(1), 5–15.
11. Criado, F. J. (2011). Aortic dissection: A 250-year perspective. *Texas Heart Institute Journal, 38*(6), 694–700.
12. Currie, G. P., Alluri, R., Christie, G. L., & Legge, J. S. (2007). Pneumothorax: An update. *Postgraduate Medical Journal, 83*(981), 461–465.
13. Davis, K. A., & Johansson, E. (2014). *Diaphragm Anatomy and Function: Advanced Concepts* (1st ed.). Wiley-Blackwell.
14. Donley, E. R., Holme, M. R., & Loyd, J. W. (2022). Anatomy, thorax, wall movements. In *StatPearls*. StatPearls Publishing. Retrieved from: https://www.ncbi.nlm.nih.gov/books/NBK535366/ (accessed on 3 July 2024).
15. Drake, R. L., Vogl, W., Mitchell, A. W. M., & Gray, H. (2019). *Gray's Anatomy for Students* (4th ed.). Elsevier.
16. Ganong, W. F. (2019). *Review of Medical Physiology* (26th ed.). McGraw-Hill Education.
17. Glenesk, N. L., Rahman, S., & Lopez, P. P. (2023). Anatomy, thorax, intercostal nerves. In *StatPearls*. StatPearls Publishing. Retrieved from: https://www.ncbi.nlm.nih.gov/books/NBK500021/ (accessed on 3 July 2024).
18. Hussain, A., & Burns, B. (2023). Anatomy, thorax, wall. In *StatPearls*. StatPearls Publishing. Retrieved from: https://www.ncbi.nlm.nih.gov/books/NBK459338/ (accessed on 3 July 2024).
19. Ilahi, M., St Lucia, K., & Ilahi, T. B. (2023). Anatomy, thorax, thoracic duct. In *StatPearls*. StatPearls Publishing. Retrieved from: https://www.ncbi.nlm.nih.gov/books/NBK482317/ (accessed on 3 July 2024).
20. Jung, H. O. (2012). Pericardial effusion and pericardiocentesis: Role of echocardiography. *Korean Circulation Journal, 42*(11), 725–734.
21. Kalamchi, L., & Valle, C. (2023). Embryology, vertebral column development. In *StatPearls*. StatPearls Publishing.

22. Kardong, K. V. (2015). *Vertebrates: Comparative Anatomy, Function, Evolution* (7th ed.). McGraw-Hill Education.
23. Keith, L. (2015). *Functional Anatomy of the Thorax* (1st ed.). Cambridge University Press.
24. Kenny, B. J., & Bordoni, B. (2022). Neuroanatomy, cranial nerve 10 (vagus nerve). In *StatPearls*. StatPearls Publishing.
25. Kocbek, L., & Rakuša, M. (2018). Common trunk of the posterior intercostal arteries from the thoracic aorta: Anatomical variation, frequency, and importance in individuals. *Surgical and Radiologic Anatomy, 40*(4), 465–470.
26. Kuo, K., & Kim, A. M. (2023). Rib fracture. In *StatPearls*. StatPearls Publishing.
27. Lazopoulos, A., Barbetakis, N., Lazaridis, G., Baka, S., Mpoukovinas, I., Karavasilis, V., & Zarogoulidis, P. (2015). Open thoracotomy for pneumothorax. *Journal of Thoracic Disease, 7*(Suppl 1), S50–S55.
28. Lumb, A. B. (2016). *Nunn's Applied Respiratory Physiology* (8th ed.). Elsevier.
29. Marta, M. J., Falcão, L. M., Saavedra, J. A., & Ravara, L. (2003). A case of complete situs inversus. *Revista Portuguesa de Cardiologia, 22*(1), 91–104.
30. Mathew, P., & Bordoni, B. (2023). Embryology, heart. In *StatPearls*. StatPearls Publishing.
31. McMinn, R. M. H., & Hutchings, R. T. (1998). *A Color Atlas of Human Anatomy* (2nd ed.). Mosby.
32. Moore, K. L., Dalley, A. F., & Agur, A. M. R. (2013). *Clinically Oriented Anatomy* (7th ed.). Lippincott Williams & Wilkins.
33. Moorman, A., Webb, S., Brown, N. A., Lamers, W., & Anderson, R. H. (2003). Development of the heart: (1) Formation of the cardiac chambers and arterial trunks. *Heart, 89*(7), 806–814.
34. Myers, T. W. (2014). *Anatomy Trains: Myofascial Meridians for Manual and Movement Therapists* (3rd ed.). Elsevier.
35. Netter, F. H. (2014). *Atlas of Human Anatomy* (6th ed.). Saunders.
36. Oliver, K. A., & Ashurst, J. V. (2023). Anatomy, thorax, phrenic nerves. In *StatPearls*. StatPearls Publishing.
37. Peterson, L. J., & Boorman, R. S. (2002). *Thoracic Surgery Atlas* (1st ed.). Saunders.
38. Polcaro, L., Charlick, M., & Daly, D. T. (2023). Anatomy, head and neck: Brachial plexus. In *StatPearls*. StatPearls Publishing.
39. Rehman, S., & Bacha, D. (2023). Embryology, pulmonary. In *StatPearls*. StatPearls Publishing.
40. Remien, K., & Jan, A. (2023). Anatomy, head and neck, thymus. In *StatPearls*. StatPearls Publishing.
41. Reser, D., Caliskan, E., Tolboom, H., Guidotti, A., & Maisano, F. (2015). Median sternotomy. *Multimedia Manual of Cardiothoracic Surgery, 2015*.
42. Rivard, A. B., Galarza-Paez, L., & Peterson, D. C. (2023). Anatomy, thorax, breast. In *StatPearls*. StatPearls Publishing.
43. Rizvi, S., Wehrle, C. J., & Law, M. A. (2023). Anatomy, thorax, mediastinum superior and great vessels. In *StatPearls*. StatPearls Publishing.
44. Rohen, J. W., Yokochi, C., & Lütjen-Drecoll, E. (2016). *Color Atlas of Anatomy: A Photographic Study of the Human Body* (8th ed.). Lippincott Williams & Wilkins.

45. Sagristà-Sauleda, J., Mercé, A. S., & Soler-Soler, J. (2011). Diagnosis and management of pericardial effusion. *World Journal of Cardiology, 3*(5), 135–143.

46. Seigel, G. (2018). *Essential Clinical Anatomy* (5th ed.). Lippincott Williams & Wilkins.

47. Shahoud, J. S., Kerndt, C. C., & Burns, B. (2023). Anatomy, thorax, internal mammary (internal thoracic) arteries. In *StatPearls*. StatPearls Publishing.

48. Snell, R. S. (2012). *Clinical Anatomy by Regions* (9th ed.). Lippincott Williams & Wilkins.

49. Standring, S. (2020). *Gray's Anatomy: The Anatomical Basis of Clinical Practice* (42nd ed.). Elsevier.

50. Stoddard, N., Heil, J. R., & Lowery, D. R. (2023). Anatomy, thorax, mediastinum. In *StatPearls*. StatPearls Publishing.

51. Tang, A., & Bordoni, B. (2023). Anatomy, thorax, muscles. In *StatPearls*. StatPearls Publishing.

52. Wang, J., Li, J., Liu, G., & Deslauriers, J. (2011). Nerves of the mediastinum. *Thoracic Surgery Clinics, 21*(2), 239–249, ix.

53. West, J. B. (2016). *Respiratory Physiology: The Essentials* (10th ed.). Lippincott Williams & Wilkins.

54. White, H. J., & Soos, M. P. (2023). Anatomy, thorax, superior vena cava. In *StatPearls*. StatPearls Publishing.

55. Williamson, A. J., & Shermetaro, C. (2023). Unilateral vocal cord paralysis. In *StatPearls*. StatPearls Publishing.

56. Yoganathan, A. P., & Chandran, K. B. (2010). *Cardiovascular Fluid Dynamics: Clinical Applications* (1st ed.). Springer.

57. Zugibe, F. T., & Zugibe, J. B. (2005). *The Diaphragm and Its Relationship to Respiratory Disease* (1st ed.). CRC Press.

58. International Agency for Research on Cancer. *GLOBOCAN 2020: New Global Cancer Data|UICC*. 2020. [(accessed on 16 March 2022)]. Available online: https://www.uicc.org/news/globocan-2020-new-global-cancer-data

59. Bruggmoser G., Bauchowitz S., Canters R., Crezee H., Ehmann M., Gellermann J., Lamprecht U., Lomax N., Messmer M., Ott O., et al. Guideline for the clinical application, documentation and analysis of clinical studies for regional deep hyperthermia. *Strahlenther. Und Onkol.* 2012;**188**:198–211. doi: 10.1007/s00066-012-0176-2.

60. Datta N.R., Puric E., Klingbiel D., Gomez S., Bodis S. Hyperthermia and Radiation Therapy in Locoregional Recurrent Breast Cancers: A Systematic Review and Meta-analysis. *Int. J. Radiat. Oncol.* 2016;**94**:1073–1087. doi: 10.1016/j.ijrobp.2015.12.361.

61. Sawai H., Kurimoto M., Suzuki Y., Yamaguchi Y., Murata A., Suganuma E., Yamamoto K., Kuzuya H., Ueno S., Koide S., et al. Efficacy of Hyperthermia in Treatment of Recurrent Metastatic Breast Cancer After Long-Term Chemotherapy: A Report of 2 Cases. *Am. J. Case Rep.* 2020;**21**:1–10. doi: 10.12659/AJCR.926647.

62. Dooley W.C., Vargas H.I., Fenn A.J., Tomaselli M.B., Harness J.K. Focused Microwave Thermotherapy for Preoperative Treatment of Invasive Breast Cancer: A Review of Clinical Studies. *Ann. Surg. Oncol.* 2010;**17**:1076–1093. doi: 10.1245/s10434-009-0872-z.

63. Zhu L., Altman M.B., Laszlo A., Straube W., Zoberi I., Hallahan D.E., Chen H. Ultrasound

Hyperthermia Technology for Radiosensitization. *Ultrasound Med. Biol.* 2019;**45**:1025–1043. doi: 10.1016/j.ultrasmedbio.2018.12.007.

64. Rossmanna C., Haemmerich D. Review of Temperature Dependence of Thermal Properties, Dielectric Properties, and Perfusion of Biological Tissues at Hyperthermic and Ablation Temperatures. *Crit. Rev. Biomed. Eng.* 2014;**42**:467–492. doi: 10.1615/CritRevBiomedEng.2015012486.
65. Evans S.S., Repasky E.A., Fisher D.T. Fever and the thermal regulation of immunity: The immune system feels the heat. *Nat. Rev. Immunol.* 2015;**15**:335–349. doi: 10.1038/nri3843.
66. van den Tempel N., Horsman M.R., Kanaar R. Improving efficacy of hyperthermia in oncology by exploiting biological mechanisms. *Int. J. Hyperth.* 2016;**32**:446–454. doi: 10.3109/02656736.2016.1157216.
67. Pennes H.H. Analysis of Tissue and Arterial Blood Temperatures in the Resting Human Forearm. *J. Appl. Physiol.* 1948;**1**:93–122. doi: 10.1152/jappl.1948.1.2.93.
68. Farrugia L., Bonello J., Sammut C. Dielectric properties of breast: A review; Proceedings of the 12th European Conference on Antennas and Propagation (EuCAP 2018); London, UK. 9–13 April 2018;
69. Lazebnik M., Popovic D., McCartney L., Watkins C.B., Lindstrom M.J., Harter J., Sewall S., Ogilvie T., Magliocco A., Breslin T.M., et al. A large-scale study of the ultrawideband microwave dielectric properties of normal, benign and malignant breast tissues obtained from cancer surgeries. *Phys. Med. Biol.* 2007;**52**:6093–6115. doi: 10.1088/0031-9155/52/20/002.
70. Yaffe M.J., Byng J.W., Boyd N.F. 21-Quantitative Image Analysis for Estimation of Breast Cancer Risk. In: Bankman I.N., editor. *Handbook of Medical Imaging.* Biomedical Engineering, Academic Press; San Diego, CA, USA: 2000. pp. 323–340.
71. Tsuyna Mammary Gland. Vector Illustration Showing Cross Section of Female Breast with the Names of the Constituent Parts Isolated on White Background. Digital Image. [(accessed on 12 April 2022)]. Available online: https://www.shutterstock.com/image-vector/mammary-gland-vector-illustration-showing-cross-1550556230
72. American Cancer Society Breast Density and Your Mammogram Report; American Cancer Society: Atlanta, GA, USA, Online Resource. [(accessed on 8 March 2022)]. Available online: https://www.cancer.org/cancer/breast-cancer/screening-tests-and-early-detection/mammograms/breast-density-and-your-mammogram-report.html
73. The Evolution of Breast Density Scales and Algorithms|Densitas. [(accessed on 11 October 2021)]. Available online: https://densitas.health/blog/breast-density-scales
74. Winchester D.J., Winchester D.P. *American Cancer Society Atlas of Clinical Oncology: Breast Cancer.* B.C. Decker; Hamilton, ON, Canada: 2000.
75. Types of Breast Cancer: Common, Rare and More Varieties|CTCA. [(accessed on 30 September 2021)]. Available online: https://www.cancercenter.com/cancer-types/breast-cancer/types
76. Inflammatory Breast Cancer: Symptoms, Treatment, Survival Rates, and More|CTCA. [(accessed on 30 September 2021)]. Available online: https://www.cancercenter.com/cancer-types/breast-cancer/types/rare-breast-cancer-types/inflammatory-breast-cancer
77. Standring S., editor. *Gray's Anatomy: The Anatomical Basis of Clinical Practice.* 41st ed. Elsevier; Amsterdam, The Netherlands: 2016.

78. Huang H.W., Horng T.L. *Heat Transfer and Fluid Flow in Biological Processes.* Elsevier; Boston, FL, USA: 2015. Bioheat Transfer and Thermal Heating for Tumor Treatment; pp. 1–42.

79. Hasgall P., Di Gennaro F., Baumgartner C., Neufeld E., Lloyd B., Gosselin M., Payne D., Klingenböck A., Kuster N. *IT'IS Database for Thermal and Electromagnetic Parameters of Biological Tissues (Version 4.1)* Elsevier; Boston, FL, USA: 2022.

80. Duck F.A. *Physical Properties of Tissues.* Elsevier; London, UK: 1990.

81. Erdmann W.S., Gos T. Density of trunk tissues of young and medium age people. *J. Biomech.* 1990;**23**:945–947. doi: 10.1016/0021-9290(90)90360-F.

82. Poppendiek H., Randall R., Breeden J., Chambers J., Murphy J. Thermal conductivity measurements and predictions for biological fluids and tissues. *Cryobiology.* 1967;**3**:318–327. doi: 10.1016/S0011-2240(67)80005-1.

83. Huang H., Wu S. The evaluation of mass densities of the human body in vivo from CT Scans. *Comput. Biol. Med.* 1976;**6**:337–343. doi: 10.1016/0010-4825(76)90070-6.

84. Mendlowitz M. The Specific Heat of Human Blood. *Science.* 1948;**107**:97–98. doi: 10.1126/science.107.2769.97.

85. Blake A.S., Petley G.W., Deakin C.D. Effects of changes in packed cell volume on the specific heat capacity of blood: Implications for studies measuring heat exchange in extracorporeal circuits. *Br. J. Anaesth.* 2000;**84**:28–32. doi: 10.1093/oxfordjournals.bja.a013376.

86. Du T., Zhu L., Levine K.M., Tasdemir N., Lee A.V., Vignali D.A.A., Houten B.V., Tseng G.C., Oesterreich S. Invasive lobular and ductal breast carcinoma differ in immune response, protein translation efficiency and metabolism. *Sci. Rep.* 2018;**8**:7205. doi: 10.1038/s41598-018-25357-0.

87. Hammerstein G.R., Miller D.W., White D.R., Masterson M.E., Woodard H.Q., Laughlin J.S. Absorbed Radiation Dose in Mammography. *Radiology.* 1979;**130**:485–491. doi: 10.1148/130.2.485.

88. Woodard H.Q., White D.R. The composition of body tissues. *Br. J. Radiol.* 1986;**59**:1209–1218. doi: 10.1259/0007-1285-59-708-1209.

89. Gautherie M. Thermopathology of breast cancer: Measurement and analysis of in vivo temperature and blood flow. *Ann. N. Y. Acad. Sci.* 1980;**335**:383–415. doi: 10.1111/j.1749-6632.1980.tb50764.x.

90. González F.J. Thermal simulation of breast tumors. *Rev. Mex. Fís.* 2007;**53**:323–326.

91. Jiang L., Zhan W., Loew M.H. Modeling static and dynamic thermography of the human breast under elastic deformation. *Phys. Med. Biol.* 2011;**56**:187–202. doi: 10.1088/0031-9155/56/1/012.

92. Bowman H. Heat Transfer and Thermal Dosimetry. *J. Microw. Power.* 1981;**16**:121–133. doi: 10.1080/16070658.1981.11689231.

93. Converse M., Bond E., Veen B., Hagness C. A computational study of ultra-wideband versus narrowband microwave hyperthermia for breast cancer treatment. *IEEE Trans. Microw. Theory Tech.* 2006;**54**:2169–2180. doi: 10.1109/TMTT.2006.872790.

94. Johns P.C., Yaffe M.J. X-ray characterisation of normal and neoplastic breast tissues. *Phys. Med. Biol.* 1987;**32**:675–695. doi: 10.1088/0031-9155/32/6/002.

95. McIntosh R.L., Anderson V. A comprehensive tissue properties database provided for the

thermal assessment of a human at rest. *Biophys. Rev. Lett.* 2010;**5**:129–151. doi: 10.1142/S1793048010001184.

96. Ng E.Y.K., Sudharsan N.M. An improved three-dimensional direct numerical modelling and thermal analysis of a female breast with tumour. *Proc. Inst. Mech. Eng. Part H J. Eng. Med.* 2001;**215**:25–37. doi: 10.1243/0954411011533508.

97. Bezerra L., Ribeiro R., Lyra P., Lima R. An empirical correlation to estimate thermal properties of the breast and of the breast nodule using thermographic images and optimization techniques. *Int. J. Heat Mass Transf.* 2020;**149**:119215. doi: 10.1016/j.ijheatmasstransfer.2019.119215.

98. Chanmugam A., Hatwar R., Herman C. Thermal analysis of cancerous breast model. *Int. Mech. Eng. Concgress Expo.* 2012 doi: 10.1115/IMECE2012-88244.

99. Amri A., Saidane A., Pulko S. Thermal analysis of a three-dimensional breast model with embedded tumour using the transmission line matrix (TLM) method. *Comput. Biol. Med.* 2011;**41**:76–86. doi: 10.1016/j.compbiomed.2010.12.002.

100. He Y., Shirazaki M., Liu H., Himeno R., Sun Z. A numerical coupling model to analyze the blood flow, temperature, and oxygen transport in human breast tumor under laser irradiation. *Comput. Biol. Med.* 2006;**36**:1336–1350. doi: 10.1016/j.compbiomed.2005.08.004.

101. Singh S., Bhowmik A., Repaka R. Radio Frequency Ablation of Malignant Breast Tumor: A Numerical Study; Proceedings of the 23rd National Heat and Mass Transfer Conference and 1st International ISHMT-ASTFE Heat and Mass Transfer Conference IHMTC2015; Thiruvananthapuram, India. 17–20 December 2015; pp. 1–8.

102. Mitra S., Balaji C. A neural network based estimation of tumour parameters from a breast thermogram. *Int. J. Heat Mass Transf.* 2010;**53**:4714–4727. doi: 10.1016/j.ijheatmasstransfer.2010.06.020.

103. Bakker J.F., Paulides M.M., Obdeijn I.M., van Rhoon G.C., van Dongen K.W.A. An ultrasound cylindrical phased array for deep heating in the breast: Theoretical design using heterogeneous models. *Phys. Med. Biol.* 2009;**54**:3201–3215. doi: 10.1088/0031-9155/54/10/016.

104. Zastrow E., Hagness S.C., Van Veen B.D. 3D computational study of non-invasive patient-specific microwave hyperthermia treatment of breast cancer. *Phys. Med. Biol.* 2010;**55**:3611–3629. doi: 10.1088/0031-9155/55/13/003.

105. Nguyen P.T., Abbosh A., Crozier S. Microwave Hyperthermia for Breast Cancer Treatment Using Electromagnetic and Thermal Focusing Tested on Realistic Breast Models and Antenna Arrays. *IEEE Trans. Antennas Propag.* 2015;**63**:4426–4434. doi: 10.1109/TAP.2015.2463681.

106. Curto S., Prakash P. Design of a compact antenna with flared groundplane for a wearable breast hyperthermia system. *Int. J. Hyperth.* 2015;**31**:726–736. doi: 10.3109/02656736.2015.1063170.

107. Li Y., Fahimi B. Thermal analysis of multiple-antenna-excited breast model for breast cancer detection; Proceedings of the 2016 38th Annual International Conference of the IEEE Engineering in Medicine and Biology Society (EMBC); Orlando, FL, USA. 16–20 August 2016; pp. 1058–1061.

108. Werner J., Buse M. Temperature profiles with respect to inhomogeneity and geometry of the human body. *J. Appl. Physiol.* 1988;**65**:1110–1118. doi: 10.1152/jappl.1988.65.3.1110.

109. Gosalia K., Weiland J., Humayun M., Lazzi G. Thermal Elevation in the Human Eye and Head Due to the Operation of a Retinal Prosthesis. *IEEE Trans. Biomed. Eng.* 2004;**51**:1469–1477.

doi: 10.1109/TBME.2004.827548.

110. Johnson R. A thermodynamic method for investigation of radiation induced changes in the microcirculation of human tumors. *Int. J. Radiat. Oncol.* 1976;**1**:659–670. doi: 10.1016/0360-3016(76)90148-6.

111. Ekstrand V., Wiksell H., Schultz I., Sandstedt B., Rotstein S., Eriksson A. Influence of electrical and thermal properties of RF ablation of breast cancer: Is the tumour preferentially heated? *BioMed. Eng. Online.* 2005;**4**:1–16. doi: 10.1186/1475-925X-4-41.

112. Beaney R.P. Positron emission tomography in the study of human tumors. *Semin. Nucl. Med.* 1984;**14**:324–341. doi: 10.1016/S0001-2998(84)80006-9.

113. Wilson C.B., Lammertsma A.A., McKenzie C.G., Sikora K., Jones T. Measurements of Blood Flow and Exchanging Water Space in Breast Tumors Using Positron Emission Tomography: A Rapid and Noninvasive Dynamic Method. *Cancer Res.* 1992;**52**:1592–1597.

114. Robinson M.P., Richardson M.J., Green J.L., Preece A.W. New materials for dielectric simulation of tissues. *Phys. Med. Biol.* 1991;**36**:1565–1571. doi: 10.1088/0031-9155/36/12/002.

115. Giering K., Lamprecht I., Minet O. Specific heat capacities of human and animal tissues. *Laser-Tissue Interact. Tissue Opt.* 1996;**2624**:188–197. doi: 10.1117/12.229547.

116. Mankoff D.A., Dunnwald L.K., Gralow J.R., Ellis G.K., Charlop A., Lawton T.J., Schubert E.K., Tseng J., Livingston R.B. Blood flow and metabolism in locally advanced breast cancer: Relationship to response to therapy. *J. Nucl. Med.* 2002;**43**:500–509.

117. Hamilton G. *Ph.D. Thesis.* University of Glasgow; Glasgow, UK: 1998. Investigations of the Thermal Properties of Human and Animal Tissues.

118. Singh M., Singh T., Soni S. Pre-operative Assessment of Ablation Margins for Variable Blood Perfusion Metrics in a Magnetic Resonance Imaging Based Complex Breast Tumour Anatomy: Simulation Paradigms in Thermal Therapies. *Comput. Methods Programs Biomed.* 2021;**198**:105781. doi: 10.1016/j.cmpb.2020.105781.

119. Valvano J.W., Cochran J.R., Diller K.R. Thermal conductivity and diffusivity of biomaterials measured with self-heated thermistors. *Int. J. Thermophys.* 1985;**6**:301–311. doi: 10.1007/BF00522151.

120. Heath T.L. *The Works of Archimedes.* Cambridge University Press; Cambridge, UK: 1897.

121. Cooper T.E., Trezek G. Correlation of thermal properties of some human tissue with water content. *Aerosp. Med.* 1971;**42**:24–28.

122. Riedel L. Kalorimetrische Untersuchungen Uber das Gefrieren von Seefischen. *Kältetechnik.* 1956;**8**:374–377.

123. Riedel L. Kalorimetrische Untersuchungen übr das Gefrieren von Fleisch. *Kältetechnik.* 1957;**9**:38–40.

124. Gautherie M., Bourjat P., Quenneville Y., Gros C. Heat production capacity in breast epitheliomas. 1. Determination by intratumor thermometry and cutaneous infrared thermography. *Rev. Eur. D'études Clin. Biol.* 1972;**17**:776–783.

125. Priebe L. Heat transport in homogeneously and isotropically perfused tissue. In: Hardy J., Gagge A., Stolwijk J.A.J., editors. *Physiological and Behavioral Temperature Regulation.* Springfield, III; Oxford, UK: 1970. pp. 272–280.

126. Gautherie M., Quenneville Y., Gros C.M. Metabolic heat production, growth rate and prognosis of early breast carcinomas. *Biomedicine.* 1975;**22**:328–336.

127. Paulides M.M., Rodrigues D.B., Bellizzi G.G., Sumser K., Curto S., Neufeld E., Montanaro H., Kok H.P., Dobsicek Trefna H. ESHO benchmarks for computational modeling and optimization in hyperthermia therapy. *Int. J. Hyperth.* 2021;**38**:1425–1442. doi: 10.1080/02656736.2021.1979254.

128. Fedrov S. GetData Graph Digitizer-Graph Digitizing Software. 2013. [(accessed on 21 February 2022)]. Available online: http://getdata-graph-digitizer.com/download.php

129. Beaney R.P., Jones T., Lammertsma A.A., Mckenzie C.G., Halnan K.E. Positron Emission Tomography for in-Vivo Measurement of Regional Blood Flow, Oxygen Utilisation, and Blood Volume in Patients With Breast Carcinoma. *Lancet.* 1984;**323**:131–134. doi: 10.1016/S0140-6736(84)90063-1.

130. Vaupel P. Tumor blood flow. In: Mollis M., Vaupel P., editors. *Blood Perfusion and Microenvironment of Human Tumors: Implications for Clinical Raiooncology.* Springfield; Berlin, Germany: 1998. pp. 41–46.

131. Erdmann B., Lang J., Seebass M. Optimization of temperature distributions for regional hyperthermia based on a nonlinear heat transfer model. *Ann. N. Y. Acad. Sci.* 1998;**858**:36–46. doi: 10.1111/j.1749-6632.1998.tb10138.x.

132. Shih T.C., Kou H.S., Lin W.L. The impact of thermally significant blood vessels in perfused tumor tissue on thermal dose distributions during thermal therapies. *Int. Commun. Heat Mass Transf.* 2003;**30**:975–985. doi: 10.1016/S0735-1933(03)00156-8.

133. Shitzer A., Stroschein L.A., Vital P., Gonzalez R.R., Pandolf K.B. Numerical Analysis of an Extremity in a Cold Environment Including Countercurrent Arterio-Venous Heat Exchange. *J. Biomech. Eng.* 1997;**119**:179–186. doi: 10.1115/1.2796078.

134. Diller K.R. *Advances in Heat Transfer.* Volume 22. Elsevier; Amsterdam, The Netherlands: 1992. Modeling of Bioheat Transfer Processes at High and Low Temperatures; pp. 157–357.

135. Lang J., Erdmann B., Seebass M. Impact of nonlinear heat transfer on temperature control in regional hyperthermia. *IEEE Trans. Biomed. Eng.* 1999;**46**:1129–1138. doi: 10.1109/10.784145.

136. Sohrab B., Farzan G., Ashkan B., Amin J. Ultrasound Thermotherapy of Breast: Theoretical Design of Transducer and Numerical Simulation of Procedure. *Jpn. J. Appl. Phys.* 2006;**45**:1856–1863. doi: 10.1143/JJAP.45.1856.

137. Çetingül M.P., Herman C. A heat transfer model of skin tissue for the detection of lesions: Sensitivity analysis. *Phys. Med. Biol.* 2010;**55**:5933–5951. doi: 10.1088/0031-9155/55/19/020.

138. Fujita S., Tamazawa M., Kuroda K. Effects of blood perfusion rate on the optimization of RF-capacitive hyperthermia. *IEEE Trans. Biomed. Eng.* 1998;**45**:1182–1186. doi: 10.1109/10.709562.

139. Elming P., Sørensen B., Oei A., Franken N., Crezee J., Overgaard J., Horsman M. Hyperthermia: The Optimal Treatment to Overcome Radiation Resistant Hypoxia. *Cancers.* 2019;**11**:60. doi: 10.3390/cancers11010060.

140. Vaupel P., Kallinowski F., Okunieff P., Review H.T.A. Blood Flow, Oxygen and Nutrient Supply, and Metabolic Microenvironment of Human Tumors: A Review. *Cancer Res.* 1989;**49**:6449–6465.

141. Shibata H.R. *Ph.D. Thesis.* McGill University; Montreal, QC, Canada: 1967. Blood Flow to Tumours.

142. Chen L., Zeng T., Pan X., Zhang Y.H., Huang T., Cai Y.D. Identifying Methylation Pattern and Genes Associated with Breast Cancer Subtypes. *Int. J. Mol. Sci.* 2019;20:4269. doi: 10.3390/ijms20174269.

143. Frick C., Rumgay H., Vignat J., Ginsburg O., Nolte E., Bray F., Soerjomataram I. Quantitative estimates of preventable and treatable deaths from 36 cancers worldwide: A population-based study. *Lancet Glob. Health.* 2023;11:1700–1712. doi: 10.1016/S2214-109X(23)00406-0.

144. Intabli H., Gee J.M., Oesterreich S., Yeoman M.S., Allen M.C., Qattan A., Flint M.S. Glucocorticoid-induced loss of estrogen receptor alpha gene methylation and restoration of sensitivity to fulvestrant in triple-negative breast cancer. *Gene.* 2023;851:147022. doi: 10.1016/j.gene.2022.147022.

145. Khadela A., Chavda V.P., Soni S., Megha K., Pandya A.J., Vora L. Anti-Androgenic Therapies Targeting the Luminal Androgen Receptor of a Typical Triple-Negative Breast Cancer. *Cancers.* 2022;15:233. doi: 10.3390/cancers15010233.

146. Łukasiewicz S., Czeczelewski M., Forma A., Baj J., Sitarz R., Stanisławek A. Breast Cancer—Epidemiology, Risk Factors, Classification, Prognostic Markers, and Current Treatment Strategies—An Updated Review. *Cancers.* 2021;13:4287. doi: 10.3390/cancers13174287.

147. Caleça T., Ribeiro P.C., Vitorino M., Menezes M., Alves M.S., Mendes A.D., Vicente R., Negreiros I., Faria A., Costa D.A. Breast Cancer Survivors and Healthy Women: Could Gut Microbiota Make a Difference? "BiotaCancerSurvivors": A Case-Control Study. *Cancers.* 2023;15:594. doi: 10.3390/cancers15030594.

148. Abbas A., Witte T., Patterson W.L.I., Fahrmann J.F., Guo K., Hur J., Hardman W.E., Georgel P.T. Epigenetic Reprogramming Mediated by Maternal Diet Rich in Omega-3 Fatty Acids Protects From Breast Cancer Development in F1 Offspring. *Front. Cell Dev. Biol.* 2021;9:1517. doi: 10.3389/fcell.2021.682593.

149. Chen M., Li S., Srinivasasainagendra V., Sharma M., Li Z., Tiwari H., Tollefsbol T.O., Li Y. Maternalsoybean genistein on prevention of later-life breast cancer through inherited epigenetic regulations. *Carcinogenesis.* 2022;43:190–202. doi: 10.1093/carcin/bgac009.

150. Cui J., Sachaphibulkij K., Teo W.S., Lim H.M., Zou L., Ong C.N., Alberts R., Chen J., Lim L.H.K. Annexin-A1 deficiency attenuates stress-induced tumor growth via fatty acid metabolism in mice: An Integrated multiple omics analysis on the stress- microbiome-metabolite-epigenetic-oncology (SMMEO) axis. *Theranostics.* 2022;12:3794–3817. doi: 10.7150/thno.68611.

151. El-Sayed A., Aleya L., Kamel M. Microbiota and epigenetics: Promising therapeutic approaches? *Environ. Sci. Pollut. Res. Int.* 2021;28:49343–49361. doi: 10.1007/s11356-021-15623-6.

152. Plaza-Díaz J., Álvarez-Mercado A.I., Ruiz-Marín C.M., Reina-Pérez I., Pérez-Alonso A.J., Sánchez-Andujar M.B., Torné P., Gallart-Aragón T., Sánchez-Barrón M.T., Lartategui S.R., et al. Association of breast and gut microbiota dysbiosis and the risk of breast cancer: A case-control clinical study. *BMC Cancer.* 2019;19:495. doi: 10.1186/s12885-019-5660-y.

153. Bobin-Dubigeon C., Luu H.T., Leuillet S., Lavergne S.N., Carton T., Le Vacon F., Michel C., Nazih H., Bard J.-M. Faecal Microbiota Composition Varies between Patients with Breast Cancer and Healthy Women: A Comparative Case-Control Study. *Nutrients.* 2021;13:2705. doi: 10.3390/nu13082705.

154. Klann E., Williamson J.M., Tagliamonte M.S., Ukhanova M., Asirvatham J.R., Chim H., Yaghjyan L., Mai V. Microbiota composition in bilateral healthy breast tissue and breast tumors. *Cancer Causes Control.* 2020;31:1027–1038. doi: 10.1007/s10552-020-01338-5.
155. Sharma M., Tollefsbol T.O. Combinatorial epigenetic mechanisms of sulforaphane, genistein and sodium butyrate in breast cancer inhibition. *Exp. Cell Res.* 2022;416:113160. doi: 10.1016/j.yexcr.2022.113160.
156. Wu H., Ganguly S., Tollefsbol T.O. Modulating Microbiota as a New Strategy for Breast Cancer Prevention and Treatment. *Microorganisms.* 2022;10:1727. doi: 10.3390/microorganisms10091727.
157. Skvortsova K., Stirzaker C., Taberlay P. The DNAmethylation landscape in cancer. *Essays Biochem.* 2019;63:797.
158. Rotondo J.C., Mazziotta C., Lanzillotti C., Tognon M., Martini F. Epigenetic Dysregulations in Merkel Cell Polyomavirus-Driven Merkel Cell Carcinoma. *Int. J. Mol. Sci.* 2021;22:11464. doi: 10.3390/ijms222111464.
159. Chen M., Li S., Arora I., Yi N., Sharma M., Li Z., Tollefsbol T.O., Li Y. Maternal soy bean diet on prevention of obesity related breast cancer through early-life gut microbiome and epigenetic regulation. *J. Nutr. Biochem.* 2022;110:109119. doi: 10.1016/j.jnutbio.2022.109119.
160. Arora I., Sharma M., Li S., Crowley M., Crossman D.K., Li Y., Tollefsbol T.O. An integrated analysis of the effects of maternal broccoli sprouts exposure on transcriptome and methylome in prevention of offspring mammary cancer. *PLoS ONE.* 2022;17:e0264858. doi: 10.1371/journal.pone.0264858.
161. Bowers L.W., Doerstling S.S., Shamsunder M.G., Lineberger C.G., Rossi E.L., Montgomery S.A., Coleman M.F., Gong W., Parker J.S., Howell A., et al. Reversing the genomic, epigenetic and triple negative breast cancer-enhancing effects of obesity. *Cancer Prev. Res.* 2022;15:581. doi: 10.1158/1940-6207.CAPR-22-0113.
162. Li S., Chen M., Wu H., Li Y., Tollefsbol T.O. Maternal Epigenetic Regulation Contributes to Prevention of Estrogen Receptor–negative Mammary Cancer with Broccoli Sprout Consumption. *Cancer Prev. Res.* 2020;13:449–462. doi: 10.1158/1940-6207.CAPR-19-0491.
163. Byrd D.A., Vogtmann E., Wu Z., Han Y., Wan Y., Clegg-Lamptey J., Yarney J., Wiafe-Addai B., Wiafe S., Awuah B., et al. Associations of fecal microbial profiles with breast cancer and nonmalignant breast disease in the Ghana Breast Health Study. *Int. J. Cancer.* 2021;148:2712–2723. doi: 10.1002/ijc.33473.
164. Hoskinson C., Zheng K., Gabel J., Kump A., German R., Podicheti R., Marino N., Stiemsma L.T. Composition and Functional Potential of the Human Mammary Microbiota Priorto and Following Breast Tumor Diagnosis. *mSystems.* 2022;7:e0148921. doi: 10.1128/msystems.01489-21.
165. Aarnoutse R., Hillege L.E., Ziemons J., De Vos-Geelen J., de Boer M., Aerts E.M.E.R., Vriens B.E.P.J., van Riet Y., Vincent J., van de Wouw A.J., et al. Intestinal microbiota in postmenopausal breast cancer patients and controls. *Cancers.* 2021;13:6200. doi: 10.3390/cancers13246200.
166. Rosean C.B., Bostic R.R., Ferey J.C.M., Feng T.Y., Azar F.N., Tung K.S., Dozmorov M.G., Smirnova E., Bos P.D., Rutkowski M.R. Preexisting commensal dysbiosis is a host-intrinsic regulator of tissue inflammation and tumor cell dissemination in hormone receptor–positive breast cancer. *Cancer Res.* 2019;79:3662–3675. doi: 10.1158/0008-5472.CAN-18-3464.

167. Semaan J., El-Hakim S., Ibrahim J.N., Safi R., Elnar A.A., El Boustany C. Comparative effect of sodium butyrate and sodium propionate on proliferation, cell cycle and apoptosis in human breast cancer cells MCF-7. *Breast Cancer.* 2020;27:696–705. doi: 10.1007/s12282-020-01063-6.

168. Sharma M., Arora I., Stoll M.L., Li Y., Morrow C.D., Barnes S., Berryhill T.F., Li S., Tollefsbol T.O. Nutritional combinatorial impact on the gut microbiota and plasma short-chain fatty acids levels in the prevention of mammary cancer in Her 2/neu estrogen receptor-negative transgenic mice. *PLoS ONE.* 2020;15:e0234893. doi: 10.1371/journal.pone.0234893.

169. Paul B., Barnes S., Demark-Wahnefried W., Morrow C., Salvador C., Skibola C., Tollefsbol T.O. Influences of Diet and the Gut Microbiome on Epigenetic Modulation in Cancer and Other Diseases. *Clin. Epigenetics.* 2015;7:112. doi: 10.1186/s13148-015-0144-7.

170. Ou X., Tan Y., Xie J., Yuan J., Deng X., Shao R., Song C., Cao X., Xie X., He R., et al. Methylation of GPRC5A Promotes Liver Metastasis and Docetaxel Resistance through Activating MTOR Signaling Pathway in Triple Negative Breast Cancer. *Drug Resist. Updates.* 2024;73:101063. doi: 10.1016/j.drup.2024.101063.

171. Xie J., Liu M., Deng X., Tang Y., Zheng S., Ou X., Tang H., Xie X., Wu M., Zou Y. Gut Microbiota Reshapes Cancer Immunotherapy Efficacy: Mechanisms and Therapeutic Strategies. *iMeta.* 2024;3:e156. doi: 10.1002/imt2.156.

172. Tsugane S. Why Has Japan Become the World's Most Long-Lived Country: Insights from a Food and Nutrition Perspective. *Eur. J. Clin. Nutr.* 2020;75:921–928. doi: 10.1038/s41430-020-0677-5.

173. Carlos-Reyes Á., López-González J.S., Meneses-Flores M., Gallardo-Rincón D., Ruíz-García E., Marchat L.A., la Vega H.A.-D., de la Cruz O.N.H., Lopez-Camarillo C. Dietary Compounds as Epigenetic Modulating Agents in Cancer. *Front. Genet.* 2019;10:79. doi: 10.3389/fgene.2019.00079.

174. Xavier M.J., Roman S.D., Aitken R.J., Nixon B. Transgenerational inheritance: How impacts to the epigenetic and genetic information of parents affect offspring health. *Hum. Reprod. Update.* 2019;25:519–541. doi: 10.1093/humupd/dmz017.

175. Yurko-Mauro K., Van Elswyk M., Teo L. A Scoping Review of Interactions between Omega-3 LongChain Polyunsaturated Fatty Acids and Genetic Variation in Relation to Cancer Risk. *Nutrients.* 2020;12:1647. doi: 10.3390/nu12061647.

176. Feigelson H.S., Caan B., Weinmann S., Leonard A.C., Powers J.D., Yenumula P.R., Arterburn D.E., Koebnick C., Altaye M., Schauer D.P. Bariatric Surgery is Associated With Reduced Risk of Breast Cancer in Both Premenopausal and Postmenopausal Women. *Ann. Surg.* 2020;272:1053–1059. doi: 10.1097/SLA.0000000000003331.

177. Wieërs G., Belkhir L., Enaud R., Leclercq S., Philippart de Foy J.M., Dequenne I., de Timary P., Cani P.D. How Probiotics Affect the Microbiota. *Front. Cell Infect. Microbiol.* 2020;9:454. doi: 10.3389/fcimb.2019.00454.

178. Parida S., Sharma D. The Microbiome–Estrogen Connection and Breast Cancer Risk. *Cells.* 2019;8:1642. doi: 10.3390/cells8121642.

179. Laborda-Illanes A., Sanchez-Alcoholado L., Dominguez-Recio M.E., Jimenez-Rodriguez B., Lavado R., Comino-Méndez I., Alba E., Queipo-Ortuño M.I. Breast and Gut Microbiota Action Mechanisms in Breast Cancer. *Cancers.* 2020;12:2465. doi: 10.3390/cancers12092465.

180. Alvandi E., Wong W.K.M., Joglekar M.V., Spring K.J., Hardikar A.A. Short-chain fatty acid concentrations in the incidence and risk-stratification of colorectal cancer: A systematic review and meta-analysis. *BMC Med.* 2022;20:323. doi: 10.1186/s12916-022-02529-4.

181. Wang G., Yu Y., Wang Y.Z., Wang J.J., Guan R., Sun Y., Shi F., Gao J., Fu X.L. Role of SCFAs in gut microbiome and glycolysis for colorectal cancer therapy. *J. Cell Physiol.* 2019;234:17023–17049. doi: 10.1002/jcp.28436.

182. Jia X., Zheng Y., Guo Y., Chen K. Sodium butyrate and panobinostat induce apoptosis of chronic myeloid leukemia cells via multiple pathways. *Mol. Genet. Genomic Med.* 2019;7:613. doi: 10.1002/mgg3.613.

183. Li Z., Wang D., Chen X., Wang W., Wang P., Hou P., Li M., Chu S., Qiao S., Zheng J., et al. PRMT1-Mediated EZH2 Methylation Promotes Breast Cancer Cell Proliferation and Tumorigenesis. *Cell Death Dis.* 2021;12:1080. doi: 10.1038/s41419-021-04381-5.

184. Chen C., Li H. The Inhibitory Effect of Gut Microbiota and Its Metabolites on Colorectal Cancer. *J. Microbiol. Biotechnol.* 2020;30:1607–1613. doi: 10.4014/jmb.2002.02032.

185. Mikó E., Kovács T., Sebő É., Tóth J., Csonka T., Ujlaki G., Sipos A., Szabó J., Méhes G., Bai P. Microbiome-Microbial Metabolome Cancer Cell Interactions in Breast Cancer-Familiar, but Unexplored. *Cells.* 2019;8:293. doi: 10.3390/cells8040293.

186. Jotshi A., Sukla K.K., Haque M.M., Bose C., Varma B., Koppiker C.B., Joshi S., Mishra R. Exploring the Human Microbiome—A Step Forward for Precision Medicine in Breast Cancer. *Cancer Rep.* 2023;6:e1877. doi: 10.1002/cnr2.1877.

187. Stewman C., Vitanzo P.C., Harwood M.I. Neurologic Thoracic Outlet Syndrome: Summarizing a Complex History and Evolution. *Curr. Sports Med. Rep.* 2014;13:100–106. doi: 10.1249/JSR.0000000000000038.

188. Bordoni B., Varacallo M. *Anatomy, Head and Neck, Scalenus Muscle.* StatPearls; Treasure Island, FL, USA: 2021.

189. Laulan J., Fouquet B., Rodaix C., Jauffret P., Roquelaure Y., Descatha A. Thoracic Outlet Syndrome: Definition, Aetiological Factors, Diagnosis, Management and Occupational Impact. *J. Occup. Rehabil.* 2011;21:366–373. doi: 10.1007/S10926-010-9278-9.

190. Freischlag J., Orion K. Understanding Thoracic Outlet Syndrome. *Scientifica.* 2014;2014:248163. doi: 10.1155/2014/248163.

191. Masocatto N.O., Da-Matta T., Prozzo T.G., Couto W.J., Porfirio G. Thoracic Outlet Syndrome: A Narrative Review. *Rev. Col. Bras. Cir.* 2019;46:e20192243. doi: 10.1590/0100-6991E-20192243.

192. Janák D., Novotný K., Roček M., Rohn V. Thoracic Outlet Syndrome: A Significant Family Genetic Phenotypic Presentation. *Prague Med. Rep.* 2016;117:117–123. doi: 10.14712/23362936.2016.12.

193. Goeteyn J., Pesser N., van Nuenen B., van Sambeek M., Teijink J. Familial Predisposition of Thoracic Outlet Syndrome: Does a Familial Syndrome Exist? Report of Cases and Review of Literature. *Acta Chir. Belg.* 2021;121:211–214. doi: 10.1080/00015458.2019.1675970.

194. Hooper T.L., Denton J., McGalliard M.K., Brismée J.M., Sizer P.S. Thoracic Outlet Syndrome: A Controversial Clinical Condition. Part 1: Anatomy, and Clinical Examination/Diagnosis. *J. Man. Manip. Ther.* 2010;18:74–83. doi: 10.1179/106698110X12640740712734.

195. Illig K.A., Rodriguez-Zoppi E., Bland T., Muftah M., Jospitre E. The Incidence of Thoracic Outlet Syndrome. *Ann. Vasc. Surg.* 2021;70:263–272. doi: 10.1016/j.avsg.2020.07.029.

196. Otoshi K., Kikuchi S., Kato K., Sato R., Igari T., Kaga T., Shishido H., Konno S., Koga R., Furushima K., et al. The Prevalence and Characteristics of Thoracic Outlet Syndrome in High School Baseball Players. *Health.* 2017;9:1223–1234. doi: 10.4236/HEALTH.2017.98088.

197. Maru S., Dosluoglu H., Dryjski M., Cherr G., Curl G.R., Harris L.M. Thoracic Outlet Syndrome in Children and Young Adults. *Eur. J. Vasc. Endovasc. Surg.* 2009;38:560–564. doi: 10.1016/j.ejvs.2009.06.015.

198. Balderman J., Abuirqeba A.A., Eichaker L., Pate C., Earley J.A., Bottros M.M., Jayarajan S.N., Thompson R.W. Physical Therapy Management, Surgical Treatment, and Patient-Reported Outcomes Measures in a Prospective Observational Cohort of Patients with Neurogenic Thoracic Outlet Syndrome. *J. Vasc. Surg.* 2019;70:832–841. doi: 10.1016/J.JVS.2018.12.027.

199. Sanders R.J., Hammond S.L., Rao N.M. Diagnosis of Thoracic Outlet Syndrome. *J. Vasc. Surg.* 2007;46:601–604. doi: 10.1016/j.jvs.2007.04.050.

200. Henry B.M., Vikse J., Sanna B., Taterra D., Gomulska M., Pękala P.A., Tubbs R.S., Tomaszewski K.A. Cervical Rib Prevalence and Its Association with Thoracic Outlet Syndrome: A Meta-Analysis of 141 Studies with Surgical Considerations. *World Neurosurg.* 2018;110:e965–e978. doi: 10.1016/J.WNEU.2017.11.148.

201. Connolly M.R., Auchincloss H.G. Anatomy and Embryology of the Thoracic Outlet. *Thorac. Surg. Clin.* 2021;31:1–10. doi: 10.1016/j.thorsurg.2020.09.007.

202. Kitsis C.K., Marino A.J., Krikler S.J., Birch R. Late Complications Following Clavicular Fractures and Their Operative Management. *Injury.* 2003;34:69–74. doi: 10.1016/S0020-1383(02)00169-9.

203. Sanders R.J. *Thoracic Outlet Syndrome.* Springer; London, UK: 2013. Anatomy of the Thoracic Outlet and Related Structures; pp. 17–24.

204. Paraskevas G., Natsis K., Ioannidis O., Papaziogas B., Kitsoulis P., Spanidou S. Accessory Muscles in the Lower Part of the Anterior Compartment of the Arm That May Entrap Neurovascular Elements. *Clin. Anat.* 2008;21:246–251. doi: 10.1002/ca.20608.

205. Weber A.E., Criado E. Relevance of Bone Anomalies in Patients with Thoracic Outlet Syndrome. *Ann. Vasc. Surg.* 2014;28:924–932. doi: 10.1016/j.avsg.2013.08.014.

206. Aignatoaei A.M., Moldoveanu C.E., Caruntu I.D., Giusca S.E., Vicoleanu S.P., Nedelcu A.H. Incidental Imaging Findings of Congenital Rib Abnormalities—A Case Series and Review of Developmental Concepts. *Folia Morphol.* 2018;77:386–392. doi: 10.5603/FM.a2017.0080.

207. Jones M.R., Prabhakar A., Viswanath O., Urits I., Green J.B., Kendrick J.B., Brunk A.J., Eng M.R., Orhurhu V., Cornett E.M., et al. Thoracic Outlet Syndrome: A Comprehensive Review of Pathophysiology, Diagnosis, and Treatment. *Pain. Ther.* 2019;8:5–18. doi: 10.1007/S40122-019-0124-2.

208. Sanders R.J., Hammond S.L. Management of Cervical Ribs and Anomalous First Ribs Causing Neurogenic Thoracic Outlet Syndrome. *J. Vasc. Surg.* 2002;36:51–56. doi: 10.1067/MVA.2002.123750.

209. Gruber W. Ueber Die Halsrippen des Menschen Vergleichend-Anatomischen Remerkungen. *Scientia.* 1869;2:7–27.

210. Paton G.J., Billings B.K. Cervical Rib Synostosis to the First Rib: A Rare Anatomic Variation. *World Neurosurg.* 2020;138:187–192. doi: 10.1016/j.wneu.2020.03.009.

211. Walden M.J., Adin M.E., Visagan R., Viertel V.G., Intrapiromkul J., Maluf F., Patel N.V., Alluwaimi F., Lin D., Yousem D.M. Cervical Ribs: Identification on MRI and Clinical Relevance. *Clin. Imaging.* 2013;37:938–941. doi: 10.1016/j.clinimag.2013.01.005.

212. Hardy A., Pougès C., Wavreille G., Behal H., Demondion X., Lefebvre G. Thoracic Outlet Syndrome: Diagnostic Accuracy of MRI. *Orthop. Traumatol. Surg. Res.* 2019;105:1563–1569. doi: 10.1016/j.otsr.2019.09.020.

213. White R., Hollier L. *Vascular Surgery: Basic Science and Clinical Correlations.* John Wiley & Sons; Hoboken, NJ, USA: 2008.

214. Todd T.W. The Relations of the Thoracic Operculum Considered in Reference to the Anatomy of Cervical Ribs of Surgical Importance. *J. Anat. Physiol.* 1911;45:293–304.

215. Sanders R.J., Hammond S.L., Rao N.M. Thoracic Outlet Syndrome: A Review. *Neurologist.* 2008;14:365–373. doi: 10.1097/NRL.0b013e318176b98d.

216. Chang C.S., Chwei-Chin Chuang D., Chin S.C., Chang C.J. An Investigation of the Relationship between Thoracic Outlet Syndrome and the Dimensions of the First Rib and Clavicle. *J. Plast. Reconstr. Aesthetic Surg.* 2011;64:1000–1006. doi: 10.1016/j.bjps.2011.03.017.

217. Gharagozloo F., Meyer M., Tempesta B., Strother E., Margolis M., Neville R. Proposed Pathogenesis of Paget-Schroetter Disease: Impingement of the Subclavian Vein by a Congenitally Malformed Bony Tubercle on the First Rib. *J. Clin. Pathol.* 2012;65:262–266. doi: 10.1136/jclinpath-2011-200479.

218. Gharagozloo F., Meyer M., Tempesta B.J., Margolis M., Strother E.T., Tummala S. Robotic En Bloc First-Rib Resection for Paget-Schroetter Disease, a Form of Thoracic Outlet Syndrome: Technique and Initial Results. *Innovations.* 2012;7:39–44. doi: 10.1097/imi.0b013e3182542ab3.

219. Gharagozloo F., Meyer M., Tempesta B., Gruessner S. Robotic Transthoracic First-Rib Resection for Paget-Schroetter Syndrome. *Eur. J. Cardiothorac. Surg.* 2019;55:434–439. doi: 10.1093/ejcts/ezy275.

220. Gharagozloo F., Atiquzzaman N., Meyer M., Tempesta B., Werden S. Robotic First Rib Resection for Thoracic Outlet Syndrome. *J. Thorac. Dis.* 2021;13:6141–6154. doi: 10.21037/jtd-2019-rts-04.

221. Lindgren K.A., Leino E., Lepäntalo M., Paukku P. Recurrent Thoracic Outlet Syndrome after First Rib Resection. *Arch. Phys. Med. Rehabil.* 1991;72:208–210.

222. Gelabert H.A., Jabori S., Barleben A., Kiang S., O'Connell J., Jimenez J.C., DeRubertis B., Rigberg D. Regrown First Rib in Patients with Recurrent Thoracic Outlet Syndrome. *Ann. Vasc. Surg.* 2014;28:933–938. doi: 10.1016/j.avsg.2014.01.004.

223. De Figueiredo M.J.P.S.S., dos Reis Braga S., Akkari M., Prado J.C.L., Santili C. Congenital Pseudarthrosis of the Clavicle. *Rev. Bras. Ortop.* 2012;47:21. doi: 10.1016/S2255-4971(15)30341-4.

224. Lozano P., Díaz M., Riera R., Gomez F.T. Venous Thoracic Outlet Syndrome Secondary to Congenital Pseudoarthrosis of the Clavicle. Presentation in the Fourth Decade of Life. *Eur. J. Vasc. Endovasc. Surg.* 2003;25:592–593. doi: 10.1053/ejvs.2002.1864.

225. Hahn K., Shah R., Shalev Y., Schmidt D.H., Bajwa T. Congenital Clavicular Pseudoarthrosis

Associated with Vascular Thoracic Outlet Syndrome: Case Presentation and Review of the Literature. *Cathet Cardiovasc. Diagn.* 1995;35:321–327. doi: 10.1002/ccd.1810350409.

226. Khu K., Midha R. Clavicle Pseudarthrosis: A Rare Cause of Thoracic Outlet Syndrome. *Can. J. Neurol. Sci.* 2010;37:863–865. doi: 10.1017/S0317167100051581.
227. Bargar W.L., Marcus R.E., Ittleman F.P. Late Thoracic Outlet Syndrome Secondary to Pseudarthrosis of the Clavicle. *J. Trauma.* 1984;24:857–859. doi: 10.1097/00005373-198409000-00016.
228. Watson H.I., Hopper G.P., Kovacs P. Congenital Pseudarthrosis of the Clavicle Causing Thoracic Outlet Syndrome. *BMJ Case Rep.* 2013;2013:bcr2013010437. doi: 10.1136/bcr-2013-010437.
229. Heyn J., Ozimek A., Sadeghi-Azandaryani M., Bürklein D., Steckmeier B. Thoracic Outlet Syndrome Caused by a Pseudoaneurysm after Pseudarthrosis of the Clavicle. *Eur. J. Trauma. Emerg. Surg.* 2008;34:511–514. doi: 10.1007/s00068-008-7126-9.
230. Makhoul R.G., Machleder H.I. Developmental Anomalies at the Thoracic Outlet: An Analysis of 200 Consecutive Cases. *J. Vasc. Surg.* 1992;16:534–545. doi: 10.1016/0741-5214(92)90161-Z.
231. Collins R.M., Bhana J., Patricios J.S., Du Plessis A., Veller M., Schultz D., Janse Van Rensburg D.C. Thoracic Outlet Syndrome in a Patient with Absent Scalenus Anterior Muscle. *Clin. J. Sport. Med.* 2014;24:268–270. doi: 10.1097/JSM.0000000000000006.
232. Valera-Calero J.A., Gómez-Sánchez S., Fernández-de-las-Peñas C., Plaza-Manzano G., Sánchez-Jorge S., Navarro-Santana M.J. A Procedure for Measuring Anterior Scalene Morphology and Quality with Ultrasound Imaging: An Intra- and Inter-Rater Reliability Study. *Ultrasound Med. Biol.* 2023;49:1817–1823. doi: 10.1016/j.ultrasmedbio.2023.04.005.
233. McNamara K.P., Greene K.A., Tooze J.A., Dang J., Khattab K., Lenchik L., Weaver A.A. Neck Muscle Changes Following Long-Duration Spaceflight. *Front. Physiol.* 2019;10:1115. doi: 10.3389/fphys.2019.01115.
234. Weaver M.L., Hicks C.W., Fritz J., Black J.H., Lum Y.W. Local Anesthetic Block of the Anterior Scalene Muscle Increases Muscle Height in Patients with Neurogenic Thoracic Outlet Syndrome. *Ann. Vasc. Surg.* 2019;59:28–35. doi: 10.1016/j.avsg.2019.01.023.
235. Greene K.A., Tooze J.A., Lenchik L., Weaver A.A. Change in Lumbar Muscle Size and Composition on MRI with Long-Duration Spaceflight. *Ann. Biomed. Eng.* 2022;50:816–824. doi: 10.1007/s10439-022-02968-3.
236. Thomas G.I., Jones T.W., Stavney L.S., Manhas D.R. The Middle Scalene Muscle and Its Contribution to the Thoracic Outlet Syndrome. *Am. J. Surg.* 1983;145:589–592. doi: 10.1016/0002-9610(83)90098-3.
237. Paraskevas G., Ioannidis O., Papaziogas B., Natsis K., Spanidou S., Kitsoulis P. An Accessory Middle Scalene Muscle Causing Thoracic Outlet Syndrome. *Folia Morphol.* 2007;66:194–197.
238. Natsis K., Totlis T., Didagelos M., Tsakotos G., Vlassis K., Skandalakis P. Scalenus Minimus Muscle: Overestimated or Not? An Anatomical Study. *Am. Surg.* 2013;79:372–374. doi: 10.1177/000313481307900425.
239. Machleder H.I., Moll F., Verity M.A. The Anterior Scalene Muscle in Thoracic Outlet Compression Syndrome: Histochemical and Morphometric Studies. *Arch. Surg.* 1986;121:1141–1144. doi: 10.1001/archsurg.1986.01400100047009.
240. Stott C.F. A Note on the Scalenus Minimus Muscle. *J. Anat.* 1928;62:359–361.

241. Savgaonkar M.G., Chimmalgi M., Kulkarni U.K. Anatomy of Inter-Scalene Triangle and Its Role in Thoracic Outlet Compression Syndrome. *J. Anat. Soc. India.* 2006;55:52–55.

242. Sanli E.C., Aktekin M., Kurtoglu Z. A Case of Large Scalenus Minimus Muscle. *Neurosciences.* 2007;12:336–337.

243. Ulusoy O.L., Alis D., Oz A., Barlas S.B., Sokmen B.K., Sever S., Mutlu A., Colakoglu B. The Prevalence and Characteristics of the Subclavius Posticus Muscle in the Adult Population on MRI. *Surg. Radiol. Anat.* 2018;40:1141–1145. doi: 10.1007/s00276-018-2065-6.

244. Akita K., Ibukuro K., Yamaguchi K., Heima S., Sato T. The Subclavius Posticus Muscle: A Factor in Arterial, Venous or Brachial Plexus Compression? *Surg. Radiol. Anat.* 2000;22:111–115. doi: 10.1007/s00276-000-0111-6.

245. Cogar A.C., Johnsen P.H., Potter H.G., Wolfe S.W. Subclavius Posticus: An Anomalous Muscle in Association with Suprascapular Nerve Compression in an Athlete. *Hand.* 2015;10:76–79. doi: 10.1007/s11552-014-9652-8.

246. Sam Y., Park S., Kim C.S. Absence of the Subclavius Muscle with Contralateral Subclavius Posticus Muscle: First Imaging Report. *Clin. Imaging.* 2018;49:54–57. doi: 10.1016/J.CLINIMAG.2017.10.008.

247. Asghar A., Narayan R.K., Satyam A., Naaz S. Prevalence of Anomalous or Ectopic Insertion of Pectoralis Minor: A Systematic Review and Meta-Analysis of 4146 Shoulders. *Surg. Radiol. Anat.* 2021;43:631–643. doi: 10.1007/s00276-020-02610-8.

248. Le Double A.F. *Traité des Variations du Système Musculaire de l' Homme.* Schleicher Frères; Paris, France: 1897.

249. Homsi C., Rodrigues M.B., Silva J.J., Stump X., Morvan G. Aspect Échographique Des Anomalies d'insertion Du Muscle Pectoralis Minor (Petit Pectoral) [Anomalous Insertion of the Pectoralis Minor Muscle: Ultrasound Findings] *J. Radiol.* 2003;84:1007–1011. (In French)

250. Dumontier C., Sautet A., Gagey O., Apoil A. Rotator Interval Lesions and Their Relation to Coracoid Impingement Syndrome. *J. Shoulder Elb. Surg.* 1999;8:130–135. doi: 10.1016/S1058-2746(99)90005-8.

251. Lee S.J., Ha D.H., Lee S.M. Unusual Variation of the Rotator Interval: Insertional Abnormality of the Pectoralis Minor Tendon and Absence of the Coracohumeral Ligament. *Skelet. Radiol.* 2010;39:1205–1209. doi: 10.1007/s00256-010-0926-0.

252. Lee C.B., Choi S.J., Ahn J.H., Ryu D.S., Park M.S., Jung S.M., Shin D.R. Ectopic Insertion of the Pectoralis Minor Tendon: Inter-Reader Agreement and Findings in the Rotator Interval on MRI. *Korean J. Radiol.* 2014;15:764–770. doi: 10.3348/kjr.2014.15.6.764.

253. Leonhard V., Smith R., Caldwell G., Smith H.F. Anatomical Variations in the Brachial Plexus Roots: Implications for Diagnosis of Neurogenic Thoracic Outlet Syndrome. *Ann. Anat.* 2016;206:21–26. doi: 10.1016/j.aanat.2016.03.011.

254. Leonhard V., Caldwell G., Goh M., Reeder S., Smith H.F. Ultrasonographic Diagnosis of Thoracic Outlet Syndrome Secondary to Brachial Plexus Piercing Variation. *Diagnostics.* 2017;7:40. doi: 10.3390/diagnostics7030040.

255. Roos D.B. Congenital Anomalies Associated with Thoracic Outlet Syndrome. Anatomy, Symptoms, Diagnosis, and Treatment. *Am. J. Surg.* 1976;132:771–778. doi: 10.1016/0002-9610(76)90456-6.

256. Tokat A.O., Atınkaya C., Fırat A., Apaydın N., Tekdemir İ., Güngör A. Cadaver analysis of thoracic outlet anomalies. *Turk. J. Thorac. Cardiovasc. Surg.* 2011;19:72–76.

257. Chavhan G.B., Batmanabane V., Muthusami P., Towbin A.J., Borschel G.H. MRI of Thoracic Outlet Syndrome in Children. *Pediatr. Radiol.* 2017;47:1222–1234. doi: 10.1007/s00247-017-3854-5.

258. Baltopoulos P., Tsintzos C., Prionas G., Tsironi M. Exercise-Induced Scalenus Syndrome. *Am. J. Sports Med.* 2008;36:369–374. doi: 10.1177/0363546507312166.

259. Bortolani E., Miani S., D'Armini A., Gallo E., Morbidelli A. Role of Anterior Scalene Muscle Hypertrophy in Thoracic Outlet Syndrome. *Minerva Chir.* 1989;44:1305–1309.

260. Qaja E., Honari S., Rhee R. Arterial Thoracic Outlet Syndrome Secondary to Hypertrophy of the Anterior Scalene Muscle. *J. Surg. Case Rep.* 2017;2017:rjx158. doi: 10.1093/jscr/rjx158.

261. Farina R., Foti P.V., Iannace F.A., Conti A., Ferlito A., Conti A., Pennisi M., Santonocito S., Basile A. Thoracic Outlet Syndrome: A Rare Case with Bilateral Cervical Ribs and Bilateral Anterior Scalene Hypertrophy. *J. Ultrasound.* 2021;24:331–336. doi: 10.1007/s40477-019-00418-w.

262. Telford E.D., Mottershead S. Pressure at the Cervico-Brachial Junction; an Operative and Anatomical Study. *J. Bone Jt. Surg. Br.* 1948;30B:249–265. doi: 10.1302/0301-620X.30B2.249.

263. Aziz S., Straehley C.J., Whelan T.J. Effort-Related Axillosubclavian Vein Thrombosis. A New Theory of Pathogenesis and a Plea for Direct Surgical Intervention. *Am. J. Surg.* 1986;152:57–61. doi: 10.1016/0002-9610(86)90141-8.

264. Kunkel J.M., Machleder H.I. Treatment of Paget-Schroetter Syndrome. A Staged, Multidisciplinary Approach. *Arch. Surg.* 1989;124:1153–1158. doi: 10.1001/archsurg.1989.01410100055010.

265. Hackenberg Booksellers ABAA . *Medico-Surgical Tributes to Harold Brunn; a Series of Essays on Various Aspects of Surgery and Medicine Written by His Pupils and Friends.* University of California Press; Berkeley, CA, USA: 1942. [(accessed on 13 December 2022)]. Available online: https://www.abebooks.com/Medico-surgical-Tributes-Harold-Brunn-Series-Essays/49473238/bd

266. Yin J., Qi Z., Chen Y., Chen Y. A Case Report of Membranous Occlusion of the Subclavian Vein: A Rare Cause of McCleery Syndrome. *Ann. Transl. Med.* 2021;9:78. doi: 10.21037/atm-20-2862.

267. Wiley A.P., Freischlag J.A. Delay in Diagnosis for Two Patients with McCleery Syndrome. *Vasc. Endovasc. Surg.* 2023;57:501–503. doi: 10.1177/15385744231154085.

268. Garraud T., Pomares G., Daley P., Menu P., Dauty M., Fouasson-Chailloux A. Thoracic Outlet Syndrome in Sport: A Systematic Review. *Front. Physiol.* 2022;13:1189. doi: 10.3389/fphys.2022.838014.

269. Chandra V., Little C., Lee J.T. Thoracic Outlet Syndrome in High-Performance Athletes. *J. Vasc. Surg.* 2014;60:1012–1018. doi: 10.1016/j.jvs.2014.04.013.

270. Beteck B., Shutze W., Richardson B., Shutze R., Tran K., Dao A., Ogola G.O., Pearl G. Comparison of Athletes and Nonathletes Undergoing Thoracic Outlet Decompression for Neurogenic Thoracic Outlet Syndrome. *Ann. Vasc. Surg.* 2019;54:269–275. doi: 10.1016/j.avsg.2018.05.049.

271. Sancho-González I., Bonilla-Hernández M.V., Ibañez-Muñoz D., Vicente-Campos D., Chicharro J.L. Upper Extremity Deep Vein Thrombosis in a Triathlete: Again Intense Endurance Exercise as a Thrombogenic Risk. *Am. J. Emerg. Med.* 2017;35:808.e1–808.e3. doi: 10.1016/j.ajem.2016.12.023.

272. Lutter C., Monasterio E., Schöffl V. Rock Climbing-Related Subclavian Vein Thrombosis. *Case Rep.* 2015;2015:bcr2015212021. doi: 10.1136/bcr-2015-212021.

273. Leung Y.F., Chung O.M., Ip P.S., Wong A., Wai Y.L. An Unusual Case of Thoracic Outlet Syndrome Associated with Long Distance Running. *Br. J. Sports Med.* 1999;33:279–281. doi: 10.1136/bjsm.33.4.279.

274. Ijaopo R., Oguntolu V., Da Costa D., Garnham A., Hobbs S. A Case of Paget-Schroetter Syndrome (PSS) in a Young Judo Tutor: A Case Report. *J. Med. Case Rep.* 2016;10:63. doi: 10.1186/s13256-016-0848-0.

275. Smith T.M., Sawyer S.F., Sizer P.S., Brismée J.M. The Double Crush Syndrome: A Common Occurrence in Cyclists with Ulnar Nerve Neuropathy—A Case-Control Study. *Clin. J. Sport. Med.* 2008;18:55–61. doi: 10.1097/JSM.0b013e31815c1d7a.

276. Zakaria A., Gill J., Nishi L.M., Nadwodny J., Pujalte G.G.A. Soccer Player with Unusual Right Shoulder and Arm Pain and Swelling. *J. Prim. Health Care.* 2020;12:181–183. doi: 10.1071/HC19101.

277. Cho Y.J., Lee H.J., Gong H.S., Rhee S.H., Park S.J., Baek G.H. The Radiologic Relationship of the Shoulder Girdle to the Thorax as an Aid in Diagnosing Neurogenic Thoracic Outlet Syndrome. *J. Hand Surg.* 2012;37:1187–1193. doi: 10.1016/j.jhsa.2012.02.022.

278. Hudson N., Starr M.R., Esdaile J.M., Fitzcharles M.A. Diagnostic Associations with Hypermobility in Rheumatology Patients. *Br. J. Rheumatol.* 1995;34:1157–1161. doi: 10.1093/rheumatology/34.12.1157.

279. Levine N.A., Rigby B.R. Thoracic Outlet Syndrome: Biomechanical and Exercise Considerations. *Healthcare.* 2018;6:68. doi: 10.3390/healthcare6020068.

280. Atasoy E. Thoracic Outlet Compression Syndrome. *Orthop. Clin. N. Am.* 1996;27:265–303. doi: 10.1016/S0030-5898(20)32074-5.

281. Cheng S.W.K., Stoney R.J. Supraclavicular Reoperation for Neurogenic Thoracic Outlet Syndrome. *J. Vasc. Surg.* 1994;19:565–572. doi: 10.1016/S0741-5214(94)70027-3.

282. Sanders R.J., Haug C.E., Pearce W.H. Recurrent Thoracic Outlet Syndrome. *J. Vasc. Surg.* 1990;12:390–400. doi: 10.1016/0741-5214(90)90040-H.

283. Demaree C.J., Wang K., Lin P.H. Thoracic Outlet Syndrome Affecting High-Performance Musicians Playing Bowed String Instruments. *Vascular.* 2017;25:329–332. doi: 10.1177/1708538116671064.

284. Franklin G.M. Work-Related Neurogenic Thoracic Outlet Syndrome: Diagnosis and Treatment. *Phys. Med. Rehabil. Clin. N. Am.* 2015;26:551–561. doi: 10.1016/j.pmr.2015.04.004.

285. Pascarelli E.F., Hsu Y.P. Understanding Work-Related Upper Extremity Disorders: Clinical Findings in 485 Computer Users, Musicians, and Others. *J. Occup. Rehabil.* 2001;11:1–21. doi: 10.1023/A:1016647923501.

286. Sällström J., Schmidt H. Cervicobrachial Disorders in Certain Occupations, with Special Reference to Compression in the Thoracic Outlet. *Am. J. Ind. Med.* 1984;6:45–52. doi: 10.1002/ajim.4700060107.

287. Hagberg M., Wegman D.H. Prevalence Rates and Odds Ratios of Shoulder-Neck Diseases in Different Occupational Groups. *Br. J. Ind. Med.* 1987;44:602. doi: 10.1136/oem.44.9.602.

288. Trenor C.C., Fisher J.G., Khan F.A., Sparks E.A., Duzan J., Harney K., Dillon B., Menard M., Modi B.P. Paget-Schroetter Syndrome in 21 Children: Outcomes after Multidisciplinary Care. *J. Pediatr.* 2015;166:1493–1497. doi: 10.1016/j.jpeds.2015.03.030.

289. Dintaman J., Watson C., Fox C.J., Hoover N., Roberts S., Gillespie D.L. Case of Adolescent with Paget-Schroetter Syndrome and Underlying Thrombophilia Due to an Elevated Lipoprotein (A) *Pediatr. Blood Cancer.* 2007;49:1036–1038. doi: 10.1002/pbc.20790.

290. Conard J., Horellou M.H., Van Dreden P., Lecompte T., Samama M. Thrombosis and Pregnancy in Congenital Deficiencies in AT III, Protein C or Protein S: Study of 78 Women. *Thromb. Haemost.* 1990;63:319–320. doi: 10.1055/s-0038-1645218.

291. Sayinalp N., Özcebe O.I., Kirazli Ş., Do⍰an R., Dündar S.V., Gürgey A. Paget-Schroetter Syndrome Associated with FV:Q506 and Prothrombin 20210A—A Case Report. *Angiology.* 1999;50:689–692. doi: 10.1177/000331979905000811.

292. Adekoya O. A Case of Upper Limb Venous Thrombosis in Paget-Schroetter Syndrome. *Cureus.* 2021;13:e13187. doi: 10.7759/cureus.13187.

293. Tchaikovski S.N., Rosing J. Mechanisms of Estrogen-Induced Venous Thromboembolism. *Thromb. Res.* 2010;126:5–11. doi: 10.1016/j.thromres.2010.01.045.

294. Curry P., Fitchett D., Stubbs W. The Pill and the Thoracic Outlet and Bilateral Carpal Tunnel Syndromes. *J. Natl. Med. Assoc.* 1981;73:995.

295. Cramer A.C.M., McLean A.W., Ahari J. Upper Extremity Deep Venous Thrombosis and Pulmonary Embolus after Ovarian Hyperstimulation. *Case Rep.* 2016;2016:bcr2016216719. doi: 10.1136/bcr-2016-216719.

296. Alderman D.B., Kwass W. Vascular Complications of Cervical Rib. *Conn. Med.* 1978;42:156–158.

297. Kommareddy A., Zaroukian M.H., Hassouna H.I. Upper Extremity Deep Venous Thrombosis. *Semin. Thromb. Hemost.* 2002;28:89–99. doi: 10.1055/s-2002-20567.

298. Stricker S.J., Sowers D.K., Sowers J.R., Sirridge M.S. "Effort Thrombosis" of the Subclavian Vein Associated with Oral Contraceptives. *Ann. Emerg. Med.* 1981;10:596–599. doi: 10.1016/S0196-0644(81)80201-6.

299. Valanejad S.M., Davis K.A. Direct Oral Anticoagulants in Select Patients with Hypercoagulable Disorders. *Ann. Pharmacother.* 2021;55:891–901. doi: 10.1177/1060028020968551.

300. Ellison D.W., Wood V.E. Trauma-Related Thoracic Outlet Syndrome. *J. Hand Surg. Br.* 1994;19:424–426. doi: 10.1016/0266-7681(94)90203-8.

301. Schwartzman R.J. Brachial Plexus Traction Injuries. [(accessed on 28 December 2022)];*Hand Clin.* 1991 7:547–556. doi: 10.1016/S0749-0712(21)01105-7. Available online: https://pubmed.ncbi.nlm.nih.gov/1658012/

302. Ide M., Ide J., Yamaga M., Takagi K. Symptoms and Signs of Irritation of the Brachial Plexus in Whiplash Injuries. *J. Bone Jt. Surg. Br.* 2001;83:226–229. doi: 10.1302/0301-620X.83B2.0830226.

303. Sanders R.J., Jackson C.G.R., Banchero N., Pearce W.H. Scalene Muscle Abnormalities in Traumatic Thoracic Outlet Syndrome. *Am. J. Surg.* 1990;159:231–236. doi: 10.1016/S0002-9610(05)80269-7.

304. Kai Y., Oyama M., Kurose S., Inadome T., Oketani Y., Masuda Y. Neurogenic Thoracic Outlet Syndrome in Whiplash Injury. *J. Spinal Disord.* 2001;14:487–493. doi: 10.1097/00002517-200112000-00004.

305. Crotti F.M., Carai A., Carai M., Sgaramella E., Sias W. Post-Traumatic Thoracic Outlet Syndrome (TOS) *Acta Neurochir. Suppl.* 2005;92:13–15. doi: 10.1007/3-211-27458-8_3.

306. Alexandre A., Corò L., Azuelos A., Pellone M. Thoracic Outlet Syndrome Due to Hyperextension-Hyperflexion Cervical Injury. *Acta Neurochir. Suppl.* 2005;92:21–24. doi: 10.1007/3-211-27458-8_5.

307. Mailis A., Papagapiou M., Vanderlinden R.G., Campbell V., Taylor A. Thoracic Outlet Syndrome after Motor Vehicle Accidents in a Canadian Pain Clinic Population. *Clin. J. Pain.* 1995;11:316–324. doi: 10.1097/00002508-199512000-00009.

308. Dubuisson A., Lamotte C., Foidart-Dessalle M., Nguyen Khac M., Racaru T., Scholtes F., Kaschten B., Lénelle J., Martin D. Post-Traumatic Thoracic Outlet Syndrome. *Acta Neurochir.* 2012;154:517–526. doi: 10.1007/s00701-011-1269-x.

309. Mulder S., Greenwood F.A., Brooks C.E. Posttraumatic Thoracic Outlet Syndrome. *J. Trauma Inj. Infect. Crit. Care.* 1973;13:706–715. doi: 10.1097/00005373-197308000-00006.

310. Casbas L., Chauffour X., Cau J., Bossavy J.P., Midy D., Baste J.C., Barret A. Post-Traumatic Thoracic Outlet Syndromes. *Ann. Vasc. Surg.* 2005;19:25–28. doi: 10.1007/s10016-004-0151-1.

311. Woods W.W., Diego S. Thoracic Outlet Syndrome. *West. J. Med.* 1978;128:9.

312. Weinberg H., Nathan H., Magora F., Robin G.C., Aviad I. Arthritis of the First Costovertebral Joint as a Cause of Thoracic Outlet Syndrome. *Clin. Orthop. Relat. Res.* 1972;86:159–163. doi: 10.1097/00003086-197207000-00023.

313. Feinberg J.H., Nguyen E.T., Boachie-Adjei K., Gribbin C., Lee S.K., Daluiski A., Wolfe S.W. The Electrodiagnostic Natural History of Parsonage-Turner Syndrome. *Muscle Nerve.* 2017;56:737–743. doi: 10.1002/mus.25558.

314. Seror P. Neuralgic Amyotrophy. An Update. *Jt. Bone Spine.* 2017;84:153–158. doi: 10.1016/j.jbspin.2016.03.005.

315. Chang K.Z., Likes K., Davis K., Demos J., Freischlag J.A. The Significance of Cervical Ribs in Thoracic Outlet Syndrome. *J. Vasc. Surg.* 2013;57:771–775. doi: 10.1016/j.jvs.2012.08.110.

316. Huang J.H., Zager E.L., McGillicuddy J.E., Benzel E.C., Adelson P.D., Kline D.G. Thoracic Outlet Syndrome. *Neurosurgery.* 2004;55:897–903. doi: 10.1227/01.NEU.0000137333.04342.4D.

317. Kuhn J.E., Lebus V.G.F., Bible J.E. Thoracic Outlet Syndrome. *J. Am. Acad. Orthop. Surg.* 2015;23:222–232. doi: 10.5435/JAAOS-D-13-00215.

318. Burt B.M. Thoracic Outlet Syndrome for Thoracic Surgeons. *J. Thorac. Cardiovasc. Surg.* 2018;156:1318–1323.e1. doi: 10.1016/j.jtcvs.2018.02.096.

319. Goeteyn J., Pesser N., Houterman S., van Sambeek M.R.H.M., van Nuenen B.F.L., Teijink J.A.W. Surgery Versus Continued Conservative Treatment for Neurogenic Thoracic Outlet Syndrome: The First Randomised Clinical Trial (STOPNTOS Trial) *Eur. J. Vasc. Endovasc. Surg.* 2022;64:119–127. doi: 10.1016/j.ejvs.2022.05.003.

320. Lindgren K.A. Conservative Treatment of Thoracic Outlet Syndrome: A 2-Year Follow-Up. *Arch. Phys. Med. Rehabil.* 1997;78:373–378. doi: 10.1016/S0003-9993(97)90228-8.

321. Warrick A., Davis B. Neurogenic Thoracic Outlet Syndrome in Athletes—Nonsurgical Treatment Options. *Curr. Sports Med. Rep.* 2021;20:319–326. doi: 10.1249/JSR.0000000000000854.

Chapter

THE MEDIASTINAL STRUCTURES, PLEURA, AND LUNGS

3

Contents

Introduction

The lungs, pleura, and mediastinum are vital organs of the thoracic cavity that are involved in breathing and general thoracic function. The pleurae of the lungs on either side, the sternum anteriorly, the spine posteriorly, and the diaphragm inferiorly define the borders of the mediastinum, the central compartment of the thoracic cavity. It contains many nerves and lymphatic tissues, as well as the heart, great vessels, trachea, esophagus, and thymus. The superior and inferior sections of the mediastinum are separated, and the inferior is further divided into anterior, middle, and posterior regions. Particular organs and structures are located in each subdivision. For example, the heart and pericardium are located in the middle mediastinum, and the esophagus, thoracic duct, and descending aorta are located in the posterior mediastinum.

The pleural cavities are formed by the pleurae, which are serous membranes that surround the lungs and line the thoracic cavity. The two layers that make up these membranes are the parietal pleura, which lines the thoracic wall, diaphragm, and mediastinum, and the visceral pleura, which adheres to the lung surface. There is a tiny quantity of lubricating fluid in the pleural cavity, which is the potential gap between these layers, allowing the lungs to glide smoothly during breathing. The main breathing organs, the lungs, are responsible for gas exchange. They are divided by fissures into two lobes in the left lung (upper and lower) and three in the right lung (upper, middle, and lower). They are located on either side of the mediastinum. The trachea, which divides into the left and right main bronchi and smaller bronchioles and alveoli where gas exchange takes place, is the pathway through which air enters the lungs. Understanding the functional relationships of these structures is essential for effective respiratory mechanics. The pleura ensures minimal friction during lung expansion and contraction, while the mediastinum provides a protected pathway for blood, oxygen, and nutrients. Since the lungs are where carbon dioxide and oxygen are exchanged, they are crucial for maintaining homeostasis. It is important to comprehend the anatomy and functions of the pleura, lungs, and mediastinal structures in order to diagnose and treat thoracic diseases and disorders.

A two-layered membranous pleural sac is formed when a serous membrane folds back on itself, forming a pleura. The outer layer adheres to the chest wall and is referred to as the parietal pleura. The lungs, blood vessels, nerves, and bronchi are all covered by the inner layer, which is known as the visceral pleura. There is no anatomical connection between the right and left pleural cavities (Adeyinka et al., 2023) (Figure 3.1).

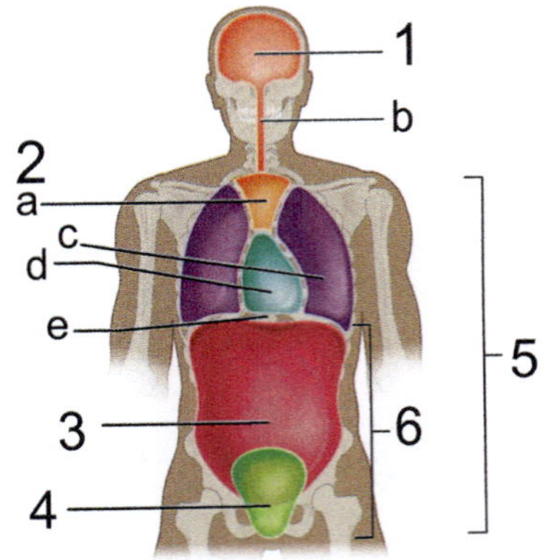

Figure 3.1. *Mediastinal divisions. The mediastinum can be divided into the following areas: superior mediastinum, anterior mediastinum, middle mediastinum, posterior mediastinum, superior compartment, and inferior compartment.*

Source: By OpenStax – https://cnx.org/contents/FPtK1zmh@8.25:fEI3C8Ot@10Version 8.25 from the Textbook OpenStax Anatomy and Physiology Published May 18, 2016, CC BY 3.0; https://commons.wikimedia.org/w/index.php?curid=64286603.

With the addition of pleural fluid, the lung pleura allows for easy movement of the lungs and inflation during breathing.

A central space in the thoracic cavity situated between the lung pleural sacs is known as the mediastinum (see Image). The transverse section of the thorax, or mediastinum. The superior and inferior portions make up its two main sections. The anterior, middle, and posterior portions make up the remaining inferior portion. Particular groups of structures are found in each region of the mediastinum (Volpe et al., 2023).

1. Superior Mediastinum:
   - **Organs:** Thymus, trachea, esophagus.
   - **Arteries:** Aortic arch, brachiocephalic trunk, left

common carotid artery, left subclavian artery.
- **Veins and Lymphatics:** superior vena cava, brachiocephalic vein, thoracic duct.
- **Nerves:** Vagus nerve, left recurrent laryngeal nerve, cardiac nerve, phrenic nerve.

2. Anterior Mediastinum:
   - Organs: Thymus.
   - Arteries: Small arterial branches.
   - Veins and Lymphatics: Small branches.
   - Nerves: None.
3. Middle Mediastinum:
   - **Organs:** Heart, pericardium.
   - **Arteries:** Ascending aorta, pulmonary trunk, pericardiophrenic arteries.
   - **Veins and Lymphatics:** Superior vena cava, azygos vein, pulmonary vein, pericardiophrenic vein.
   - **Nerve:** Phrenic.
4. Posterior Mediastinum:
   - **Organs:** Esophagus.
   - **Arteries:** Thoracic aorta.
   - **Veins and Lymphatics:** Azygos vein, hemiazygos vein, thoracic duct.
   - **Nerve:** The vagus nerve.

Orientation and Directional Terms

Term	Definition	Illustration
Lungs	The lungs and respiratory system allow us to breathe. They bring oxygen into our bodies (called inspiration, or inhalation) and send carbon dioxide out (called expiration, or exhalation). This exchange of oxygen and carbon dioxide is called respiration.	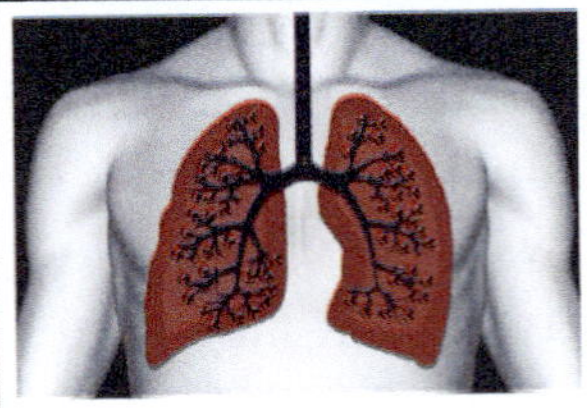
Pleura	A pleura is a serous membrane that folds back on itself to form a two-layered membranous pleural sac. The outer layer is called the parietal pleura and attaches to the chest wall. The inner layer is called the visceral pleura and covers the lungs, blood vessels, nerves, and bronchi.	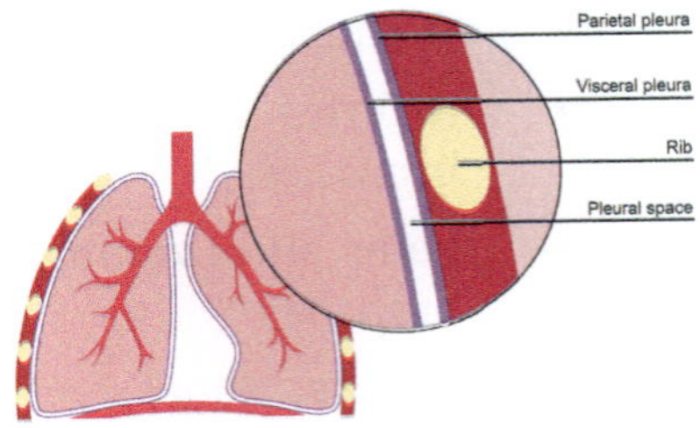
Mediastinum	Mediastinum is the central compartment of the thoracic cavity. Surrounded by loose connective tissue, it is an undelineated region that contains a group of structures within the thorax, namely the heart and its vessels, the esophagus, the trachea, the phrenic and cardiac nerves, the thoracic duct, the thymus and the lymph nodes of the central chest.	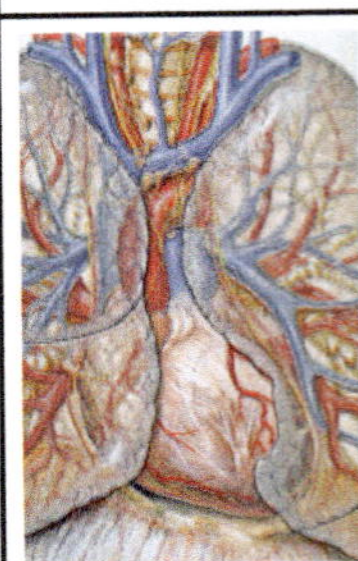
Aortic Arch	The aortic arch has three main branches on its superior aspect. The first, and largest, branch of the arch of the aorta is the brachiocephalic trunk, which is to the right and slightly anterior to the other two branches and originates behind the manubrium of the sternum.	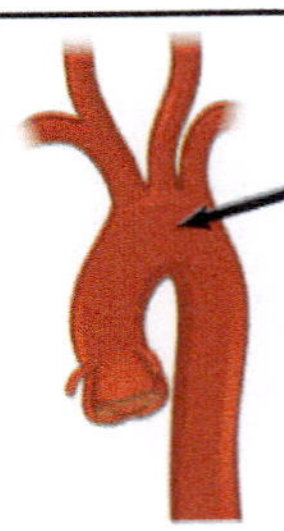
Brachiocephalic veins	Brachiocephalic veins are major veins in the upper chest, formed by the union of the ipsilateral internal jugular vein and subclavian vein (the so-called venous angle) behind the sternoclavicular joint.	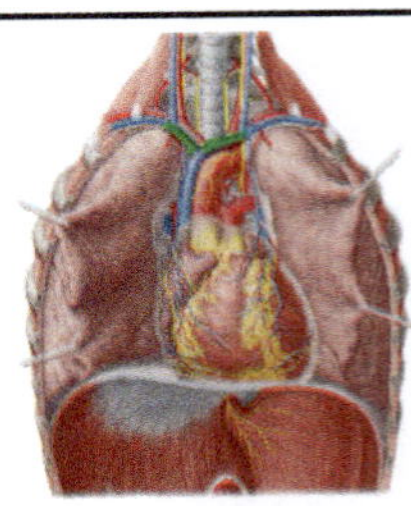

3.1. The Mediastinal Structures

3.1.1. The Aorta

The left ventricle is the source of the major artery trunk of the systemic circulation, which ascends momentarily before reversing course and passing over the left lung's root to descend through the thorax and abdomen. It is separated descriptively into an abdominal part, a descending thoracic part, an ascending part, and an arch.

3.1.1.1. The Ascending Aorta

The ascending aorta is a broad, five-centimeter-long vessel. It starts below the level of the sternal angle at the aortic orifice behind the third right costal cartilage and ascends to the right, around the pulmonary trunk, to the sternal angle. An aortic sinus, or dilatation, is located at the base of the aortic valve above each of the semilunar valvules.

3.1.1.1.1. Relations

A common sheath of serous pericardium surrounds the ascending aorta, while the fibrous pericardium encloses the pulmonary trunk. The sternum is anterior to its lower portion, which is behind the right ventricle's infundibulum and the pulmonary trunk's origin. The right pulmonary artery, right main bronchus, and left atrium are located posteriorly, ascending from below. The pulmonary trunk and left auricle are located on its left, while the superior vena cava and right auricle are located on its right.

3.1.1.1.2. Branches

The right and left coronary arteries arise from the anterior and left posterior aortic sinuses.

3.1.1.1.3. Aortic Arch

The aortic arch ascends from the sternal angle behind the manubrium, then descends to the left side of the fourth thoracic vertebra before arching backward and to the left over the left lung root. The head, neck, and upper limbs are supplied by three arteries that emerge from the convexity of the arch (Figure 3.2).

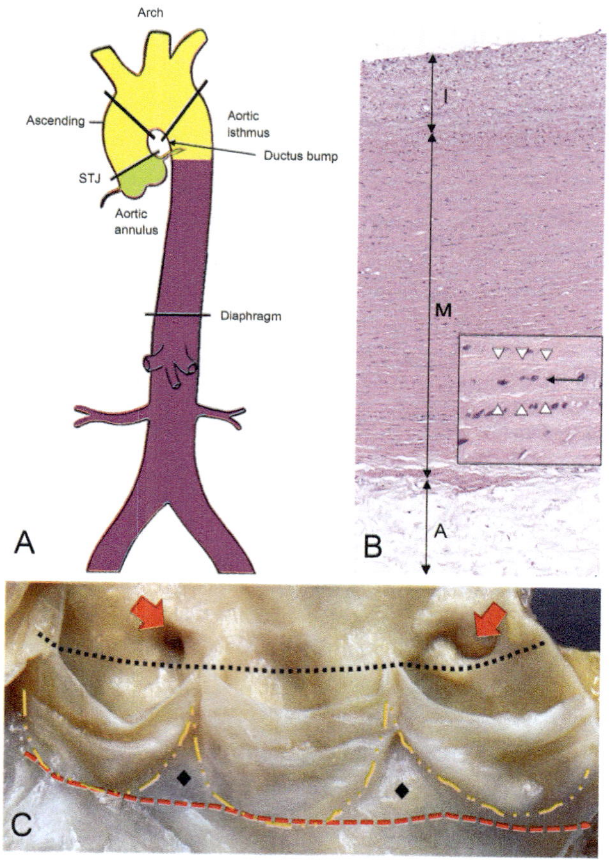

Figure 3.2. *Topographic anatomy and normal histology of the aorta.*

Source: di Gioia, C. R. T., Ascione, A., Carletti, R., & Giordano, C., (2023). Thoracic aorta: Anatomy and pathology. Diagnostics, 13(13), 2166. https://doi.org/10.3390/diagnostics13132166.

(A) Diagram of the aorta with different colors reflecting the different histogenesis of the SMCs of the tunica media: SMCs of the aortic root derive from the secondary heart field (lateral plate mesoderm) (green); SMCs of ascending aorta and the arch derive from the neural crests (ectoderm) (yellow); SMCs of the descending and abdominal aorta derive from the somites of the paraxial mesoderm (purple). SMCs = smooth muscle cells. (B) Histological anatomy of the descending aorta with tunica intima (I), media (M), and adventitia (A). The mild fibrous intimal thickening is a typical age-related change. The normal lamellar architecture of the tunica media is preserved and showed at higher magnification in the insert, with its elastic laminae (white arrowheads) and the intervening smooth muscle cells (black arrow) (Hematoxylin and eosin, original magnification 10×; insert: 40×). And (C) the aortic root is the segment between the annulus (red dashed line) and the Sino tubular junction (black dotted line) and comprises the sinuses of Valsalva with the aortic cusps (outlined with the orange dashed line), the origin of the coronary arteries (red arrows), and the intercuspal triangles (black diamonds).

3.1.1.1.4. Relations

The left phrenic nerve, left vagus nerve, mediastinal pleura, and lung are located to its left. The superior vena cava, trachea, left recurrent laryngeal nerve, esophagus, thoracic duct, and fourth thoracic vertebra are located to its right. It passes inferiorly through the ligamentum arteriosum, the left main bronchus, and the bifurcation of the pulmonary trunk. Its trio of branches are superior. The ligamentum arteriosum, a fibrous remnant of the ductus arteriosus, connects the arch inferiorly to the left pulmonary artery. The ligamentum and arch are passed around by the left recurrent laryngeal nerve as it travels posteriorly. The ligamentum and the cardiac plexus are closely related. In front of the arch, one may find thymus gland remnants.

3.1.1.1.5. Branches

The brachiocephalic artery, the first branch, originates behind the manubrium and ascends to the right sternoclavicular joint, where it splits into the right subclavian and right common carotid arteries, the two terminal branches.

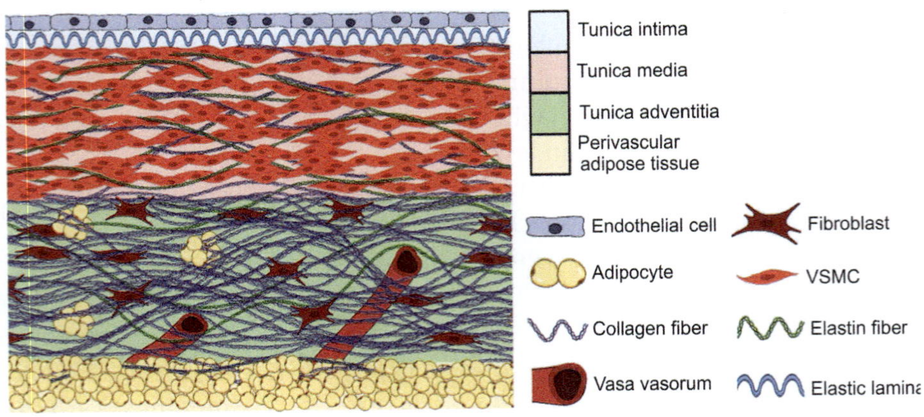

Figure 3.3. *Layers of aortic wall.*

Source: Domagała, D., Data, K., Szyller, H., Farzaneh, M., Mozdziak, P., Woźniak, S., Zabel, M., Dzięgiel, P., & Kempisty, B., (2024). Cellular, molecular, and clinical aspects of aortic aneurysm – Vascular physiology and pathophysiology. Cells, 13(3), 274. https://doi.org/10.3390/cells13030274.

The trachea is located posteriorly, and the left brachiocephalic vein and thymus divide it from the manubrium anteriorly. The superior vena cava and right brachiocephalic vein are located to its right, while the left common carotid artery is located to its left. The brachiocephalic artery is the point from which the left common carotid artery emerges. It then ascends along the left side of the trachea and enters the neck. After emerging from behind the left common carotid artery, the left subclavian artery curves leftward, passing over the left pleura's dome, the left sternoclavicular joint, and the first rib (Figure 3.3).

3.1.1.2. The Descending Aorta

The descending aorta emerges from the left side of the fourth thoracic vertebra, slopes medially toward the front of the twelfth, and becomes the abdominal aorta after passing through the diaphragm.

3.1.1.2.1. Relations

The left lung root, the pericardium-covered left atrium, the esophagus, and the diaphragm are located anteriorly, descending from above. The 4th through the 12th thoracic vertebrae are located posteriorly. Its right side is in contact with the esophagus above and the right lung and pleura below, while its left side is in contact with the left pleura and lung. On its right side are the azygos vein and thoracic duct.

3.1.1.2.2. Branches

These include the diaphragmatic arteries, two or three small bronchial arteries, several small esophageal arteries, the third through 11th posterior intercostal arteries, and a pair of subcostal arteries (Figure 3.4).

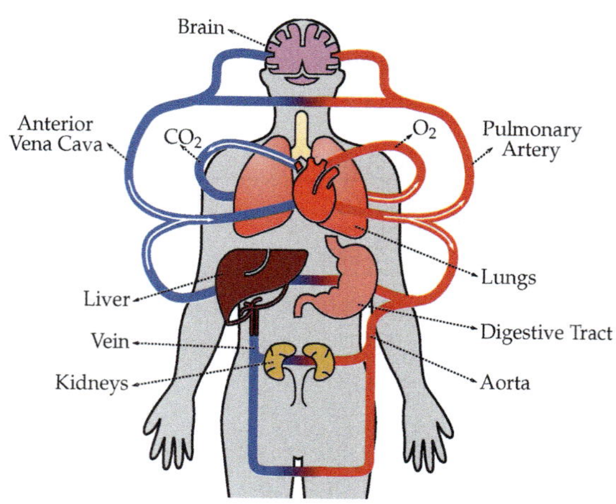

Figure 3.4. *Diagram of the circulatory system.*

Source: Syed, F., Khan, S., & Toma, M., (2023). Modeling dynamics of the cardiovascular system using fluid-structure interaction methods. Biology, 12(7), 1026. https://doi.org/10.3390/biology12071026.

3.1.2. The Pulmonary Trunk

This broad, roughly 5-centimeter-long vessel begins at the pulmonary orifice and ascends posteriorly to the left of the aorta before terminating at the point where the left and right pulmonary arteries split apart beneath the aortic arch's concavity. It is located in front of the pericardium's transverse sinus and is enclosed within a common sleeve of serous pericardium with the ascending aorta. Its base is surrounded by both coronary arteries and both auricles. Radiological techniques make it convenient to study these mediastinal structures (Table 3.1).

Table 3.1. *The International Thymic Malignancy Interest Group (ITMIG) Classification of Mediastinal Compartments*

Compartment	Boundaries
Prevascular	Anterior: Sternum
	Posterior: Anterior surface of pericardium as it wraps around the heart
	Superior: Thoracic inlet
	Inferior: Diaphragm
	Lateral: Mediastinal pleura
Visceral	Anterior: Posterior boundaries of prevascular compartment
	Posterior: Vertical line connecting a point on each thoracic vertebral body 1 cm posterior to its anterior margin
	Superior: Thoracic inlet
	Inferior: Diaphragm
Paravertebral	Anterior: Posterior boundaries of the visceral compartment
	Posterolateral: Vertical line against the posterior margin of the chest wall at the lateral margin of the transverse process of the thoracic spine
	Superior: Thoracic inlet
	Inferior: Diaphragm

Source: Ahuja, J., Strange, C. D., Agrawal, R., Erasmus, L. T., & Truong, M. T., (2023). Approach to imaging of mediastinal masses. Diagnostics, 13(20), 3171. https://doi.org/10.3390/diagnostics13203171.

3.1.2.1. Branches

The ascending aorta, superior vena cava, esophagus, and right main bronchus are the pathways that the right pulmonary artery uses to reach the right lung hilus. The descending aorta and lung hilus of the left pulmonary artery are passed in front of each other. It is joined to the lower part of the aortic arch by the ligamentum arteriosum. The bronchi and bronchioles are followed by pulmonary artery branches (Stauffer et al., 2023; Volpe & Makaryus, 2023).

3.1.3. The Great Veins

The pulmonary veins are a pair of small, broad vessels that are located anteriorly and inferiorly to the artery in the hilum of each lung.

3.1.3.1. Brachiocephalic Veins

The internal jugular and subclavian veins of each side unite to form the brachiocephalic veins, which after a brief course unite to form the superior vena cava behind the right side of the manubrium. This formation occurs behind the sternoclavicular joint. The right phrenic nerve runs lateral to the approximately 3-centimeter-long right brachiocephalic vein, descending behind the right margin of the manubrium anterolateral to the brachiocephalic artery. The longer brachiocephalic vein on the left descends obliquely behind the manubrium, above the aortic arch, and in front of the trachea and its three major branches (Figure 3.5).

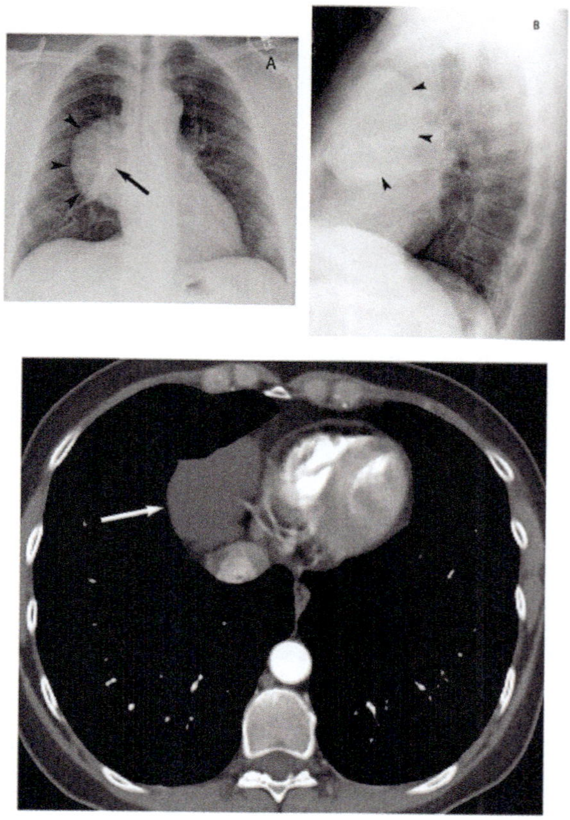

Figure 3.5. *Mediastinal masses.*

Note: (a) Hilum overlay sign. Chest radiograph posteroanterior view (A) shows well-marginated mass over right hilum (arrowheads). Hilar vessels (arrow) are seen through the mass, suggesting the mass is either anterior or posterior to the hilum. Chest radiograph lateral view (B) confirms the anterior location of the mass (arrowheads). (b) Pericardial cyst. CT shows a fluid attenuating structure (10 Hounsfield units) in the prevascular mediastinum at the right anterior cardio phrenic angle (arrow).

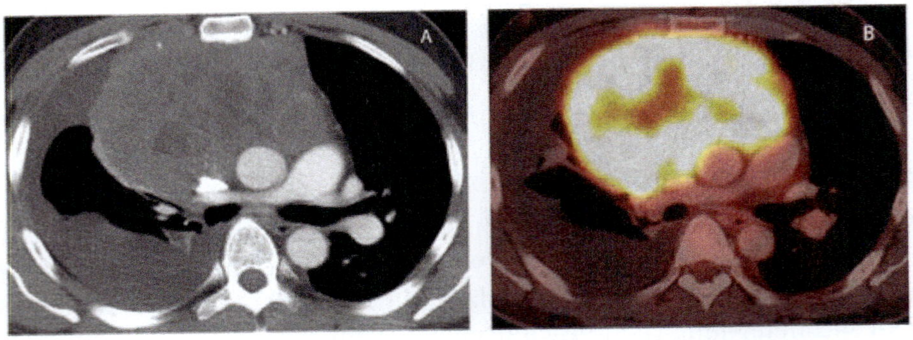

(c) Primary mediastinal lymphoma. CT (A) shows large heterogeneous soft tissue mass in the prevascular mediastinum. The mass is hypermetabolic on FDG PET-CT (B). Biopsy showed diffuse large B cell lymphoma.

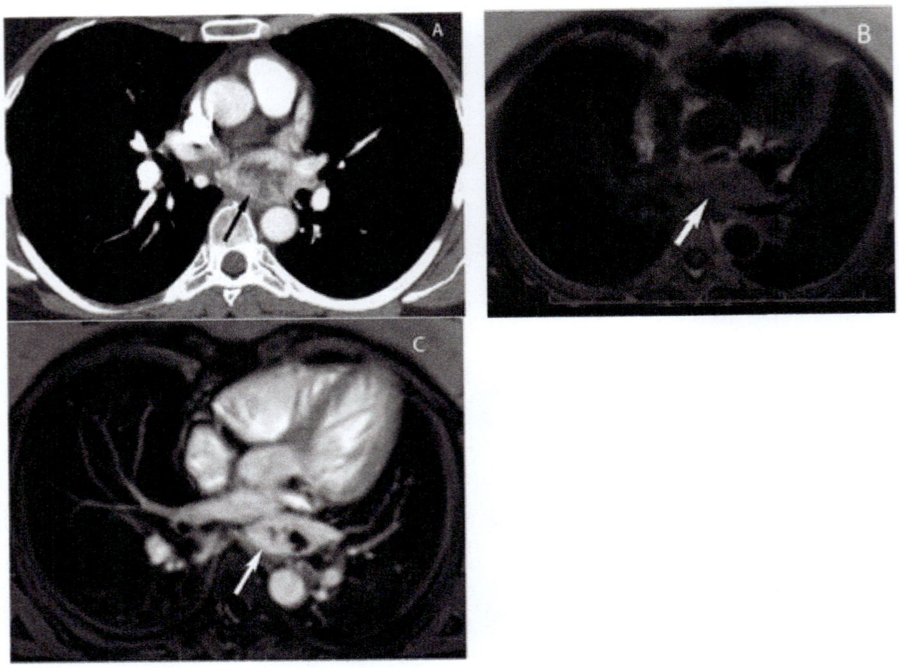

(d) Paraganglioma. CT (A) shows a hyper vascular mass with central necrosis in the visceral mediastinum behind the left atrium. MRI ((B) and (C)) shows the mass is hyperintense compared to muscle upon black blood double inversion MRI (arrow in (B)) and hyper vascular upon post-gadolinium imaging (arrow in (C)).

Source: *Ahuja, J., Strange, C. D., Agrawal, R., Erasmus, L. T., & Truong, M. T., (2023). Approach to imaging of mediastinal masses. Diagnostics, 13(20), 3171. https://doi.org/10.3390/diagnostics13203171.*

3.1.3.1.1. Branches

These are the inferior thyroid veins, which combine in front of the trachea and empty into the left brachiocephalic vein, the internal thoracic vein, which empties into the anterior chest wall, and the vertebral veins, which drain the neck muscles. The smaller right lymph duct empties into the right brachiocephalic vein, while the thoracic duct empties into the left brachiocephalic vein.

3.1.3.2. Superior Vena Cava

The two brachiocephalic veins unite behind the right border of the manubrium to form the superior vena cava, which is 1.5 cm wide and roughly 7 cm long. It then descends behind the sternum's body and enters the right atrium at the level of the third costal cartilage. It is valveless.

3.1.3.2.1. Relations

Its lower half is located anteriorly to the right lung root and behind the right lung, pleura, and manubrium, covered by a fibrous and serous pericardium. It is lateral to the right lung and pleura, and medial to the ascending aorta and right brachiocephalic artery. The azygos vein, its sole tributary, enters posteriorly.

A catheter can be inserted into the internal jugular or subclavian vein via the superior vena cava into the right atrium to measure the right atrial pressure, which is crucial for the management of critically ill patients (central venous pressure line). When a tumor obstructs the superior vena cava, the venous blood inside it is diverted into the chest wall's subcutaneous veins and then into the anterior abdominal wall's veins. The blood that has been diverted then flows into the IVC and azygos vein system.

3.1.3.3. Azygos Vein

The azygos vein, which is located to the right of the aorta, emerges from the abdomen in front of the second lumbar vertebra and enters the chest through the aortic aperture in the diaphragm. It moves up the posterior mediastinum of the vertebral bodies. It crosses the right lung root anteriorly at the level of the fourth thoracic vertebra before entering the superior vena cava.

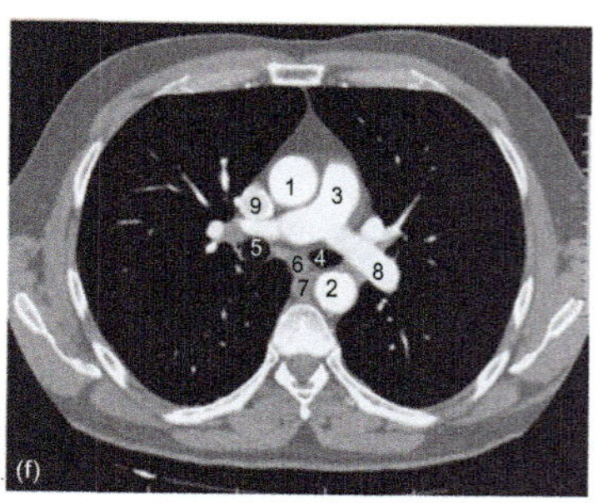

III

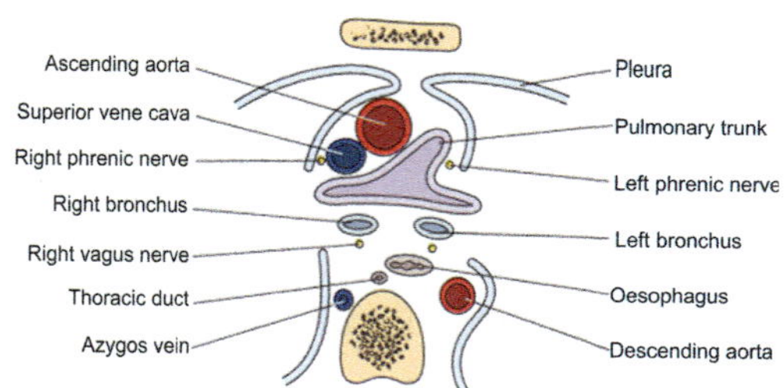

(g)

3.1.3.3.1. Branches

It drains the right bronchial veins and the intercostal spaces along with the smaller left-sided hemiazygos vein. The intrathoracic course of the inferior vena cava is extremely brief. It enters the right atrium straight after piercing the diaphragm's central tendon (Stauffer et al., 2023; Volpe & Makaryus, 2023).

3.1.4. Nerves

3.1.4.1. The Phrenic Nerves

The ventral rami of C3, C4, and C5 are the source of the phrenic nerves, which exit the neck through the thorax in front of each lung root. The right phrenic nerve descends on the pericardium over the superior, inferior, and right atrial veins before entering the thorax lateral to the right brachiocephalic vein and passing through the diaphragm's caval opening. The mediastinal pleura covers it laterally throughout. The left phrenic nerve descends over the left ventricle and pericardium, passing between the left subclavian artery and left brachiocephalic vein before penetrating the left diaphragm. Lateral mediastinal pleura covers it.

The diaphragm receives motor function from both nerves, which also supply sensory branches to the pericardium, peritoneum, mediastinal, and diaphragmatic pleura. The skin above the shoulder tip, which is supplied by nerves derived from the C4 spinal segment, including the phrenic nerve, is the traditional site of pain resulting from inflammation of the diaphragmatic pleura.

3.1.4.2. The Vagus Nerves

The right vagus originates from the right brachiocephalic artery posterolaterally entering the thorax. It then descends laterally to the trachea beneath the mediastinal pleura to the rear of the right main bronchus, where it branches into the esophageal plexus and the pulmonary plexus.

Between the left common carotid and subclavian arteries, the left vagus enters the thorax. It then descends across the left side of the aortic arch, giving rise to its recurrent laryngeal branch, and exits behind the left lung root to the esophagus. The two vagi combine to form the esophageal plexus, which gives rise to the anterior and posterior gastric nerves (also known as the anterior and posterior vagal trunks). These nerves contain fibers from both the sympathetic and vagal branches, and they descend to pass through the diaphragm's esophageal opening. The nerves supply the pancreas, liver, stomach, duodenum, and other viscera. They also branch out to other viscera through the celiac plexus.

3.1.4.2.1. Branches

Ascending between the trachea and esophagus into the neck, the left recurrent laryngeal nerve winds around the ligamentum arteriosum and aortic arch. It then provides cardiac branches to the cardiac plexus as well as branches to the pulmonary and esophageal plexuses.

3.1.5. The Thymus

The thymus is a bilobed mass of lymphoid tissue that extends posteriorly to the manubrium and is located in front of the trachea. It might spread to the upper thorax and lower neck. Though it is variable in size and may extend below the aortic arch to the anterior mediastinum, it is larger at birth and atrophies after puberty. Thymomas, which are tumors that grow in the thymus and may be linked to myasthenia gravis, can occasionally develop and need to be surgically removed.

3.1.6. The Esophagus

The cricoid cartilage marks the beginning of the esophagus. Its cervical segment descends through the thorax primarily to the left of the midline after lying in the midline on the prevertebral fascia. At the level of the tenth thoracic vertebra, it first curves forward in its lower part, piercing the diaphragm encircled by fibers of its right crus. Its total length is 25 cm, with its intraabdominal portion measuring approximately 2 cm (Figure 3.6).

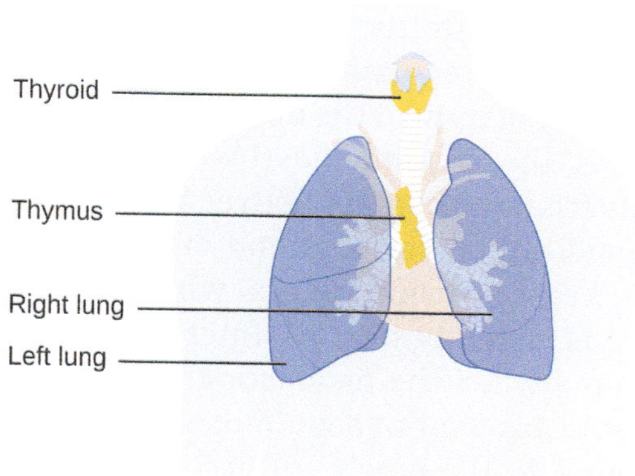

Figure 3.6. *Chest the thymus.*

Source: By Cancer Research UK – Original email from CRUK, CC BY-SA 4.0; https://commons.wikimedia.org/w/index.php?curid=34334288.

3.1.6.1. Relations

The left recurrent laryngeal nerve is located in the groove between the trachea and the vertebral column in the upper mediastinum, which is situated between the former and the latter. The azygos and hemiazygos veins, the thoracic duct, and the aorta divide it from the vertebral column below. Anteriorly, the left bronchus crosses it below the trachea, and the pericardium separates it from the left atrium below this. The aortic arch, the subclavian artery, and the descending aorta divide it from mediastinal pleura on the left, from above. The azygos vein and mediastinal pleura cover it on the right. The pleura is in contact with its lower portion.

3.1.6.2. Lymphatic Drainage

The thoracic portion empties into the tracheobronchial and posterior mediastinal nodes, the abdominal portion empties into the left gastric nodes, and the cervical esophagus empties into the deep cervical lymph nodes. To obtain a radiological examination of the esophagus, the patient is made to swallow barium. It typically exhibits mild constrictions where the left bronchus and aortic arch cross it, as well as when it goes through the diaphragm. Patients with heart failure will exhibit an enlarged left atrium that appears to be compressing their esophagus. By using endoscopy, its luminal surface can be examined more closely. It is easier to perform esophagoscopy, whether using a rigid or flexible esophagoscope, if you know that the adult esophagus originates 15 cm from the incisor teeth and that the esophagogastric junction is typically 40 cm from that point.

3.1.7. The Thoracic Trachea and Bronchi

The trachea begins in the neck just below the cricoid cartilage, running down the center and entering the superior mediastinum. At the level of the 5th thoracic vertebra, it splits into two main bronchi. In the chest, the left recurrent laryngeal nerve runs in the groove between the trachea and esophagus.

Its walls, like those of the main bronchi, are strengthened by U-shaped incomplete rings of cartilage. Anteriorly, the brachiocephalic artery and the left brachiocephalic vein cross it; on its left lie the common carotid and subclavian arteries, and below them the aortic arch; on the right, the right vagus nerve and azygos vein separate it from the pleura.

The tracheal bifurcation (carina) lies at the level of the sternal angle and the lower border of the 4th thoracic vertebra, anterior to the esophagus and to the right of the pulmonary trunk bifurcation.

3.1.7.1. The Extrapulmonary Bronchi

The bifurcation is where the left and right main bronchi originate. They then go laterally to enter the lung's hilus, where they split to form the intrapulmonary bronchial tree. With a length of 3 cm, the right bronchus is more vertical and wider than the left. Before it enters the hilus, the right upper lobe bronchus emerges.

3.1.7.1.1. Relations

The aortic arch is located above the left pulmonary artery, which divides the left atrium from the carina anteriorly. The descending thoracic aorta and the esophagus are located posteriorly. The trachea is visible on chest X-rays as a radiolucent (dark) structure that descends backward and slightly to the right in the upper mediastinum because it contains air. It could be dislodged or compressed by the thyroid gland's enlargement. Lung cancer that has spread to other areas or enlargement of the tracheobronchial lymph nodes may cause the carina to widen or distort. Inhaled foreign bodies typically travel more frequently to the right bronchus, which is wider and more vertical. Through endoscopy, the trachea and proximal bronchi can be directly viewed. A radio-opaque medium is applied, e.g., lipiodol into the bronchi allowing for the acquisition of a bronchial tree radiograph. Blood-stained sputum, bronchial blockage, ulceration, and bleeding are typical symptoms of bronchial cancer (Stauffer et al., 2023; Volpe & Makaryus, 2023).

3.2. The Pleura

The pleura is a fibroelastic serous membrane that forms a sac on either side of the chest and is lined by squamous epithelium. Each pleural sac is a sealed space that encloses a lung. The visceral (pulmonary) pleura covers the lungs, while the parietal pleura lines the chest wall. These two pleural layers can easily glide on top of each other because they are separated by a thin layer of serous fluid and are continuous around the root of the lung. The surface tension of the fluid and the negative pressure in the thoracic cavity prevent the layers from separating. Consequently, air must be inhaled, causing the lung to expand along with the thoracic cage. The lateral surface of the mediastinum, the upper surface of the diaphragm, the costal cartilages, and the ribs are all lined with parietal pleura. It forms the cervical dome of pleura above the thoracic inlet into the neck; inferiorly, it forms the costodiaphragmatic recess, a narrow gutter around the margin of the diaphragm; anteriorly, it forms the costomediastinal recess, which results from the contact between the left costal and mediastinal surfaces and extends in front of the heart. Visceral pleura, which covers the lung and extends into its interlobar fissures, is formed when the mediastinal pleura invests the main bronchi and pulmonary vessels and continues to the lung's surface.

It is important to observe the pleural sacs' surface markings. The upper limit is located approximately 3 cm above the medial third of the clavicle on both sides. From this point on, the pleural reflection lines descend behind the sternoclavicular joints and nearly meet at the level of the second costal cartilage in the midline.

The right pleural reflection continues down, close to the midline, to the sixth costal cartilage at the fourth costal cartilage, while the left pleura diverges laterally and descends along the lateral border of the sternum to the sixth costal cartilage.

The pleural reflections now travel laterally behind the costal margin on both sides, passing over the tips of the transverse processes and approximately 3 cm from the midline to reach the eighth rib in the midclavicular line, the tenth rib in the midaxillary line, and along the paravertebral line and the 12th rib.

The parietal pleura is extensively supplied by branches of the somatic intercostal and phrenic nerves, whereas the visceral pleura lacks pain fibers. The pulmonary pleura's lymph travels to the lung's superficial plexus before arriving at the hilar nodes. The diaphragmatic, posterior mediastinal, and parasternal nodes receive the parietal pleura's drainage. The pleural sac is a potential space that can fill with fluid or air under pathological conditions.

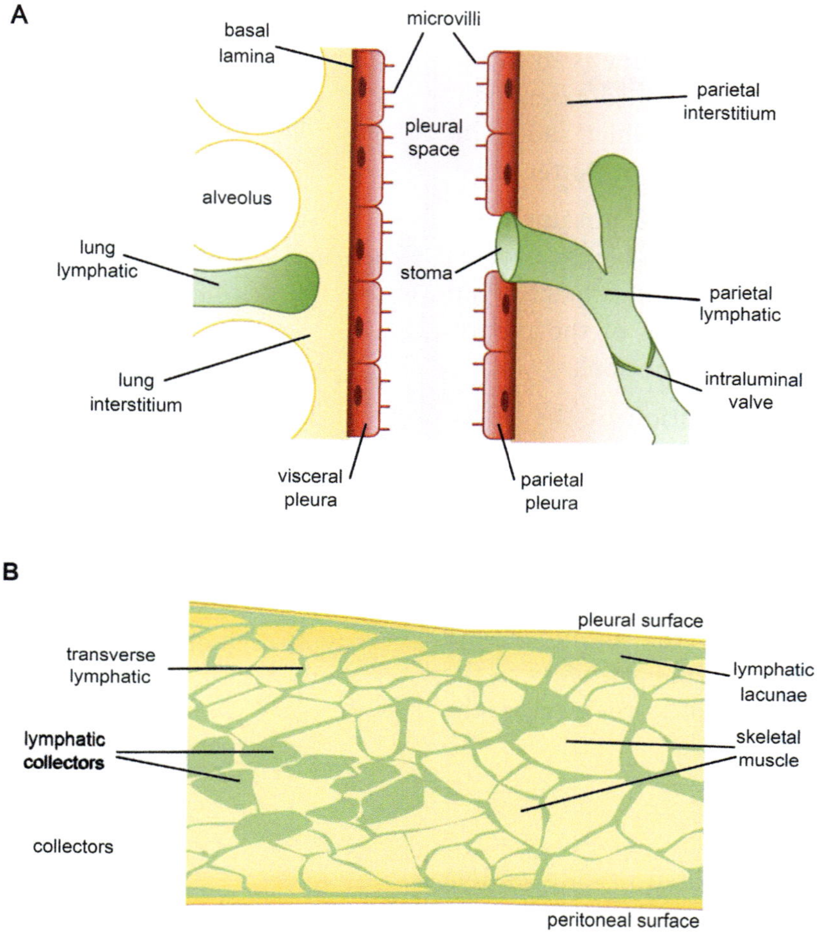

Figure 3.7. (A) Anatomical arrangement of parietal and visceral pleurae and the pleural space among them. Lymphatic stomata open directly into the pleural cavity. (B) Drawing of rat diaphragm cross section showing the reciprocal anatomical relationship among pleural and peritoneal submesothelial lymphatic lacunae, the transverse lymphatic network, and central lymphatic collectors (green). Skeletal muscle fiber bundles are shown in yellow and provide a strong extrinsic mechanical support to lymph propulsion during spontaneous breathing.

Source: Solari, E., Marcozzi, C., Ottaviani, C., Negrini, D., & Moriondo, A., (2022). Draining the pleural space: Lymphatic vessels facing the most challenging task. Biology, 11(3), 419. https://doi.org/10.3390/biology11030419.

It can fill with blood following an intrathoracic hemorrhage (hemothorax), with pus or inflammatory exudate (pleural effusion) following a pyothorax, or with air following a pneumothorax caused by a ruptured lung bulla or chest wall trauma that has torn the lung. Lung expansion may be impeded by a pleural cavity that has become enlarged. A needle or tube attached to an underwater seal can be inserted into the seventh intercostal space in the midaxillary line to drain fluid from the pleural cavity. If the needle is inserted below this point, there is a chance that it will puncture both the underlying liver or spleen and the diaphragm. It is best to place the needle along the top of the rib, avoiding the vessels that are located in the subcostal groove, to prevent damage to the neurovascular bundle. The safest method for aspirating air in an emergency is to insert a needle into the second or third intercostal space in the midclavicular line, which should be connected to an underwater seal or flutter valve.

Pleural specimens can be obtained for histological analysis using punch biopsy needles inserted through the intercostal space. Pain from pleurisy, or inflammation of the pleura, is exacerbated by breathing motions.

The cutaneous distribution of the nerve supplying the pain receives a referral from sensory fibers located within the parietal pleura. Therefore, inflammation of the diaphragmatic pleura refers to the area supplied by the nerve root (C4) from which the phrenic nerve originates, i.e., the tip of the shoulder, and inflammation of the costal pleura refers to the chest wall or, in the case of lower nerves, the upper abdominal wall.

3.3. The Lungs

These two organs are situated in independent pleural sacs that are joined to the mediastinum at the hila. Their composition is elastic and sponge-like, allowing them to mold to the curves of the thoracic cavity. About 620 g makes up the right lung and 560 g makes up the left. Radiating shadows from blood vessels and denser shadows at the hilus, caused by hilar lymph nodes, give them a characteristic mottled appearance on radiographs where lung tissue is clear. The outline of the heart, the inferior vena cava, and the normal aortic arch (knuckle) can all be seen on a PA chest X-ray. Details of the mediastinal structures can be seen in a lateral view (Figures 3.8 and 3.9).

The base of each lung rests on the diaphragm, and the apex is located in the root of the neck. The base is divided from the lateral convex costal surface and the medial concave mediastinal surface by a sharp inferior border. The lung root structures are situated in the center of the base, encircled by a cuff of pleura.

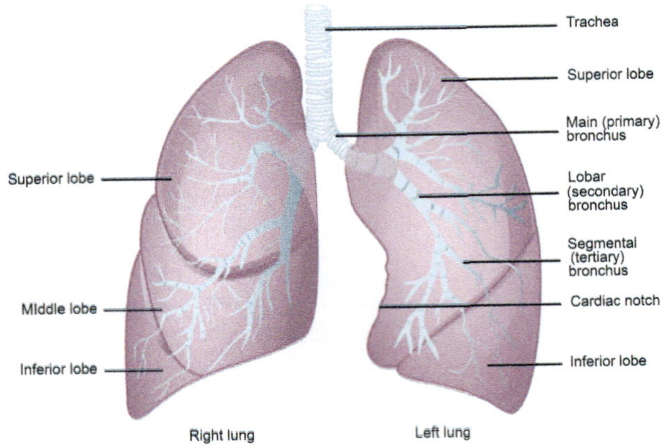

Figure 3.8. *The lungs.*

Source: https://courses.lumenlearning.com/suny-ap2/chapter/the-lungs/.

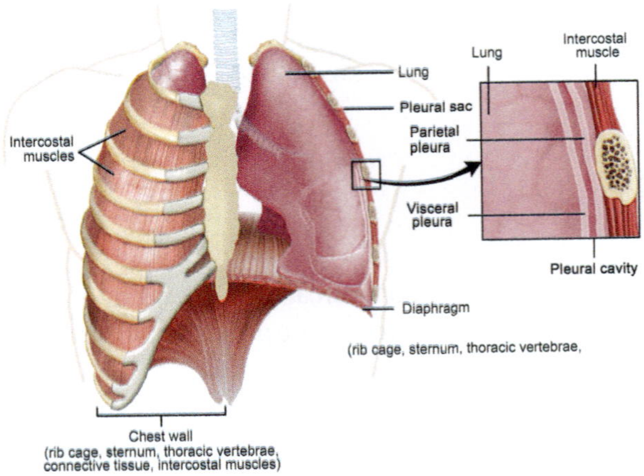

Figure 3.9. *The pleura.*

Source: https://courses.lumenlearning.com/suny-ap2/chapter/the-lungs/.

The left ventricle of the heart is accommodated by the deeper concavity of the left lung. The rounded posterior border of each lung is located in the paravertebral sulcus, while the left lung's anterior border is deeply indented by the heart to form the cardiac notch.

Each lung has fissures that go deep into the

tissue that divides it. The left lung is divided into an upper and lower lobe by an oblique fissure, and the right lung is divided into an upper, middle, and lower lobe by an oblique and horizontal fissure. A line drawn around the chest wall from the third thoracic vertebra's spine to the sixth costochondral junction can be used to identify each side's oblique fissure. A horizontal line that connects the fourth right costal cartilage to the previously drawn oblique line indicates the horizontal fissure. The majority of the posterior and inferior borders are made up of the lower lobes of both lungs, which are located below and behind the oblique fissure. The apex and the majority of the mediastinal and costal surfaces are located in the upper lobe of the left lung, which is situated above and anterior to the oblique fissure. The horizontal fissure splits the corresponding portion of the right lung into a large upper lobe and a smaller anterior wedge-shaped middle lobe that is located deep to the right breast. The lingula, the left-sided counterpart of the middle lobe, is a slender anteroinferior section of the left upper lobe located next to the cardiac notch. There are sometimes extra lobes present, and fissures can be partial or nonexistent (Stauffer et al., 2023; Volpe & Makaryus, 2023).

The pleural cuff encloses the pulmonary artery, pulmonary veins, pulmonary nerve plexus, lymph nodes, and main bronchus in the hilum, or root, of each lung. The pulmonary ligament is an inferior, narrow extension of the cuff. The two veins are anterior and below the bronchus, which is located behind the pulmonary artery.

3.3.1. The Intrapulmonary Bronchi and Bronchopulmonary Segments

Aspiration of foreign bodies is more common on the right side due to the right side's hilum being shorter, wider, and more vertical than the left. Each main bronchus descends to enter the lung. Every main bronchus splits into lobar bronchi, which split into segmental bronchi, each of which supplies a segment of the bronchopulmonary system. There are 10 such segments in each lung. Before the hilum, the right upper lobe bronchus splits into the apical, anterior, and posterior segmental bronchi after leaving the lung substance. It originates from the right main bronchus.

Beyond this, the medial and lateral segmental bronchi split off from the middle lobe bronchus. After reaching the lower lobe, the right main bronchus continues and splits into the apical, anterior, medial, lateral, and posterior basal segmental bronchi. The anterior and inferior segmental bronchi of the left upper lobe bronchus pass to the lingula. The bronchus splits into five segments after emerging from the lung's main bronchus. The left bronchus continues to the lower lobe, where it splits into five segmental bronchi just like the right side does. Every segmental bronchus is separated into bronchopulmonary segments, which are functionally separate units of lung tissue with their own vascular supply. Along with pseudostratified columnar epithelium and mucous glands, the walls of the bronchi are lined with smooth muscle and hyaline cartilage. The nonciliated columnar epithelium lining their slender terminal branches, the bronchioles, is devoid of cartilage.

Aspiration is particularly dangerous in comatose or anesthetized patients, since the most vulnerable area of the lung is the posterior part. The highest and most posterior segmental bronchi supply the apical segment of the lower lobe; consequently, aspiration pneumonia most frequently occurs in this segment (especially the right).

3.3.1.1. Relations

With the exception of inferiorly, where the lower lung border (costodiaphragmatic recess) lies approximately two intercostal spaces above the pleural reflection, and anteriorly, where the anterior border of the left lung lies approximately three centimeters lateral to the pleural reflection (costomediastinal recess), the lung borders closely follow the lines of pleural reflection on the chest wall. The diaphragm divides the base from the liver, stomach, and spleen on the left, and the right lobe of the liver on the right. The costal surfaces are connected to the thoracic wall. The suprapleural membrane, a fibrous sheet that runs from the transverse process of the seventh cervical vertebra to the inner border of the first rib, covers the apex of the pleura, which is covered by the dome of the pleura. The membrane is covered by the subclavian vessels arch. The sympathetic trunk and the anterior primary ramus of the first thoracic nerve, which travel to the brachial plexus, are located posteriorly on the first rib's neck.

On each side, the medial relations are different. A large concavity for the left ventricle and a groove for the aortic arch, which passes in front of the hilum, are located on the left. The lung is in contact with the left subclavian artery, left common carotid artery, left brachiocephalic vein, and the esophagus above the arch, going from anterior to posterior. The inferior vena cava has a shorter groove below, and the superior vena cava has a continuous groove above the shallow concavity for the right atrium that is located in front of the hilum. The azygos vein curves forward above the hilum, grooving the lung. With the exception of the location where the azygos vein divides it from the lung, the esophagus and the posterior border are in contact along its whole length. The esophagus is situated between the trachea and the superior vena cava.

3.3.1.2. Blood Supply

The bronchial arteries, which are branches of the descending aorta, supply blood to the lung tissue. Part of this blood is returned to the heart through the pulmonary veins. The azygos or hemiazygos veins drain other bronchial veins. The pulmonary artery's branches follow the bronchial tree, delivering low-oxygen blood to the alveoli. The upper and lower pulmonary veins are formed by veins that emerge from the alveolar capillary network and follow the bronchi. A pulmonary embolism could be lethal. It is brought on by big blood clots (thrombi) that start in the pelvic or leg deep veins, get dislodged, and travel through the heart's right ventricle to lodge in and block the pulmonary trunk or, worse, the large or segmental pulmonary arteries. As a result, a portion or lobe of the lung that is ventilated but no longer receives blood perfusion has a partial or total blockage of its arterial supply. Acute respiratory distress and cyanosis occur if the embolus obstructs the main pulmonary artery, and death frequently occurs within a few minutes. Segmental emboli result in pulmonary infarcts, which, if they are small, heal in a few weeks and kill lung tissue.

3.3.2. Lymphatic Drainage

This is caused by a deep plexus of vessels that accompany the bronchi, as well as a superficial subpleural lymph plexus. The tracheobronchial nodes surrounding the tracheal bifurcation (carina) receive drainage from both groups' hilar (bronchopulmonary) nodes, which in turn drain to the mediastinal lymph trunks.

3.3.3. Nerve Supply

Parasympathetic (bronchoconstrictor) fibers from the vagus nerve and sympathetic (bronchodilator) fibers from the upper thoracic segments supply the lungs. The latter supply the cough reflex's afferent fibers, which are crucial for expelling mucus and other inhaled particles. Both use the pulmonary plexuses to supply the lungs. Chest radiographs can identify abnormal collections of air or fluid in the pleural space and provide precise localization of lung disease. The definition of pulmonary lesions can be enhanced by CT and MRI scans, which can also be used to direct tiny biopsy needles inserted percutaneously toward suspicious lesions. The bronchial tree can be drawn out using radio-opaque contrast material, and radioisotopes help determine how well the lung tissue is ventilated and perfused. Understanding the bronchopulmonary segments' architecture directly aids in the excision of pulmonary segments for localized disease. This information is also applied to the efficient drainage of infected lung segments through physical therapy.

3.4. Lymphatic Drainage of the Thorax

The lymph vessels of the thoracic viscera and those draining the chest wall are the two groups of lymph vessels in the thorax. Both shallow and deep systems drain the chest wall. Similar to the breast vessels, the superficial vessels empty into the pectoral and central groups of axillary lymph nodes. There is some communication between the opposing side's vessels.

The vessels draining the deeper chest wall drain to the:

- Parasternal nodes alongside the internal thoracic artery, whose efferents drain to the broncho mediastinal lymph trunk.
- Intercostal nodes lying at the back of the intercostal spaces, whose efferents drain to the right lymph duct and the thoracic duct.
- Diaphragmatic nodes on the upper surface of the diaphragm, whose efferents drain to parasternal and posterior mediastinal nodes and, through the diaphragm, to communicate with those draining the upper surface of the liver.

The thoracic viscera drain to the:

- The anterior mediastinal nodes are located in front of the brachiocephalic veins and are responsible for draining the anterior mediastinum. They connect to the tracheobronchial nodes through their efferent vessels.
- The trachea and main bronchi, which drain the heart, lungs, and trachea, are accompanied by tracheobronchial nodes. Their efferents combine with the anterior mediastinal nodes' efferents to form the broncho mediastinal trunk, which joins the thoracic duct on the left and the right lymph duct on the right.
- Posterior mediastinal nodes, alongside the esophagus. Their efferents pass into the thoracic duct.

The thoracic duct and the smaller right lymph duct return lymph to the bloodstream. The thoracic duct, which is roughly 45 cm long, originates in the abdomen as the cisterna chyli continues and enters the thorax through the diaphragm's aortic opening to the right of the aorta. Alongside the azygos vein, it ascends behind and to the right of the esophagus before turning left and passing in front of the fifth thoracic vertebra. It curves laterally behind the carotid sheath at the level of the seventh cervical vertebra, then forward to enter the left brachiocephalic vein's origin. Through its junction with the left jugular and subclavian lymph trunks, as well as the left broncho mediastinal lymph trunk, it transports lymph from the left half of the thorax and below the diaphragm, as well as from the head and neck.

The union of the right jugular, subclavian, and broncho mediastinal lymph trunks forms the right lymph duct, a brief vessel located in the neck. Transporting lymph from the right side of the head, neck, and thorax, it enters the right brachiocephalic vein's origin. The abnormal accumulation of lymph in the pleural cavity is called a chylothorax. The most common cause of this is surgical damage, which can arise from extensive surgery in the posterior mediastinum, a left-sided subclavian venous puncture, or surgery at the root of the neck. Less frequently, a filarial parasite infection or malignant infiltration can obstruct the thoracic duct, resulting in a chylothorax (Table 3.2).

Table 3.2. *Classification of Interstitial Lung Diseases (ILDs) Used in the Child-EU Register*

Category	Specifier	Subcategories (Major Examples)	
Lung only (native parenchymal) disorders.	Developmental	• Diffuse (A1) • Alveolar capillary dysplasia, misalign pulmonary veins (ACDMPV) • Congenital alveolar dysplasia (CAD)	• Alveolarization (A2) • Pulmonary hypoplasia • Pulmonary hypoplasia associated with diaphragmatic hernia • Chronic lung disease of prematurity (BPD-cLD)
–	–	• Infant tachypnea (A3) • Chronic tachypnea of infancy (CTI) (usual, aberrant) • Neuroendocrine cell hyperplasia of infancy (NEHI) • Pulmonary interstitial glycogenosis (PIG)	• Surfactant region (A4) • Chronic pneumonitis of infancy (CPI) • Surfactant protein B deficiency • Other surfactant dysfunction disorders • Undefined ILD in mature neonate • Undefined ILD in almost (gest. age 30–36 weeks) mature neonate
–	All ages	• ABCA3 deficiency • Surfactant protein C deficiency • Lipoid pneumonitis, cholesterol pneumonia • Nonspecific interstitial pneumonia (NSIP) • Idiopathic pulmonary fibrosis (IPF)/Usual interstitial pneumonitis (UIP) • Cryptogenic organizing pneumonia (COP)	• Acute interstitial pneumonia (AIP) • Desquamative interstitial pneumonia (DIP) • Idiopathic pleuro-parenchymal fibroelastosis • Eosinophilic pneumonitis • Undefined ILD in NON-neonate • Unclassifiable idiopathic interstitial pneumonias

Systemic disease related disorders	Immuno competent	• Collagen vascular/ connective tissue related disorders (CTD-ILD) • Eosinophilic granulomatosis with polyangiitis (EGPA, Churg Strauss) • Granulomatosis with polyangiitis (GPA, Wegener) • Metabolic disorders • Disorders related to chromosomal abnormalities • Aminoacyl-tRNA synthetase (-ARS) deficiency • Birt-Hogg-Dube syndrome • Granulomatous diseases	• Diffuse alveolar hemorrhage due to vasculitic disorders • ITGA3 (Integrin α3) mutations with kidney, lung, skin disease • Niemann-Pick disease • Nkx2.1 gene defect (brain-thyroid-lung syndrome) • Lysin uric proteinuria • PAP secondary to associated diseases • Sarcoidosis • TBX4 mutation (small patella syndrome) • Hoyeral Hreidasson Syndrome (congenital dyskeratosis) • Telomere-related-diseases
–	Immuno deficient	• Phagocyte-PAP.CSF2RA or CSF2RB (PAP due to GMCSF receptor deficiency)	• Phagocyte-GATA2 def (MonoMac syndrome). GATA2
–	Transplanted	• Chronic allograft dysfunction, idiopathic pneumonia syndrome	–
–	Immune-dysregulated	• Autoimmune pulmonary alveolar proteinosis (PAP) • Antisynthetase syndrome • Celiac disease/ pulmonary hemorrhage (Lane-Hamilton) • Anti-basement membrane antibody disease (Goodpasture) • Granulomatous lymphocytic interstitial lung disease (GLILD)	• Follicular bronchitis/ bronchiolitis • Lymphocytic interstitial pneumonia (LIP) • Interstitial pneumonia with auto-immune features (IPAF) • ZNFX1 deficiency • Immune-dysregulated Hermansky Pudlak syndrome

–	Auto-inflammatory	• COPA defect • STING-associated vasculopathy, infantile-onset. TMEM173	• OAS1 deficiency • Other interferonopathies
Exposure related disorders	Non-infectious	• Exogen allergic alveolitis/hypersensitivity pneumonitis • Drug induced ILD • Pneumoconiosis	• Radiation lung injury • Respiratory bronchiolitis-interstitial lung disease (RB-ILD) • Occupational lung diseases
–	Infectious	• Infectious/post-infectious bronchiolitis obliterans (PIBO) • Diffuse pan bronchiolitis	• Mac-Leod-Swyer-James-Syndrome
Vascular disorders	–	• Diffuse pulmonary (alveolar) hemorrhage (DPH) • Idiopathic pulmonary hemorrhage (hemosiderosis) (IPH) with or without associated features • Pulmonary capillaritis	• Pulmonary capillary hemangiomatosis (PCH) • Pulmonary vena-occlusive disease • Lymphangiomatosis

Source: Griese, M., (2022). Etiologic classification of diffuse parenchymal (interstitial) lung diseases. Journal of Clinical Medicine, 11(6), 1747. https://doi.org/10.3390/jcm11061747.

3.5. Autonomic Nervous System

The cardiac, pulmonary, and esophageal plexuses—all of which receive contributions from the sympathetic and parasympathetic nervous systems—provide the autonomic nerve supply to the thoracic viscera. Part of the ligamentum arteriosum and the tracheal bifurcation support the cardiac plexus. Together, the components function as a single, cohesive whole. They receive parasympathetic branches from both vagi as well as branches from the cervical and upper thoracic sympathetic ganglia. The coronary arteries connect the plexus's branches to the heart's conducting system. The pulmonary plexus receives branches from the cardiac plexus as well. Each lung has a pulmonary plexus surrounding its root, which supplies the lung substance and has branches from both vagi and the upper four cervical ganglia.

The lower esophagus is surrounded by a network called the esophageal plexus. It receives branches from both vagi and the upper cervical ganglia. It provides nourishment to the esophagus, and upon crossing the lower esophagus, the left and right vagal trunks arise and descend alongside the esophagus, emerging as the anterior and posterior gastric nerves, respectively, into the abdomen. Behind the parietal pleura, each thoracic sympathetic trunk is positioned beside the spinal column. It is continuous with the lumbar sympathetic trunk below and the cervical trunk above. It typically has 12 ganglia, each of which is supplied by a thoracic nerve. However, on the neck of the first rib, half of the first thoracic ganglion is fused to the 7th cervical to form a larger stellate ganglion. Every ganglion receives preganglionic fibers from its matching spinal nerve in the form of a white ramus communicantes, and it returns postganglionic fibers in the form of a gray ramus communicantes to that nerve.

The upper limb is subjected to sympathetic denervation (sympathectomy) in order to dilate cutaneous blood vessels or prevent sweating. The procedure involves the surgical excision of the second and third thoracic ganglia. In order to maintain sympathetic innervation to the head and neck and stop Horner's syndrome from developing, the first ganglion is left intact.

Unilateral ptosis, flushed and dry skin on the same side of the face, enophthalmos, and a small pupil (meiosis) are the characteristics of the syndrome. The upper cervical trunk is damaged, which results in the syndrome. Stellate ganglion blocks or surgical excision are two possible causes, but the most common cause is cancerous infiltration from the lung's apex (Stauffer et al., 2023; Volpe & Makaryus, 2023).

The sympathetic trunk supplies:

- Rami communicantes to each of its spinal nerves;
- Branches to the cardiac, pulmonary, and esophageal plexuses from the upper four ganglia;
- Branches to form the greater, lesser and least splanchnic nerves. These descend medial to the sympathetic chain and enter the abdomen by piercing the diaphragmatic crura. They contribute branches to the coeliac and other preaortic ganglia.

A Closer Look

Pleural Fluid Testing

Pleural fluid testing is a critical diagnostic tool used to evaluate the pleural space, the cavity between the lungs and the chest wall. This fluid can accumulate due to various pathological conditions, and analyzing its properties helps in diagnosing the underlying cause. The procedure typically involves thoracentesis, where a needle is inserted into the pleural space to withdraw fluid for analysis. Key tests include gross examination, biochemical analysis, cytology, microbiological cultures, and specific disease markers (Table 3.3).

Table 3.3. *Clinical and Biological PROMISE Scores*

Variable Clinical PROMISE Score		Points Biological PROMISE Score	
Previous chemotherapy	No	0	0
	Yes	4	3
Previous radiotherapy	No	0	0
	Yes	2	2
Hemoglobin (g/dL)	≥16	0	0
	14 to <16	1	1
	12 to <14	2	2
	10 to <12	3	3
	<10	4	4
Serum white blood cell count (10^9 cells/L)	<4	0	0
	4 to <6.3	2	2
	6.3 to <10	4	4
	10 to <15.8	7	7
	≥15.8	10	9
C-reactive protein (IU/L)	<3	0	0
	3 to <10	3	3
	10 to <32	5	5
	32 to <100	8	8
	≥100	11	10

ECOG performance status	0–1	0	0
	2–4	7	7
Cancer type	Mesothelioma	0	0
	All other types of cancer	4	5
	Lung	5	6
TIMP1 (ng/mg protein)	<40	n/a	0
	40 to <160	n/a	1
	≥160	n/a	2
Total score and corresponding 3-month mortality			
Group (3-month mortality)		Clinical score	Biological score
A: <25%		0–20	0–20
B: 25% to <50%		21–27	21–28
C: 50% to <75%		28–35	29–37
D: ≥75%		>35	>37

Source: Jacobs, B., Sheikh, G., Youness, H. A., Keddissi, J. I., & Abdo, T., (2022). Diagnosis and management of malignant pleural effusion: A decade in review. Diagnostics, 12(4), 1016. https://doi.org/10.3390/diagnostics12041016. Adapted from: Psallidas et al. [Psallidas I.,et al. 2018].

The gross examination involves assessing the color, clarity, and odor of the fluid. Normal pleural fluid is clear and pale yellow, while variations can indicate different pathologies. For example, bloody fluid might suggest trauma, malignancy, or pulmonary embolism, whereas milky fluid could indicate chylothorax, often due to lymphatic system disruption. Turbidity can signal the presence of cells, protein, or infection.

Biochemical tests are essential in distinguishing between transudates and exudates, classifications that provide clues to the underlying cause. Transudates are typically due to systemic factors like heart failure or cirrhosis, leading to fluid leakage, while exudates result from local factors such as infection, malignancy, or inflammatory conditions causing increased capillary permeability. Key measurements include protein levels, lactate dehydrogenase (LDH), glucose, pH, and amylase. The Light criteria, which compare protein and LDH levels in pleural fluid to serum, help differentiate transudates from exudates: pleural fluid is considered an exudate if the protein level is greater than 0.5 times that of serum or the LDH level is more than 0.6 times that of serum.

Cytological analysis involves examining the fluid for malignant cells, which can indicate cancers like lung, breast, or lymphoma that have metastasized to the pleura. The presence of abnormal cells guides oncologists in staging the disease and planning treatment. Additionally, the differential cell count can help identify the nature of pleural effusions; for instance, a predominance of neutrophils suggests bacterial infection, while lymphocytosis might point to tuberculosis or malignancy.

Microbiological cultures are crucial in diagnosing infectious causes of pleural effusion. Samples are cultured to detect bacterial, fungal, or mycobacterial organisms. This step is vital in cases of suspected empyema, a collection of pus in the pleural space, where prompt identification and treatment of the causative pathogen are essential. Specific disease markers and additional tests might be employed based on the clinical suspicion.

Table 3.4. *Overview of the Most Common Malignant Diseases Associated with Malignant Pleural Effusion (MPE)*

Malignancy	General Median Survival in Days (95% CI)	Histologic Subtype	Prevalence (%)
Lung cancer	74 (60 to 92)	–	–
	–	Lung adenocarcinoma	29–37
	–	Small cell carcinoma of the lung	6–9
Breast cancer	192 (133 to 271)	–	–
	–	Breast adenocarcinoma	8–40
Gynecological malignancy	230 (97 to 279)	–	–
		Ovarian adenocarcinoma	18–20
Gastrointestinal cancer	61 (44 to 73)	–	–
	–	Gastric adenocarcinoma	2
	–	Colorectal	1
	–	Renal cell carcinoma	1
	–	Pancreatic adenocarcinoma	3
Hematological malignancy	218 (160 to 484)	–	–
	–	Lymphoma	3–16
Skin cancer	43 (23 to 72)	–	–
	–	Melanoma	5–6
Mesothelioma	339 (267 to 422)	–	–
		Malignant mesothelioma	1–6
Sarcoma	44 (19 to 76)	Sarcoma	1–3

Source: Skok, K., Hladnik, G., Grm, A., & Crnjac, A., (2019). Malignant pleural effusion and its current management: A review. Medicina, 55(8), 490. https://doi.org/10.3390/medicina55080490.

For example, adenosine deaminase (ADA) levels are measured in suspected tuberculosis cases, while rheumatoid factor and antinuclear antibody tests can be used for rheumatologic diseases. Tumor markers like carcinoembryonic antigen (CEA) and CA 15–3 might be tested when malignancy is suspected (Table 3.4).

Pleural fluid testing, therefore, provides a comprehensive diagnostic approach, integrating multiple analyses to pinpoint the cause of pleural effusions. It is a pivotal component of patient evaluation, offering insights that guide treatment decisions and improve patient outcomes. The interplay of biochemical, cytological, and microbiological data helps clinicians navigate complex cases, ensuring that underlying conditions are accurately identified and appropriately managed (Table 3.5).

Table 3.5. *Summary of Current Recommendations ATS/STS/STR to Treat Patients with MPE*

SL. No.	PICO	Recommendations
1.	In patients with known or suspected MPE, should thoracic US be used to guide pleural interventions?	Yes.
2.	In patients with known or suspected MPE who are asymptomatic, should pleural drainage be performed?	Pleural drainage is not recommended to be performed in this type of patients.
3.	Should the management of patients with symptomatic known or suspected MPE be guided by large-volume thoracentesis and pleural manometry?	Yes, large-volume thoracentesis is recommended, as the contribution of thoracentesis prevails over potential complications.
4.	In patients with symptomatic MPE with known or suspected expandable lung and no prior definitive therapy, should IPCs or chemical pleurodesis be used as a first-line definitive pleural intervention for management of dyspnea?	Yes, IPC or chemical pleurodesis are used as a first-line definitive pleural intervention for the management of dyspnea.
5.	In patients with symptomatic MPE undergoing talc pleurodesis, should talc poudrage or talc slurry be used?	Yes, there was no evidence of differences in efficacy between them.
6.	In patients with symptomatic MPE with non-expandable lung, failed pleurodesis, or loculated effusion, should an IPC or chemical pleurodesis be used?	The method of choice is the use of IPC as it is associated with a shorter hospitalization period.
7.	In patients with IPC-associated infection (cellulitis, tunnel infection, or pleural infection), should medical therapy alone or medical therapy and catheter removal be used?	Firstly, causative treatment without removing IPC. In case there is no improvement (e.g., persistent infection), the removal of IPC is recommended.

Note: Summarized after Feller-Kopman et al. [Sterman D.H., et al. 2018].

Abbreviations: US: Ultrasound; IPC: indwelling pleural catheter; P: patient, problem or population; I: intervention; C: comparison, control, or comparator; and O: outcome.

Source: *Skok, K., Hladnik, G., Grm, A., & Crnjac, A., (2019). Malignant pleural effusion and its current management: A review. Medicina, 55(8), 490. https://doi.org/10.3390/medicina55080490.*

Summary

- The pleurae are serous membranes that envelop the lungs and line the thoracic cavity, forming the pleural cavities. These membranes consist of two layers: the visceral pleura, which is adherent to the lung surface, and the parietal pleura, which lines the thoracic wall, diaphragm, and mediastinum.
- The ascending aorta is enclosed in a sheath of serous pericardium common to it and the pulmonary trunk within the fibrous pericardium. Its lower part lies behind the infundibulum of the right ventricle and the origin of the pulmonary trunk, and above this the sternum is anterior.
- The right pulmonary artery passes to the right lung hilus behind the ascending aorta and superior vena cava, and in front of the esophagus and right main bronchus. The left pulmonary artery passes in front of the left bronchus and descends to the aorta to its lung hilus.
- The pulmonary veins are paired short, wide vessels lying in the hilus of each lung, anterior and inferior to the artery.
- The azygos vein is formed in the abdomen in front of the 2nd lumbar vertebra and passes into the chest via the aortic opening in the diaphragm, lying to the right of the aorta.
- The right vagus enters the thorax posterolateral to the right brachiocephalic artery and descends lateral to the trachea under the mediastinal pleura to the back of the right main bronchus, where it gives branches, first to the pulmonary plexus and then to the esophageal plexus.
- The cervical esophagus drains to the deep cervical lymph nodes, the thoracic portion drains to the tracheobronchial and posterior mediastinal nodes, and its abdominal portion to the left gastric nodes.
- The right and left main bronchi arise at the bifurcation and descend laterally to enter the hilus of the lung, where they divide to form the intrapulmonary bronchial tree.
- The pleura is a fibroelastic serous membrane lined by squamous epithelium forming a sac on each side of the chest. Each pleural sac is a closed cavity invaginated by a lung. Parietal pleura lines the chest wall and visceral (pulmonary) pleura covers the lungs (Stauffer et al., 2023; Volpe & Makaryus, 2023).

References

1. Adeyinka, A., & Pierre, L. (2023). Air leak. In *StatPearls*. StatPearls Publishing.
2. Cho, T. H., Kim, S. H., O, J., Kwon, H. J., Kim, K. W., & Yang, H. M. (2021). Anatomy of the thoracic paravertebral space: 3D micro-CT findings and their clinical implications for nerve blockade. *Regional Anesthesia and Pain Medicine, 46*(8), 699–703. https://doi.org/10.1136/rapm-2021-102676.
3. Ferreiro, L., Toubes, M. E., San José, M. E., Suárez-Antelo, J., Golpe, A., & Valdés, L. (2020). Advances in pleural effusion diagnostics. *Expert Review of Respiratory Medicine, 14*(1), 51–66. https://doi.org/10.1080/17476348.2020.1685392.

4. Ghigna, M. R., & Thomas de Montpreville, V. (2021). Mediastinal tumours and pseudo-tumours: A comprehensive review with emphasis on multidisciplinary approach. *European Respiratory Review, 30*(162), 200309. https://doi.org/10.1183/16000617.0309-2020.

5. Gilday, C., Odunayo, A., & Hespel, A. M. (2021). Spontaneous pneumothorax: Pathophysiology, clinical presentation and diagnosis. *Topics in Companion Animal Medicine, 45*, 100563. https://doi.org/10.1016/j.tcam.2021.100563.

6. Hu, K., Chopra, A., Kurman, J., & Huggins, J. T. (2021). Management of complex pleural disease in the critically ill patient. *Journal of Thoracic Disease, 13*(8), 5205–5222. https://doi.org/10.21037/jtd-20-2921.

7. Isaka, T., Mitsuboshi, S., Maeda, H., Kikkawa, T., Oyama, K., Murasugi, M., Kanzaki, M., & Onuki, T. (2020). Anatomical analysis of the left upper lobe of lung on three-dimensional images with focusing the branching pattern of the subsegmental veins. *Journal of Cardiothoracic Surgery, 15*(1), 273. https://doi.org/10.1186/s13019-020-01310-4.

8. Stauffer, C. M., Meshida, K., Bernor, R. L., Granite, G. E., & Boaz, N. T. (2023). Anatomy, thorax, pericardiacophrenic vessels. In *StatPearls*. StatPearls Publishing.

9. Tran, J., Haussner, W., & Shah, K. (2021). Traumatic pneumothorax: A review of current diagnostic practices and evolving management. *Journal of Emergency Medicine, 61*(5), 517–528. https://doi.org/10.1016/j.jemermed.2021.07.029.

10. Volpe, J. K., & Makaryus, A. N. (2023). Anatomy, thorax, heart and pericardial cavity. In *StatPearls*. StatPearls Publishing.

Chapter 4

THE ABDOMEN

Contents

Introduction

The abdomen is a vital region of the human body where essential organs and structures are located for digestion, metabolism, and various bodily functions. In clinical terms, the abdomen is divided into quadrants or regions to assist in diagnosing and treating medical conditions. The four quadrants – right upper, right lower, left upper, and left lower – are determined by lines intersecting at the umbilicus. Alternatively, nine regions can be identified using specific planes. The abdominal cavity is surrounded by the diaphragm above and the pelvic inlet below and is enclosed by muscular and fascial layers known as the abdominal wall. This cavity houses important organs such as the stomach, liver, gallbladder, pancreas, spleen, intestines, kidneys, and adrenal glands, each of which serves a critical function in maintaining the body's balance. The peritoneum, a serous membrane, lines the abdominal cavity and covers most of the abdominal organs, creating the peritoneal cavity. This cavity is divided into the greater and lesser sacs, with distinct roles in reducing friction, supporting organs, and facilitating the passage of blood vessels, lymphatics, and nerves.

Understanding the anatomy of the abdomen is crucial for clinical practice, particularly in diagnosing abdominal pain, masses, and organ dysfunction. Common clinical conditions include appendicitis, cholecystitis, pancreatitis, and various forms of hernias. Advanced imaging techniques like ultrasound, CT scans, and MRI play an essential role in abdominal diagnostics, allowing detailed visualization of organ structure and pathology.

Surgical interventions, such as laparotomies and laparoscopic surgeries, rely heavily on precise anatomical knowledge to avoid complications and ensure effective treatment. Furthermore, understanding referred pain patterns from abdominal organs aids in the comprehensive assessment of patients presenting with abdominal symptoms.

The abdomen's complex anatomy and the critical functions of its organs make it a focal point in clinical medicine. Mastery of abdominal anatomy is essential for healthcare professionals to accurately diagnose, treat, and manage a wide array of medical conditions.

Orientation and Directional Terms

Term	Definition	Illustration
Abdomen	The abdomen is the frontal body cavity between the chest and pelvis that holds vital organs like the stomach, kidneys, bladder, liver, and intestines. Informally called the belly or stomach region, the abdomen is made up of protective tissues, membranes, and muscles.	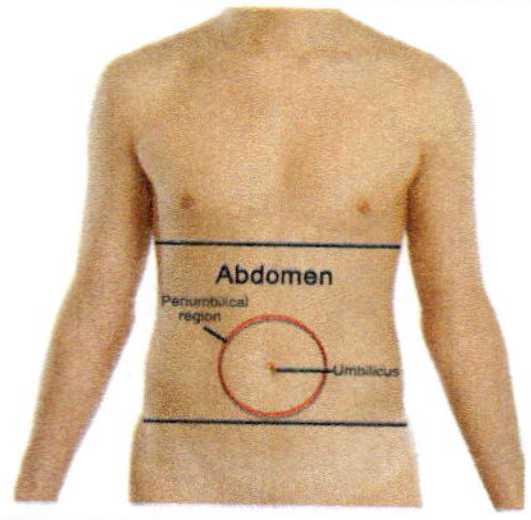
Digestive system	Digestive system includes the mouth, pharynx (throat), esophagus, stomach, small intestine, large intestine, rectum, and anus. It also includes the salivary glands, liver, gallbladder, and pancreas, which make digestive juices and enzymes that help the body digest food and liquids.	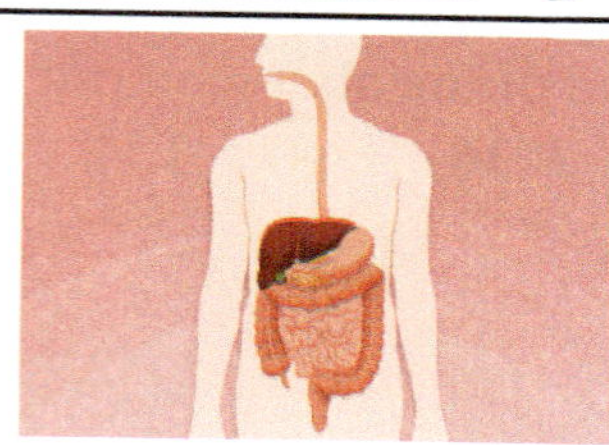
Peritoneum	Peritoneum is a membrane, a sheet of smooth tissue that lines your abdominopelvic cavity and surrounds your abdominal organs. It pads and insulates your organs, helps hold them in place and secretes a lubricating fluid to reduce friction when they rub against each other.	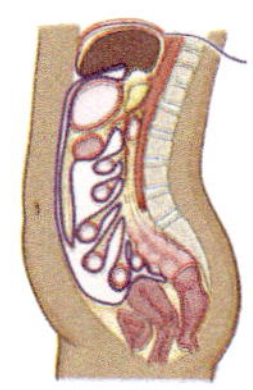
Pseudomyxoma peritonei (PMP)	Pseudomyxoma peritonei (PMP) is a rare tumour that grows slowly and causes a build-up of mucin (a jelly-like substance) in the abdomen and pelvis, giving rise to the name "jelly belly". PMP often starts in the appendix but can also start in other organs such as the large bowel and ovary.	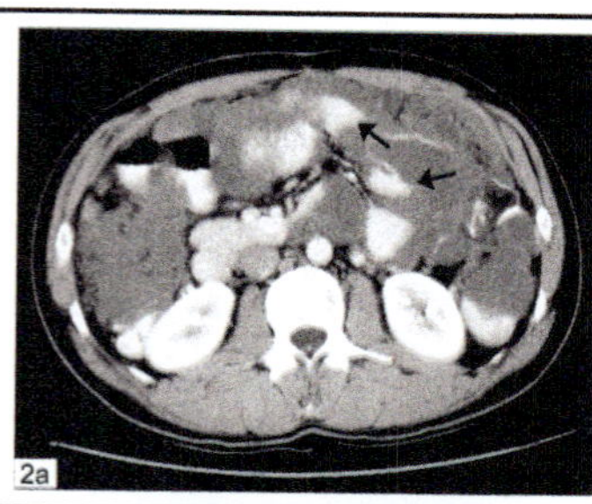
Kocher incision	The Kocher incision is a subcostal incision on the right side of the abdomen used for open exposure of the gallbladder and biliary tree. This incision is just inferior and parallel to the subcostal margin. Unlike the midline incision, it is not an avascular plane.	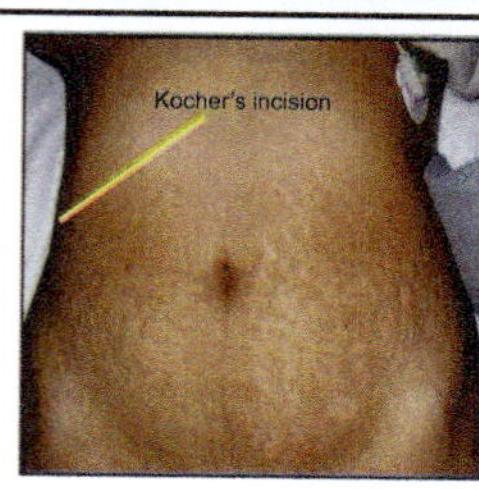

4.1. An Overview of the Abdomen

The stomach, kidneys, bladder, liver, and intestines are among the essential organs housed in the abdomen, which is the frontal body cavity situated between the chest and pelvis. The abdomen, also referred to colloquially as the "belly" or "stomach region," is composed of muscles, membranes, and protective tissues. Your body couldn't sustain and safeguard the organs required for bowel movements, urination, and digestion without the abdomen (Wade et al., 2023).

Since the abdomen is home to a variety of organs, illnesses affecting these organs frequently result in abdominal pain. Almost everyone has stomach pain occasionally from gas, constipation, or stomach viruses. On the other hand, pancreatitis, appendicitis, and kidney stones are among the medical disorders that can be indicated by abdominal pain (Patterson et al., 2023). The tissues and fluid of the abdomen can also be directly impacted by cancer and other abdominal conditions (Mehta, 2016) (Figure 4.1).

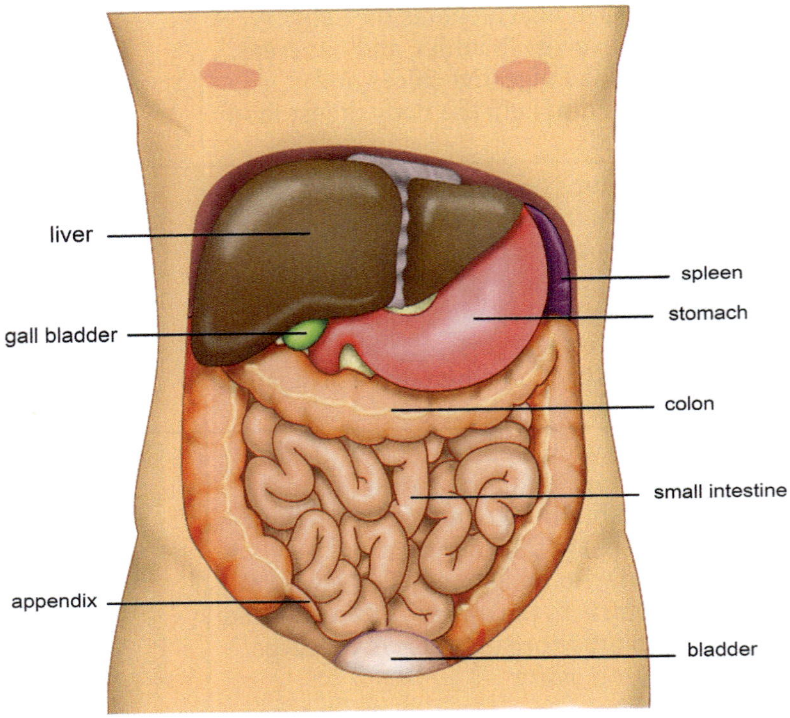

Figure 4.1. *Anatomy of the abdomen.*

Source: By Tvanbr – Own work, Public Domain; https://commons.wikimedia.org/w/index.php?curid=11625998.

The abdomen is a body cavity—a hollow, fluid-filled space that holds organs and other bodily structures. Organs inside the abdomen include:

- Digestive system organs like the stomach, small intestine, large intestine (colon), pancreas, appendix, liver, and gallbladder.
- Lymphatic system organs like the spleen and lymph vessels.

- Urinary system organs like the kidneys, ureters (tubes that carry urine), and bladder.
- Reproductive organs like the uterus, ovaries, and fallopian tubes.
- Blood vessels (arteries and veins).
- Parasympathetic and sympathetic nerves.

4.1.1. Structure

The majority of the body's trunk is made up of the vertically oval abdomen, which is the largest cavity in the body. The abdominal cavity is filled with fluid, which helps cushion and lubricate the organs to allow for friction-free movement. The organs that comprise the abdominal wall are covered by tissues, muscles, and membranes. Layers of the abdomen include (Kim et al., 2017):

1. **Peritoneum:** This thin membrane covers the inside of the abdominal cavity (parietal peritoneum) and the organs (visceral peritoneum). Along with ligaments, a large double layer of the peritoneum (the mesentery) attaches abdominal organs together or to the rear abdominal wall.
2. **Preperitoneal Adipose Tissue:** This fatty tissue creates a pad that covers the abdominal cavity. It also fills in space that doesn't contain organs.
3. **Areolar Tissue:** This loose connective tissue made from collagen fibers and elastic tissue helps connect skin to muscles. It also gives the abdomen structure to help support the body and protect organs.
4. **Transversalis Fascia:** This thin layer of connective tissue lines the abdominal cavity to help support organs and muscles in the abdomen.
5. **Transversus Abdominis:** As the deepest abdominal muscle layer, the transversus abdominis helps protect organs by holding them in place and stabilizing the abdomen and lower back.
6. **Obliques:** These twin muscles are located on the right and left of the waist, surrounding the six-pack muscles. The internal and external obliques help the trunk twist left and right.
7. **Superficial Fascia:** This stringy connective tissue surrounds organs and other structures in the abdomen, flexing and stretching to help your abdominal muscles and tissue move.
8. **Subcutaneous Tissue:** This deep layer of fatty and connective tissue allows your skin to move over other tissues and muscles. It also helps absorb shock to protect your abdominal organs and muscles.

4.1.2. Location

The area of the lower torso that faces forward is where the abdomen is situated. This cavity is located above the top of your pelvis and directly beneath your lungs in your chest. Your lungs and abdomen are divided by a muscle group known as the diaphragm. Your spine and back muscles are situated behind the abdominal cavity (Wade et al., 2023).

The vagus nerve, the principal nerve of the parasympathetic nervous system, runs from the neck to the abdomen. The parasympathetic nervous system aids in regulating immune response, heart rate, and digestion, among other bodily processes. Many blood vessels in the abdomen connect to the circulatory system.

Blood is transported from the heart to the digestive system's organs via the aorta. Blood is transferred from the abdomen to your lower extremities by the inferior vena cava, which then returns the blood to your heart (Tucker et al., 2023).

4.1.3. Anatomical Variations

Birth defects can cause the abdominal wall to develop abnormally, causing openings where organs protrude out of the body. Birth defects that affect the anatomy of the abdomen include gastroschisis and omphalocele. Gastroschisis is a defect in the abdominal wall that causes the large and small intestines to push through, usually to the right of the belly button. There is no membrane covering the exposed organs.

Omphalocele, also known as exomphalos, is when organs like the intestines, stomach, and liver push through an opening in the center of the abdominal wall—where the umbilical cord meets the abdomen. A membrane covers the opening and organs.

4.1.3.1. What Does the Abdomen Do?

The abdomen's function as a body cavity is to house and safeguard the digestive, urinary, endocrine, exocrine, circulatory, and female reproductive systems' essential internal organs. Together, the layers of muscle, tissue, and membrane support and shield these organs from external damage so they don't fall out of the cavity (Wade et al., 2023).

Additionally, the abdomen helps to support and shield a growing fetus. To make room for the expanding uterus, the muscles in the abdomen flex and the organs press up against the top of the cavity during pregnancy. The nervous, lymphatic, and circulatory systems are all connected to the abdominal organs through the abdomen. To transport blood to and from organs and support their function, blood vessels branch out throughout the abdomen (Tucker et al., 2023). Your abdomen's lymph vessels function as channels to remove lymph that is left over after blood passes through your organs. White blood cells found in lymph, a transparent fluid, aid in the removal of waste products, germs, and aberrant cells that can cause illness (Michael et al., 2023). The abdomen is a passageway for sympathetic and parasympathetic nervous system nerves that enter organs. Under stress, the sympathetic nervous system becomes more active and activates to regulate your fight-or-flight response. To redirect energy and activate liver energy stores, the nerves in the abdomen aid in slowing down digestion. Your body receives signals from the parasympathetic nervous system to relax and to begin digesting and urinating (Wade et al., 2023).

4.1.4. Associated Conditions

Abdominal health conditions frequently impact particular organs, the abdominal cavity, or its walls. Although gas is usually the cause of abdominal bloating or swelling, it can also indicate a more serious illness. The most common health problem pertaining to the abdomen is abdominal pain.

4.1.4.1. Abdominal Wall and Cavity Conditions

Health conditions that directly affect the abdominal wall and cavity include:

1. **Hernia:** A small sac that forms when the small intestine pushes through a hole, tear, or weak area in the abdominal wall's muscle. An incisional hernia can occur after abdominal surgery. An umbilical hernia forms around the belly button when the muscle doesn't fully close after birth.
2. **Ascites:** This fluid buildup between

the abdominal lining and organs causes the abdomen to swell. Scarring of the liver (cirrhosis) usually causes ascites (Chiejina et al., 2023).

3. **Peritonitis:** A condition where the peritoneum—the membrane that covers the abdomen and its organs—becomes inflamed or infected. Symptoms can include abdominal pain, swelling, fever, and vomiting. A hole in a digestive tract organ or bile leaking into the abdominal cavity can cause this dangerous condition.
4. **Abdominal Adhesions:** These bands of scar-like tissue inside the abdomen form between organs or between organs and the abdominal wall. Adhesions can happen after abdominal surgery and cause the intestines and other abdominal organs to twist or compress enough to cause blockages.
5. **Abdominal Distension:** This abdominal swelling, or distention, makes your abdominal region larger than usual. Overeating, fluid buildup, or intestinal or bowel blockages can cause it.

4.1.4.2. Abdominal Cancers and Related Conditions

Cancer and related conditions that affect the abdomen include:

1. **Peritoneal Mesothelioma:** This rare cancer affects the peritoneum lining in the abdominal cavity. Asbestos exposure—a carcinogenic fibrous mineral once used in building materials—causes this cancer (Kim et al., 2017).

2. **Pseudomyxoma Peritonei (PMP):** This is a condition where cancerous growths fill the abdominal cavity with jelly-like fluid. PMP is caused by cancers in the abdomen—like stomach, colon, pancreatic, or ovarian cancer (Yu et al., 2023).

2. **Peritoneal Carcinomatosis:** This is cancer that has spread to the peritoneum from other cancers like those of the colon/rectum, pancreas, stomach, ovaries, and gallbladder (Szadkowska et al., 2023).

3. **Mesenteric Panniculitis (Sclerosing Mesenteritis):** This rare condition is often associated with cancer. It causes inflammation of the mesentery—folds of peritoneum tissue at the back of the abdomen. Over time, it can scar abdominal tissues. It can also cause abdominal swelling and chronic or intermittent abdominal pain (Alsuhaimi et al., 2022).

4.1.4.3. Abdominal Organ Conditions

Other conditions that cause abdominal pain and issues are related to organs inside the abdomen. Some common conditions affecting abdominal organs include:

1. **Appendicitis:** Inflammation of the appendix causes on-and-off pain in the middle of the abdomen. The pain eventually travels to the lower right side of the abdomen, where the appendix is located.
2. **Gallstones:** These blockages in the gallbladder can cause colicky pain and digestive issues.
3. **Pancreatitis:** This swelling of the pancreas can cause pain on the left side of the abdomen.

4. **Kidney Stones:** Mineral deposits from the kidneys create blockages in the urethra (the tube that lets urine release from your body), making urinating difficult and painful.
5. **Intestinal Colic:** This is when hardened feces, food, scar tissue, tumors, polyps, or inflamed tissue create partial or complete blockage in the intestines. It causes cramp-like abdominal pain.
6. **Bowel Obstruction:** A blockage in the small or large bowel can prevent stool from passing, causing pain in the upper abdomen and near the belly button.

4.1.5. Diagnostic Testing

To diagnose abdominal issues, a healthcare provider will typically consider your symptom history, perform a physical examination, and run diagnostic tests. Tests that help diagnose abdomen-related health issues include:

1. **Blood Tests:** Drawing blood and testing it in a lab can identify infections or organ problems.
2. **Urine Tests (Urinalysis):** This test examines a person's urine for pH level, appearance, abnormal substances, proteins, and bacteria.
3. **Stool Tests:** Examining a stool sample with or without a microscope can help diagnose digestive tract system issues.
4. **Abdominal X-Ray:** This imaging test uses electromagnetic waves to take pictures of the inside of the abdomen and its organs. It can identify blockages or injuries.
5. **Transabdominal Ultrasound:** This imaging test uses sound waves to see inside the abdomen and look at organs and blood vessels. It can help identify tumors, organ abnormalities, and kidney stones.
6. **Endoscopy:** This test inserts a tube with a tiny camera called an endoscope into your mouth or rectum to look inside your digestive tract. This test can help identify issues with your intestines or stomach.
7. **Barium Enema:** This special type of X-ray looks at the large intestine. Barium sulfate is inserted into the rectum during the test to help highlight specific areas of the colon.
8. **Computerized Tomography (CT) Scan:** An imaging test that creates pictures of the abdomen from different angles. CT scans give a three-dimensional view of the abdomen to identify injury, fluid, tumors, infections, blood clots, and internal bleeding (Flynn & Vickerton, 2023; Mikhael & Khan, 2024; Wade & Streitz, 2023).

4.2. Surface Anatomy and Surface Markings

The xiphoid. The costal margin has a distinct step at the tip of the 9th costal cartilage. It runs from the 7th costal cartilage at the xiphoid to the tip of the 12th rib, though it is frequently difficult to feel.

The iliac crest terminates at the front of the body at the anterior superior spine, where the inguinal ligament (Poupart's ligament) extends downward and inward towards the pubic tubercle. Locate this tubercle by feeling for it directly and by tracing along the adductor longus tendon (which is tightened by flexing, abducting, and externally rotating the thigh) to its attachment point at the tubercle. Feel the firm vas deferens between thumb and finger where it is located at the scrotal neck within the spermatic cord. By using your fingertip to invaginate the scrotal skin, you can feel the external inguinal ring as you trace the vas upward and observe that it passes medially to the pubic tubercle.

4.2.1. Vertebral Levels

- **L1** – the transpyloric plane of Addison lies halfway between the suprasternal notch and the pubis, or approximately a hand's breadth below the xiphoid. This plane passes through the pylorus, the pancreatic neck, the duodenojejunal flexure, the fundus of the gallbladder, the tip of the 9th costal cartilage (felt as a distinct 'step'), and the hila of the kidneys. It also corresponds to the level of termination of the spinal cord.
- **L3** – the subcostal plane, a line joining the lowest point of the thoracic cage on each side, which is the inferior margin of the 10th rib. It passes through the origin of the inferior mesenteric artery.
- **L4** – the plane of the iliac crests. This corresponds to the level of the bifurcation of the aorta. It is also a useful landmark in performing a lumbar puncture since it is well below the level of the termination of the spinal cord, which is approximately at L1.
- The umbilicus is an inconstant landmark. In the healthy adult, it lies at the junction of the L3 and L4 vertebrae. It is lower in the infant and, naturally, when the abdomen is pendulous. It is higher in late pregnancy.

4.2.2. Surface Markings

Although the positions of the abdominal viscera vary, the following structures' surface markings have clinical significance (Figure 4.2).

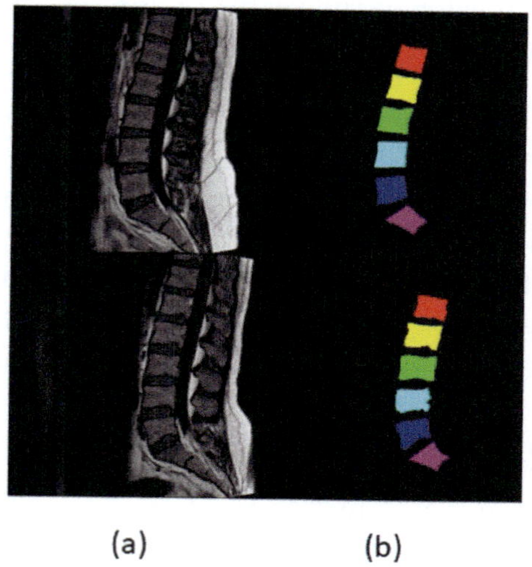

Figure 4.2. *Lumbar spine.*

Source: Mushtaq, M., Akram, M. U., Alghamdi, N. S., Fatima, J., & Masood, R. F., (2022). Localization and edge-based segmentation of lumbar spine vertebrae to identify the deformities using deep learning models. Sensors, 22(4), 1547. https://doi.org/10.3390/s22041547.

4.2.2.1. Liver

The lower border of the liver can just be felt in a normal subject, particularly during deep inspiration. It stretches from the tip of the right 10th rib to the left 5th intercostal space in the midclavicular line. The upper border is formed by a line that on each side passes through the fifth intercostal space.

4.2.2.2. Spleen

This underlies the 9th, 10th, and 11th ribs posteriorly on the left side commencing 2 in

(5 cm) from the midline. It is about the size of the subject's cupped hand.

4.2.2.3. Gallbladder

When the fingers are run along the costal margin, the fundus of the gallbladder can be easily identified as a distinct "step" at the tip of the 9th costal cartilage, which is where the lateral border of the rectus abdominis crosses the costal margin.

4.2.2.4. Pancreas

The level of the pancreatic neck above the spinal column is defined by the transpyloric plane. Imagine the head moving downward and to the right, and the body and tail moving upward and to the left, starting from this landmark.

4.2.2.5. Aorta

This terminates just to the left of the midline at the level of the iliac crest at L4; a pulsatile swelling below this level may thus be an iliac, but cannot be an aortic aneurysm.

4.2.2.6. Kidneys

Occasionally, the thin subject may feel the lower pole of the normal right kidney during deep inspiration. The kidney's hilum is located anteriorly, four fingerbreadths from the midline, on the transpyloric plane. The kidney's upper pole extends deep to the 12th rib on the posterior side. Normally, the right kidney extends 2.5 cm (2 in) shorter than the left. The kidney outlines can be projected onto the anterior or posterior abdominal walls using these landmarks. Only the aorta is palpable in the majority of us; in some perfectly normal thin people, especially women, the lower pole of the right kidney and the sigmoid colon, if full of feces, can be felt (Flynn & Vickerton, 2023; Mikhael & Khan, 2024; Wade & Streitz, 2023).

4.3. The Fasciae and Muscles of the Abdominal Wall

4.3.1. Fasciae of the Abdominal Wall

The superficial fascia only covers the trunk; there is no deep fascia present. (If there were, we probably wouldn't be able to breathe deeply or eat a big meal!) This creates a deeper fibrous layer (of Scarpa) and a superficial fatty layer (of Camper) in the lower abdomen. The fibrous layer merges with the deep fascia of the upper thigh, reaches into the penis and scrotum (also known as labia majora), and continues into the perineum as Colles' fascia. The fatty layer is continuous with the superficial fat of the rest of the body. It is connected laterally to the pubis rami and ischium in the perineum, as well as posteriorly to the perineal body and membrane. These attachments allow blood and urine to seep into the scrotum, perineum, and penis before entering the lower abdomen deep into the fibrous fascial plane in the event of a rupture of the urethral bulb. However, extravasation of fluid into the lower limb is prevented by the fascia's attachment to the deep fascia of the upper thigh.

4.3.1.1. Nerve Supply

The segmental nerve supply of the abdominal muscles and the overlying skin is derived from T7 to L1. This distribution can be mapped out approximately if it is remembered that the umbilicus is supplied by T10 and the groin and scrotum by L1 (via the ilio-inguinal and iliohypogastric nerves).

4.3.2. The Muscles of the Anterior Abdominal Wall

Because of the way that their anatomy serves as the foundation for abdominal incisions, these are extremely important practically. The fifth, sixth, and seventh costal cartilages form the rectus abdominis, which extends 3 inches (7.5 cm) horizontally and inserts itself into the pubic crest for a length of 1 inch (2.05 cm).

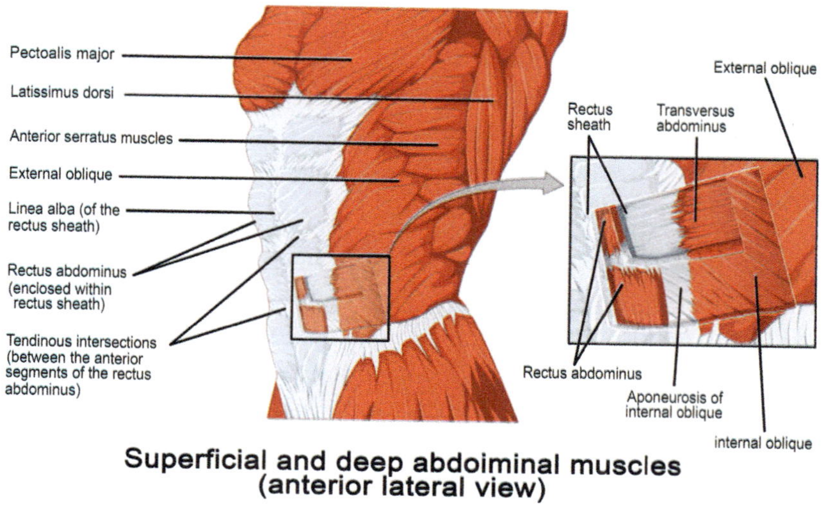

Figure 4.3. *Muscles of the abdomen. The anterior abdominal muscles include the medially located rectus femoris, which is covered by a sheet of connective tissue called the Linea alba. On the flanks of the body, medial to the rectus femoris, the abdominal wall is composed of three layers. The external oblique muscles form the outermost layer, while the internal oblique muscles form the middle layer, and the transverses abdominus forms the innermost layer.*

Source: https://courses.lumenlearning.com/suny-ap1/chapter/axial-muscles-of-the-abdominal-wall-and-thorax/.

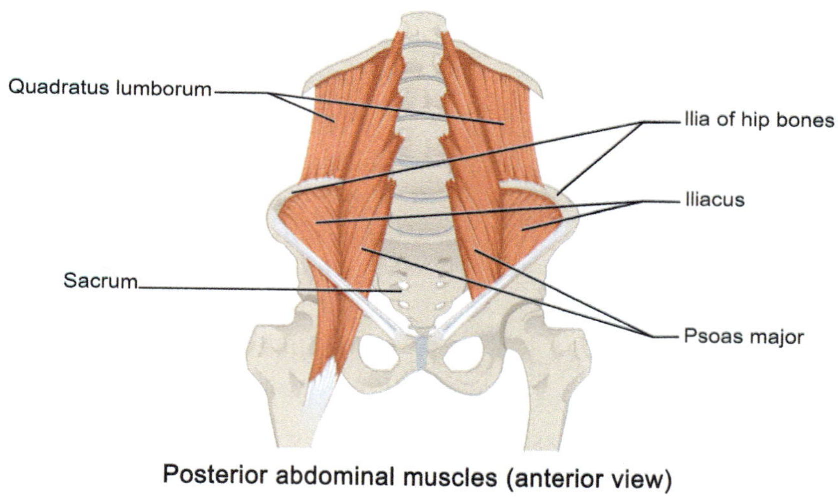

Figure 4.4. *The muscles of the lower back move the lumbar spine but also assist in femur movements.*

Source: https://courses.lumenlearning.com/suny-ap1/chapter/axial-muscles-of-the-abdominal-wall-and-thorax/.

There are three constant transverse tendinous intersections at the tip of the xiphoid, the umbilicus, and halfway between; sporadically, there is a fourth intersection below the umbilicus. These intersections only occur on the muscle's anterior surface, where they attach to the anterior rectus sheath. Consequently, the rectus muscle is entirely free behind because they are absent posteriorly. The rectus is punctured by vessels from the superior epigastric artery and vein at each intersection. The aponeurotic expansions of the lateral abdominal muscles play a major role in forming the sheath that houses the rectus (Figures 4.3 and 4.4).

i. Above the costal margin, the anterior sheath comprises the external oblique aponeurosis only; posteriorly lie the costal cartilages.

ii. From the costal margin to a point halfway between the umbilicus and pubis, the external oblique and the anterior part of the internal oblique aponeurosis form the anterior sheath. Posteriorly lie the posterior part of this split internal oblique aponeurosis and the aponeurosis of the transversus abdominis.

iii. Below a point halfway between the umbilicus and pubis, all the aponeuroses pass in front of the rectus so that the anterior sheath here comprises the tendinous expansions of all three oblique muscles blended together. The posterior wall at this level is made up of the only other structures available—the transversalis fascia (the thickened extraperitoneal fascia of the lower abdominal wall) and peritoneum.

The lower border of the posterior aponeurotic part of the rectus sheath is where the arcuate line of Douglas marks the posterior junction between (b) and (c). Here, the inferior epigastric artery and vein from the external iliac vessels enter the sheath and anastomose with the superior epigastric vessels, terminal branches of the internal thoracic artery and vein. The rectus sheaths join in the midline to create the linea alba, which extends from the xiphoid to the pubic symphysis.

The transverse, internal, and external oblique muscles make up the lateral muscles of the abdominal wall. These share their neurovascular bundles running between the second and third layer with the external, internal, and innermost intercostals, the three layers of muscle that make up the chest wall. They are crucial from a clinical standpoint because they form the inguinal canal and the rectus sheath, and they have to be divided to make lateral abdominal incisions.

When one considers that they occupy the space between the iliac crest below, the costal margin above, and the lumbar muscles covered by lumbar fascia behind, their attachments become more easily remembered. As previously mentioned, they form the rectus sheath medially and then merge into the linea alba from the xiphoid to the pubic crest.

The obliquus externus abdominis (external oblique) arises from the outer surfaces of the lower eight ribs and fans out into the xiphoid, linea alba, the pubic crest, pubic tubercle, and the anterior half of the iliac crest. From the pubic tubercle to the anterior superior iliac spine, its lower border forms the aponeurotic inguinal ligament of Poupart.

The lumbar fascia, the anterior two-thirds of the iliac crest, and the lateral two-thirds of the inguinal ligament are the sources of the obliquus internus abdominis, also known as the internal oblique. It is inserted into the pubic crest, linea alba, and the lowest six costal cartilages. The transversus abdominis is derived from the lumbar fascia, the anterior two-thirds of the iliac crest, the lateral one-third of the inguinal ligament, and the lowest six costal cartilages (which interdigitate with the diaphragm). It is inserted into the pubic crest and the linea alba. Keep in mind that the transversus passes transversely, the internal oblique passes upwards and forwards, and the external oblique passes downward and forward. Additionally, take note of the fact that the deeper two muscles originate posteriorly from the lumbar fascia, whereas the external oblique has its posterior border free.

4.3.3. The Anatomy of Abdominal Incisions

Making incisions to reveal the intraperitoneal structures is an indication of the operator's expertise. While they need maximum access, they also aim to leave a scar that, if placed in an inconspicuous crease, will cause the least harm to the abdominal wall's muscles and nerve supply. The lateral abdominal muscles receive their nerve supply from a richly communicating network, meaning that severing one or two of these nerves and splitting the muscle fibers will not result in any clinically significant side effects. Nonetheless, there is minimal cross-communication in the segmental nerve supply that innervates the rectus, so injury to these nerves needs to be prevented whenever possible. The numerous anastomoses between the blood vessels supplying the abdominal muscles mean that damage from operative incisions is of no practical importance.

4.3.3.1. Midline Incision

The linea alba is cut through during the midline incision. This fibrous structure is relatively wide superiorly, but it becomes almost hairline below the umbilicus, making it difficult for the surgeon to locate the precise point of cleavage between the recti at this level. Made entirely of fibrous tissue, it offers a nearly bloodless line that can be used to quickly and, if needed, open the abdomen from Dan in the north to Beersheba in the south!

4.3.3.2. Paramedian Incision

The anterior rectus sheath is opened, the rectus is shifted laterally, and the posterior sheath and peritoneum are then incised. The paramedian incision is made 1 in (2.5 cm) to 1.5 in (4 cm) lateral and parallel to the midline. One benefit of this incision is that the rectus slides back into place to cover and shield the peritoneal scar after the peritoneum is sutured. The anterior sheath adheres to the rectus muscle at its tendinous intersections, necessitating the sheath's dissection from the muscle at each location and the division of a segmental vessel at each. Once this is done, the rectus can be freely slid laterally out of the posterior sheath. As we have seen, below the pubis and umbilicus, the posterior sheath and peritoneum form a tough membrane that is composed only of transversalis fascia and peritoneum, losing its aponeurotic component. Below this point, the membrane is much thinner and more fatty. The inferior epigastric vessels are visible in the posterior sheath, passing beneath the arcuate line of Douglas. A low paramedian incision is typically necessary for the division of these vessels.

4.3.3.3. The Transrectus Incision

The rectus muscle may occasionally split along the paramedian incision's path. It is best to avoid making this incision because the rectus receives its nerve supply laterally, depriving the muscle medial to the incision of its innervation and causing it to atrophy.

4.3.3.4. Subcostal Incision

The subcostal (Kocher) incision is used for spleen exposure on the left side and biliary surgery on the right. Starting from the midline, the skin incision extends parallel to the costal margin and 1 in (2.5 cm) below it. The posterior sheath with underlying adherent peritoneum is incised, the rectus is cut, and the anterior rectus sheath is opened.

The larger and more significant 9th nerve, located in the lateral region of the wound, is preserved, but the tiny 8th intercostal nerve branch that leads to the rectus is sacrificed. Very little retracts from the divided rectus muscle, which is held in place by the intersections above and below. After that, fibrous tissue heals it. When a patient has a large subcostal angle, this incision is useful. Generally, the paramedian incision is preferred when this angle is narrow.

4.3.3.5. The Muscle Split or Gridiron Approach to the Appendix

The McBurney's point oblique skin incision, which is located two-thirds of the way laterally from the umbilicus to the anterior superior iliac spine, is becoming less common. Instead, people prefer to make an almost transverse incision in the line where the skin crease forwards from the anterior spine, 1 in (2.25 cm) above it.

The external oblique's aponeurosis is cut in the direction of its fibers, which is medially and obliquely downward. The internal oblique and transversus muscles are then divided in the direction of their fibers and retract without the need for division. These muscles snap back together when the incision is closed, leaving the abdominal wall essentially intact.

4.3.3.6. Transverse and Oblique Incisions

Cuts through the lateral abdominal muscles heal without causing weakness and do not harm their richly anastomosing nerve supply. They are helpful, for instance, in exposing the caecum or the sigmoid colon, as well as in repositioning the peritoneum medially to expose extraperitoneal structures like the sympathetic chain, ureter, and external iliac vessels.

4.3.3.7. Thoraco-Abdominal Incisions

The diaphragm can be cut, an extensive exposure of the upper abdomen and thorax can be achieved, and an upper paramedian or upper oblique abdominal incision can be extended through the eighth or ninth intercostal space. For instance, this is used to remove growths from the upper stomach or lower esophagus on the left, and to resect the right liver lobe on the right.

4.3.3.8. Paracentesis Abdominis

It is possible to remove intraperitoneal fluid collections using a cannula that is inserted through the abdominal wall. After using a catheter to empty the bladder, the cannula is inserted via a trocar either lateral to McBurney's point (where there is no risk of puncturing the inferior epigastric vessels) or through the midline (where the linea alba is comparatively bloodless).

Because the trocar tip pushes the gut coils away and they are mobile, the gut coils are not in danger during this procedure. It is also possible to insert cannulae for laparoscopic surgery using these two landmarks.

4.3.4. The Inguinal Canal

This canal is a representation of the testis and cord's oblique passage through the lower abdominal wall (the round ligament in the female). Given the significance of this area in the diagnosis and treatment of hernias, questions about its anatomy are likely asked during examinations more frequently than any other. The canal is 4 cm (1.5 in) long. It lies parallel to and directly above the inguinal ligament as it descends and medially between the internal and external inguinal rings (Figure 4.5).

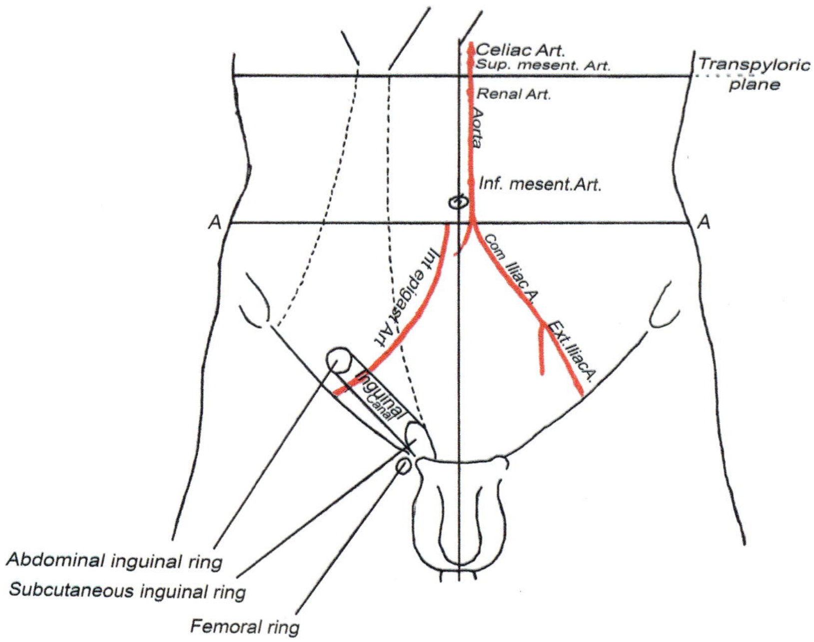

Figure 4.5. *The inguinal canal.*

Source: By Henry Vandyke Carter – Henry Gray, (1918). Anatomy of the human body (see "Book" section below) Bartleby.com: Gray's Anatomy, Plate 1227, Public Domain; https://commons.wikimedia.org/w/index.php?curid=564843.

4.3.4.1. Relations

- **Anteriorly** – the skin, superficial fascia and the external oblique aponeurosis cover the full length of the canal; the internal oblique covers its lateral one-third.
- **Posteriorly** – the conjoint tendon forms the posterior wall of the canal medially, the transversalis fascia laterally. (The conjoint tendon represents the fused common insertion of the internal oblique and transversus into the pubic crest and pectineal line.)
- **Above** – arch the lowest fibers of the internal oblique and transversus abdominis.
- **Below** – lies the inguinal ligament.

The spermatic cord pushes through the transversalis fascia at the internal (or deep) ring, dragging a covering that forms the internal spermatic fascia with it. The inferior epigastric arteries that ascend from the external iliac vein and artery divide this ring medially. The external (or superficial) ring is located directly above and medial to the pubic tubercle. It is a V-shaped defect in the external oblique aponeurosis. The cord carries the external spermatic fascia from the ring's margins as it passes through this opening. The round ligament and the ilio-inguinal nerve in females, as well as the spermatic cord in males, are transmitted through the inguinal canal. The spermatic cord comprises (Figure 4.6):

1. **Three Layers of Fascia** – the external spermatic, from the external oblique aponeurosis; the cremasteric, from the

internal oblique aponeurosis (containing muscle fibers termed the cremaster muscle); the internal spermatic, from the transversalis fascia;

2. **Three Arteries:** The testicular (from the aorta); the cremasteric (from the inferior epigastric artery); the artery of the vas (from the inferior vesical artery);
3. **Three Veins:** The pampiniform plexus of veins (draining the right testis into the inferior vena cava and the left into the left renal vein), and the cremasteric vein and vein of the vas, which accompany their corresponding arteries.
4. **Three Nerves:** The nerve to the cremaster (from the genito-femoral nerve); sympathetic fibers from T10–11 spinal segments; the ilio-inguinal nerve (strictly, on and not in the cord);
5. **Three Other Structures:** The vas deferens, lymphatics of the testis, which pass to the para-aortic lymph nodes and, pathologically present as the third structure, a patent processus vaginalis in patients with an indirect inguinal hernia!

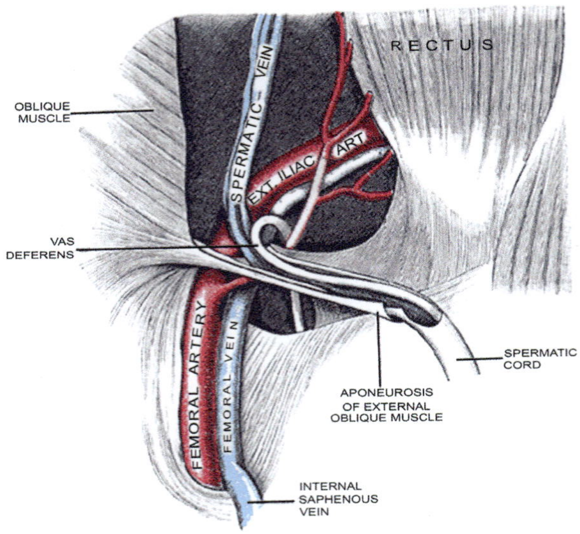

Figure 4.6. *Scheme of the spermatic cord and its contents, in transverse section.*

Source: By Henry Vandyke Carter – Henry Gray, (1918). Anatomy of the human body (see "Book" section below) Bartleby.com: Gray's Anatomy, Plate 1146, Public Domain; https://commons.wikimedia.org/w/index.php?curid=567115.

4.3.4.2. Clinical Features

If it is sufficiently large, an indirect inguinal hernia can emerge through the external ring and descend into the scrotum after passing through the internal ring and along the canal. Should the hernia be reducible, it can be entirely managed by applying pressure with the fingertip over the internal ring, which is located 0.5 inches (12 mm) above the point where the femoral artery passes beneath the inguinal ligament, i.e., 12 mm or 0.5 in above the femoral pulse. Halfway between the anterior superior iliac spine and the symphysis pubis, at the mid-inguinal point, is where this pulse can be felt.

A femoral hernia emerging from the femoral canal lies below and lateral to the pubic tubercle; if the hernia protrudes through the external ring, it can be felt to lie above and medial to this landmark. A direct inguinal hernia penetrates the inguinal canal's posterior wall straight forward. Digital pressure applied immediately above the femoral pulse does not control it because it lies medial to the internal ring. Every now and then, a direct hernia gets big enough to squeeze through the external ring and into the scrotal neck. Because this is so uncommon, a scrotal hernia is typically thought to be an indirect hernia.

An indirect hernia sac will pass laterally and a direct hernia medially to the inferior epigastric vessels, which define the medial edge of the internal ring. This is the only surefire method to identify the problem while it is in operation. Both a direct and an indirect hernia frequently coexist; they protrude like a pair of pantaloons from either side of the inferior epigastric vessels (Flynn & Vickerton, 2023; Mikhael & Khan, 2024; Wade & Streitz, 2023).

4.4. Peritoneal Cavity

The embryo's primitive coelomic cavity's endothelium gives rise to the thoracic pleura and the abdominal peritoneum. Each is invaginated by ingrowing viscera, which result in the visceral and parietal layers, respectively, being tightly packed into a serous-lined cavity and covered by a serous membrane.

The female peritoneal cavity is perforated by the uterine tube openings, which could provide a route for external infection, while the male peritoneal cavity is completely closed. It is best to start at one location and trace this membrane in an imaginary round trip of the abdominal cavity to review the intricate peritoneal attachments. The parietal peritoneum, which is located beneath the umbilicus on the anterior abdominal wall, is a handy place to start. Except for the shallow ridges created by the obliterated fetal urachus (the obliterated umbilical arteries passing from the bladder to the umbilicus), the obliterated umbilical arteries passing from the internal iliac arteries to the umbilicus, and the lateral umbilical folds (the peritoneum covering the inferior epigastric vessels), the membrane is smooth at this level (Figure 4.7).

The falciform ligament sweeps upward and slightly to the right of the midline to reach the liver from the posterior aspect of the umbilicus, where a cicatrix is typically felt and visible. The ligamentum teres (the severed fetal left umbilical vein) enters the groove between the liver's left lobe and quadrate lobe within the ligament's free border. There are other places where the peritoneum sweeps over the inferior aspect of the diaphragm, reflecting onto the liver (where the upper and lower coronary ligaments of the liver define a bare area) and onto the right margin of the abdominal esophagus. Following its encirclement of the liver, the peritoneum descends to the lesser curve of the stomach from the porta hepatis in the form of a double sheet known as the lesser omentum. Once more, it divides to enclose this organ, reorganizes at its larger curve, loops down, and then rises once more to join the transverse colon's length, forming the greater omentum, which resembles an apron. This peritoneum, in turn, encloses the transverse colon. The transverse mesocolon then travels upward and backward to join the anterior aspect of the pancreas to the posterior abdominal wall (Figure 4.8).

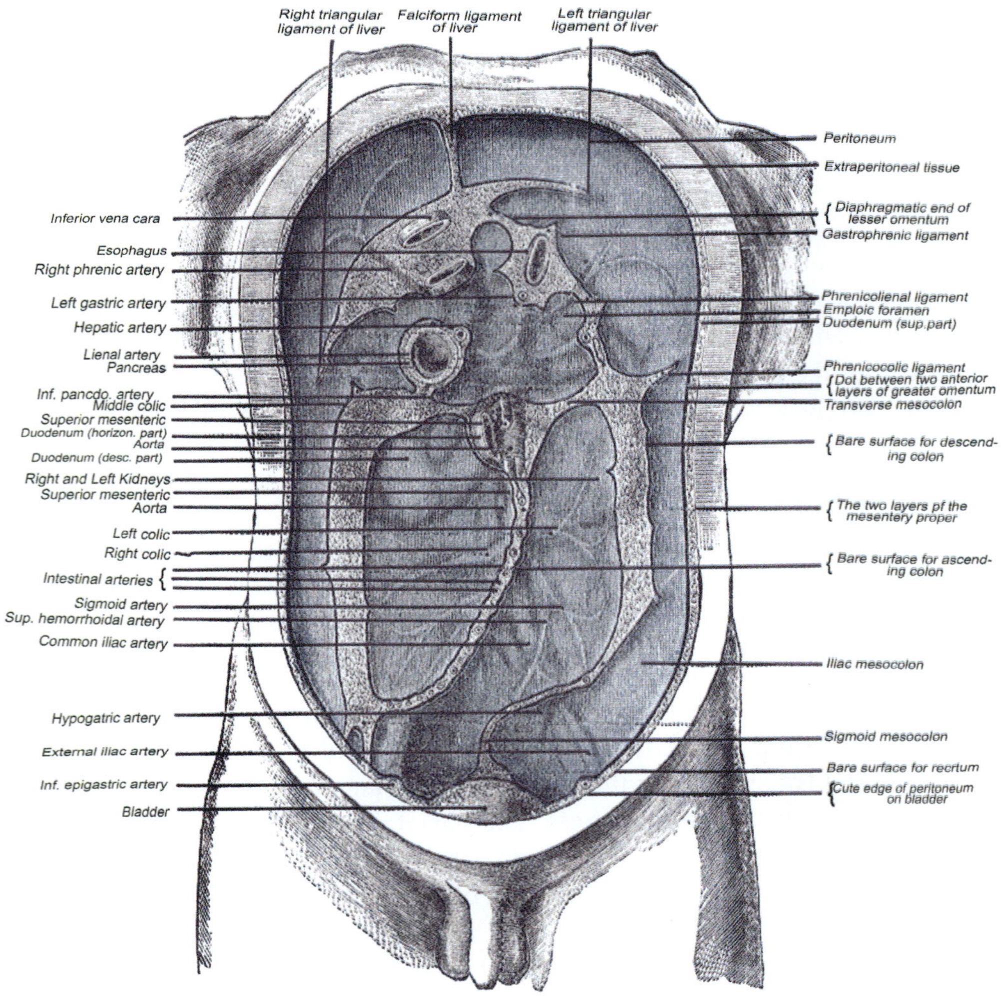

Figure 4.7. *The peritoneal cavity.*

Source: By Henry Vandyke Carter – Henry Gray, (1918). Anatomy of the human body (see "Book" section below) Bartleby.com: Gray's Anatomy, Plate 1040, Public Domain; https://commons.wikimedia.org/w/index.php?curid=566987.

This double peritoneal sheet splits again at the base of the transverse mesocolon; the upper leaf crosses the posterior abdominal wall upward to reflect on the liver (at the bare area), while the lower leaf crosses the posterior abdominal wall lower to cover the pelvic viscera and to reconnect with the anterior wall's peritoneum. However, this posterior layer is broken up by its reflection along an oblique line that forms the small intestine's mesentery. This line runs from the duodenojejunal flexure, which is located above and to the left, to the ileocecal junction, which is located below and to the right. The lymph drainage and vascular supply of the contained viscera are carried by the mesocolon, the smaller intestine's mesentery, and the greater and lesser omenta. The large pouch that extends between the layers of the greater omentum and lies behind the stomach and lesser omentum is known as the lesser sac. Normally, this space is obliterated. The spleen, which is joined by the gastrosplenic and lienorenal ligaments, forms its left wall (Figure 4.9).

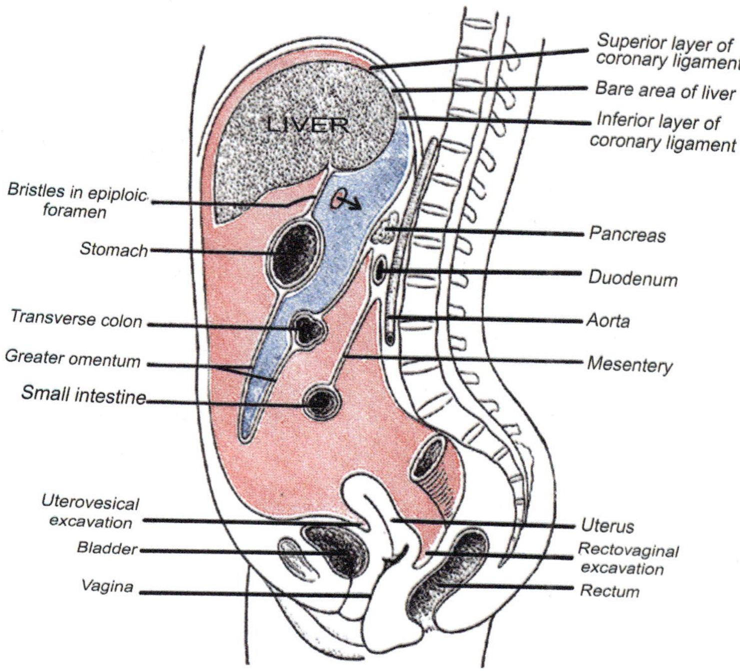

Figure 4.8. *The peritoneal cavity.*

Source: By Henry Vandyke Carter – Henry Gray, (1918). Anatomy of the human body (see "Book" section below) Bartleby.com: Gray's Anatomy, Plate 1035, Public Domain; https://commons.wikimedia.org/w/index.php?curid=566980

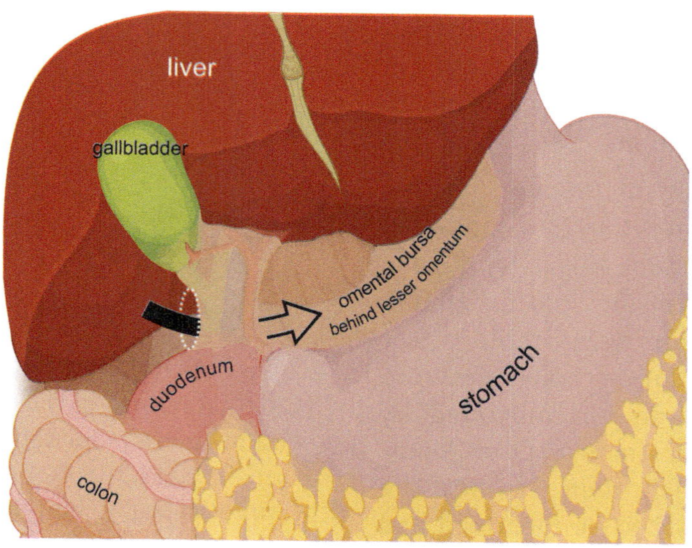

Figure 4.9. *The foramen of Winslow.*

Source: By Olek Remesz (wiki-pl: Orem, commons: Orem) – Own work, CC BY-SA 3.0; https://commons.wikimedia.org/w/index.php?curid=27670622.

The right extremity of the sac opens into the main peritoneal cavity via the epiploic foramen or foramen of Winslow, whose boundaries are as follows:

1. **Anteriorly:** The free edge of the lesser omentum, containing the common bile duct to the right, hepatic artery to the left, and portal vein posteriorly.
2. **Posteriorly:** The inferior vena cava.
3. **Inferiorly:** The 1st part of the duodenum, over which runs the hepatic artery before ascending into the anterior wall of the foramen.
4. **Superiorly:** The caudate process of the liver.

4.4.1. Clinical Features

1. Occasionally, a loop of intestine passes through the foramen of Winslow into the lesser sac and becomes strangulated by the edges of the foramen. Notice that none of these important boundaries can be incised to release the strangulation; the bowel must be decompressed by a needle to allow its reduction.
2. It is important for the surgeon that the hepatic artery can be compressed between his index finger within the foramen of Winslow and his thumb on its anterior wall. If the cystic artery is torn during cholecystectomy, hemorrhage can be controlled by this maneuver (named after James Pringle), which then enables the damaged vessel to be identified and secured.

4.4.2. Intraperitoneal Fossae

A number of fossae occur within the peritoneal cavity into which loops of bowel may become caught and strangulated (Figure 4.10). Those of importance are:

1. The lesser sac via the foramen of Winslow, described above;
2. Para duodenal fossa—between the duodenojejunal flexure and the inferior mesenteric vessels;
3. Retrocecal fossa—in which the appendix frequently lies;
4. Intersigmoid fossa—formed by the inverted V attachment of the mesosigmoid.

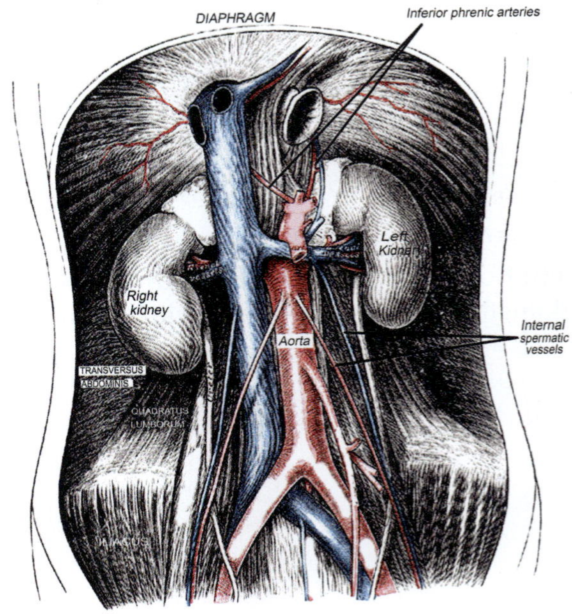

Figure 4.10. *The diaphragm.*

Source: By Henry Vandyke Carter – Henry Gray, (1918). Anatomy of the human body (see "Book" section below) Bartleby.com: Gray's Anatomy, Plate 531, Public Domain; https://commons.wikimedia.org/w/index.php?curid=541100.

4.4.3. The Subphrenic Spaces

There are several possible spaces formed below the diaphragm in relation to the liver's attachments.

Adhesions may wall off one or more of these spaces inferiorly, causing a subphrenic abscess to fill with pus. Five divisions are considered to be clinically significant. The falciform ligament divides the right and left subphrenic spaces, which are located between the diaphragm and the liver. Beneath the liver are the right and left subhepatic spaces. The liver is located above and the posterior abdominal wall behind the right, which is known as the Morison pouch. It connects anteriorly to the right subphrenic space around the anterior liver lobe margin, and both open into the general peritoneal cavity below, where an infection may spread from a perforated peptic ulcer or appendix, for example. The lesser sac, or left subhepatic space, connects to the right through the Winslow foramen. A pseudocyst of the pancreas may form from it filling with fluid due to an injury or inflammation to the pancreas, or from a perforation in the stomach's posterior wall. The liver's exposed region and the diaphragm are separated by the right extraperitoneal space. It may develop directly from a liver abscess or from retroperitoneal infections. The drainage of posterior subphrenic abscesses is accomplished by making an incision through the 12th rib's bed. The abscess cavity is then accessible by passing a finger between the liver and the diaphragm, upward and forward. An incision made below and parallel to the costal margin can also be used to drain a pus collection that is anteriorly positioned beneath the diaphragm. These days, percutaneous drainage of intra-abdominal fluid collections can frequently be carried out under CT or ultrasonography guidance (Flynn & Vickerton, 2023; Mikhael & Khan, 2024; Wade & Streitz, 2023).

4.5. The Gastrointestinal Tract

4.5.1. The Stomach

The stomach varies greatly in size and shape, but it generally has a J shape. Even within the same person, its shape varies depending on whether it is full or empty, the position of the body, and the phase of respiration. It tends to be high and transverse in the obese short subject and to be elongated in the asthenic individual. The stomach is composed of the anterior and posterior surfaces, the greater and lesser curvatures, and the cardia and pylorus orifices.

The stomach forms the dome-shaped gastric fundus, which protrudes to the left, above the level of the cardia. The stomach's body leads to a narrow section known as the pyloric antrum that is located just before the pylorus, between the cardia and the pylorus. An identifiable notch on the lesser curvature known as the incisura angularis indicates the location of the junction between the body and the pyloric antrum. The constant vein (of Mayo) that crosses the pylorus at this level and an external constriction indicate the junction with the duodenum.

The pyloric lumen is encircled by the readily palpable thickened sphincter. The pyloric sphincter is a physiological mechanism in addition to an anatomical structure. The cardia, on the other hand, lacks a distinct anatomical sphincter despite being competent (gastric contents do not flow out of your mouth if you stand on your head). Although the precise mechanism underlying the cardiac sphincter's action is still unknown, the following theories have been put forth and are backed by some experimental and clinical data (Figure 4.11).

1. Mucosal folds at the esophagogastric junction act as a valve.
2. The acute angle of entry of the esophagus into stomach produces a valvelike effect.
3. The circular muscle of the lower esophagus is a physiological, as distinct from an anatomical, sphincter.

4. The arrangement of the muscle fibers of the stomach around the cardia acts either as a sphincter or else maintains the acute angle of entry of esophagus into the stomach.
5. The right crus of the diaphragm acts as a 'pinch-cock' to the lower esophagus as it pierces this muscle.
6. The positive intra-abdominal pressure compresses the walls of the short segment of intra-abdominal esophagus.

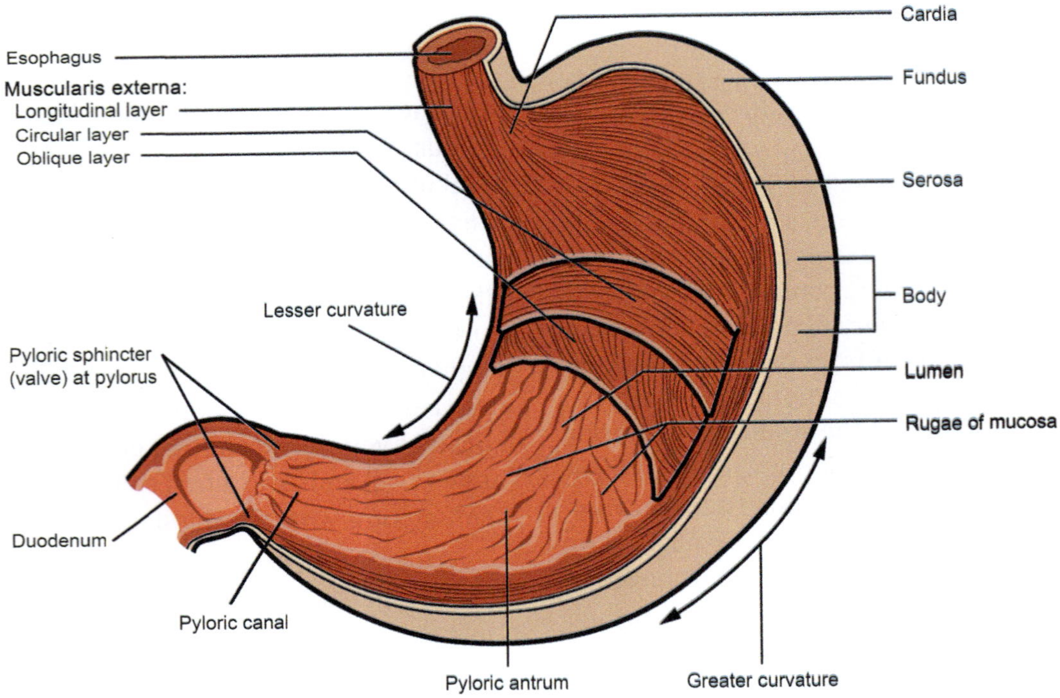

Figure 4.11. *The stomach and its subdivisions.*

Source: By OpenStax College – Anatomy & Physiology, Connexions Web site. http://cnx.org/content/col11496/1.6/, CC BY 3.0; https://commons.wikimedia.org/w/index.php?curid=30148437.

4.5.1.1. Relations of the Stomach

1. **Anteriorly:** The abdominal wall, the left costal margin, the diaphragm and the left lobe of the liver.
2. **Posteriorly:** The lesser sac, which separates the stomach from the pancreas, transverse mesocolon, left kidney, left suprarenal, the spleen and the splenic artery.
3. **Superiorly:** The left dome of the diaphragm.

The lesser omentum is attached along the lesser curvature of the stomach, the greater omentum along the greater curvature. These omenta contain the vascular and lymphatic supply of the stomach (Figures 4.12–4.14).

The arterial supply to the stomach is extremely rich and comprises:

- the left gastric artery—from the coeliac axis;
- the right gastric artery—from the hepatic artery;

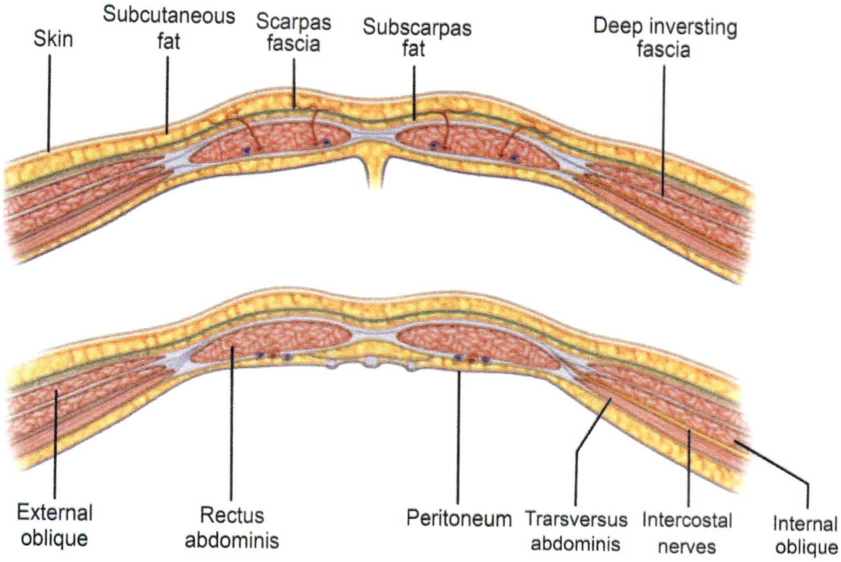

Figure 4.12. *Composition of the abdominal wall is shown.*

Source: Kriener, K., Lala, R., Homes, R. A. P., Finley, H., Sinclair, K., Williams, M. K., Midwinter, M. J., (2023). Mechanical characterization of the human abdominal wall using uniaxial tensile testing. Bioengineering, 10(10), 1213. https://doi.org/10.3390/bioengineering10101213.

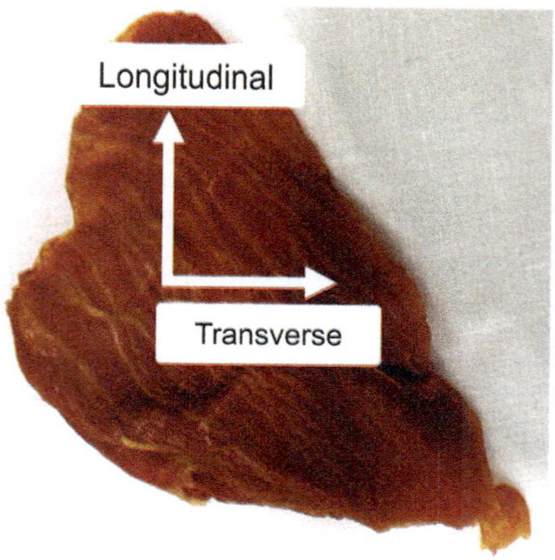

Figure 4.13. *Example of the external oblique muscle extracted in its in vivo orientation.*

Source: Kriener, K., Lala, R., Homes, R. A. P., Finley, H., Sinclair, K., Williams, M. K., & Midwinter, M. J., (2023). Mechanical characterization of the human abdominal wall using uniaxial tensile testing. Bioengineering, 10(10), 1213. https://doi.org/10.3390/bioengineering10101213.

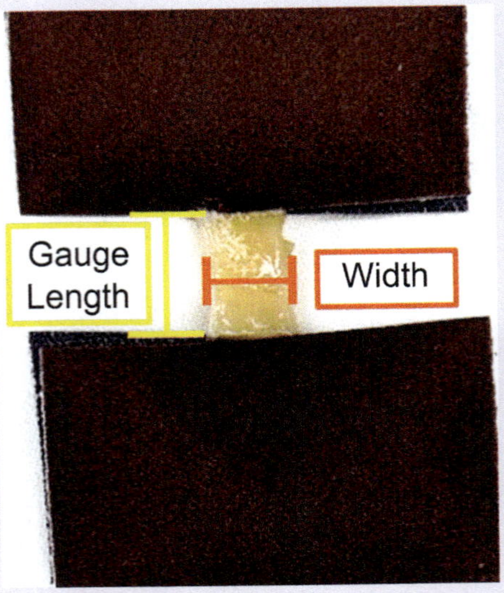

Figure 4.14. *A sample of parietal peritoneum adhered to grit paper. An example of locations for gauge length and width measurements are shown in this figure.*

Source: Kriener, K., Lala, R., Homes, R. A. P., Finley, H., Sinclair, K., Williams, M. K., & Midwinter, M. J., (2023). Mechanical characterization of the human abdominal wall using uniaxial tensile testing. Bioengineering, 10(10), 1213. https://doi.org/10.3390/bioengineering10101213.

- Area I drains along the right and left gastric vessels to the aortic nodes.
- Area II drains to the sub-pyloric and thence aortic nodes via lymphatics along the right gastro-epiploic vessels.
- Area III drains via lymphatics along the splenic vessels to the suprapancreatic nodes and thence to aortic nodes.
- the right gastro-epiploic artery—from the gastroduodenal branch of the hepatic artery;
- the left gastro-epiploic artery—from the splenic artery;
- the short gastric arteries—from the splenic artery.

The corresponding veins drain into the portal system. The lymphatic drainage of the stomach accompanies its blood vessels. The stomach can be divided into three drainage zones.

- **Area I:** The superior two-thirds of the stomach drain along the left and right gastric vessels to the aortic nodes.
- **Area II:** The right two-thirds of the inferior one-third of the stomach drain along the right gastro-epiploic vessels to the sub-pyloric nodes and thence to the aortic nodes.
- **Area III:** The left one-third of the greater curvature of the stomach drains along the short gastric and splenic vessels lying in the gastrosplenic and lienorenal ligaments, then, via the suprapancreatic nodes, to the aortic group.

One of the main issues in treating stomach cancer is the extensive lymphatic drainage and the technical impossibility of its total removal. Removing the spleen, the gastrosplenic and lienorenal ligaments, as well as the pancreatic body and tail, can address the involvement of the nodes along the splenic vessels. By removing the greater omentum, lymph nodes within the gastro-epiploic vessels are eliminated. However, the growth might be irreversible if the pancreatic head and the nodes surrounding the aorta are affected.

4.5.2. The Vagal Supply to the Stomach

The esophageal hiatus allows the anterior and posterior vagi to enter the abdomen. The larger posterior nerve is located at a slight distance from the stomach wall, while the anterior nerve is located near to it. Along with a sizable hepatic branch, the anterior vagus supplies branches to the cardia and stomach's lesser curve (Figure 4.15).

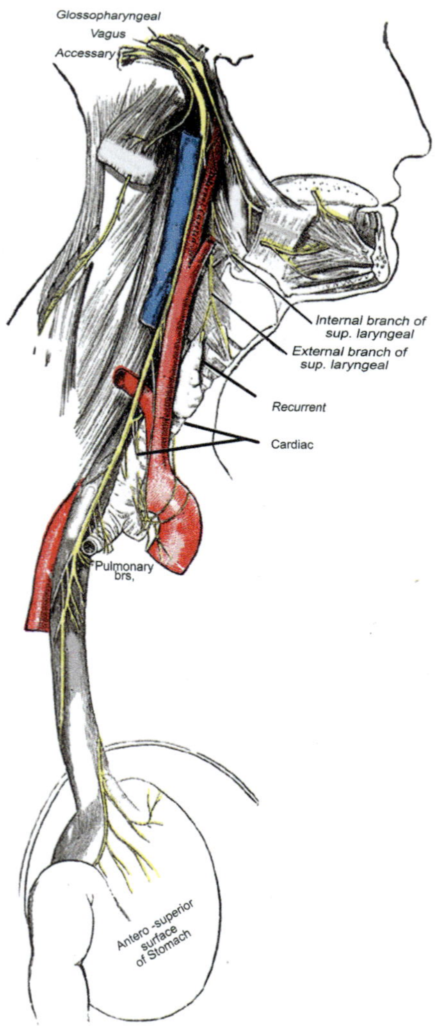

Figure 4.15. *The vagal supply to the stomach.*

Source: By Henry Vandyke Carter – Henry Gray, (1918). Anatomy of the human body (see "Book" section below) Bartleby.com: Gray's Anatomy, Plate 793, Public Domain; https://commons.wikimedia.org/w/index.php?curid=526636.

Although the majority of the nerve forms the celiac branch, the posterior vagus gives branches to the anterior and posterior parts of the stomach's body. This travels via the celiac ganglion along the left gastric artery before being distributed to the pancreas, the midtransverse colon, and the intestine. For a surgeon, the precise pathway taken by the vagal fibers to reach the stomach is crucial. The anterior and posterior nerves of Latarjet, which are the anterior and posterior peritoneal attachments of the lesser omentum, are where the gastric divisions of the anterior and posterior vagi enter the stomach at the cardia. They then descend along the lesser curvature. Because the anterior and posterior gastric nerves send terminal branches to the stomach, which supply the stomach's acid-secreting body while maintaining the pyloric innervation, can be divided (a procedure known as a highly selective vagotomy). The motor and secretory nerve supply to the stomach is provided by the vagus nerve. A pyloroplasty (to enlarge the pyloric exit and render the pyloric sphincter incompetent) or a gastrojejunostomy (to drain the stomach into the proximal small intestine) must always be performed in conjunction with total vagotomy because, when divided, the neurogenic (reflex) gastric acid secretion is abolished but the stomach is simultaneously rendered atonic so that it empties only with difficulty. By keeping the Latarjet nerve intact, it is possible to prevent drainage and preserve the pyloric antrum's innervation and function (very selective vagotomy).

4.5.2.1. Clinical Features

1. Back pain may be referred from a pancreas that is eroding due to a posterior gastric ulcer or cancer. A direct posterior relation, an ulcer into the splenic artery, can result in torrential bleeding.
2. The transverse mesocolon may be intimately connected to the stomach or greater omentum due to adhesions that may span the lesser sac. In these cases, there is a risk of injury to the middle colic vessels when the stomach is mobilized for a gastrectomy.
3. Radiology of the stomach. A simple erect abdominal film shows a gas bubble in the stomach fundus beneath the left diaphragm. Once the patient has ingested radio-opaque contrast material, such as barium sulfate, the stomach can be observed and its shape, position, and movements examined. These investigations have primarily revealed the wide variations in the position and shape of the stomach that we have already discussed. The opaque meal can be forced to press against the cardia by tipping the subject head-down; this will show that the sphincter mechanism is ineffective as barium will regurgitate into the esophagus.
4. Gastroscopy. Using a gastroscope, the mucosa of the air-inflated stomach can be examined in a living subject. The duodenum can be examined, the pancreatic and common bile ducts can be intubated for retrograde contrast-enhanced radiological study, and the entire stomach mucosa can be viewed with a modern fiber-optic instrument (Figure 4.16).

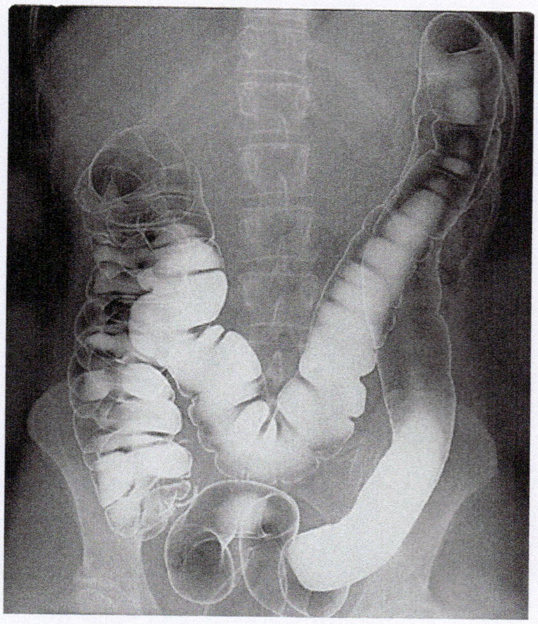

Figure 4.16. *Tracing the barium meal X-ray of the stomach.*

Source: By The original uploader was Glitzy queen00 at English Wikipedia. Own work by the original uploader, Public Domain; https://commons.wikimedia.org/w/index.php?curid=26525379.

4.5.3. The Duodenum

The duodenum forms a C-shaped curve around the head of the pancreas and measures 10 inches (25 cm) in length. Initially, it is fully surrounded by peritoneum for approximately 1 inch (2.5 cm) from its connection to the pylorus. However, it then transitions to being a retroperitoneal organ, with only partial coverage by the serous membrane.

4.5.3.1. Relations

The duodenum is segmented into four sections for descriptive purposes (Figures 4.17 and 4.18):

- The first part (2 in (5 cm)) ascends from the gastroduodenal junction, overlapped by the liver and gall bladder. Immediately posterior to it lie the portal vein, common bile duct, and gastroduodenal artery which separate it from the inferior vena cava.
- The second part (3 in (7.5 cm)) descends in a curve around the head of the pancreas. It is crossed by the transverse colon and lies on the right kidney and ureter. Halfway along, its posteromedial aspect enters the common opening of the bile duct and main pancreatic duct (of Wirsung) onto an eminence called the duodenal papilla. This common opening is guarded by the sphincter of Oddi. The subsidiary pancreatic duct (of Santorini) opens into the duodenum a little above the papilla.
- The third part (4 in (10 cm)) runs transversely to the left, crossing the inferior vena cava, the aorta, and the third lumbar vertebra. It is itself crossed anteriorly by the root of the mesentery and the superior mesenteric vessels. Its upper border hugs the pancreatic head.
- The fourth part (1 in (2.5 cm)) ascends upwards and to the left to end at the duodenojejunal junction. It is surprisingly easy for the surgeon to confuse this with the ileocecal junction, a mistake which may be disastrous. He confirms the identity of the duodenal termination by the presence of the suspensory ligament of Treitz, which is a well-marked peritoneal fold descending from the right crus of the diaphragm to the duodenal termination, and by visualizing the inferior mesenteric

vein which descends from behind the pancreas immediately to the left of the duodenojejunal junction.

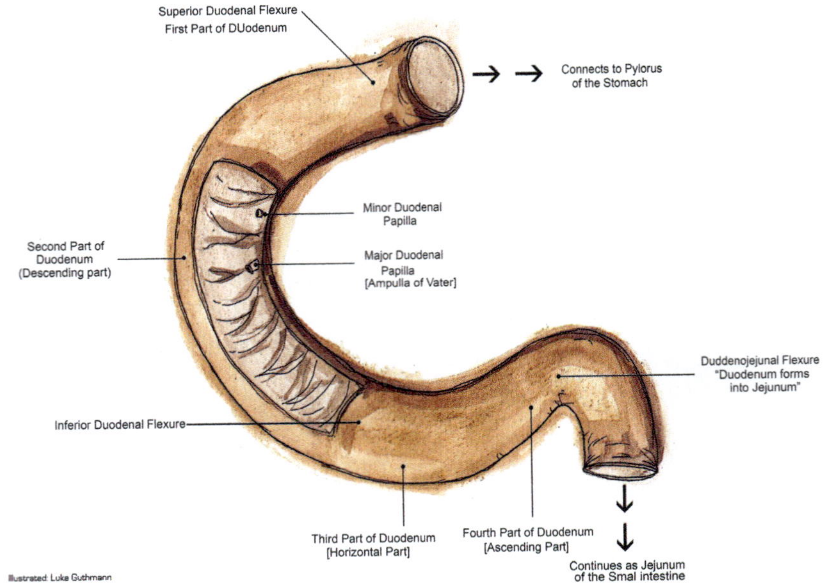

Figure 4.17. *The relations of the duodenum.*

Source: By Luke Guthmann – Own work, CC BY-SA 3.0; https://commons.wikimedia.org/w/index.php?curid=29376911.

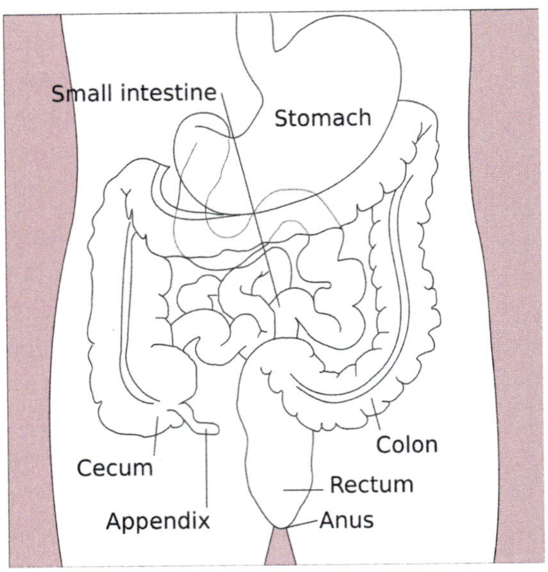

Figure 4.18. *The duodenum.*

Source: By Indolences created it on the English Wikipedia. This SVG image was created by Medium69. Cette image SVG a été créée par Medium69.Please credit this: William Crochot – US PD picture, Public Domain; https://commons.wikimedia.org/w/index.php?curid=1521879.

4.5.3.2. Blood Supply of the Duodenum

The inferior pancreaticoduodenal artery begins as the first branch of the superior mesenteric artery, while the superior pancreaticoduodenal artery emerges from the gastroduodenal artery. These blood vessels supply both the duodenum and the pancreatic head, which are curved in the same direction. It's interesting to note that, at the level of the duodenal papilla, their anastomosis symbolizes the point where the mid-gut, supplied by the superior mesenteric artery, and the fore-gut, supplied by the coeliac artery, converge.

4.5.3.3. Clinical Features

- The liver and gallbladder overlap the first segment of the duodenum and can adhere to or even become ulcerated by a duodenal ulcer. Additionally, a gallstone may develop an ulcer from the gallbladder's fundus into the duodenum. The gallstone may then cause intestinal blockage (gallstone ileus) by impacting in the lower ileum as it passes through the gut.
- Being the closest organ to the duodenum, the pancreas is easily infected by a posterior duodenal ulcer. If the patient has pain that extends to the dorsolumbar region, this should be suspected. Severe bleeding occurs when such an ulcer erodes the gastroduodenal artery.
- A duodenum scarred by severe ulceration may require extensive dissection to avoid damaging the common bile duct, which runs approximately 1 inch (2.25 cm) behind the duodenum's first portion. The duodenum's second portion may sustain damage during the right hemicolectomy due to the colon's hepatic flexure. Similarly, this portion of the duodenum is directly behind the right kidney, which could be damaged during a right nephrectomy.
- Radiology of the duodenum: After ingesting a barium meal, the duodenal cap, appearing as a triangular shadow, becomes visible within a few minutes. The duodenum contracts every few seconds, pushing out the contents of the cap which is then quickly refilled. This area is where most duodenal ulcers are found, with the possibility of seeing an ulcer filled with barium or scar tissue causing deformities in the cap. The rest of the duodenum can also be observed, with a floccular shadow due to the mucosa's rugose arrangement.
- Kocher's maneuver, which involves cutting the peritoneum lateral to the second part of the duodenum and creating an avascular plane between these structures and the posterior abdominal wall, is how the duodenum, the head of the pancreas, and the common bile duct are mobilized.

4.5.4. Small Intestine

The average length of the small intestine is approximately 24 feet (6.5 meters), although it can range from 10 to 33 feet (3–10 meters) in different subjects. A completely normal life can be maintained after resection of up to one-third or even half of the small intestine; survival has been documented with as little as 18 in (45 cm) of small intestine remaining. The superior mesenteric vessels, lymph nodes that drain the small intestine, and autonomic nerve fibers are all found in the mesentery of the small intestine, which extends 6 inches (15 cm) from the posterior abdominal wall to the right sacroiliac joint. It starts at the duodenojejunal junction, which is to the left of the second lumbar vertebra.

The jejunum refers to the upper portion of the small intestine, while the ileum is the lower portion. The two are not clearly different from one another, and this division is purely conventional. Nonetheless, the bowel does change characteristics from top to bottom. The surgeon can ascertain the level of a small intestine loop during an operation by referring to the following points.

1. The jejunum has a thicker wall as the circular folds of mucosa (valvulae conniventes) are larger and thicker more proximally.
2. The proximal small intestine is of greater diameter than the distal.
3. The jejunum tends to lie at the umbilical region, the ileum in the suprapubic region and pelvis.
4. The mesentery becomes thicker and more fat-laden from above downwards.
5. The mesenteric vessels form only one or two arcades to the jejunum, with long and relatively infrequent terminal branches passing to the gut wall. The ileum is supplied by shorter and more numerous terminal vessels arising from complete series of three, four or even five arcades.

4.5.5. Large Intestine

The large intestine is subdivided, for descriptive purposes, into (Figure 4.19):

- Caecum with the appendix vermiformis;
- Ascending colon (5–8 in (12–20 cm));
- Hepatic flexure;
- Transverse colon (18 in (45 cm));
- Splenic flexure;
- Descending colon (9–12 in (22–30 cm));
- Sigmoid colon (5–30 in (12–75 cm), average 15 in (37 cm));
- Rectum (5 in (12 cm));
- Anal canal (1.5 in (4 cm)).

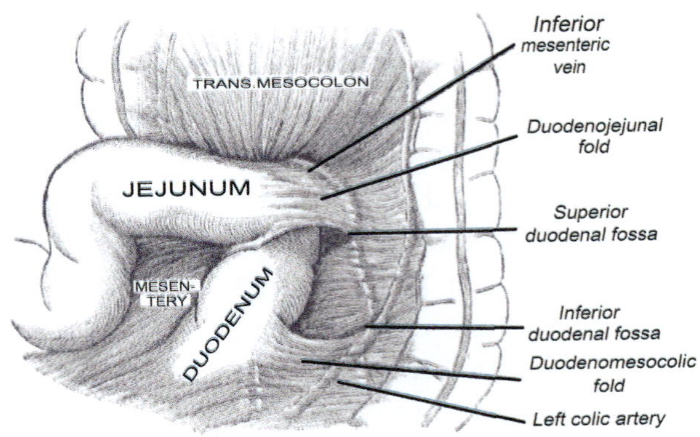

Figure 4.19. *The jejunum.*

Source: By Henry Vandyke Carter – Henry Gray, (1918). Anatomy of the human body (see "Book" section below) Bartleby.com: Gray's Anatomy, Plate 1041, Public Domain; https://commons.wikimedia.org/w/index.php?curid=545181.

The average length of the large bowel is about 5 feet (1.5 meters), though it can vary greatly among subjects. The colon has distinctive fat-filled peritoneal tags called appendices epiploic dispersed throughout its surface, but not the appendix, cecum, or rectum. These are particularly abundant in the colon of the sigmoid. The taeniae coli mark the colon and cecum, but not the appendix or rectum. These three flattened bands start at the appendix's base and extend all the way through the large intestine, ending at the rectosigmoid junction. They make up the majority of the long bowel's longitudinal muscle. The colon condenses into its characteristic sacculated shape because the taeniae are roughly a foot shorter than the gut to which they are attached. When the large bowel is enlarged, these sacculation's can be seen on an abdominal plain radiograph as incomplete septa protruding into the gas shadow. In contrast, the transverse mucosal folds of the valvulae conniventes produce complete transverse lines across the bowel shadow on the radiograph of a distended small intestine.

4.5.5.1. Peritoneal Attachments

Both the transverse colon and the sigmoid have fully developed peritoneum; the former can be easily recognized by its attachment to the greater omentum. While the descending and ascending colons stick to the posterior abdominal wall directly, they lack a mesocolon. In rare cases, the ascending colon does have a mesocolon. It is possible for the caecum to be fully peritonealized, and the appendix, which is normally free within its own mesentery, to occasionally lie extra peritoneally behind the ascending colon and caecum or attach itself to their posterior walls. In its upper third, the rectum is extraperitoneal on the posterior aspect; in its middle third, it is extraperitoneal posteriorly and laterally; and in its lower third, as it descends below the pelvic peritoneum, it is extraperitoneal fully.

4.5.6. The Appendix

The appendix is located approximately 1 inch (2.5 cm) below the ileocecal valve and originates from the posteromedial aspect of the caecum. Its length varies from 0.5 in (12 mm) to 9 in (22 cm). The caecum in a fetus directly protrudes, but its medial displacement is caused by the differential overgrowth of the lateral cecal wall. Compared to all other organs, the appendix's position varies the greatest. The appendix is usually located behind the caecum in 75% of cases.

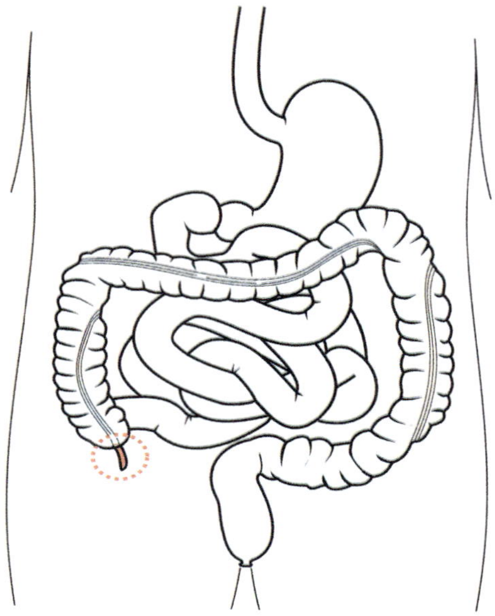

Figure 4.20. *The positions in which the appendix may lie, together with their approximate incidence.*

Source: By Olek Remesz (wiki-pl: Orem, commons: Orem) – Own work, CC BY-SA 2.5; https://commons.wikimedia.org/w/index.php?curid=2599162.

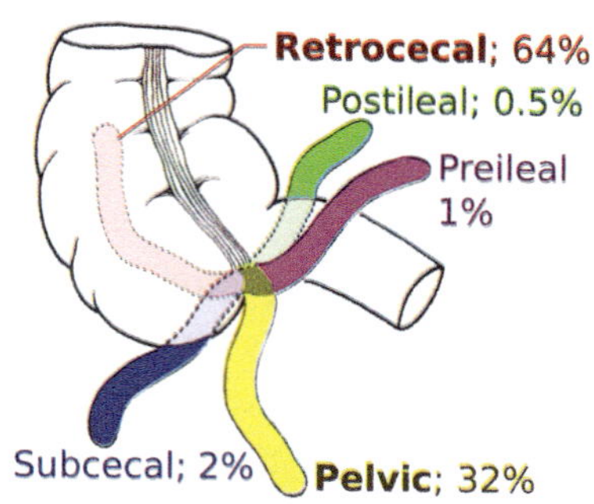

Figure 4.21. *The appendix.*

Source: *By Mikael Häggström, M.D. Author info – Reusing images – Conflicts of interest: NoneMikael Häggström, M.D. – Source image: Public Domain, CC0, https://commons.wikimedia.org/w/index.php?curid=87694884.*

Although it occasionally lies beneath the caecum's peritoneal covering, the appendix is normally fairly free in this position. The distal part of the appendix lies extra peritoneally in these situations. If the appendix is extremely long, it may stretch behind the ascending colon and abut the right kidney or the duodenum (Figures 4.20 and 4.21).

The appendix hangs down into the pelvis or lies just below the cecum in about 20% of cases. Less frequently, it lies in the right paracolic gutter, in front of the cecum, or passes in front of or behind the terminal ileum. The appendix has been known to ulcerate into the duodenum or perforate into the left paracolic gutter. It may well be said that 'the appendix is the only organ in the body that has no anatomy.'

The mesentery of the appendix, containing the appendicular branch of the ileocolic artery, descends behind the ileum as a triangular fold. Another peritoneal sheet, the ileocecal fold, passes to the appendix or to the base of the cecum from the front of the ileum. The ileocecal fold is termed the bloodless fold of Treves although, in fact, it often contains a vessel and, if cut, proves far from bloodless.

4.5.6.1. Clinical Features

- The appendix lumen is often entirely obliterated in the elderly, despite being relatively wide in infants. It is therefore not abnormal that appendicitis should be rare at the two extremes of life, since obstruction of the lumen is the typical precipitating cause of acute appendicitis.
- The appendix's whole vascular supply is represented by the appendicular artery. It travels distally along the wall of the appendix after initially running along the edge of the appendicular mesentery. An acute appendix infection may cause thrombosis in this artery, which can lead to gangrene developing quickly and a perforation later on. This is not the case with acute cholecystitis, where the liver bed's abundant collateral vascular supply guarantees that gallbladder gangrene is rare, even in the event that the cystic artery thromboses.
- Typically, an incision through the muscle splitting the right iliac fossa is used to perform an appendicectomy. The caecum is inserted into the wound, and if the appendix is not immediately apparent, it can be found by following the taeniae coli, which fuse at the appendix's base. It may be challenging to raise the appendix into the incision when the caecum is extraperitoneal; this can be overcome by first mobilizing the caecum by making incisions along the lateral and inferior borders of the nearly avascular peritoneum.
- The appendix mesentery, containing the appendicular vessels, is firmly tied and divided, the appendix base tied, the appendix removed, and its stump invaginated into the caecum.

4.5.7. The Rectum

The length of the rectum is 5 in (12 cm). It starts in front of the sacrum's third segment and finishes at the prostate's apex or the lower vaginal quarter, where it enters the anal canal. The rectum is curved in humans to fit into the sacral hollow, but it is straight in lower mammals—thus the name. Additionally, it exhibits three lateral inflections that project left, right, and left from above downward, and are capped by the Houston valves.

4.5.7.1. Relations

The rectum's primary relationships are significant. They are crucial for the local spread of rectal growths, must be seen when performing a rectal examination, and play a significant role in the surgical excision of the rectum. The middle sacral artery, the sacrum, and the coccyx are located posteriorly. They are divided from it by extraperitoneal connective tissue, which also contains lymphatics and rectal vessels. Growths spreading posteriorly from the rectum may involve the lower sacral nerves, which emerge from the anterior sacral foramina and cause excruciating sciatic pain.

The pouch of Douglas lies between the rectum and either the bladder or the uterus, and the upper two-thirds of the rectum are covered by the peritoneum. These coils of small intestine are related to the pouch. The vagina in women and the prostate, bladder base, and seminal vesicles in men are located in front of the lower one-third. The plane of dissection that must be pursued in order to excise the rectum is formed by a layer of fascia (Denon Villiers) that divides it from the anterior structures. The levator ani provides lateral support for the rectum (Table 4.1).

Table 4.1. *The Criteria for the Diagnosis and Staging of Appendiceal Adenocarcinomas*

T Category	T Criteria
TX	Primary tumor cannot be assessed.
T0	No evidence of primary tumor.
Tis	Carcinoma *in situ* (intramucosal carcinoma; invasion of the lamina propria or extension into but not through the muscularis mucosae).
Tis (LAMN)	Low-grade appendiceal mucinous neoplasm confined by the muscularis propria. Acellular mucin or mucinous epithelium may invade the muscularis propria. T1 and T2 are not applicable to LAMN. Acellular mucin or mucinous epithelium that extends into the subserosa or serosa should be classified as T3 or T4a, respectively.
T1	Tumor invades the submucosa (through the muscularis mucosa but not into the muscularis propria).
T2	Tumor invades the muscularis propria.
T3	Tumor invades through the muscularis propria into the subserosa or the mesoappendix.
T4	Tumor invades the visceral peritoneum, including the acellular mucin or mucinous epithelium involving the serosa of the appendix or mesoappendix, and/or directly invades adjacent organs or structures.
T4a	Tumor invades through the visceral peritoneum, including the acellular mucin or mucinous epithelium involving the serosa of the appendix or serosa of the mesoappendix.
T4b	Tumor directly invades or adheres to adjacent organs or structures.

Note: The criteria for the diagnosis and staging of appendiceal adenocarcinomas, according to the AJCC Staging Manual (2017) [Amin M.B.,et al. 2017] and WHO Classification of Tumors of the Digestive System (2019) [10]: definition of the primary tumor (T).

N Category	N Criteria
NX	Regional lymph nodes cannot be assessed.
N0	No regional lymph node metastasis.

N1	One to three regional lymph nodes are positive (tumor in lymph node measuring ≥ 0.2 mm), or any number of tumor deposits is present, and all identifiable lymph nodes are negative.
N1a	One regional lymph node is positive.
N1b	Two or three regional lymph nodes are positive.
N1c	No regional lymph nodes are positive, but there are tumor deposits in the subserosa or mesentery.
N2	Four or more regional lymph nodes are positive.

Note: The criteria for the diagnosis and staging of appendiceal adenocarcinomas, according to the AJCC Staging Manual (2017) [Amin M.B.,et al. 2017] and WHO Classification of Tumors of the Digestive System (2019) [Nagtegaal I.D.,2020]: definition of regional lymph node (N).

M Category	M Criteria
M0	No distant metastasis.
M1	Distant metastasis.
M1a	Intraperitoneal acellular mucin, without identifiable tumor cells in the disseminated peritoneal mucinous deposits.
M1b	Intraperitoneal metastasis only, including peritoneal mucinous deposits containing tumor cells.
M1c	Metastasis to sites other than the peritoneum.

Note: The criteria for the diagnosis and staging of appendiceal adenocarcinomas, according to the AJCC Staging Manual (2017) [Amin M.B.,et al. 2017] and WHO Classification of Tumors of the Digestive System (2019) [Nagtegaal I.D.,2020]: definition of distant metastasis (M).

G	G Definition
GX	Grade cannot be assessed.
G1	Well-differentiated.
G2	Moderately differentiated.
G3	Poorly differentiated.

Note: The criteria for the diagnosis and staging of appendiceal adenocarcinomas, according to the AJCC Staging Manual (2017) [Amin M.B.,et al. 2017] and WHO Classification of Tumors of the Digestive System (2019) [Nagtegaal I.D.,2020]: definition of histologic grade (G).

TNM	Grade	Stage Group
Tis N0 M0	–	0
Tis(LAMN) N0 M0	–	0
T1 N0 M0	–	I
T2 N0 M0	–	I
T3 N0 M0	–	IIA
T4a N0 M0	–	IIB
T4b N0 M0	–	IIC
T1 N1 M0	–	IIIA
T2 N1 M0	–	IIIA
T3 N1 M0	–	IIIB
T4 N1 M0	–	IIIB
T(any) N2 M0	–	IIIC
T(any) N(any) M1a	–	IVA
T(any) N(any) M1b	G1	IVA
T(any) N(any) M1b	G2, G3, or GX	IVB
T(any) N(any) M1c	Any G	IVC

Note: The criteria for the diagnosis and staging of appendiceal adenocarcinomas, according to the AJCC Staging Manual (2017) [Amin M.B.,et al. 2017] and WHO Classification of Tumors of the Digestive System (2019) [Nagtegaal I.D.,2020]: AJCC prognostic stage groups.

Source: Constantin, M., Petrescu, L., Mătanie, C., Vrancianu, C. O., Niculescu, A. G., Andronic, O., & Bolocan, A., (2023). The vermiform appendix and its pathologies. Cancers, 15(15), 3872. https://doi.org/10.3390/cancers15153872.

4.5.8. The Anal Canal

The anal orifice is the end of the 1.5-inch (4-cm) anal canal, which extends from the rectum downward and backward. The mid-anal canal is the point where the ectoderm of the cutaneous invagination, known as the proctodaeum, and the endoderm of the hindgut converge. Imperforate anus is caused by the separating membrane failing to break down.

- The upper half is lined by columnar epithelium, which is connected at their distal extremities by folds that resemble valves and consists of vertical columns of mucosa, known as the columns of Morgagni. The lower half is lined by squamous epithelium. Thus, an adenocarcinoma of the upper anal canal is different from a squamous tumor arising from the lower part.
- The inferior rectal vessels, which originate from the internal pudendal and ultimately the internal iliac vessels, supply blood to the lower half of the anal canal, while the superior rectal vessels supply blood to the upper half. As a result of their communication, the two venous systems create one of the anastomoses connecting the portal and systemic circulations.
- The lymphatics above this mucocutaneous junction drain along the superior rectal vessels to the lumbar nodes, whereas below this line, drainage is to the inguinal nodes. A carcinoma of the rectum that invades the lower anal canal may thus metastasize to the groin nodes.
- The somatic inferior rectal nerve, a terminal branch of the pudendal nerve, supplies the lower part of the anal canal; the autonomic plexuses supply the upper part. As a result, the lower canal is sensitive to the prick of a hypodermic needle, but injecting sclerosant fluid into an internal hemorrhoid by inserting the needle through the upper canal's mucosa causes no pain.

4.5.8.1. The Anal Sphincter

A complex muscle arrangement that forms the walls of the anal canal functions as a potent sphincter mechanism. This comprises:

- the internal anal sphincter, of involuntary muscle, which continues above with the circular muscle coat of the rectum;
- the external anal sphincter, of voluntary muscle, which surrounds the internal sphincter and which extends further downwards and curves medially to occupy a position below and slightly lateral to the lower rounded edge of the internal sphincter, close to the skin of the anal orifice. The lowermost, or subcutaneous, portion of the external sphincter is traversed by a fan-shaped expansion of the longitudinal muscle fibers of the anal canal which continue above with the longitudinal muscle of the rectal wall. At its upper end, the external sphincter fuses with the fibers of the levator ani.

The anorectal ring is the muscle ring that is located slightly over an inch from the anal margin when performing a digital rectal examination. This indicates the junction of the anal canal and rectum, as well as the deep portion of the external sphincter where it merges with the internal sphincter and levator ani. The anal canal is connected anteriorly to the perineal body that divides it from the lower vagina in females and the bulb of the urethra in males, laterally to the ischiorectal fossae containing fat, and posteriorly to the fibrous tissue that separates it from the coccyx (anococcygeal body). Because it relates to the anal canal rather than the rectum, the ischiorectal fossa is now more correctly known as the ischioanal fossa.

4.5.8.2. Rectal Examination

The following structures can be palpated by the finger passed per rectum in the normal patient:

- **Both Sexes:** The anorectal ring (see above), coccyx and sacrum, ischiorectal fossae, ischial spines.
- **Male:** Prostate, rarely the healthy seminal vesicles.
- **Female:** Perineal body, cervix, occasionally the ovaries.

Abnormalities which can be detected include:

- **Within the Lumen:** Fecal impaction, foreign bodies.
- **In the Wall:** Rectal growths, strictures, granulomata, etc., but not hemorrhoids unless these are thrombosed.
- **Outside the Rectal Wall:** Pelvic bony tumors, abnormalities of the prostate or seminal vesicle, distended bladder, uterine or ovarian enlargement, collections of fluid or neoplastic masses in the pouch of Douglas.

Do not be deceived by foreign objects placed in the vagina. The commonest are a tampon or a pessary. During parturition, dilatation of the cervical os can be assessed by rectal examination since it can be felt quite easily through the rectal wall.

4.5.8.3. Clinical Features

4.5.8.3.1. Hemorrhoids

A dilation of the superior rectal vein is called hemorrhoids, or piles. They are first contained in the anal canal (1st degree), then they progressively enlarge, prolapse during defecation (2nd degree), and ultimately stay prolapsed through the anal orifice (3rd degree). The anatomic components of each pile are as follows: terminal branches of the corresponding superior rectal artery; a covering of anal canal mucosa and submucosa; and a venous plexus draining into one of the superior rectal veins (Table 4.2).

Table 4.2. *Chosen Aspects of Comparative Analysis of Human Perianal Crohn's Disease (PCD) and Canine Anal Furunculosis (AF)*

		Humans – Perianal Crohn's Disease	**Dogs – Anal Furunculosis**	**References**
Symptoms	Association of perianal disease with bowel inflammation.	Established. Only about 5% of patients with perianal CD do not have concurrent luminal form of CD.	Probable. Around 39% of dogs with diagnosed AF do not present histological symptoms of colitis or endoscopic signs of proctitis.	[Pogacnik J.S., et al. 2019]

	Perianal symptoms	Fissures, skin tags, ulcers, abscesses, true fistulas with two openings, anal strictures.	Perianal blind sinuses, ulcerations, fistulas communicating with anal sac or anorectum (the incidence of true fistulas with two openings not established).	[Panés J., et al. 2017]
Response to Pharmacologic Therapy	Antibiotics	Proven to reduce drainage of perianal fistulas, not to induce healing, recommended as adjunctive therapy.	Efficacy not proven, sometimes used as adjunctive therapy.	[Panés J., et al. 2017]
	Cyclosporine (CsA)	Efficacy not proven—not recommended.	Proven efficacy—recommended.	[Gecse K.B., et al. 2014]
	Thiopurine derivatives (i.e., azathioprin).	Moderate efficacy—recommended.	Moderate efficacy based on scant data, sometimes used if CsA therapy is not possible (due to economic reasons or availability problems).	[Dejaco C., et al. 2003]
	Anti-TNF	Proven efficacy—recommended.	Not tested, caninized anti-TNF not available.	[Shehab M., et al. 2022]
Pathogenesis	Genetic factors	The role of genes encoding MHC molecules (generally for CD)—confirmed.	The role of genes encoding MHC molecules (DLA-DRB1)—confirmed.	[Mahdi B.M. 2015]
		The role of SNPs in *NOD2* (one of PPRs) (specifically in pCD) – confirmed.	The role of SNPs in chosen PPRs (including NOD2) failed to be confirmed.	[Schnitzler F., et al. 2015]
		The role of TNF pathway genes (specifically for pCD)—confirmed.	The role of TNF pathway not confirmed.	[Kaur M., et al. 2016]
		The role of other genes associated with cell adhesion, extracellular matrix, scaffolding proteins or autophagy indicated (specifically for pCD).	6 non-synonymous SNPs identified to be related to AF. The most significantly associated genes were *ADAMTS16* and *CTNND2*.	[Kaur M., et al. 2016]
	Intestinal microbiota	Association of gut microbiota with pCD confirmed. Dichotomy of microbiome into dysbiotic and non-dysbiotic reported.	Association of gut microbiota with AF confirmed. Dichotomy of microbiome into dysbiotic and non-dysbiotic reported.	[Lloyd-Price J., et al. 2019]

	Disturbances in T cell mediated immunity.	Association of abnormal T cell response with pCD confirmed. Excessive Th1 response; Excessive Th17 response.	Association of abnormal T cell response with AF confirmed. Excessive Th1 response; role of Th17 response not studied.	[Maggi L., et al. 2013]
	Metallo-proteinases (MMPs).	Elevated expression of MMP-2, MMP-9, and MMP-13 in pCD fistulas.	Elevated expression of *MMP9* and *MMP13* but not *MMP2* in perianal tissue of dogs with AF.	[Altadill A., et al. 2012]
	Epithelial-to-mesenchymal transition.	The EMT process confirmed to be involved in the formation of CD-related fistulas.	The association of EMT process and AF not studied.	[Siegmund B., et al. 2016]

Source: Burdzinska, A., Galanty, M., Więcek, S., Dabrowski, F. A., Lotfy, A., & Sadkowski, T., (2022). The intersection of human and veterinary medicine – A possible direction towards the improvement of cell therapy protocols in the treatment of perianal fistulas. International Journal of Molecular Sciences, 23(22), 13917. https://doi.org/10.3390/ijms232213917.

It would be more accurate to refer to the so-called "thrombosed external pile" as a perianal hematoma instead of the tiny, tense hemorrhage at the anal margin brought on by a subcutaneous vein rupture.

4.5.8.4. Perianal Abscesses

These can be found subcutaneously beneath perianal skin, submucosally beneath the anal mucosa, or within the ischiorectal (-anal) fossa, or, for anatomical precision, the ischio. Abscesses can occasionally be found deep to the pelvic peritoneum, beside the rectum, and above the levator ani.

4.5.8.5. Fistulae

Anal fistulae usually result from rupture of perianal abscesses. They are classified anatomically and may be:

- **Submucous:** Confined to the tissues immediately below the anal mucosa;
- **Subcutaneous:** Confined to the perianal skin;
- **Low-Level:** Passing through the lower part of the superficial sphincter (most common);
- **High-Level:** Passing through the deeper part of the superficial sphincter;
- **Anorectal:** This which has its track passing above the anorectal ring and which may or may not open into the rectum.

In laying open fistulae in ano, it is essential to preserve the anorectal ring if fecal incontinence is to be avoided. The lower part of the sphincter, on the other hand, can be divided quite safely without this risk.

4.5.8.6. Fissure in Ano

More than 90% of these anal mucosal tears occur posteriorly in the midline. The insertion of the superficial component of the external anal sphincter posteriorly into the coccyx is most likely the anatomical basis for this; between the two limbs of the V that is thus formed, the mucosa is relatively unsupported and may therefore be torn at this site by a hard fecal mass (Tables 4.3–4.5).

Table 4.3. *Evidence of Biologic and Small Molecule Therapy in Perianal Fistulizing Crohn's Disease (pCD)*

Therapy	Evidence to Date in pCD
Anti-TNF	Present et al. showed a 50% reduction in fistula drainage in 68% of patients in the Infliximab 5 mg/kg induction dose cohort compared to 26% of patients treated with the placebo ($p = 0.002$) [Present D.H., et al. 1999]. The ACCENT II trial then went on to show that maintenance IFX for a period of 54 weeks was superior to the placebo in patients who responded to induction therapy [Sands B.E., et al. 2004]. At week 54, 36% of patients in the IFX maintenance group had a complete absence of draining fistulas compared with 19% in the placebo group ($p = 0.009$) [Sands B.E., et al. 2004]. Furthermore, multiple retrospective studies have assessed the benefit of Infliximab including higher serum levels (ranging from >7.2 to >20) [Yarur A.J., et al. 2017, Davidov Y., et al. 2017, Papamichael K., et al. 2021] corresponding to improved clinical and radiological remission outcomes [Yarur A.J., et al. 2017, Davidov Y., et al. 2017, Papamichael K., et al. 2021, De Gregorio M., et al. 2022, Zhu M., et al. 2021, Plevris N., et al. 2020, Strik A.S., et al. 2019]. In the subgroup analysis of the CHARM study, fistula healing was seen in approximately 60% of patients after two years of Adalimumab therapy [Colombel J.F., et al. 2007]. In the CHOICE trial, 39% of patients who had complete fistula healing due to Adalimumab therapy were primary or secondary non-responders to Infliximab [Lichtiger S., et al. 2010]. However, the ACCESS study suggested that fistula healing rates in Adalimumab-treated patients were much higher for Infliximab-naïve patients than Infliximab-experienced patients (60% versus 28%, respectively; $p < 0.01$) [Panaccione R., et al. 2011]. Similar to studies of Infliximab in pCD, higher Adalimumab serum levels correlated with improved fistula outcomes [Plevris N., et al. 2020, Strik A.S., et al. 2019]. Furthermore, local intra-fistula Anti-TNF injections have also been trialed in small pilot studies with mixed results and a lack of long-term data [Adegbola S.O., et al. 2017].
Ustekinumab	A subgroup analysis of the pivotal studies of Ustekinumab in CD (UNITI-1, UNITI-2 and CERTIFI) showed complete fistula resolution in 25% of all pooled Ustekinumab patients at week 8 compared to only 14% of the pooled placebo group patients with active fistula ($p = 0.073$) [Sands B.O., et al. 2017]. In addition, a post-hoc pooled of the STARDUST and SEAVUE studies showed an overall 50% of patients receiving Ustekinumab had clinical fistula healing at the end of the study with no impact of trough levels or dosing intervals seen in the small numbers of patients studied (17 and 12, respectively) [Laurent P., et al. 2022]. A Dutch nationwide prospective observational cohort study of 28 patients showed 36% complete clinical resolution after 24 weeks of treatment in patients who had prior anti-TNF exposure [Biemans V.B.C., et al. 2020]. The Bio-LAP multicenter study from the GETAID group showed clinical success at 6 months (as assessed by the physician's judgment without additional medical or surgical treatment) occurred in 38.5% (57/148) of patients. In this study, 33% of patients (29/88) with setons at Ustekinumab initiation had successful removal [Chapuis-Biron C., et al. 2020].

	Finally, a recent retrospective analysis showed that in patients who had received at least 16 weeks of Ustekinumab therapy, clinical remission and response rates were 40.7% and 63.0%, respectively. The study also went on to show radiological healing observed in 44.8% [Chapuis-Biron C., et al. 2020]. An Ustekinumab trough concentration over 2.11 μg/mL was correlated with a higher likelihood of perianal fistula clinical remission [Yao J., et al. 2023].
Vedolizumab	The GETAID Bio-LAP study also assessed 102 patients with active perianal disease treated with Vedolizumab, in whom success was reached in 23 patients (23%). Among patients with setons at initiation, 9/61 (15%) had a successful removal [Chapuis-Biron C., et al. 2020]. The ENTERPRISE study was a randomized trial evaluating the effectiveness of two different 22-week Vedolizumab treatment regimens in pCD with 78.6% of the patients having had previous Anti-TNF exposure [Schwartz D.A., et al. 2021]. Unfortunately, the study was ceased prematurely due to recruitment challenges resulting in low patient counts and as a result, all analyses were descriptive. In the standard dosing group, 9/14 patients (64%) showed ≥50% reduction from the baseline in the number of draining perianal fistulae at week 30 [Schwartz D.A., et al. 2021]. In contrast, only 6/14 patients (43%) in the group that received an additional week 10 dose achieved ≥50% reduction in drainage [Schwartz D.A., et al. 2021].
Small molecules	Filgotinib, a selective JAK1 inhibitor, has shown good efficacy in pCD in the Phase II DIVERGENCE 2 study. The proportion of patients who achieved a combined fistula response at week 24 was numerically higher in the FIL 200 mg group (47.1%; 90% confidence interval [CI]: 26.0–68.9) than in the PBO group (25.0%; 90% CI: 7.2–52.7) [Reinisch W., et al. 2022]. Upadacitinib (UPA), another selective JAK1 inhibitor, has shown some promise in its pivotal studies. The subgroup analysis of U-EXCEL, U-EXCEED, and U-ENDURE studies showed that 124 patients had perianal fistulas. Of these, the proportion of patients who achieved the complete resolution of draining and ≥50% reduction in draining was higher with UPA vs placebo at week 12 (47.7% vs. 9.1%; p = 0.002 and 50.0% vs. 13.6%; p = 0.004). However, the response was not statistically significant at week 52 [Colombel J.F., et al. 2023].

Source: Anandabaskaran, S., Hanna, L., Iqbal, N., Constable, L., Tozer, P., & Hart, A., (2023). Where are we and where to next? – The future of perianal Crohn's disease management. Journal of Clinical Medicine, 12(19), 6379. https://doi.org/10.3390/jcm12196379.

Table 4.4. *Summary of Selected Studies of Medical Therapy in Fistulizing Crohn's Disease*

Study (Year)	Study Design	No.	Fistula Type (%)	Intervention and/or Comparator	Study Endpoint (Duration)	Main Result
Infliximab (IFX)						
Present et al. (1999)	RCT	94	Perianal (90%) Abdominal (10%)	IFX (56) vs. PBO (29)	Fistula response: 50% closure, fistula remission: 100% closure (18 months).	Fistula response rate: IFX 62% vs. PBO 26% (p = 0.002) fistula remission rate: IFX 46% vs. PBO 13% (p = 0.001).
Sands (2004) (ACCENT II)	RCT	282	Perianal (87%), abdominal (11%), rectovaginal (8%).	IFX (96) vs. PBO (99)	Time to the loss of response in maintenance phase (14 and 54 weeks).	IFX > 40 weeks vs. PBO 14 weeks (p < 0.001), complete response rate at 54 weeks: (IFX 36% vs. PBO 19%, p = 0.009).
West et al. (2004)	RCT	24	Perianal (100%)	IFX + CIP (11) vs. IFX + PBO (13)	Response: 50% reduction in the number of draining fistulas (18 weeks).	The higher response rate in IFX + CIP; 73% vs. IFX + PBO; 39%, p = 0.12.
Bouguen et al. (2013)	Retrospective	156	Perianal (100%)	IFX + AZA (90) vs. IFX alone (66)	Fistula closure (five years)	Combined therapy was associated with an increased rate of fistula closure (HR 2.58, 1.16–5.6; p = 0.02).

Zhu et al. (2021)	Retrospective	178	Perianal (100%)	IFX (178)	Clinical and radiological (MRI) (135 weeks).	Clinical remission and response: 55.1% and 26.4%, radiological remission and response: 38.2% and 34.3%, respectively.
Lee et al. (2018)	Meta-analysis	432	Perianal and non-perianal fistulas.	Six studies anti-TNFs (267) vs. PBO (165).	Fistula remission and response.	Induction remission rates; anti-TNFs 34% (90/267) vs. PBO 16% (26/165). Pooled RR: 2.01 (95% CI, 1.36–2.97, p < 0.001). In the maintenance therapy, fistula remission: anti-TNFs 35% (43/124) vs. PBO 18% (23/129), pooled RR: 1.94 (95% CI, 1.25–3.02, p = 0.003).
Adalimumab (ADA)						
Hanauer et al. (2006) (Classic I)	RCT	32	Perianal, enterocutaneous (NS)	ADA (26) vs. PBO (6)	Response: 50% closure, remission: 100% closure (4 weeks).	No significant difference in fistula healing rates ADA vs. PBO.

Sandborn et al. (2007) (GAIN)	RCT	45	Perianal, abdominal (NS)	ADA (20) vs. PBO (25)	Response: 50% closure, remission 100% closure (4 weeks).	No difference in fistula response: ADA 15% vs. PBO 20% and remission: ADA 5% vs. PBO 8%.
Colombel et al. (2009) (CHARM)	RCT and post hoc	117	Perianal (97%), abdominal (3%).	ADA (70) vs. PBO (47)	Fistula healing (100% closure) (two years).	At 26 weeks: ADA 30% vs. PBO 13%, $p = 0.043$, and at 52 weeks: ADA 33% vs. PBO 13%, $p = 0.016$, and 90% of patients who had fistula healing maintained healing until two years.
Dewint et al. (2014) (ADAFI)	RCT	76	Perianal (100%)	ADA + CIP (36) vs. ADA (34)	Fistula response: 50% closer, remission: 100% closure (12 and 24 weeks).	Fistula response at 12 weeks: ADA + CIP 71% and ADA + PBO 47%, $p = 0.047$ and remission: ADA + CIP 65% and ADA + PBO 33%, $p = 0.009$. The response was not maintained at 24 weeks.
Lichtiger et al. (2010) (CHOICE)	Phase IIIb single-arm	88	Perianal (93%), enterocutaneous (13%)	ADA (88)	Fistula healing: 100% closure (36 weeks).	Fistula healing rate: 39% during a follow-up visit (4–36 weeks).

Castaño-Milla et el. (2015)	Retrospective	46	Perianal (100%)	ADA (46)	Fistula healing and response (6 and 12 months).	Fistula responses: 72% and 49% of patients at 6 and 12 months, respectively.
Ji & Takano (2017)	Retrospective	47	Perianal (100%)	ADA (16) vs. IFX (31)	Recurrence-free and disease progression (two years).	No significant difference between IFX 83.9% vs. ADA 62.5%, p = 0.09.
Ustekinumab (UST)						
Sand (2017) (UNITI-1, UNITI-2, CERTIFI)	Post hoc analysis	238	Perianal (100%)	UST (161) vs. PBO (77)	Fistula healing: 100% closure, response: 50% closure (8 weeks).	Fistula healing: UST 24.7% vs. 14.1% PBO (p = 0.073); no significant fistula response between the groups.
Chapuis-Biron et al. (2020) (LioLAP)	Retrospective	207	Perianal (100%)	UST 207	Success rate: no need for surgical or additional treatment (52 weeks).	In patients with active fistula, success rate: 38.5% (57/148), successful seton removal: 33% (29/88), and recurrence-free survival: 75.1%.
Ma et al. (2017)	Retrospective	45	Perianal (100%)	UST (45)	Completed healing on imaging (12 months)	31.1% of patients achieved complete radiologic healing (MRI or contrast-enhanced pelvic ultrasound).

Biemans et al. (2020)	Prospective observational	28	Perianal (100%)	UST (28)	Fistula response and remission (24 weeks).	Complete clinical remission: 35.7% and clinical response: 14.3%.
Attauabi et al. (2020)	Meta-analysis	396	Perianal (100%)	Nine studies UST (396)	Fistula response and remission (52 weeks).	The pooled fistula response: 41.0%, 39.7%, and 55.9% at weeks 8, 24, and 52, respectively. Pooled fistula remission: 17.1%, 17.7%, and 16.7% at week 8, 24, and 52, respectively.
Brewer et al. (2021)	Meta-analysis	209	Perianal (100%)	25 studies UST (209)	Fistula response (6 and 12 months).	Clinical response: 44% and 53.9% at 6 and 12 months, respectively.
Vedolizumab (VDZ)						
Feagan et al. (2018) (GEMINI 2)	Post hoc analysis	57	Perianal (79%), NS (21%)	VDZ (39) vs. PBO (18)	Fistula closure; no drainage (14 and 52 weeks).	Fistula closure at week 14: VDZ 28% vs. PBO 11% (ARR: 17.1%; 95% CI, −11.4 to 43.9). At week 52: VDZ 33% vs. PBO 11% (ARR: 19.7%; 95% CI, −8.9 to 46.2).

Chapuis-Biron et al. (2020)	Retrospective	151	Perianal (100%)	VDZ (151)	Clinical remission, seton removal and recurrence rate (6 months).	In patients with active fistula, clinical remission: 22.5%, successful seton removal: 9/61 (15%), and in patients with inactive fistula, the perianal disease recurrence: 30.6%.
Ayoub et al. (2022)	Meta-analysis	198	Perianal (100%)	Four studies VDZ (198)	Complete and partial fistula healing.	The pooled complete healing rate: 27.6% (95% CI, 18.9–37.3%), pooled partial healing rate: 34.9% (95% CI, 23.2–47.7%).
Filgotinib (FIL)						
Reinish et al. (2022) (DIVERG-ENCE2)	RCT	57	Perianal (100%)	Filgotinib (42) vs. PBO (15)	Combined clinical and MRI response/ remission (24 weeks).	Fistula response was numerically higher in the FIL 200 mg group (47.1%; CI: 26.0–68.9) vs. PBO group (25.0%; CI: 7.2–52.7). Fistula remission (FIL 200 mg (47.1%; CI: 26.0–68.9) vs. PBO (16.7%; CI: 3.0–43.8)).

Therapeutic Drug Monitoring (TDM)						
Papamichael et al. (2021)	Post hoc of the ACCENT-II	282	Perianal (87%), abdominal (11%), rectovaginal (8%).	IFX level high vs. low	Fistula remission (54 weeks)	The higher post-induction IFX levels were associated with remission (OR: 2.05; 95% CI: 1.10–3.82). IFX level of 15 mg/mL at week 6 and 7.2 mg/mL at week 14 stratified early fistula remission.
Yarur et al. (2017)	Observational	117	Perianal (100%)	TDM level high vs. low	Fistula healing (29 weeks)	IFX levels: patients with healing: 15.8 ug/mL vs. no healing: 4.4 ug/mL, $p < 0.001$. The cut-off > 10.1 mcg/mL and >20.3 mcg/mL predict fistula healing 3- and 8-fold, respectively.
Gregorio et al. (2021)	Retrospective	193	Perianal (100%)	TDM level in active vs. remission.	Radiologic response on MRI (2.1 years ADA, 2.5 years IFX).	Anti-TNF levels in patients with MRI remission vs. active disease: IFX; 7.4 vs. 3.9 mg/mL; and ADA; 9.8 vs. 6.2 mg/mL.

Source: *Wetwittayakhlang, P., Al-Khoury, A., Hahn, G. D., & Lakatos, P. L., (2022). The optimal management of fistulizing Crohn's disease: Evidence beyond randomized clinical trials. Journal of Clinical Medicine, 11(11), 3045. https://doi.org/10.3390/jcm11113045.*

Abbreviations: RCT: Randomized controlled trial; TNF: tumor necrosis factor; IFX: infliximab; ADA: adalimumab; VDZ: vedolizumab; UST: ustekinumab; FIL: filgotinib; CIP: ciprofloxacin; AZA: azathioprine; PBO: placebo; TDM: therapeutic drug monitoring; ARR: absolute risk reduction;

HR: hazard ratio; OR: odds ratio; and NS: non-specified.

4.5.9. Arterial Supply of the Intestine

The gastrointestinal tract arises from the fore-, mid-, and hindgut; each has a distinct vascular supply, albeit one that anastomoses with its neighbor. The stomach and duodenum up to the bile duct entry comprise the foregut, which is supplied by branches of the celiac axis that emerge from the aorta at the T12 vertebral level. The midgut is supplied by the superior mesenteric artery, which emerges from the aorta at L1, and stretches from the mid-duodenum to the distal transverse colon.

- the inferior pancreaticoduodenal artery;
- jejunal and ileal branches—supplying the bulk of the small intestine;
- the ileocolic artery, supplying terminal ileum, caecum, and commencement of ascending colon and giving off an appendicular branch to the appendix—the most commonly ligated intra-abdominal artery;
- the right colic artery—supplying the ascending colon;
- the middle colic artery—supplying the transverse colon.

The hind-gut receives its supply from the inferior mesenteric artery, arising from the aorta at L3 and giving the following branches:

i. **The Left Colic Artery** – supplying the descending colon;

ii. **The Sigmoid Branches** – supplying the sigmoid;

iii. **The Superior Rectal Artery** – supplying the rectum.

Since every branch of the superior and inferior mesenteric arteries anastomoses with its neighbor both above and below, the gastrointestinal canal is actually lined with a continuous vascular arcade.

4.5.10. The Portal System of Veins

The portal venous system transports blood from the pancreas, the spleen, the gallbladder, and its ducts to the liver through the abdominal portion of the alimentary canal (apart from the anal canal). The superior and inferior mesenteric arteries listed above, as well as the branches of the coeliac, are accompanied by the distal branches of this system; the arrangement varies proximally. To reach the splenic vein behind the pancreas, the inferior mesenteric vein rises above the location of its artery.

After joining the splenic vein behind the pancreatic neck in the transpyloric plane, the superior mesenteric vein becomes the portal vein. This vein then ascends into the anterior wall of the foramen of Winslow, behind the first portion of the duodenum, and ends up in the porta hepatis. Here, the portal vein splits into the left and right branches and becomes smaller, forming capillaries that run between the liver's lobules. The hepatic vein's radicles, which empty into the inferior vena cava, are where these capillaries drain.

4.5.10.1. Connections Between the Portal and Systemic Venous Systems

The hepatic vein and inferior vena cava are the normal routes via which portal venous blood empties into the systemic venous circulation after passing through the liver as previously mentioned. This pathway may be blocked by a variety of causes which are classified into:

- **Prehepatic** – e.g., thrombosis or congenital obliteration of the portal vein;

- **Hepatic** – e.g., cirrhosis of the liver;
- **Posthepatic** – e.g., congenital stenosis of the hepatic veins.

Portal venous pressure increases (portal hypertension) and collateral pathways between the portal and systemic venous systems become available if obstruction from any of these sources takes place.

These communications are:

1. Between the esophageal branch of the left gastric vein and the esophageal veins of the azygos system (these esophageal varices are the cause of the severe hematemesis that may occur in portal hypertension);
2. Between the superior rectal branch of the inferior mesenteric vein and the inferior rectal veins draining into the internal iliac vein via its internal pudendal tributary;
3. Between the portal branches in the mesentery and mesocolon and retroperitoneal veins communicating with the renal, lumbar, and phrenic veins;
4. Between the portal branches in the liver and the veins of the abdominal wall via veins passing along the falciform ligament from the umbilicus (which may result in the formation of a cluster of dilated veins which radiate from the navel and which are called the caput Medusae);
5. Between the portal branches in the liver and the veins of the diaphragm across the bare area of the liver.

The remarkable dilatation of every channel available between the two systems during operations on patients with portal hypertension is a striking characteristic that makes the procedures time-consuming and bloody.

4.5.11. Lymph Drainage of the Intestine

The small and large intestines have comparatively uniform lymph node arrangements. Many small nodes on or near the intestinal wall empty into larger, intermediately positioned nodes along the vessels in the mesentery or mesocolon, which then empty into clusters of nodes close to the superior and inferior mesenteric artery origins. Efferent vessels connect from these and empty into the cisterna chyli. Every bowel segment has a lymphatic drainage field that roughly matches its blood supply. Therefore, the lymph nodes draining the area will be removed by high ligation of the vessels to the involved segment of bowel along with removal of a wide surrounding segment of mesocolon. For a transverse colon growth, for instance, a large wedge of the transverse mesocolon would be excised, along with the division of the middle colic vessels.

4.5.12. The Structure of the Alimentary Canal

The mucosa that makes up the alimentary canal is separated from the submucosa by the muscularis mucosae, the muscle coat, and the serosa, which is absent in extraperitoneal gut regions.

The mucosa of the esophagus and lower anal canal is columnar in other places and stratified squamous in the former. This transition is very abrupt at the cardio-esophageal junction, though the lower esophagus may occasionally have columnar epithelium lining it. Simple glands that resemble crypts protrude from the gastric mucosa into the muscularis mucosae. The hormone gastrin and mucus are present in the alkaline juice secreted by the pyloric antrum. The stomach's body secretes both pepsin and hydrochloric acid (HCl), with the latter coming from the oxyntic cells that are tightly positioned between the surface cells. Additionally, the stomach mucosa secretes intrinsic factor.

Along with having glands resembling crypts, the mucosa of the duodenum and small intestine projects into the lumen of the colon through villous processes, significantly increasing its surface area. The duodenum is characterized by its crypts, which penetrate deeply into the muscularis mucosae and open into a vast network of acini in the submucosa that are known as Brunner's glands.

There are no villi in the mucosa of the large intestine; goblet cells that secrete mucus line the mucosa almost entirely. There are two layers to the muscle coat of the alimentary tract: an outer longitudinal layer and an inner circular layer. This muscle is voluntary in the upper two-thirds of the esophagus and at the anal margin, but involuntary elsewhere. An innermost oblique coat of muscle reinforces the stomach wall, and the colon is distinguished by the condensation of its longitudinal layer into three taeniae coli. The Meissner and Auerbach autonomic nerve plexuses are located in the submucosal layer and between the circular and longitudinal muscle coats, respectively.

4.5.13. The Development of the Intestine and Its Congenital Abnormalities

The primitive endodermal tube of the gut is divided into:

1. The foregut (supplied by the celiac axis) extends as far as the entry of the bile duct into the duodenum;
2. The midgut (supplied by the superior mesenteric artery) continues as far as the distal transverse colon;
3. The hindgut (supplied by the inferior mesenteric artery) extends thence to the ectodermal part of the anal canal.

Recanalization occurs after the gut wall's lumen is completely destroyed in an early stage due to rapid proliferation. As the smaller sac develops, the foregut rotates, causing the stomach's original right wall to form its posterior surface and its original left wall to form its anterior surface. The vagi lie anteriorly and posteriorly at the esophageal hiatus because they rotate with the stomach.

The duodenum swings to the right due to this rotation, and the organ's mesentery then combines with the posterior abdominal wall's peritoneum; this blending process is known as zygosis. In the 5-week fetus, the mid-gut grows quickly, eventually becoming too big to fit inside the abdomen and herniating into the cord. The yolk sac and the vitello-intestinal duct are connected to the apex of this herniated bowel, but even at this early stage of fetal life, this connection is already reduced to a fibrous strand.

The superior mesenteric artery forms the axis of this herniated loop of gut, separating the caudal and cephalic limbs. The caudal segment differentiates into the terminal 2 feet (62 cm) of the ileum, the caecum, and the colon up to the point where the left and middle thirds of the transverse colon converge. The cephalic element develops into the proximal small intestine. A bud that forms on the caudal segment marks the location of the caecum's subsequent formation; it's possible that this bud postpones the caudal limb's return in favor of the cephalic gut during the herniated bowel's subsequent reduction. This return of the bowel to the abdominal cavity starts at 10 weeks. The cephalic limb now lies to the right and the caudal limb to the left as the mid-gut loop first rotates 90° counter-clockwise.

The head comes back first, moving left and upward into the area that the large liver had previously vacated. This mid-gut pushes the hind-gut, or definitive distal colon, over to the left and passes behind the superior mesenteric artery, which crosses the third portion of the duodenum in the process. The caecum is located directly below the liver, and the caudal limb returns to its only remaining location, which is superficial to and above the small intestine.

The caecum moves into its final position in the right iliac fossa, pulling the colon along with it. As a result, the transverse colon ends up in front of the superior mesenteric vessels and the small intestine. The mesenteries of the ascending and descending parts of the colon eventually merge with the peritoneum of the posterior abdominal wall through a process called zygosis. This fusion has significant importance in surgery. When mobilizing the right or left colon, a cut is made along this avascular zygosis line next to the bowel, allowing it to be moved along with its mesocolon and blood supply. Similarly, the duodenum, head of the pancreas, and end of the common bile duct can be mobilized without bleeding by cutting the peritoneum along the right side of the duodenum—known as Kocher's maneuver (Flynn & Vickerton, 2023; Mikhael & Khan, 2024; Wade & Streitz, 2023).

Numerous anomalies may occur in the highly complex developmental process (Table 4.6):

1. Atresia or stenosis of the bowel may result from failure of recanalization of the lumen. Another cause of this may be damage to the blood supply to the bowel within the fetal umbilical hernia with consequent ischemic changes. Imperforate anus.
2. Meckel's diverticulum represents the remains of the embryonic Vitello intestinal duct (communication between the primitive mid-gut and yolk sac) and is, therefore, always on the anti-mesenteric border of the bowel. As an approximation to the truth, it can be said to occur in 2% of subjects, twice as often in males as females, to be situated at 2 feet (62 cm) from the ileocecal junction, and to be 2 in (5 cm) long. In fact, it may occur anywhere from 6 in (15 cm) to 12 feet (3.5 m) from the terminal ileum and vary from a tiny stump to a 6 in (15 cm) long sac. Occasionally, the diverticulum ends in a whip-like solid strand.

   In addition to the most common form, a diverticulum, this duct can also continue as a band or fistula joining the intestine to the umbilicus, as a cyst hanging from the ileum's anti-mesenteric border, or as a "raspberry tumor" at the umbilicus, formed by the red mucosa of a persistent diverticulum's umbilical extremity pouting at the navel.

   The diverticulum's lining may have small clusters of peptic epithelium composed of oxyntic cells that secrete acid. This can lead to peptic ulcers in the surrounding intestinal lining, which may result in bleeding or perforation.
3. The caecum may not properly descend, causing the peritoneal fold that usually seals it to pass across the duodenum in the right iliac fossa, resulting in a neonatal intestinal obstruction. This can leave the mesentery of the small intestine as a narrow pedicle, leading to volvulus of the entire small intestine (neonatal volvulus).

4. Sometimes, there is a reversed rotation where the transverse colon moves behind the superior mesenteric vessels, with the duodenum in front of them. This can lead to extrinsic duodenal obstruction caused by a peritoneal fold.
5. Exomphalos is the persistence of the mid-gut herniation at the umbilicus after birth.

Table 4.6. *Examples of Analyses of Geospatial Multivariable Regression Models*

Ø **Geospatial Multivariable Regression Models for Esophageal Stenosis or Atresia:**

Parameter Values			**Model Parameters**		
Parameter	**Estimate (C.I.)**	***p*-Value**	**Parameter**	Value	Significance
Additive					
Rate ~ Alcohol + Tobacco + LM.Cannabis_x_Daily.Interpol._x_Resin.THC + LM.Cannabis_x_Resin.THC + Resin + LM.Cannabis_x_Herb.THC_x_Daily.Interpol. + Resin + Cocaine + Income + Amphetamines					
Cocaine	0.33 (0.19, 0.47)	5.32×10^{-6}	rho	−0.3908	0.0290
			lambda	0.3247	0.0679
Interactive					
Rate ~ Tobacco * LM.Cannabis_x_Daily.Interpol._x_Resin.THC * Resin + Resin + LM.Cannabis + Alcohol + Cocaine + Income + Amphetamines					
Cocaine	0.33 (0.19, 0.47)	5.32×10^{-6}	rho	−0.3908	0.0290
			lambda	0.3247	0.0679
2 Lags					
*Rate ~ Tobacco + LM.Cannabis_x_Daily.Interpol._x_Resin.THC * Resin + LM.Cannabis_x_Resin.THC + LM.Cannabis + Alcohol + Cocaine + Income + Amphetamines*					
Resin	−1.59 (−2.96, −0.22)	0.0232	rho	0.6439	3.16×10^{-9}
LM.Cannabis_x_Resin.THC	2.57 (1.18, 3.96)	0.0003	lambda	−0.6327	3.54×10^{-8}
Income	0 (0, 0)	0.0008			

Ø **Geospatial Multivariable Regression Models for Biliary Stenosis:**

Parameter Values			**Model Parameters**	
Parameter	**Estimate (C.I.)**	***p*-Value**	**Parameter**	**Value**
Additive				
Rate ~ Alcohol + Tobacco + LM.Cannabis_x_Resin.THC + Daily.Interpol. + LM.Cannabis_x_Daily.Interpol._x_Resin.THC + LM.Cannabis_x_Herb.THC_x_Daily.Interpol. + Amphetamines + Cocaine				
Alcohol	0.03 (0, 0.05)	0.0209	Least Squares	

Amphetamines	−0.12 (−0.18, −0.06)	7.15×10^{-5}	S.D.	0.2286
Cocaine	0.19 (0.12, 0.26)	8.01×10^{-8}		
Income	0 (0, 0)	0.0375		
Interactive				
*Rate ~ Tobacco * Daily.Interpol. + LM.Cannabis_x_Herb.THC_x_Daily.Interpol. + LM.Cannabis_x_Resin.THC + LM.Cannabis_x_Daily.Interpol._x_Resin.THC + Alcohol + Cocaine + Income + Amphetamines*				
Alcohol	0.03 (0, 0.05)	0.0209	Least Squares	
Amphetamines	−0.12 (−0.18, −0.06)	7.15×10^{-5}	S.D.	0.2286
Cocaine	0.19 (0.12, 0.26)	8.01×10^{-8}		
Income	0 (0, 0)	0.0375		
2 Lags				
*Rate ~ Tobacco + Daily.Interpol. * LM.Cannabis_x_Daily.Interpol._x_Resin.THC + LM.Cannabis_x_Herb.THC_x_Daily.Interpol. + LM.Cannabis_x_Resin.THC + Alcohol + Cocaine + Income + Amphetamines*				
Amphetamines	−0.1 (−0.17, −0.03)	0.00509	Least Squares	
Cocaine	0.23 (0.16, 0.31)	8.87×10^{-10}	S.D.	0.2362

Table Key: As in Table 4.1.

Ø **Geospatial Multivariable Regression Models for Small Intestinal Stenosis or Atresia:**

Parameter Values			**Model Parameters**		
Parameter	**Estimate (C.I.)**	***p*-Value**	**Parameter**	**Value**	**Significance**
Additive					
Rate ~ Alcohol + Tobacco + Daily.Interpol. + LM.Cannabis_x_Daily.Interpol._x_Resin.THC + LM.Cannabis_x_Resin.THC + LM.Cannabis_x_Herb.THC_x_Daily.Interpol. + Herb + Cocaine + Income + Amphetamines					
LM.Cannabis_x_Resin.THC	1.23 (0.31, 2.15)	0.0086	rho	0.5992	6.25×10^{-9}
Herb	4.6 (1.41, 7.79)	0.0047	lambda	−0.5627	8.47×10^{-7}
Interactive					
*Rate ~ Tobacco + Daily.Interpol. * LM.Cannabis_x_Daily.Interpol._x_Resin.THC + LM.Cannabis_x_Herb.THC_x_Daily.Interpol. + LM.Cannabis_x_Resin.THC + Alcohol + Cocaine + Income + Amphetamines*					
LM.Cannabis_x_Daily.Interpol._x_Resin.THC	−2.96 (−5.61, −0.31)	0.0288	rho	0.65254	4.55×10^{-14}
LM.Cannabis_x_Resin.THC	2.22 (0.12, 4.32)	0.0378	lambda	−0.5878	8.56×10^{-9}
Alcohol	0.06 (0.01, 0.11)	0.0150			
Income	0 (0, 0)	0.0012			

Daily.Interpol.: LM.Cannabis_x_Daily. Interpol._x_Resin.THC	75.9 (15.73, 136.07)	0.0135			
2 Lags					
*Rate ~ Tobacco * Daily.Interpol. + LM.Cannabis_x_Daily.Interpol._x_Resin.THC + LM.Cannabis_x_Herb. THC_x_Daily.Interpol. + LM.Cannabis_x_Resin.THC + Alcohol + Cocaine + Income + Amphetamines*					
Daily.Interpol.	64.7 (5.51, 123.89)	0.0324	rho	0.71746	$<2.2 \times 10^{-16}$
Alcohol	0.12 (0.07, 0.17)	0.0000	lambda	−0.68322	8.10×10^{-13}
Income	0 (0, 0)	0.0005			

Table Key: As in Table 4.1.

Ø **Geospatial Multivariable Regression Models for Anorectal Stenosis or Atresia:**

Parameter Values			**Model Parameters**		
Parameter	**Estimate (C.I.)**	***p*-Value**	**Parameter**	Value	Significance
Additive					
Rate ~ Alcohol + Tobacco + LM.Cannabis_x_Daily.Interpol._x_Resin.THC + LM.Cannabis_x_Herb.THC_x_Daily.Interpol. + LM.Cannabis_x_Resin.THC + Daily.Interpol. + Cocaine + Income + Amphetamines					
LM.Cannabis_x_Herb. THC: LM.Cannabis_x_Daily. Interpol._x_Resin.THC	1.66 (0, 3.31)	0.0495	rho	0.6082	2.32×10^{-10}
LM.Cannabis_x_Herb.THC_x_ Daily.Interpol.	−5.86 (−9.81, −1.92)	0.0036	lambda	−0.4807	5.90×10^{-5}
Resin	2.05 (0.6, 3.5)	0.0055			
Herb	6.38 (2.61, 10.15)	0.0009			
Cocaine	0.44 (0.27, 0.61)	1.98×10^{-7}			
Interactive					
*Rate ~ Tobacco * Resin + Herb + LM.Cannabis_x_Daily.Interpol._x_Resin.THC * LM.Cannabis_x_Herb. THC_x_Daily.Interpol. + Alcohol + Cocaine + Income + Amphetamines*					
Tobacco	−0.06 (−0.1, −0.01)	0.0122	rho	0.6082	2.32×10^{-10}
Resin	−9.07 (−14.7, −3.44)	0.0016	lambda	−0.4807	5.90×10^{-5}

Cocaine	0.15 (0.01, 0.3)	0.0374			
Income	0 (0, 0)	0.0002			
Tobacco: Resin	0.42 (0.21, 0.63)	6.62×10^{-5}			
2 Lags					
*Rate ~ Tobacco * Resin + Herb +LM.Cannabis_x_Herb.THC_x_Daily.Interpol. + LM.Cannabis_x_Daily.Interpol._x_Resin.THC + Alcohol + Cocaine + Income + Amphetamines*					
Resin	−5.33 (−9.86, −0.8)	0.0210	rho	−0.4204	0.0284
Income	0 (0, 0)	1.20×10^{-5}	lambda	0.4484	0.013
Tobacco: Resin	0.24 (0.07, 0.41)	0.0049			

Table Key: As in Table 4.1.

Source: *Reece, A. S., & Hulse, G. K., (2023). Congenital gastrointestinal anomalies in Europe 2010–2019: A geo-spatiotemporal and causal inferential study of epidemiological patterns in relationship to cannabis- and substance exposure. Gastroenterology Insights, 14(1), 64–109. https://doi.org/10.3390/gastroent14010007.*

4.6. The Gastrointestinal Adnexae: Liver, Gall Bladder, and Its Ducts, Pancreas, and Spleen

4.6.1. The Liver

The body's largest organ is the liver. It is connected to the diaphragm, which divides it from the pleura, lungs, pericardium, and heart, by virtue of its domed upper surface. Its postero-inferior, or visceral, surface bears the gallbladder and is abutted by the stomach, duodenum, colon's hepatic flexure, the right kidney, and the suprarenal canal.

The liver is divided into a larger right and small left lobe, separated superiorly by the falciform ligament and postero-inferiorly by an H-shaped arrangement of fossae:

- **Anteriorly and to the Right** – the fossa for the gall bladder;
- **Posteriorly and to the Right** – the groove in which the inferior vena cava lies embedded;
- **Anteriorly and to the Left** – the fissure containing the ligamentum teres;
- **Posteriorly and to the Left** – the fissure for the ligamentum venosum.

The porta hepatis is the crossbar of the H-shaped liver. Between the limbs of this H, two subsidiary lobes can be found on the visceral aspect of the liver – the quadrate lobe in front and the caudate lobe behind. The ligamentum teres is the leftover tissue from the left umbilical vein in utero, which carries blood from the placenta to the fetus. The ligamentum venosum is the fibrous remnants of the fetal ductus venosus, which bypasses the liver and connects the left umbilical vein to the inferior vena cava. The grooves for these ligaments and the inferior vena cava follow the pathway of a fetal venous trunk and are continuous in the adult liver.

Lying in the porta hepatis (which is 2 in (5 cm) long) are:

i. the common hepatic duct - anteriorly;

ii. the hepatic artery - in the middle;

iii. the portal vein - posteriorly.

As well as these, autonomic nerve fibers (sympathetic from the coeliac axis and parasympathetic from the vagus), lymphatic vessels and lymph nodes are found there (Figure 4.22).

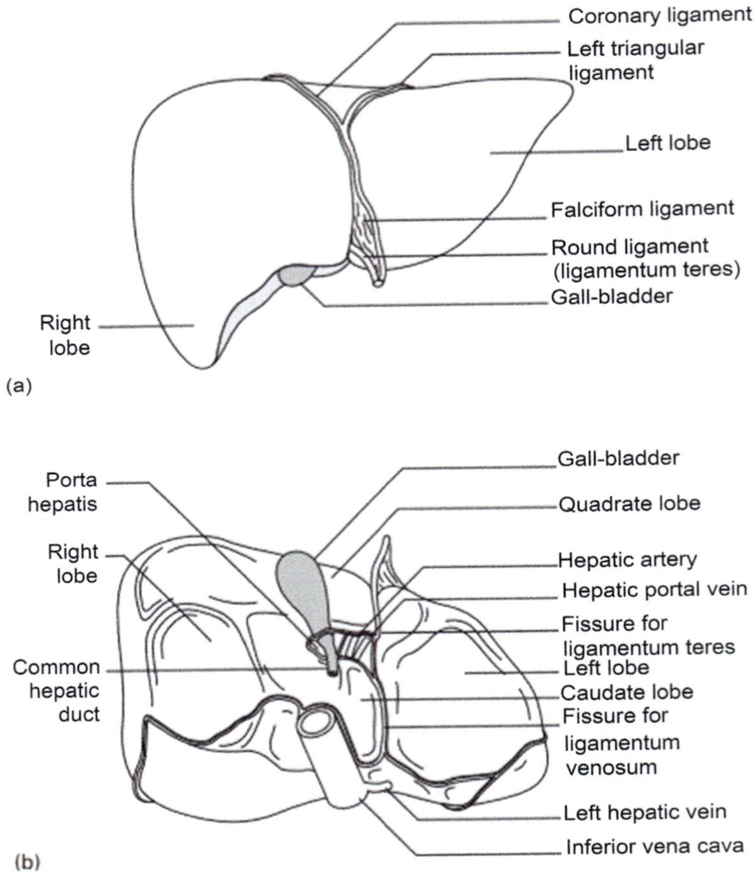

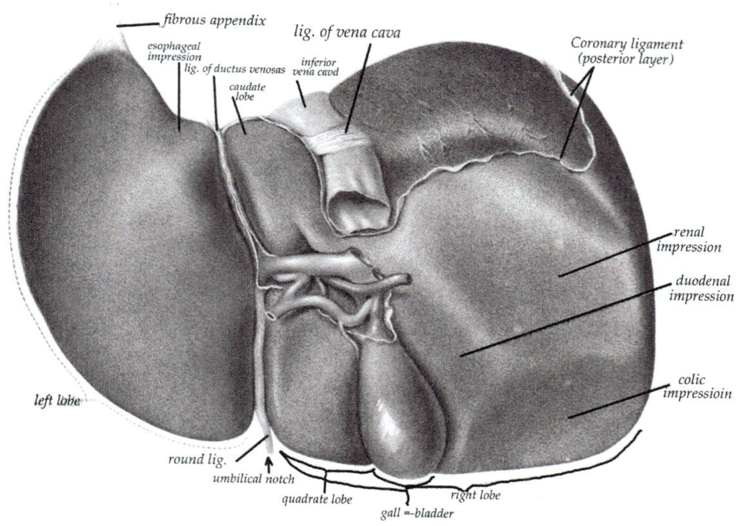

Figure 4.22. *The liver and its subdivisions.*

Source: By Dr. Johannes Sobotta – Sobotta's Atlas and Textbook of Human Anatomy, 1906, Public Domain; https://commons.wikimedia.org/w/index.php?curid=29901575.

4.6.1.1. Peritoneal Attachments

The liver is mostly surrounded by a protective layer called the peritoneum, except for a small area at the back that is not covered. This area is separated from the diaphragm by the upper and lower layers of the coronary ligament. On the right side, these layers come together to form the right triangular ligament. The falciform ligament runs from the umbilicus to the liver, slightly off-center to the right, and contains the ligamentum teres along its edge. The ligamentum teres goes into a groove on the underside of the liver, while the falciform ligament goes over the liver's dome and splits. Its right part connects to the upper layer of the coronary ligament, while the left part becomes the long, narrow left triangular ligament. This left triangular ligament connects to the lesser omentum near the top of the fissure for the ligamentum venosum. The lesser omentum starts at the openings of the portal vein and the ligamentum venosum, and extends as a sheet to attach along the lesser curve of the stomach.

4.6.1.2. Structure

The liver is composed of lobules, each containing a central vein that drains into the hepatic vein and eventually into the inferior vena cava. Portal canals between the lobules contain branches of the hepatic artery and portal vein, which both connect to the central vein through sinusoids within the lobule. Additionally, the portal canals house branches of the hepatic duct, which collect bile from the liver lobules.

4.6.1.3. Segmental Anatomy

This gross anatomical descriptive term, which has no morphological significance, refers to the division of the liver into a right and left lobe. It is marked by a line that runs from the falciform ligament's attachment on the anterior surface to the fissures for the ligamentum teres and ligamentum venosum on the posterior surface. The true morphological and physiological division of the liver is into the right and left lobes, which are separated by a plane that passes through the inferior vena cava and the gallbladder fossa, according to studies on the distribution of the hepatic blood vessels and ducts. These two lobes have independent biliary drainage systems and their own arterial and portal venous blood supplies, despite the absence of any discernible line separating them on the liver's dome. The caudate lobe splits partially to the left and partially to the right lobe in this morphological division, which is located to the right of the gross anatomical plane. The quadrate lobe becomes a part of the left morphological lobe of the liver in this division.

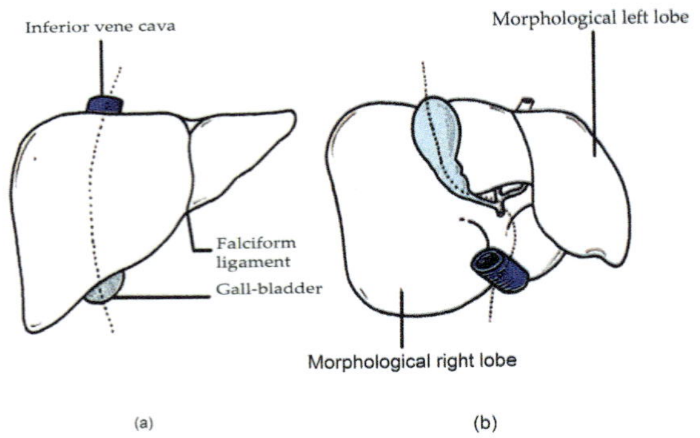

The right and left morphological lobes of the liver can be divided into several segments, with four segments in each lobe. While students may not need to memorize these details, hepatic surgeons must have a thorough understanding of these segments, including their individual blood supply and biliary drainage, especially when performing a partial liver resection. The hepatic artery, portal vein, and bile duct split into right and left branches at the hilum of the liver, with minimal communication between the divisions on each side. These branches extend laterally from the porta hepatis and spread upwards and downwards throughout the liver, defining the distinct morphological left and right lobes (Figure 4.23).

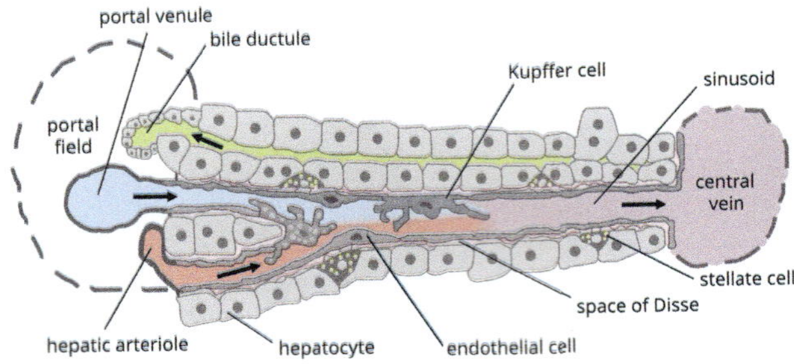

Figure 4.23. *Cells.*

Source: By Originally by Frevert, U., Engelmann, S., Zougbédé, S., Stange, J., Ng, B., et al., (n.d.). Converted to SVG by Viacheslav Vtyurin who was hired to do so by User: Eug. – Based on the research article "Intravital Observation of Plasmodium berghei Sporozoite Infection of the Liver," PLoS Biology, doi: 10.1371/journal.pbio.0030192.g011, CC BY 2.5; https://commons.wikimedia.org/w/index.php?curid=14388642.

4.6.1.4. The Hepatic Veins

These massive veins are distributed somewhat differently from the previously described portal, hepatic artery, and bile duct systems. The right, central, and left hepatic veins are the three main veins in the liver. These drain into the inferior vena cava at the superior margin of the liver by passing both upward and backward. The left hepatic vein and the central hepatic vein often meet close to their terminations, though this is not always the case. In certain specimens, the drainage may occur straight into the cava. Furthermore, tiny hepatic venous branches emerge directly from the liver's substance and join the vena cava at a greater distance from the primary hepatic veins. During a right hepatic lobectomy, these obtrude upon the surgeon even though they are not of great functional importance.

The right, middle, and left thirds of the liver are roughly corresponded to the three drainage zones of the three main hepatic veins. The boundaries of the zones drained by the left and middle hepatic veins line up with the plane delineated by the falciform ligament. Regretfully for the surgeon, the right hepatic resection procedure is complicated by the middle hepatic vein's location right at the line of the liver's principal plane between its left and right morphological lobes (Flynn & Vickerton, 2023; Mikhael & Khan, 2024; Wade & Streitz, 2023).

4.6.2. The Biliary System

The common hepatic duct (1.5 in/4 cm) is formed when the left and right hepatic ducts unite in the porta hepatis. This forms the common bile duct (4 in (10 cm)) by joining with the cystic duct (1.5 in (4 cm)), which drains the gallbladder. Starting approximately 1 in (4 cm) above the duodenum, the common bile duct travels behind it before emerging at a papilla on the medial aspect of the duodenum's second portion. In this course, the common duct is buried in the substance of the pancreas or lies in a groove in the posterior aspect of the organ.

The sphincter of Oddi protects the ampulla of Vater, the opening of which in the duodenum is where the common duct termination usually connects to the main pancreatic duct (of Wirsung). Periodically, the pancreatic and bile ducts open into the duodenum independently.

The common hepatic duct and the supraduodenal part of the common bile duct lie in the free edge of the lesser omentum where they are related as follows (Figure 4.24):

- **Bile Duct** – anterior to the right;
- **Hepatic Artery** – anterior to the left;
- **Portal Vein** – posterior;
- **Inferior Vena Cava** – still more posterior, separated from the portal vein by the foramen of Winslow.

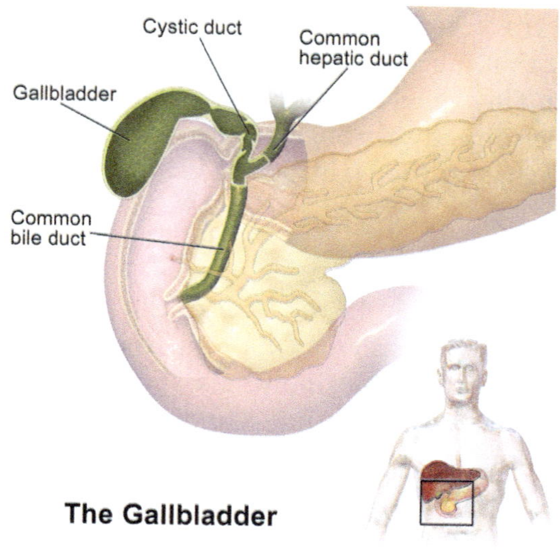

Figure 4.24. *The gall bladder.*

Source: By BruceBlaus – Own work, CC BY-SA 4.0; https://commons.wikimedia.org/w/index.php?curid=44926476.

4.6.3. The Gall Bladder

The gallbladder typically stores around 50 ml of bile and functions as both a bile concentrator and reservoir. It is located in a depression between the right and quadrate lobes of the liver and is positioned below the duodenum and transverse colon. In cases of inflammation, the gallbladder may ulcerate into either of these neighboring structures. Anatomically, the gallbladder is divided into the fundus, body, and neck, with the neck connecting to the cystic duct. In enlarged or diseased gallbladders, there is often a pouch near the neck known as Hartmann's pouch, where gallstones can become trapped.

4.6.3.1. Blood Supply

The cystic artery, which is a branch of the right hepatic artery and is located in the triangle formed by the liver, cystic duct, and common hepatic duct, supplies the gallbladder. Other hepatic artery-derived vessels leave the liver and travel to the gallbladder. It's interesting to note that the cystic artery has no corresponding vein. Tiny veins originate in the gallbladder and travel directly through its bed into the liver's branches of the right portal vein.

4.6.3.2. Structure

There is muscle in the wall of the gallbladder and the sphincter of Oddi, but the remaining biliary duct system only has sporadic muscle fibers. Mucus-secreting glands and columnar cells line the mucosa's exterior.

4.6.3.3. Development

Anatomical variations in the gallbladder and ducts can be better understood by examining their embryological development. A diverticulum emerges from the ventral wall of the duodenum, giving rise to the hepatic ducts and liver. Another diverticulum branching from the side of the hepatic duct forms the gallbladder and cystic duct.

4.6.3.4. Clinical Features

- Failure to recognize the variations in the biliary system's anatomy often leads to errors in gallbladder surgery. For this reason, it's crucial to accurately identify the hepatic and cystic arteries as well as all three biliary ducts before dividing any structures or excising the gallbladder. The inferior aspect of the liver, the common hepatic duct, and the cystic duct form Calot's triangle, which is home to the cystic artery.
- By applying pressure to the hepatic artery (which produces the cystic branch) where it is located in the anterior wall of the foramen of Winslow, between the finger and thumb, bleeding during cholecystectomy can be managed (Pringle's maneuver).
- Because there is a rich secondary blood supply originating from the liver bed, gangrene of the gallbladder is uncommon even in cases of acute cholecystitis where the cystic artery becomes thrombosed. In the rare event that a gallbladder on an unusually long mesentery undergoes torsion, which will destroy both of its sources of blood supply, gangrene may result.
- Common duct stones are typically excised endoscopically with the use of a Dormia basket inserted following the division of the sphincter of Oddi. Other times, an incision in the supraduodenal section of the common bile duct is made in order to examine it. Occasionally, a stone that has struck the ampulla of Vater needs to be removed by making an incision in the duodenum's second section. When it's necessary to divide the sphincter of Oddi or remove a tumor that arises at the common bile duct's termination, this last method is also employed.

4.6.4. The Pancreas

In general, the transpyloric plane is where the pancreas is located retroperitoneally. It is broken down into the head, neck, body, and tail for descriptive purposes.

4.6.4.1. Relations

The head is located in the duodenum's C-curve, and it extends the uncinate process, which hooks posteriorly onto the superior mesenteric vessels as they pass through the mesentery's root from behind the pancreas. The inferior vena cava, the beginning of the portal vein, the aorta, the superior mesenteric vessels, the diaphragm's crura, the coeliac plexus, the left kidney, and the suprarenal gland are located posteriorly. Along the upper border of the pancreas, the splenic artery is a tortuous anatomical feature. The portal vein behind the pancreatic neck is formed by the splenic vein running behind the gland, receiving the inferior mesenteric vein and joining it with the superior mesenteric vein. The common bile duct, which empties into the second portion of the duodenum, is either embedded in the gland's substance or rests in a groove on its right extremity, rounding out this list of significant posterior relationships. The lesser sac divides the stomach from its anterior location. The pancreatic tail rests against the spleen's hilum to the left.

4.6.4.2. The Blood Supply

The pancreaticoduodenal and splenic arteries supply blood, and their corresponding veins empty into the portal system.

4.6.4.3. The Lymphatics

The groove between its head and the duodenum, the root of the superior mesenteric vessels, and its upper border are where the lymphatics empty into nodes.

4.6.4.4. Structure

In terms of macroscopy, the pancreas is lobulated and housed inside a thin capsule; these lobules are composed of serous secretory cell alveoli that empty into the principal ducts through their ductules.

The Langerhans islets, which secrete insulin, are located in between these alveoli. The pancreatic main duct (Wirsung) extends the entire length of the gland and often opens at the Vater ampulla alongside the common bile duct; on rare occasions, it empties into the duodenum on its own. After connecting with the main duct and emerging into the duodenum above it, the accessory duct (of Santorini) originates from the lower portion of the head in front of it. It occasionally disappears.

4.6.4.5. Development

A bigger dorsal diverticulum from the duodenum and a smaller ventral outpouching from the side of the common bile duct give rise to the pancreas. The superior mesenteric vessels are trapped between the ventral pouch and the lower aspect of the dorsal diverticulum as it swings around posteriorly to fuse with it. The ducts of the two formative segments of the pancreas then connect with one another. The duct of the smaller segment becomes the main duct, taking over the pancreatic flow, while the duct of the larger segment remains the accessory duct.

4.6.4.6. Clinical Features

In rare cases, duodenal obstruction may result from the two developing pancreatic segments completely encircling the duodenum's second section (known as the "annular pancreas") (Figure 4.25).

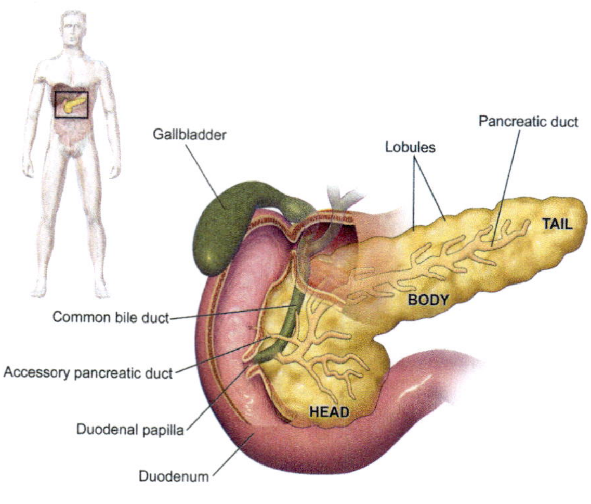

Figure 4.25. *Pancreas.*

Source: By BruceBlaus. When using this image in external sources it can be cited as: Blausen.com staff (2014). "Medical gallery of Blausen Medical, 2014." Wiki Journal of Medicine, 1(2). doi: 10.15347/wjm/2014.010. ISSN: 2002-4436. Own work, CC BY 3.0; https://commons.wikimedia.org/w/index.php?curid=28909219.

A pancreatic neoplasm that compresses the common bile duct will cause obstructive jaundice, as can be seen from the posterior relations of the pancreas. Portal or inferior vena caval obstruction may result from a large growth within the gland's body. The stomach is located anterior to the pancreas and is divided from it by the lesser sac. An acute pancreatitis-related fluid outpouring or a posterior gastric ulcer puncture can cause this sac to close off and swell, creating a pseudocyst of the pancreas. An almost full collection could encircle the abdomen.

4.6.5. The Spleen

The spleen resembles a cupped hand in size. It creates the lesser sac's left lateral extremity. The gastrosplenic ligament, which carries the left gastroepiploic and short gastric vessels, and the lienorenal ligament, which carries the splenic vessels and pancreatic tail, pass from it to the greater curvature of the stomach.

4.6.5.1. Relations

- **Posteriorly** – the left diaphragm, separating it from the pleura, left lung and the 9th, 10th and 11th ribs.
- **Anteriorly** – the stomach.
- **Inferiorly** – the splenic flexure of the colon.
- **Medially** – the left kidney.

The tail of the pancreas abuts against the hilum of the spleen through which vessels and nerves enter and leave this organ.

4.6.5.2. Blood Supply

One of the celiac axis's three principal branches is the splenic artery. The portal vein is created when the superior mesenteric vein connects with the splenic vein. (Note that the pancreas' primary blood supply also comes from the splenic vessels).

4.6.5.3. Structure

The body's largest reticulo-endothelial accumulation is found in the spleen. The peritoneum is closely attached to its thin, fibrous capsule. The splenic pulp is located between a sequence of trabeculae formed by the fibrous tissue of the capsule extending into the spleen.

4.6.5.4. Clinical Features

It is important to keep in mind the close relationship between the pancreatic tail and the splenic pedicle during a splenectomy because it is easily injured.

It is important to be aware of the close proximity of the lower ribs, the lowest part of the left lung, the pleural cavity, the left diaphragm, the left kidney, and the spleen. Injuries to the left upper abdomen can potentially damage any combination of these structures. Additionally, a stab wound to the posterior left chest may puncture the diaphragm and lacerate the spleen. The spleen, which has a thin, tense capsule, is the most commonly ruptured intra-abdominal organ by blunt trauma.

One or more accessory spleens can occur most frequently in the vicinity of the hilum, but they can also occur in the pancreatic tail, the omentum, the small bowel mesentery, the ovary, and even the testis. They affect roughly 10% of subjects and, if untreated, can lead to congenital acholuric jaundice or thrombocytopenic purpura symptoms that persist even after splenectomy (Flynn & Vickerton, 2023; Mikhael & Khan, 2024; Wade & Streitz, 2023).

A Closer Look

Gall Bladder

The gallbladder, a small pear-shaped organ located beneath the liver, plays a critical role in the digestive system. It stores and concentrates bile, a digestive fluid produced by the liver, which helps in the breakdown of fats in the small intestine. When food, especially fatty food, enters the digestive tract, the gallbladder releases bile through the bile ducts into the small intestine to aid in digestion.

Structurally, the gallbladder can be divided into three sections: the fundus, the body, and the neck, which connects to the cystic duct. This duct, in turn, joins with the hepatic duct from the liver to form the common bile duct, facilitating the flow of bile. The gallbladder wall is composed of several layers, including the mucosa, muscularis, and serosa, each contributing to its function of storing and expelling bile.

One of the primary conditions associated with the gallbladder is gallstones, which are solid particles that form from bile cholesterol and bilirubin. Gallstones can block the bile ducts, causing severe pain, inflammation, and infection, a condition known as cholecystitis. Risk factors for gallstones include obesity, high-fat diets, certain medical conditions, and genetics. Symptoms typically include intense pain in the upper right abdomen, nausea, vomiting, and jaundice.

Diagnosis of gallbladder issues often involves imaging techniques such as ultrasound, which can detect gallstones and inflammation. Other methods include HIDA scans, MRI, and CT scans, which provide detailed images of the biliary tract. Blood tests may also be conducted to check for signs of infection or bile duct obstruction.

Treatment for gallbladder conditions varies depending on the severity and type of issue. For asymptomatic gallstones, often no treatment is necessary, while symptomatic cases might require medication to dissolve the stones or surgery. Cholecystectomy, the surgical removal of the gallbladder, is a common procedure, especially in recurrent or severe cases of gallstones. This can be performed via laparoscopic surgery, which is minimally invasive, or through open surgery.

Post-cholecystectomy, most individuals can live without the gallbladder as bile flows directly from the liver to the small intestine, although some may experience changes in digestion and bowel habits. Dietary adjustments, such as eating smaller, low-fat meals, can help mitigate these effects.

The gallbladder's importance extends beyond its digestive role; its malfunction can signal broader health issues. Chronic gallbladder disease, if untreated, can lead to complications like gallbladder cancer, though rare, or secondary infections that can spread beyond the gallbladder. Thus, maintaining gallbladder health through a balanced diet, regular exercise, and prompt medical attention for symptoms is essential. Understanding the gallbladder's function and associated conditions underscores its significant, though often overlooked, role in overall digestive health.

Through advancements in diagnostic and surgical techniques, managing gallbladder diseases has become more effective, improving the quality of life for those affected by its disorders. This emphasizes the importance of awareness and early intervention in gallbladder-related health issues (Flynn & Vickerton, 2023; Mikhael & Khan, 2024; Wade & Streitz, 2023).

Summary

- The abdomen is a central region of the human body, housing vital organs and structures crucial for digestion, metabolism, and various bodily functions. Clinically, the abdomen is divided into quadrants or regions to facilitate diagnosis and treatment.
- The abdominal cavity is bordered superiorly by the diaphragm, inferiorly by the pelvic inlet, and is enclosed by the abdominal wall, comprising muscular and fascial layers.
- The abdomen is the frontal body cavity between the chest and pelvis that holds vital organs like the stomach, kidneys, bladder, liver, and intestines. Informally called the belly or stomach region, the abdomen is made up of protective tissues, membranes, and muscles.
- Health conditions associated with the abdomen often affect specific organs or the abdominal cavity and walls. Abdominal swelling or bloating is usually a sign of gas, but it can signal a more serious condition.
- The lower border of the liver extends along a line from the tip of the right 10th rib to the left 5th intercostal space in the midclavicular line; it may just be palpable in the normal subject, especially on deep inspiration.
- The paramedian incision is placed 1 in (2.5 cm) to 1.5 in (4 cm) lateral, and parallel, to the midline; the anterior rectus sheath is opened, the rectus displaced laterally and the posterior sheath, together with peritoneum, then incised.
- The anterior and posterior vagi enter the abdomen through the esophageal hiatus. The anterior nerve lies close to the stomach wall but the posterior, and larger, nerve is at a little distance from it.
- The lumen of the appendix is relatively wide in the infant and is frequently completely obliterated in the elderly. Since obstruction of the lumen is the usual precipitating cause of acute appendicitis, it is not unnatural, therefore, that appendicitis should be uncommon at the two extremes of life.
- The rectum is 5 in (12 cm) in length. It commences anterior to the third segment of the sacrum and ends at the level of the apex of the prostate or at the lower quarter of the vagina, where it leads into the anal canal.
- The anal canal is 1.5 in (4 cm) long and is directed downwards and backward from the rectum to the end at the anal orifice. The mid-anal canal represents the junction between endoderm of the hind-gut and ectoderm of the cutaneous invagination termed the proctodaeum.

References

1. Alsuhaimi, M. A., Alshowaiey, R. A., Alsumaihi, A. S., & Aldhafeeri, S. M. (2022). Mesenteric panniculitis various presentations and management: A single institute ten years, experience. *Annals of Medicine and Surgery, 80*, 104203. https://doi.org/10.1016/j.amsu.2022.104203.
2. Chiejina, M., Kudaravalli, P., & Samant, H. (2023). Ascites. In *StatPearls*. StatPearls Publishing.

3. Flynn, W., & Vickerton, P. (2023). Anatomy, abdomen and pelvis: Abdominal wall. In *StatPearls*. StatPearls Publishing.

4. Kasırga, E. (2019). The importance of stool tests in diagnosis and follow-up of gastrointestinal disorders in children. *Turk Pediatri Ars, 54*(3), 141–148. https://doi.org/10.14744/TurkPediatriArs.2018.00483.

5. Kim, J., Bhagwandin, S., & Labow, D. M. (2017). Malignant peritoneal mesothelioma: A review. *Annals of Translational Medicine, 5*(11), 236. https://doi.org/10.21037/atm.2017.03.96.

6. Kurzweil, A., & Martin, J. (2023). Transabdominal ultrasound. In *StatPearls*. StatPearls Publishing.

7. Mehta, H. (2016). Abdominal pain. In S. S. David (Ed.), *Clinical Pathways in Emergency Medicine* (pp. 329–345). Springer India. https://doi.org/10.1007/978-81-322-2710-6_26.

8. Mikhael, M., & Khan, Y. S. (2023). Anatomy, abdomen and pelvis: Lymphatic drainage. In *StatPearls*. StatPearls Publishing.

9. Patterson, J. W., Kashyap, S., & Dominique, E. (2023). Acute abdomen. In *StatPearls*. StatPearls Publishing.

10. Szadkowska, M. A., Pałucki, J., & Cieszanowski, A. (2023). Diagnosis and treatment of peritoneal carcinomatosis - A comprehensive overview. *Polish Journal of Radiology, 88*, e89–e97. https://doi.org/10.5114/pjr.2023.125027.

11. Tucker, W. D., Shrestha, R., & Burns, B. (2023). Anatomy, abdomen and pelvis: Inferior vena cava. In *StatPearls*. StatPearls Publishing.

12. Wade, C. I., & Streitz, M. J. (2023). Anatomy, abdomen and pelvis: Abdomen. In *StatPearls*. StatPearls Publishing.

13. Yu, B., & Raj, M. S. (2023). Pseudomyxoma peritonei. In *StatPearls*. StatPearls Publishing.

14. Pogacnik J.S., Salgado G. Perianal Crohn's Disease. *Clin. Colon Rectal Surg.* 2019;32:377–385. doi: 10.1055/s-0039-1687834.

15. Gecse K.B., Bemelman W., Kamm M.A., Stoker J., Khanna R., Ng S.C., Panés J., van Assche G., Liu Z., Hart A., et al. A global consensus on the classification, diagnosis and multidisciplinary treatment of perianal fistulising Crohn's disease. *Gut.* 2014;63:1381–1392. doi: 10.1136/gutjnl-2013-306709.

16. Adegbola S.O., Pisani A., Sahnan K., Tozer P., Ellul P., Warusavitarne J. Medical and surgical management of perianal Crohn's disease. *Ann. Gastroenterol.* 2018;31:129–139. doi: 10.20524/aog.2018.0236.

17. Panes J., Reinisch W., Rupniewska E., Khan S., Forns J., Khalid J.M., Bojic D., Patel H. Burden and outcomes for complex perianal fistulas in Crohn's disease: Systematic review. *World J. Gastroenterol.* 2018;24:4821–4834. doi: 10.3748/wjg.v24.i42.4821.

18. Cao Y., Su Q., Zhang B., Shen F., Li S. Efficacy of stem cells therapy for Crohn's fistula: A meta-analysis and systematic review. *Stem Cell Res. Ther.* 2021;12:32. doi: 10.1186/s13287-020-02095-7.

19. Panés J., García-Olmo D., Van Assche G., Colombel J.F., Reinisch W., Baumgart D.C., Dignass A., Nachury M., Ferrante M., Kazemi-Shirazi L., et al. Expanded allogeneic adipose-derived mesenchymal stem cells (Cx601) for complex perianal fistulas in Crohn's disease: A phase

3 randomised, double-blind controlled trial. *Lancet.* 2016;388:1281–1290. doi: 10.1016/S0140-6736(16)31203-X.

20. Ciccocioppo R., Klersy C., Leffler D.A., Rogers R., Bennett D., Corazza G.R. Systematic review with meta-analysis: Safety and efficacy of local injections of mesenchymal stem cells in perianal fistulas. *JGH Open.* 2019;3:249–260. doi: 10.1002/jgh3.12141.
21. Johnson S., Hoch J.S., Halabi W.J., Ko J., Nolta J., Dave M. Mesenchymal Stem/Stromal Cell Therapy Is More Cost-Effective Than Fecal Diversion for Treatment of Perianal Crohn's Disease Fistulas. *Front. Immunol.* 2022;13:859954. doi: 10.3389/fimmu.2022.859954.
22. Lu S., Zhu K., Guo Y., Wang E., Huang J. Evaluation of animal models of Crohn's disease with anal fistula (Review) *Exp. Ther. Med.* 2021;22:974. doi: 10.3892/etm.2021.10406.
23. Ryska O., Serclova Z., Mestak O., Matouskova E., Vesely P., Mrazova I. Local application of adipose-derived mesenchymal stem cells supports the healing of fistula: Prospective randomised study on rat model of fistulising Crohn's disease. *Scand. J. Gastroenterol.* 2017;52:543–550. doi: 10.1080/00365521.2017.1281434.
24. Rivera-Nieves J., Bamias G., Vidrich A., Marini M., Pizarro T.T., McDuffie M.J., Moskaluk C.A., Cohn S.M., Cominelli F. Emergence of perianal fistulizing disease in the SAMP1/YitFc mouse, a spontaneous model of chronic ileitis. *Gastroenterology.* 2003;124:972–982. doi: 10.1053/gast.2003.50148.
25. Flacs M., Collard M., Doblas S., Zappa M., Cazals-Hatem D., Maggiori L., Panis Y., Treton X., Ogier-Denis E. Preclinical Model of Perianal Fistulizing Crohn's Disease. *Inflamm. Bowel Dis.* 2020;26:687–696. doi: 10.1093/ibd/izz288.
26. Bruckner R.S., Nissim-Eliraz E., Marsiano N., Nir E., Shemesh H., Leutenegger M., Gottier C., Lang S., Spalinger M.R., Leibl S., et al. Transplantation of Human Intestine Into the Mouse: A Novel Platform for Study of Inflammatory Enterocutaneous Fistulas. *J. Crohn's Colitis.* 2019;13:798–806. doi: 10.1093/ecco-jcc/jjy226.
27. Galipeau J., Sensébé L. Mesenchymal Stromal Cells: Clinical Challenges and Therapeutic Opportunities. *Cell Stem Cell.* 2018;22:824–833. doi: 10.1016/j.stem.2018.05.004.
28. Kozawa S., Sagawa F., Endo S., De Almeida G.M., Mitsuishi Y., Sato T.N. Predicting Human Clinical Outcomes Using Mouse Multi-Organ Transcriptome. *iScience.* 2020;23:100791. doi: 10.1016/j.isci.2019.100791.
29. Kol A., Arzi B., Athanasiou K.A., Farmer D.L., Nolta J.A., Rebhun R.B., Chen X., Griffiths L.G., Verstraete F.J.M., Murphy C.J., et al. Companion animals: Translational scientist's new best friends. *Sci. Transl. Med.* 2015;7:308ps321. doi: 10.1126/scitranslmed.aaa9116.
30. Hoffman A.M., Dow S.W. Concise Review: Stem Cell Trials Using Companion Animal Disease Models. *Stem Cells.* 2016;34:1709–1729. doi: 10.1002/stem.2377.
31. Ferrer L., Kimbrel E.A., Lam A., Falk E.B., Zewe C., Juopperi T., Lanza R., Hoffman A. Treatment of perianal fistulas with human embryonic stem cell-derived mesenchymal stem cells: A canine model of human fistulizing Crohn's disease. *Regen. Med.* 2016;11:33–43. doi: 10.2217/rme.15.69.
32. Arzi B., Webb T.L., Koch T.G., Volk S.W., Betts D.H., Watts A., Goodrich L., Kallos M.S., Kol A. Cell Therapy in Veterinary Medicine as a Proof-of-Concept for Human Therapies: Perspectives From the North American Veterinary Regenerative Medicine Association. *Front. Vet. Sci.* 2021;8:779109. doi: 10.3389/fvets.2021.779109.

33. Cain C.L. Canine Perianal Fistulas: Clinical Presentation, Pathogenesis, and Management. *Vet. Clin. N. Am. Small Anim. Pract.* 2019;49:53–65. doi: 10.1016/j.cvsm.2018.08.006.

34. Hermanson J.W., De Lahunta A. *Miller and Evans' Anatomy of the Dog.* American Veterinary Medical Association; Schaumburg, IL, USA: 2020. [Google Scholar]

35. Cohen R., Windsor A. *Anus: Surgical Treatment and Pathology.* Springer Science & Business Media; Berlin, Germany: 2013.

36. Seow-Choen F., Ho J.M.S. Histoanatomy of anal glands. *Dis. Colon Rectum.* 1994;37:1215–1218. doi: 10.1007/BF02257784.

37. McColl I. The comparative anatomy and pathology of anal glands. Arris and Gale lecture delivered at the Royal College of Surgeons of England on 25th February 1965. *Ann. R. Coll. Surg. Engl.* 1967;40:36–67.

38. Shabadash S.A., Zelikina T.I. [Once more about hepatoid circumanal glands of dogs. History of their discovery and reasons for revision the structural and functional data] *Izv. Akad. Nauk. Seriia Biol.* 2002;2:176–185.

39. Janssenswillen S., Roelants K., Carpentier S., de Rooster H., Metzemaekers M., Vanschoenwinkel B., Proost P., Bossuyt F. Odorant-binding proteins in canine anal sac glands indicate an evolutionarily conserved role in mammalian chemical communication. *BMC Ecol. Evol.* 2021;21:182. doi: 10.1186/s12862-021-01910-w.

40. Budsberg S.C., Spurgeon T.L., Liggitt H.D. Anatomic predisposition to perianal fistulae formation in the German shepherd dog. *Am. J. Vet. Res.* 1985;46:1468–1472.

41. GBD 2017 Inflammatory Bowel Disease Collaborators The global, regional, and national burden of inflammatory bowel disease in 195 countries and territories, 1990–2017: A systematic analysis for the Global Burden of Disease Study 2017. *Lancet Gastroenterol. Hepatol.* 2020;5:17–30. doi: 10.1016/S2468-1253(19)30333-4.

42. Killingsworth C.R., Walshaw R., Dunstan R.W., Rosser E.J., Jr. Bacterial population and histologic changes in dogs with perianal fistula. *Am. J. Vet. Res.* 1988;49:1736–1741.

43. Jamieson P.M., Simpson J.W., Kirbyand B.M., Else R.W. Association between anal furunculosis and colitis in the dog: Preliminary observations. *J. Small Anim. Pract.* 2002;43:109–114. doi: 10.1111/j.1748-5827.2002.tb00039.x.

44. House A., Gregory S.P., Catchpole B. Expression of cytokine mRNA in canine anal furunculosis lesions. *Vet. Rec.* 2003;153:354–358. doi: 10.1136/vr.153.12.354.

45. Day M.J., Weaver B.M.Q. Pathology of surgically resected tissue from 305 cases of anal furunculosis in the dog. *J. Small Anim. Pract.* 1992;33:583–589. doi: 10.1111/j.1748-5827.1992.tb01062.x.

46. Kaur M., Panikkath D., Yan X., Liu Z., Berel D., Li D., Vasiliauskas E.A., Ippoliti A., Dubinsky M., Shih D.Q., et al. Perianal Crohn�s Disease is Associated with Distal Colonic Disease, Stricturing Disease Behavior, IBD-Associated Serologies and Genetic Variation in the JAK-STAT Pathway. *Inflamm. Bowel Dis.* 2016;22:862–869. doi: 10.1097/MIB.0000000000000705.

47. Tsai L., McCurdy J.D., Ma C., Jairath V., Singh S. Epidemiology and Natural History of Perianal Crohn's Disease: A Systematic Review and Meta-Analysis of Population-Based Cohorts. *Inflamm. Bowel Dis.* 2021;28:1477–1484. doi: 10.1093/ibd/izab287.

48. de Zoeten E., Pasternak B.A., Mattei P., Kramer R.E., Kader H. Diagnosis and treatment of

perianal Crohn disease: NASPGHAN clinical report and consensus statement. *J. Pediatr. Gastroenterol. Nutr.* 2013;57:401–412. doi: 10.1097/MPG.0b013e3182a025ee.

49. House A., Catchpole B., Gregory S. Matrix metalloproteinase mRNA expression in canine anal furunculosis lesions. *Vet. Immunol. Immunopathol.* 2007;115:68–75. doi: 10.1016/j.vetimm.2006.10.018.

50. Panés J., Rimola J. Perianal fistulizing Crohn's disease: Pathogenesis, diagnosis and therapy. *Nat. Rev. Gastroenterol. Hepatol.* 2017;14:652–664. doi: 10.1038/nrgastro.2017.104.

51. Mathews K.A., Sukhiani H.R. Randomized controlled trial of cyclosporine for treatment of perianal fistulas in dogs. *J. Am. Vet. Med. Assoc.* 1997;211:1249–1253.

52. Dejaco C., Harrer M., Waldhoer T., Miehsler W., Vogelsang H., Reinisch W. Antibiotics and azathioprine for the treatment of perianal fistulas in Crohn's disease. *Aliment. Pharmacol. Ther.* 2003;18:1113–1120. doi: 10.1046/j.1365-2036.2003.01793.x.

53. Harkin K.R., Phillips D., Wilkerson M. Evaluation of Azathioprine on Lesion Severity and Lymphocyte Blastogenesis in Dogs With Perianal Fistulas. *J. Am. Anim. Hosp. Assoc.* 2007;43:21–26. doi: 10.5326/0430021.

54. Shehab M., Alrashed F., Heron V., Restellini S., Bessissow T. Comparative Efficacy of Biologic Therapies for Inducing Response and Remission in Fistulizing Crohn's Disease: Systematic Review and Network Meta-Analysis of Randomized Controlled Trials. *Inflamm. Bowel Dis.* 2022 doi: 10.1093/ibd/izac103.

55. Mahdi B.M. Role of HLA typing on Crohn's disease pathogenesis. *Ann. Med. Surg.* 2015;4:248–253. doi: 10.1016/j.amsu.2015.07.020.

56. Kennedy L.J., O'Neill T., House A., Barnes A., Kyöstilä K., Innes J., Fretwell N., Day M.J., Catchpole B., Lohi H., et al. Risk of anal furunculosis in German Shepherd dogs is associated with the major histocompatibility complex. *Tissue Antigens.* 2008;71:51–56. doi: 10.1111/j.1399-0039.2007.00964.x.

57. Schnitzler F., Friedrich M., Wolf C., Stallhofer J., Angelberger M., Diegelmann J., Olszak T., Tillack C., Beigel F., Göke B., et al. The NOD2 Single Nucleotide Polymorphism rs72796353 (IVS4+10 A>C) Is a Predictor for Perianal Fistulas in Patients with Crohn's Disease in the Absence of Other NOD2 Mutations. *PLoS ONE.* 2015;10:e0116044. doi: 10.1371/journal.pone.0116044.

58. House A.K., Gregory S.P., Catchpole B. Pattern-recognition receptor mRNA expression and function in canine monocyte/macrophages and relevance to canine anal furunuclosis. *Vet. Immunol. Immunopathol.* 2008;124:230–240. doi: 10.1016/j.vetimm.2008.03.012.

59. Massey J., Short A.D., Catchpole B., House A., Day M.J., Lohi H., Ollier W.E.R., Kennedy L.J. Genetics of canine anal furunculosis in the German shepherd dog. *Immunogenetics.* 2014;66:311–324. doi: 10.1007/s00251-014-0766-5.

60. Lloyd-Price J., Arze C., Ananthakrishnan A.N., Schirmer M., Avila-Pacheco J., Poon T.W., Andrews E., Ajami N.J., Bonham K.S., Brislawn C.J., et al. Multi-omics of the gut microbial ecosystem in inflammatory bowel diseases. *Nature.* 2019;569:655–662. doi: 10.1038/s41586-019-1237-9.

61. Maldonado-Contreras A., Ferrer L., Cawley C., Crain S., Bhattarai S., Toscano J., Ward D.V., Hoffman A. Dysbiosis in a canine model of human fistulizing Crohn's disease. *Gut Microbes.* 2020;12:1785246. doi: 10.1080/19490976.2020.1785246.

62. Maggi L., Capone M., Giudici F., Santarlasci V., Querci V., Liotta F., Ficari F., Maggi E., Tonelli F., Annunziato F., et al. CD4+CD161+ T Lymphocytes Infiltrate Crohn's Disease-Associated Perianal Fistulas and Are Reduced by Anti-TNF-α Local Therapy. *Int. Arch. Allergy Immunol.* 2013;161:81–86. doi: 10.1159/000343467.

63. Altadill A., Eiró N., González L.O., Junquera S., González-Quintana J.M., Sánchez M.R., Andicoechea A., Saro C., Rodrigo L., Vizoso F.J. Comparative analysis of the expression of metalloproteases and their inhibitors in resected crohn's disease and complicated diverticular disease. *Inflamm. Bowel Dis.* 2012;18:120–130. doi: 10.1002/ibd.21682.

64. Siegmund B., Feakins R.M., Barmias G., Ludvig J.C., Teixeira F.V., Rogler G., Scharl M. Results of the Fifth Scientific Workshop of the ECCO (II): Pathophysiology of Perianal Fistulizing Disease. *J. Crohn's Colitis.* 2016;10:377–386. doi: 10.1093/ecco-jcc/jjv228.

65. Ellison G.W. Treatment of perianal fistulas in dogs. *J. Am. Vet. Med. Assoc.* 1995;206:1680–1682.

66. Mathews K.A., Ayres S.A., Tano C.A., Riley S.M., Sukhiani H.R., Adams C. Cyclosporin treatment of perianal fistulas in dogs. *Can. Vet. J.* 1997;38:39–41.

67. Hanauer S.B., Smith M.B. Rapid closure of Crohn's disease fistulas with continuous intravenous cyclosporin A. *Am. J. Gastroenterol.* 1993;88:646–649.

68. Present D.H., Lichtiger S. Efficacy of cyclosporine in treatment of fistula of crohn's disease. *Am. J. Dig. Dis.* 1994;39:374–380. doi: 10.1007/BF02090211.

69. Hardie R.J., Gregory S.P., Tomlin J., Sturgeon C., Lipscomb V., Ladlow J. Cyclosporine treatment of anal furunculosis in 26 dogs. *J. Small Anim. Pract.* 2005;46:3–9. doi: 10.1111/j.1748-5827.2005.tb00267.x.

70. House A.K., Guitian J., Gregory S.P., Hardie R.J. Evaluation of the Effect of Two Dose Rates of Cyclosporine on the Severity of Perianal Fistulae Lesions and Associated Clinical Signs in Dogs. *Vet. Surg.* 2006;35:543–549. doi: 10.1111/j.1532-950X.2006.00187.x.

71. Doust R., Griffiths L.G., Sullivan M. Evaluation of once daily treatment with cyclosporine for anal furunculosis in dogs. *Vet. Rec.* 2003;152:225–229. doi: 10.1136/vr.152.8.225.

72. Wetwittayakhlang P., Al Khoury A., Hahn G.D., Lakatos P.L. The Optimal Management of Fistulizing Crohn's Disease: Evidence beyond Randomized Clinical Trials. *J. Clin. Med.* 2022;11:3045. doi: 10.3390/jcm11113045.

73. Rovira P., Mascarell L., Bachi P.T. The Impact of Immunosuppressive Drugs on the Analysis of T-Cell Activation. *Curr. Med. Chem.* 2000;7:673–692. doi: 10.2174/0929867003374778.

74. Archer T., Boothe D., Langston V., Fellman C., Lunsford K., Mackin A. Oral Cyclosporine Treatment in Dogs: A Review of the Literature. *J. Vet. Intern. Med.* 2013;28:1–20. doi: 10.1111/jvim.12265.

75. Khan K.J., Ullman T.A., Ford A., Abreu M.T., Abadir A., Marshall J., Talley N.J., Moayyedi P. Antibiotic Therapy in Inflammatory Bowel Disease: A Systematic Review and Meta-Analysis. *Am. J. Gastroenterol.* 2011;106:661–673. doi: 10.1038/ajg.2011.72.

76. West R.L., Van Der Woude C.J., Hansen B., Felt-Bersma R.J.F., Van Tilburg A.J.P., Drapers J.A.G., Kuipers E.J. Clinical and endosonographic effect of ciprofloxacin on the treatment of perianal fistulae in Crohn's disease with infliximab: A double-blind placebo-controlled study. *Aliment. Pharmacol. Ther.* 2004;20:1329–1336. doi: 10.1111/j.1365-2036.2004.02247.x.

77. Maeda Y., Ng S.C., Durdey P., Burt C., Torkington J., Rao P.K.D., Mayberry J., Moshkovska T.,

Stone C.D., Carapeti E., et al. Randomized clinical trial of metronidazole ointment versus placebo in perianal Crohn's disease. *Br. J. Surg.* 2010;97:1340–1347. doi: 10.1002/bjs.7121.

78. Thia K.T., Mahadevan U., Feagan B.G., Wong C., Cockeram A., Bitton A., Bernstein C.N., Sandborn W.J. Ciprofloxacin or metronidazole for the treatment of perianal fistulas in patients with Crohn's disease: A randomized, double-blind, placebo-controlled pilot study. *Inflamm. Bowel Dis.* 2009;15:17–24. doi: 10.1002/ibd.20608.
79. Lim S.Z., Chua E.W. Revisiting the Role of Thiopurines in Inflammatory Bowel Disease Through Pharmacogenomics and Use of Novel Methods for Therapeutic Drug Monitoring. *Front. Pharmacol.* 2018;9:1107. doi: 10.3389/fphar.2018.01107.
80. Tisdall P., Hunt G.B., Beck J.A., Malik R. Management of perianal fistulae in five dogs using azathioprine and metronidazole prior to surgery. *Aust. Vet. J.* 1999;77:374–378. doi: 10.1111/j.1751-0813.1999.tb10307.x.
81. Kalliolias G., Ivashkiv L.B. TNF biology, pathogenic mechanisms and emerging therapeutic strategies. *Nat. Rev. Rheumatol.* 2016;12:49–62. doi: 10.1038/nrrheum.2015.169.
82. Kobayashi T., Momoi Y., Iwasaki T. Cyclosporine A Inhibits the mRNA Expressions of IL-2, IL-4 and IFN-.GAMMA., but not TNF-.ALPHA., in Canine Mononuclear Cells. *J. Vet. Med. Sci.* 2007;69:887–892. doi: 10.1292/jvms.69.887.
83. Guan Q. A Comprehensive Review and Update on the Pathogenesis of Inflammatory Bowel Disease. *J. Immunol. Res.* 2019;2019:7247238. doi: 10.1155/2019/7247238.
84. Kopper J.J., Iennarella-Servantez C., Jergens A.E., Sahoo D.K., Guillot E., Bourgois-Mochel A., Martinez M.N., Allenspach K., Mochel J.P. Harnessing the Biology of Canine Intestinal Organoids to Heighten Understanding of Inflammatory Bowel Disease Pathogenesis and Accelerate Drug Discovery: A One Health Approach. *Front. Toxicol.* 2021;3:773953. doi: 10.3389/ftox.2021.773953.
85. Coelho L.P., Kultima J.R., Costea P.I., Fournier C., Pan Y., Czarnecki-Maulden G., Hayward M.R., Forslund S.K., Schmidt T.S.B., Descombes P., et al. Similarity of the dog and human gut microbiomes in gene content and response to diet. *Microbiome.* 2018;6:72. doi: 10.1186/s40168-018-0450-3.
86. Day M.J. Immunopathology of analfurunculosis in the dog. *J. Small Anim. Pract.* 1993;34:381–388. doi: 10.1111/j.1748-5827.1993.tb02726.x.
87. Bataille F., Klebl F., Rümmele P., Schroeder J., Farkas S., Wild P.-J., Fürst A., Hofstädter F., Schölmerich J., Herfarth H., et al. Morphological characterisation of Crohn's disease fistulae. *Gut.* 2004;53:1314–1321. doi: 10.1136/gut.2003.038208.
88. Ruffolo C., Scarpa M., Faggian D., Pozza A., Navaglia F., Dincà R., Hoxha P., Romanato G., Polese L., Sturniolo G.C., et al. Cytokine network in rectal mucosa in perianal Crohn's disease: Relations with inflammatory parameters and need for surgery. *Inflamm. Bowel Dis.* 2008;14:1406–1412. doi: 10.1002/ibd.20486.
89. Lauro M.L., Burch J.M., Grimes C.L. The effect of NOD2 on the microbiota in Crohn's disease. *Curr. Opin. Biotechnol.* 2016;40:97–102. doi: 10.1016/j.copbio.2016.02.028.
90. House A.K., Binns M.M., Gregory S.P., Catchpole B. Analysis of NOD1, NOD2, TLR1, TLR2, TLR4, TLR5, TLR6 and TLR9 genes in anal furunculosis of German shepherd dogs. *Tissue Antigens.* 2009;73:250–254. doi: 10.1111/j.1399-0039.2008.01190.x.

91. O'Sullivan S., Gilmer J.F., Medina C. Matrix Metalloproteinases in Inflammatory Bowel Disease: An Update. *Mediat. Inflamm.* 2015;2015:964131. doi: 10.1155/2015/964131.

92. Kirkegaard T., Hansen A., Bruun E., Brynskov J. Expression and localisation of matrix metalloproteinases and their natural inhibitors in fistulae of patients with Crohn's disease. *Gut.* 2004;53:701–709. doi: 10.1136/gut.2003.017442.

93. Lavini-Ramos C., Silva H.M., Soares-Schanoski A., Monteiro S.M., Ferreira L.R.P., Pacanaro A.P., Gomes S., Batista J., Faé K., Kalil J., et al. MMP9 integrates multiple immunoregulatory pathways that discriminate high suppressive activity of human mesenchymal stem cells. *Sci. Rep.* 2017;7:874. doi: 10.1038/s41598-017-00923-0.

94. Gu J.J., Hoj J., Rouse C., Pendergast A.M. Mesenchymal stem cells promote metastasis through activation of an ABL-MMP9 signaling axis in lung cancer cells. *PLoS ONE.* 2020;15:e0241423. doi: 10.1371/journal.pone.0241423.

95. Barnes A., O'Neill T., Kennedy L.J., Short A.D., Catchpole B., House A., Binns M., Fretwell N., Day M.J., Ollier W.E.R. Association of canine anal furunculosis with TNFA is secondary to linkage disequilibrium with DLA-DRB1*. *Tissue Antigens.* 2009;73:218–224. doi: 10.1111/j.1399-0039.2008.01188.x.

96. Hugot J.-P., Chamaillard M., Zouali H., Lesage S., Cézard J.-P., Belaiche J., Almer S., Tysk C., O'Morain C.A., Gassull M., et al. Association of NOD2 leucine-rich repeat variants with susceptibility to Crohn's disease. *Nature.* 2001;411:599–603. doi: 10.1038/35079107.

97. Garza-Hernandez D., Sepulveda-Villegas M., Garcia-Pelaez J., Aguirre-Gamboa R., Lakatos P.L., Estrada K., Martinez-Vazquez M., Trevino V. A systematic review and functional bioinformatics analysis of genes associated with Crohn's disease identify more than 120 related genes. *BMC Genom.* 2022;23:302. doi: 10.1186/s12864-022-08491-y.

98. Franchimont D., Vermeire S., El Housni H., Pierik M., Van Steen K., Gustot T., Quertinmont E., Abramowicz M., Van Gossum A., Devière J., et al. Deficient host-bacteria interactions in inflammatory bowel disease? The toll-like receptor (TLR)-4 Asp299gly polymorphism is associated with Crohn's disease and ulcerative colitis. *Gut.* 2004;53:987–992. doi: 10.1136/gut.2003.030205.

99. Włodarczyk M., Czerwińska K., Włodarczyk J., Fichna J., Dziki A., Dziki L. Current Overview on the Use of Mesenchymal Stem Cells for Perianal Fistula Treatment in Patients with Crohn's Disease. *Life.* 2021;11:1133. doi: 10.3390/life11111133.

100. Hass R., Kasper C., Böhm S., Jacobs R. Different populations and sources of human mesenchymal stem cells (MSC): A comparison of adult and neonatal tissue-derived MSC. *Cell Commun. Signal.* 2011;9:12. doi: 10.1186/1478-811X-9-12.

101. Jiang W., Xu J. Immune modulation by mesenchymal stem cells. *Cell Prolif.* 2020;53:e12712. doi: 10.1111/cpr.12712.

102. Wu X., Jiang J., Gu Z., Zhang J., Chen Y., Liu X. Mesenchymal stromal cell therapies: Immunomodulatory properties and clinical progress. *Stem Cell Res. Ther.* 2020;11:345. doi: 10.1186/s13287-020-01855-9.

103. Dabrowski F.A., Burdzinska A., Kulesza A., Chlebus M., Kaleta B., Borysowski J., Zolocinska A., Paczek L., Wielgos M. Mesenchymal Stem Cells from Human Amniotic Membrane and Umbilical Cord Can Diminish Immunological Response in an in vitro Allograft Model. *Gynecol. Obstet. Investig.* 2016;82:267–275. doi: 10.1159/000449199.

104. Le Blanc K., Tammik L., Sundberg B., Haynesworth S.E., Ringden O. Mesenchymal Stem Cells Inhibit and Stimulate Mixed Lymphocyte Cultures and Mitogenic Responses Independently of the Major Histocompatibility Complex. *Scand. J. Immunol.* 2003;57:11–20. doi: 10.1046/j.1365-3083.2003.01176.x.

105. Duffy M.M., Pindjakova J., Hanley S.A., McCarthy C., Weidhofer G.A., Sweeney E.M., English K., Shaw G., Murphy J.M., Barry F.P., et al. Mesenchymal stem cell inhibition of T-helper 17 cell- differentiation is triggered by cell-cell contact and mediated by prostaglandin E2 via the EP4 receptor. *Eur. J. Immunol.* 2011;41:2840–2851. doi: 10.1002/eji.201141499.

106. Luz-Crawford P., Kurte M., Bravo-Alegría J., Contreras R., Nova-Lamperti E., Tejedor G., Noël D., Jorgensen C., Figueroa F., Djouad F., et al. Mesenchymal stem cells generate a CD4+CD25+Foxp3+ regulatory T cell population during the differentiation process of Th1 and Th17 cells. *Stem Cell Res. Ther.* 2013;4:65. doi: 10.1186/scrt216.

107. Kim J., Hematti P. Mesenchymal stem cell–educated macrophages: A novel type of alternatively activated macrophages. *Exp. Hematol.* 2009;37:1445–1453. doi: 10.1016/j.exphem.2009.09.004.

108. Dymowska M., Aksamit A., Zielniok K., Kniotek M., Kaleta B., Roszczyk A., Zych M., Dabrowski F., Paczek L., Burdzinska A. Interaction between Macrophages and Human Mesenchymal Stromal Cells Derived from Bone Marrow and Wharton's Jelly—A Comparative Study. *Pharmaceutics.* 2021;13:1822. doi: 10.3390/pharmaceutics13111822.

109. Kamada N., Hisamatsu T., Okamoto S., Chinen H., Kobayashi T., Sato T., Sakuraba A., Kitazume M.T., Sugita A., Koganei K., et al. Unique CD14+ intestinal macrophages contribute to the pathogenesis of Crohn disease via IL-23/IFN-γ axis. *J. Clin. Investig.* 2008;118:2269–2280. doi: 10.1172/JCI34610.

110. Sakuraba A., Sato T., Kamada N., Kitazume M., Sugita A., Hibi T. Th1/Th17 Immune Response Is Induced by Mesenteric Lymph Node Dendritic Cells in Crohn's Disease. *Gastroenterology.* 2009;137:1736–1745. doi: 10.1053/j.gastro.2009.07.049.

111. Li Y.-P., Paczesny S., Lauret E., Poirault S., Bordigoni P., Mekhloufi F., Hequet O., Bertrand Y., Ou-Yang J.-P., Stoltz J.-F., et al. Human Mesenchymal Stem Cells License Adult $CD34^+$ Hemopoietic Progenitor Cells to Differentiate into Regulatory Dendritic Cells through Activation of the Notch Pathway. *J. Immunol.* 2008;180:1598–1608. doi: 10.4049/jimmunol.180.3.1598.

112. Cuerquis J., Romieu-Mourez R., François M., Routy J.-P., Young Y.K., Zhao J., Eliopoulos N. Human mesenchymal stromal cells transiently increase cytokine production by activated T cells before suppressing T-cell proliferation: Effect of interferon-γ and tumor necrosis factor-α stimulation. *Cytotherapy.* 2014;16:191–202. doi: 10.1016/j.jcyt.2013.11.008.

113. Hass R. Role of MSC in the Tumor Microenvironment. *Cancers.* 2020;12:2107. doi: 10.3390/cancers12082107.

114. Liang W., Chen X., Zhang S., Fang J., Chen M., Xu Y., Chen X. Mesenchymal stem cells as a double-edged sword in tumor growth: Focusing on MSC-derived cytokines. *Cell. Mol. Biol. Lett.* 2021;26:3. doi: 10.1186/s11658-020-00246-5.

115. Scharl M., Frei S., Pesch T., Kellermeier S., Arikkat J., Frei P., Fried M., Weber A., Jehle E., Rühl A., et al. Interleukin-13 and transforming growth factor β synergise in the pathogenesis of human intestinal fistulae. *Gut.* 2013;62:63–72. doi: 10.1136/gutjnl-2011-300498.

116. Carrade D.D., Borjesson D.L. Immunomodulation by mesenchymal stem cells in veterinary species. *Comp. Med.* 2013;63:207–217.

117. Luo H., Li D., Chen Z., Wang B., Chen S. Manufacturing and banking canine adipose-derived mesenchymal stem cells for veterinary clinical application. *BMC Vet. Res.* 2021;17:96. doi: 10.1186/s12917-021-02791-3.

118. Delfi I., Wood C., Johnson L., Snow M., Innes J., Myint P., Johnson W. An In Vitro Comparison of the Neurotrophic and Angiogenic Activity of Human and Canine Adipose-Derived Mesenchymal Stem Cells (MSCs): Translating MSC-Based Therapies for Spinal Cord Injury. *Biomolecules.* 2020;10:1301. doi: 10.3390/biom10091301.

119. Teshima T., Yuchi Y., Suzuki R., Matsumoto H., Koyama H. Immunomodulatory Effects of Canine Adipose Tissue Mesenchymal Stem Cell-Derived Extracellular Vesicles on Stimulated CD4+ T Cells Isolated from Peripheral Blood Mononuclear Cells. *J. Immunol. Res.* 2021;2021:2993043. doi: 10.1155/2021/2993043.

120. An J.-H., Li Q., Bhang D.-H., Song W.-J., Youn H.-Y. TNF-α and INF-γ primed canine stem cell-derived extracellular vesicles alleviate experimental murine colitis. *Sci. Rep.* 2020;10:2115. doi: 10.1038/s41598-020-58909-4.

121. Shahsavari A., Weeratunga P., Ovchinnikov D.A., Whitworth D.J. Pluripotency and immunomodulatory signatures of canine induced pluripotent stem cell-derived mesenchymal stromal cells are similar to harvested mesenchymal stromal cells. *Sci. Rep.* 2021;11:3486. doi: 10.1038/s41598-021-82856-3.

122. Torres J., Mehandru S., Colombel J.F., Peyrin-Biroulet L. Crohn's disease. *Lancet.* 2017;389:1741–1755. doi: 10.1016/S0140-6736(16)31711-1.

123. Schwartz D.A., Loftus E.V., Jr., Tremaine W.J., Panaccione R., Harmsen W.S., Zinsmeister A.R., Sandborn W.J. The natural history of fistulizing Crohn's disease in Olmsted County, Minnesota. *Gastroenterology.* 2002;122:875–880. doi: 10.1053/gast.2002.32362.

124. Ingle S.B., Loftus E.V., Jr. The natural history of perianal Crohn's disease. *Dig. Liver Dis.* 2007;39:963–969. doi: 10.1016/j.dld.2007.07.154.

125. Eglinton T.W., Barclay M.L., Gearry R.B., Frizelle F.A. The spectrum of perianal Crohn's disease in a population-based cohort. *Dis. Colon Rectum.* 2012;55:773–777. doi: 10.1097/DCR.0b013e31825228b0.

126. Hellers G., Bergstrand O., Ewerth S., Holmström B. Occurrence and outcome after primary treatment of anal fistulae in Crohn's disease. *Gut.* 1980;21:525–527. doi: 10.1136/gut.21.6.525.

127. Lightner A.L., Faubion W.A., Fletcher J.G. Interdisciplinary Management of Perianal Crohn's Disease. *Gastroenterol. Clin. N. Am.* 2017;46:547–562. doi: 10.1016/j.gtc.2017.05.008.

128. Siegmund B., Feakins R.M., Barmias G., Ludvig J.C., Teixeira F.V., Rogler G., Scharl M. Results of the Fifth Scientific Workshop of the ECCO (II): Pathophysiology of Perianal Fistulizing Disease. *J. Crohn's Colitis.* 2016;10:377–386. doi: 10.1093/ecco-jcc/jjv228.

129. American Gastroenterological Association Clinical Practice Committee American Gastroenterological Association medical position statement: Perianal Crohn's disease. *Gastroenterology.* 2003;125:1503–1507.

130. Schwartz D.A., Herdman C.R. Review article: The medical treatment of Crohn's perianal fistulas. *Aliment. Pharmacol. Ther.* 2004;19:953–967. doi: 10.1111/j.1365-2036.2004.01917.x.

131. Adegbola S.O., Dibley L., Sahnan K., Wade T., Verjee A., Sawyer R., Mannick S., McCluskey D., Bassett P., Yassin N., et al. Development and initial psychometric validation of a patient-

reported outcome measure for Crohn's perianal fistula: The Crohn's Anal Fistula Quality of Life (CAF-QoL) scale. *Gut.* 2021;70:1649–1656. doi: 10.1136/gutjnl-2019-320553.

132. Panés J., Rimola J. Perianal fistulizing Crohn's disease: Pathogenesis, diagnosis and therapy. *Nat. Rev. Gastroenterol. Hepatol.* 2017;14:652–664. doi: 10.1038/nrgastro.2017.104.
133. Schwartz D.A., Wiersema M.J., Dudiak K.M., Fletcher J.G., Clain J.E., Tremaine W.J., Zinsmeister A.R., Norton I.D., Boardman L.A., Devine R.M., et al. A comparison of endoscopic ultrasound, magnetic resonance imaging, and exam under anesthesia for evaluation of Crohn's perianal fistulas. *Gastroenterology.* 2001;121:1064–1072. doi: 10.1053/gast.2001.28676.
134. Sahni V.A., Ahmad R., Burling D. Which method is best for imaging of perianal fistula? *Abdom. Imaging.* 2008;33:26–30. doi: 10.1007/s00261-007-9309-y.
135. Siddiqui M.R., Ashrafian H., Tozer P., Daulatzai N., Burling D., Hart A., Athanasiou T., Phillips R.K. A diagnostic accuracy meta-analysis of endoanal ultrasound and MRI for perianal fistula assessment. *Dis. Colon Rectum.* 2012;55:576–585. doi: 10.1097/DCR.0b013e318249d26c.
136. Adamina M., Bonovas S., Raine T., Spinelli A., Warusavitarne J., Armuzzi A., Bachmann O., Bager P., Biancone L., Bokemeyer B., et al. ECCO Guidelines on Therapeutics in Crohn's Disease: Surgical Treatment. *J. Crohn's Colitis.* 2020;14:155–168. doi: 10.1093/ecco-jcc/jjz187.
137. Aguilera-Castro L., Ferre-Aracil C., Garcia-Garcia-de-Paredes A., Rodriguez-de-Santiago E., Lopez-Sanroman A. Management of complex perianal Crohn's disease. *Ann. Gastroenterol.* 2017;30:33–44. doi: 10.20524/aog.2016.0099.
138. Marzo M., Felice C., Pugliese D., Andrisani G., Mocci G., Armuzzi A., Guidi L. Management of perianal fistulas in Crohn's disease: An up-to-date review. *World J. Gastroenterol.* 2015;21:1394–1403. doi: 10.3748/wjg.v21.i5.1394.
139. Kaur M., Panikkath D., Yan X., Liu Z., Berel D., Li D., Vasiliauskas E.A., Ippoliti A., Dubinsky M., Shih D.Q., et al. Perianal Crohn's Disease is Associated with Distal Colonic Disease, Stricturing Disease Behavior, IBD-Associated Serologies and Genetic Variation in the JAK-STAT Pathway. *Inflamm. Bowel Dis.* 2016;22:862–869. doi: 10.1097/MIB.0000000000000705.
140. Present D.H., Rutgeerts P., Targan S., Hanauer S.B., Mayer L., van Hogezand R.A., Podolsky D.K., Sands B.E., Braakman T., DeWoody K.L., et al. Infliximab for the treatment of fistulas in patients with Crohn's disease. *N. Engl. J. Med.* 1999;340:1398–1405. doi: 10.1056/NEJM199905063401804.
141. Sands B.E., Anderson F.H., Bernstein C.N., Chey W.Y., Feagan B.G., Fedorak R.N., Kamm M.A., Korzenik J.R., Lashner B.A., Onken J.E., et al. Infliximab maintenance therapy for fistulizing Crohn's disease. *N. Engl. J. Med.* 2004;350:876–885. doi: 10.1056/NEJMoa030815.
142. Yarur A.J., Kanagala V., Stein D.J., Czul F., Quintero M.A., Agrawal D., Patel A., Best K., Fox C., Idstein K., et al. Higher infliximab trough levels are associated with perianal fistula healing in patients with Crohn's disease. *Aliment. Pharmacol. Ther.* 2017;45:933–940. doi: 10.1111/apt.13970.
143. Davidov Y., Ungar B., Bar-Yoseph H., Carter D., Haj-Natour O., Yavzori M., Chowers Y., Eliakim R., Ben-Horin S., Kopylov U. Association of Induction Infliximab Levels With Clinical Response in Perianal Crohn's Disease. *J. Crohn's Colitis.* 2017;11:549–555. doi: 10.1093/ecco-jcc/jjw182.
144. Papamichael K., Vande Casteele N., Jeyarajah J., Jairath V., Osterman M.T., Cheifetz A.S. Higher Postinduction Infliximab Concentrations Are Associated With Improved Clinical

Outcomes in Fistulizing Crohn's Disease: An ACCENT-II Post Hoc Analysis. *Am. J. Gastroenterol.* 2021;116:1007–1014. doi: 10.14309/ajg.0000000000001111.

145. De Gregorio M., Lee T., Krishnaprasad K., Amos G., An Y.K., Bastian-Jordan M., Begun J., Borok N., Brown D.J.M., Cheung W., et al. Higher Anti-tumor Necrosis Factor-α Levels Correlate With Improved Radiologic Outcomes in Crohn's Perianal Fistulas. *Clin. Gastroenterol. Hepatol.* 2022;20:1306–1314. doi: 10.1016/j.cgh.2021.07.053.

146. Zhu M., Xu X., Feng Q., Cui Z., Wang T., Yan Y., Ran Z. Effectiveness of Infliximab on Deep Radiological Remission in Chinese Patients with Perianal Fistulizing Crohn's Disease. *Dig. Dis. Sci.* 2021;66:1658–1668. doi: 10.1007/s10620-020-06398-w.

147. Plevris N., Jenkinson P.W., Arnott I.D., Jones G.R., Lees C.W. Higher anti-tumor necrosis factor levels are associated with perianal fistula healing and fistula closure in Crohn's disease. *Eur. J. Gastroenterol. Hepatol.* 2020;32:32–37. doi: 10.1097/MEG.0000000000001561.

148. Strik A.S., Löwenberg M., Buskens C.J., Gecse B.K., Ponsioen I.C., Bemelman W.A., D'Haens G.R. Higher anti-TNF serum levels are associated with perianal fistula closure in Crohn's disease patients. *Scand. J. Gastroenterol.* 2019;54:453–458. doi: 10.1080/00365521.2019.1600014.

149. Colombel J.F., Sandborn W.J., Rutgeerts P., Enns R., Hanauer S.B., Panaccione R., Schreiber S., Byczkowski D., Li J., Kent J.D., et al. Adalimumab for maintenance of clinical response and remission in patients with Crohn's disease: The CHARM trial. *Gastroenterology.* 2007;132:52–65. doi: 10.1053/j.gastro.2006.11.041.

150. Lichtiger S., Binion D.G., Wolf D.C., Present D.H., Bensimon A.G., Wu E., Yu A.P., Cardoso A.T., Chao J., Mulani P.M., et al. The CHOICE trial: Adalimumab demonstrates safety, fistula healing, improved quality of life and increased work productivity in patients with Crohn's disease who failed prior infliximab therapy. *Aliment. Pharmacol. Ther.* 2010;32:1228–1239. doi: 10.1111/j.1365-2036.2010.04466.x.

151. Panaccione R., Loftus E.V., Jr., Binion D., McHugh K., Alam S., Chen N., Guerette B., Mulani P., Chao J. Efficacy and safety of adalimumab in Canadian patients with moderate to severe Crohn's disease: Results of the Adalimumab in Canadian SubjeCts with ModErate to Severe Crohn's DiseaSe (ACCESS) trial. *Can. J. Gastroenterol.* 2011;25:419–425. doi: 10.1155/2011/724813.

152. Adegbola S.O., Sahnan K., Tozer P.J., Phillips R.K., Faiz O.D., Warusavitarne J., Hart A. Review of local injection of anti-TNF for perianal fistulizing Crohn's disease. *Int. J. Color. Dis.* 2017;32:1539–1544. doi: 10.1007/s00384-017-2899-0.

153. Sands B.O., Gasink C., Jacobstein D., Gao L.L., Johanns J., Colombel J.F., de Villiers W.J., Sandborn W.J. Fistula healing in pivotal studies of Ustekinumab in Crohn's disease. *Gastroenterology.* 2017;152:S185. doi: 10.1016/S0016-5085(17)30930-7.

154. Laurent P., Panaccione R., Gasink C., Hoops T., Izanec J.L., Ma T., Nazar M., Bravata I., Lahaye M., Irving P.M., et al. O30 Closure of perianal fistula in patients receiving ustekinumab in the SEAVUE and STARDUST trials. *Gut.* 2022;71:A17.

155. Biemans V.B.C., van der Meulen-de Jong A.E., van der Woude C.J., Löwenberg M., Dijkstra G., Oldenburg B., de Boer N.K.H., van der Marel S., Bodelier A.G.L., Jansen J.M., et al. Ustekinumab for Crohn's Disease: Results of the ICC Registry, a Nationwide Prospective Observational Cohort Study. *J. Crohn's Colitis.* 2020;14:33–45. doi: 10.1093/ecco-jcc/jjz119.

156. Chapuis-Biron C., Kirchgesner J., Pariente B., Bouhnik Y., Amiot A., Viennot S., Serrero M.,

Fumery M., Allez M., Siproudhis L., et al. Ustekinumab for Perianal Crohn's Disease: The BioLAP Multicenter Study From the GETAID. *Am. J. Gastroenterol.* 2020;115:1812–1820. doi: 10.14309/ajg.0000000000000810.

157. Yao J., Zhang H., Su T., Peng X., Zhao J., Liu T., Wang W., Hu P., Zhi M., Zhang M. Ustekinumab Promotes Radiological Fistula Healing in Perianal Fistulizing Crohn's Disease: A Retrospective Real-World Analysis. *J. Clin. Med.* 2023;12:939. doi: 10.3390/jcm12030939.

158. Chapuis-Biron C., Bourrier A., Nachury M., Nancey S., Bouhnik Y., Serrero M., Armengol-Debeir L., Buisson A., Tran-Minh M.L., Zallot C., et al. Vedolizumab for perianal Crohn's disease: A multicentre cohort study in 151 patients. *Aliment. Pharmacol. Ther.* 2020;51:719–727. doi: 10.1111/apt.15665.

159. Schwartz D.A., Peyrin-Biroulet L., Lasch K., Adsul S., Danese S. Efficacy and Safety of 2 Vedolizumab Intravenous Regimens for Perianal Fistulizing Crohn's Disease: ENTERPRISE Study. *Clin. Gastroenterol. Hepatol.* 2021;20:1059–1067.e9. doi: 10.1016/j.cgh.2021.09.028.

160. Reinisch W., Colombel J.F., D'Haens G., Rimola J., DeHaas-Amatsaleh A., McKevitt M., Ren X., Serone A., Schwartz D.A., Gecse K.B. OP18 efficacy and safety of filgotinib for the treatment of perianal fistulizing Crohn's disease: Results from the phase 2 divergence 2 study. *J. Crohn's Colitis.* 2022;16:i019–i021. doi: 10.1093/ecco-jcc/jjab232.017.

161. Colombel J.F., Irving P., Rieder F., Panaccione R., Schwartz D., Hayashi R., Zhu X., Lacerda A.P., Dubcenco E., Marced E., et al. Efficacy and safety of upadacitinib for the treatment of fistulas and fissures in patients with Crohn's disease. *J. Crohn's Colitis.* 2023;17:i620–i622. doi: 10.1093/ecco-jcc/jjac190.0621.

162. Mak J.W.Y., Tang W., Yip T.C.F., Ran Z.H., Wei S.C., Ahuja V., Kumar S., Leung W.K., Hilmi I., Limsrivilai J., et al. Stopping anti-tumour necrosis factor therapy in patients with perianal Crohn's disease. *Aliment. Pharmacol. Ther.* 2019;50:1195–1203. doi: 10.1111/apt.15547.

163. Huinink S.T.B., Thomassen D., Steyerberg E.W., Pauwels R.W.M., Casanova M.J., Bouguen G., Mak J.W.Y., Molnár T., Lobo A.J., Seidelin J.B., et al. Discontinuation of Anti-Tumour Necrosis Factor Therapy in Patients with Perianal Fistulizing Crohn's Disease: Individual Participant Data Meta-Analysis of 309 patients from 12 studies. *J. Crohn's Colitis.* 2023 doi: 10.1093/ecco-jcc/jjad118. *online ahead of print* .

164. Lee M.J., Heywood N., Sagar P.M., Brown S.R., Fearnhead N.S., pCD Collaborators Surgical management of fistulating perianal Crohn's disease: A UK survey. *Color. Dis.* 2017;19:266–273. doi: 10.1111/codi.13462.

165. Lamb C.A., Kennedy N.A., Raine T., Hendy P.A., Smith P.J., Limdi J.K., Hayee B., Lomer M.C.E., Parkes G.C., Selinger C., et al. British Society of Gastroenterology consensus guidelines on the management of inflammatory bowel disease in adults. *Gut.* 2019;68((Suppl. 3)):s1–s106. doi: 10.1136/gutjnl-2019-318484.

166. Regueiro M., Mardini H. Treatment of perianal fistulizing Crohn's disease with infliximab alone or as an adjunct to exam under anesthesia with seton placement. *Inflamm. Bowel Dis.* 2003;9:98–103. doi: 10.1097/00054725-200303000-00003.

167. Gaertner W.B., Decanini A., Mellgren A., Lowry A.C., Goldberg S.M., Madoff R.D., Spencer M.P. Does infliximab infusion impact results of operative treatment for Crohn's perianal fistulas? *Dis. Colon Rectum.* 2007;50:1754–1760. doi: 10.1007/s10350-007-9077-3.

168. Stellingwerf M.E., van Praag E.M., Tozer P.J., Bemelman W.A., Buskens C.J. Systematic review and meta-analysis of endorectal advancement flap and ligation of the intersphincteric fistula tract for cryptoglandular and Crohn's high perianal fistulas. *BJS Open.* 2019;3:231–241. doi: 10.1002/bjs5.50129.

169. Soltani A., Kaiser A.M. Endorectal advancement flap for cryptoglandular or Crohn's fistula-in-ano. *Dis. Colon Rectum.* 2010;53:486–495. doi: 10.1007/DCR.0b013e3181ce8b01.

170. Wood T., Truong A., Mujukian A., Zaghiyan K., Fleshner P. Increasing experience with the LIFT procedure in Crohn's disease patients with complex anal fistula. *Tech. Coloproctol.* 2022;26:205–212. doi: 10.1007/s10151-022-02582-4.

171. Wasmann K.A., de Groof E.J., Stellingwerf M.E., D'Haens G.R., Ponsioen C.Y., Gecse K.B., Dijkgraaf M.G.W., Gerhards M.F., Jansen J.M., Pronk A., et al. Treatment of Perianal Fistulas in Crohn's Disease, Seton Versus Anti-TNF Versus Surgical Closure Following Anti-TNF [PISA]: A Randomised Controlled Trial. *J. Crohn's Colitis.* 2020;14:1049–1056. doi: 10.1093/ecco-jcc/jjaa004.

172. Tian Z., Li Y.L., Nan S.J., Xiu W.C., Wang Y.Q. Video-assisted anal fistula treatment for complex anorectal fistulas in adults: A systematic review and meta-analysis. *Tech. Coloproctol.* 2022;26:783–795. doi: 10.1007/s10151-022-02614-z.

173. Chase T.J.G., Quddus A., Selvakumar D., Cunha P., Cuming T. VAAFT for complex anal fistula: A useful tool, however, cure is unlikely. *Tech. Coloproctol.* 2021;25:1115–1121. doi: 10.1007/s10151-021-02492-x.

174. Schwandner O. Video-assisted anal fistula treatment (VAAFT) combined with advancement flap repair in Crohn's disease. *Tech. Coloproctol.* 2013;17:221–225. doi: 10.1007/s10151-012-0921-7.

175. Adegbola S.O., Sahnan K., Tozer P.J., Strouhal R., Hart A.L., Lung P.F.C., Phillips R.K.S., Faiz O., Warusavitarne J. Symptom Amelioration in Crohn's Perianal Fistulas Using Video-Assisted Anal Fistula Treatment (VAAFT) *J. Crohn's Colitis.* 2018;12:1067–1072. doi: 10.1093/ecco-jcc/jjy071.

176. Cao D., Li W., Ji Y., Wang X., Cui Z. Efficacy and safety of FiLaC™ for perianal fistulizing Crohn's disease: A systematic review and meta-analysis. *Tech. Coloproctol.* 2022;26:775–781. doi: 10.1007/s10151-022-02682-1.

177. Senéjoux A., Siproudhis L., Abramowitz L., Munoz-Bongrand N., Desseaux K., Bouguen G., Bourreille A., Dewit O., Stefanescu C., Vernier G., et al. Fistula Plug in Fistulising Ano-Perineal Crohn's Disease: A Randomised Controlled Trial. *J. Crohn's Colitis.* 2016;10:141–148. doi: 10.1093/ecco-jcc/jjv162.

178. Grimaud J.C., Munoz-Bongrand N., Siproudhis L., Abramowitz L., Sénéjoux A., Vitton V., Gambiez L., Flourié B., Hébuterne X., Louis E., et al. Fibrin glue is effective healing perianal fistulas in patients with Crohn's disease. *Gastroenterology.* 2010;138:2275–2281.e1. doi: 10.1053/j.gastro.2010.02.013.

179. Lee M.J., Parker C.E., Taylor S.R., Guizzetti L., Feagan B.G., Lobo A.J., Jairath V. Efficacy of Medical Therapies for Fistulizing Crohn's Disease: Systematic Review and Meta-analysis. *Clin. Gastroenterol. Hepatol.* 2018;16:1879–1892. doi: 10.1016/j.cgh.2018.01.030.

180. de Groof E.J., Sahami S., Lucas C., Ponsioen C.Y., Bemelman W.A., Buskens C.J. Treatment of perianal fistula in Crohn's disease: A systematic review and meta-analysis comparing

seton drainage and anti-tumour necrosis factor treatment. *Color. Dis.* 2016;18:667–675. doi: 10.1111/codi.13311.

181. Yassin N.A., Askari A., Warusavitarne J., Faiz O.D., Athanasiou T., Phillips R.K., Hart A.L. Systematic review: The combined surgical and medical treatment of fistulizing perianal Crohn's disease. *Aliment. Pharmacol. Ther.* 2014;40:741–749. doi: 10.1111/apt.12906.
182. Gecse K.B., Sebastian S., Hertogh G.D., Yassin N.A., Kotze P.G., Reinisch W., Spinelli A., Koutroubakis I.E., Katsanos K.H., Hart A., et al. Results of the Fifth Scientific Workshop of the ECCO [II]: Clinical Aspects of Perianal Fistulizing Crohn's Disease-the Unmet Needs. *J. Crohn's Colitis.* 2016;10:758–765. doi: 10.1093/ecco-jcc/jjw039.
183. Meima-van Praag E.M., van Rijn K.L., Wasmann K.A.T.G.M., Snijder H.J., Stoker J., D'Haens G.R., Gecse K.B., Gerhards M.F., Jansen J.M., Dijkgraaf M.G.W., et al. Short-term anti-TNF therapy with surgical closure versus anti-TNF therapy in the treatment of perianal fistulas in Crohn's disease (PISA-II): A patient preference randomised trial. *Lancet Gastroenterol. Hepatol.* 2022;7:617–626. doi: 10.1016/S2468-1253(22)00088-7.
184. Tozer P., Ng S.C., Siddiqui M.R., Plamondon S., Burling D., Gupta A., Swatton A., Tripoli S., Vaizey C.J., Kamm M.A., et al. Long-term MRI-guided combined anti-TNF-α and thiopurine therapy for Crohn's perianal fistulas. *Inflamm. Bowel Dis.* 2012;18:1825–1834. doi: 10.1002/ibd.21940.
185. Chambaz M., Verdalle-Cazes M., Desprez C., Thomassin L., Charpentier C., Grigioni S., Armengol-Debeir L., Bridoux V., Savoye G., Savoye-Collet C. Deep remission on magnetic resonance imaging impacts outcomes of perianal fistulizing Crohn's disease. *Dig. Liver Dis.* 2019;51:358–363. doi: 10.1016/j.dld.2018.12.010.
186. Panés J., García-Olmo D., Van Assche G., Colombel J.F., Reinisch W., Baumgart D.C., Dignass A., Nachury M., Ferrante M., Kazemi-Shirazi L., et al. Expanded allogeneic adipose-derived mesenchymal stem cells (Cx601) for complex perianal fistulas in Crohn's disease: A phase 3 randomised, double-blind controlled trial. *Lancet.* 2016;388:1281–1290. doi: 10.1016/S0140-6736(16)31203-X.
187. Panés J., Bouma G., Ferrante M., Kucharzik T., Nachury M., de la Portilla de Juan F., Reinisch W., Selvaggi F., Tschmelitsch J., Brett N.R., et al. INSPECT: A Retrospective Study to Evaluate Long-term Effectiveness and Safety of Darvadstrocel in Patients With Perianal Fistulizing Crohn's Disease Treated in the ADMIRE-CD Trial. *Inflamm. Bowel Dis.* 2022;28:1737–1745. doi: 10.1093/ibd/izab361.
188. Geldof J., Iqbal N., LeBlanc J.F., Anandabaskaran S., Sawyer R., Buskens C., Bemelman W., Gecse K., Lundby L., Lightner A.L., et al. Classifying perianal fistulising Crohn's disease: An expert consensus to guide decision-making in daily practice and clinical trials. *Lancet Gastroenterol. Hepatol.* 2022;7:576–584. doi: 10.1016/S2468-1253(22)00007-3.
189. Scharl M., Frei S., Pesch T., Kellermeier S., Arikkat J., Frei P., Fried M., Weber A., Jehle E., Rühl A., et al. Interleukin-13 and transforming growth factor β synergise in the pathogenesis of human intestinal fistulae. *Gut.* 2013;62:63–72. doi: 10.1136/gutjnl-2011-300498.
190. Bataille F., Rohrmeier C., Bates R., Weber A., Rieder F., Brenmoehl J., Strauch U., Farkas S., Fürst A., Hofstädter F., et al. Evidence for a role of epithelial mesenchymal transition during pathogenesis of fistulae in Crohn's disease. *Inflamm. Bowel Dis.* 2008;14:1514–1527. doi: 10.1002/ibd.20590.

191. Scharl M., Weber A., Fürst A., Farkas S., Jehle E., Pesch T., Kellermeier S., Fried M., Rogler G. Potential role for SNAIL family transcription factors in the etiology of Crohn's disease-associated fistulae. *Inflamm. Bowel Dis.* 2011;17:1907–1916. doi: 10.1002/ibd.21555.

192. Frei S.M., Pesch T., Lang S., Weber A., Jehle E., Vavricka S.R., Fried M., Rogler G., Scharl M. A role for tumor necrosis factor and bacterial antigens in the pathogenesis of Crohn's disease-associated fistulae. *Inflamm. Bowel Dis.* 2013;19:2878–2887. doi: 10.1097/01.MIB.0000435760.82705.23.

193. Goffin L., Fagagnini S., Vicari A., Mamie C., Melhem H., Weder B., Lutz C., Lang S., Scharl M., Rogler G., et al. Anti-MMP-9 Antibody: A Promising Therapeutic Strategy for Treatment of Inflammatory Bowel Disease Complications with Fibrosis. *Inflamm. Bowel Dis.* 2016;22:2041–2057. doi: 10.1097/MIB.0000000000000863.

194. Kirkegaard T., Hansen A., Bruun E., Brynskov J. Expression and localisation of matrix metalloproteinases and their natural inhibitors in fistulae of patients with Crohn's disease. *Gut.* 2004;53:701–709. doi: 10.1136/gut.2003.017442.

195. Rizzo G., Rubbino F., Elangovan S., Sammarco G., Lovisa S., Restelli S., Pineda Chavez S.E., Massimino L., Lamparelli L., Paulis M., et al. Dysfunctional Extracellular Matrix Remodeling Supports Perianal Fistulizing Crohn's Disease by a Mechanoregulated Activation of the Epithelial-to-Mesenchymal Transition. *Cell. Mol. Gastroenterol. Hepatol.* 2023;15:741–764. doi: 10.1016/j.jcmgh.2022.12.006.

196. Tozer P.J., Lung P., Lobo A.J., Sebastian S., Brown S.R., Hart A.L., Fearnhead N., ENiGMA Collaboration Review article: Pathogenesis of Crohn's perianal fistula-understanding factors impacting on success and failure of treatment strategies. *Aliment. Pharmacol. Ther.* 2018;48:260–269. doi: 10.1111/apt.14814.

197. Toyonaga T., Matsushima M., Tanaka Y., Shimojima Y., Matsumura N., Kannyama H., Nozawa M., Hatakeyama T., Suzuki K., Yanagita K., et al. Microbiological analysis and endoanal ultrasonography for diagnosis of anal fistula in acute anorectal sepsis. *Int. J. Color. Dis.* 2007;22:209–213. doi: 10.1007/s00384-006-0121-x.

198. Tozer P.J., Rayment N., Hart A.L., Daulatzai N., Murugananthan A.U., Whelan K., Phillips R.K. What role do bacteria play in persisting fistula formation in idiopathic and Crohn's anal fistula? *Color. Dis.* 2015;17:235–241. doi: 10.1111/codi.12810.

199. van Onkelen R.S., Mitalas L.E., Gosselink M.P., van Belkum A., Laman J.D., Schouten W.R. Assessment of microbiota and peptidoglycan in perianal fistulas. *Diagn. Microbiol. Infect. Dis.* 2013;75:50–54. doi: 10.1016/j.diagmicrobio.2012.09.012.

200. van Onkelen R.S., Gosselink M.P., van Meurs M., Melief M.J., Schouten W.R., Laman J.D. Pro-inflammatory cytokines in cryptoglandular anal fistulas. *Tech. Coloproctol.* 2016;20:619–625. doi: 10.1007/s10151-016-1494-7.

201. Singh S., Ding N.S., Mathis K.L., Dulai P.S., Farrell A.M., Pemberton J.H., Hart A.L., Sandborn W.J., Loftus E.V., Jr. Systematic review with meta-analysis: Faecal diversion for management of perianal Crohn's disease. *Aliment. Pharmacol. Ther.* 2015;42:783–792. doi: 10.1111/apt.13356.

202. Goren I., Ian W., Reshef L., Sharar Fischler T., Pauker M., Silverman J., Dotan I., Yanai H. P683 Patients with newly diagnosed fistulizing perianal Crohn's disease have a distinct microbial signature. *J. Crohn's Colitis.* 2021;15:S602. doi: 10.1093/ecco-jcc/jjab076.803.

203. Breton J., Tanes C., Tu V., Albenberg L., Rowley S., Devas N., Hwang R., Kachelries K., Wu G.D., Baldassano R.N., et al. A Microbial Signature for Paediatric Perianal Crohn's Disease. *J. Crohn's Colitis.* 2022;16:1281–1292. doi: 10.1093/ecco-jcc/jjac032.

204. Schnitzler F., Friedrich M., Wolf C., Stallhofer J., Angelberger M., Diegelmann J., Olszak T., Tillack C., Beigel F., Göke B., et al. The NOD2 Single Nucleotide Polymorphism rs72796353 (IVS4+10 A>C) Is a Predictor for Perianal Fistulas in Patients with Crohn's Disease in the Absence of Other NOD2 Mutations. *PLoS ONE.* 2015;10:e0116044. doi: 10.1371/journal.pone.0116044.

205. Vermeire S., Pierik M., Hlavaty T., Claessens G., van Schuerbeeck N., Joossens S., Ferrante M., Henckaerts L., Bueno de Mesquita M., Vlietinck R., et al. Association of organic cation transporter risk haplotype with perianal penetrating Crohn's disease but not with susceptibility to IBD. *Gastroenterology.* 2005;129:1845–1853. doi: 10.1053/j.gastro.2005.10.006.

206. Palmieri O., Latiano A., Valvano R., D'Incà R., Vecchi M., Sturniolo G.C., Saibeni S., Peyvandi F., Bossa F., Zagaria C., et al. Variants of OCTN1-2 cation transporter genes are associated with both Crohn's disease and ulcerative colitis. *Aliment. Pharmacol. Ther.* 2006;23:497–506. doi: 10.1111/j.1365-2036.2006.02780.x.

207. Eglinton T.W., Roberts R., Pearson J., Barclay M., Merriman T.R., Frizelle F.A., Gearry R.B. Clinical and genetic risk factors for perianal Crohn's disease in a population-based cohort. *Am. J. Gastroenterol.* 2012;107:589–596. doi: 10.1038/ajg.2011.437.

208. Latiano A., Palmieri O., Cucchiara S., Castro M., D'Incà R., Guariso G., Dallapiccola B., Valvano M.R., Latiano T., Andriulli A., et al. Polymorphism of the IRGM gene might predispose to fistulizing behavior in Crohn's disease. *Am. J. Gastroenterol.* 2009;104:110–116. doi: 10.1038/ajg.2008.3.

209. Zhang M., Wang X., Jiang X., Yang X., Wen C., Zhi M., Gao X., Hu P., Liu H. Polymorphisms of the TNF Gene and Three Susceptibility Loci Are Associated with Crohn's Disease and Perianal Fistula Crohn's Disease: A Study among the Han Population from South China. *Med. Sci. Monit.* 2019;25:9637–9650. doi: 10.12659/MSM.917244.

210. Beser O.F., Conde C.D., Serwas N.K., Cokugras F.C., Kutlu T., Boztug K., Erkan T. Clinical features of interleukin 10 receptor gene mutations in children with very early-onset inflammatory bowel disease. *J. Pediatr. Gastroenterol. Nutr.* 2015;60:332–338. doi: 10.1097/MPG.0000000000000621.

211. Yang D.H., Yang S.K., Song K., Hong M., Park S.H., Lee H.S., Kim J.B., Lee H.J., Park S.K., Jung K.W., et al. TNFSF15 is an independent predictor for the development of Crohn's disease-related complications in Koreans. *J. Crohn's Colitis.* 2014;8:1315–1326. doi: 10.1016/j.crohns.2014.04.002.

212. de Ridder L., Weersma R.K., Dijkstra G., van der Steege G., Benninga M.A., Nolte I.M., Taminiau J.A., Hommes D.W., Stokkers P.C. Genetic susceptibility has a more important role in pediatric-onset Crohn's disease than in adult-onset Crohn's disease. *Inflamm. Bowel Dis.* 2007;13:1083–1092. doi: 10.1002/ibd.20171.

213. Henckaerts L., Van Steen K., Verstreken I., Cleynen I., Franke A., Schreiber S., Rutgeerts P., Vermeire S. Genetic risk profiling and prediction of disease course in Crohn's disease patients. *Clin. Gastroenterol. Hepatol.* 2009;7:972–980.e2. doi: 10.1016/j.cgh.2009.05.001.

214. Quaranta M., Burden A.D., Griffiths C.E., Worthington J., Barker J.N., Trembath R.C., Capon

F. Differential contribution of CDKAL1 variants to psoriasis, Crohn's disease and type II diabetes. *Genes Immun.* 2009;10:654–658. doi: 10.1038/gene.2009.51.

215. Song J., Zhuang Y., Zhu C., Meng H., Lu B., Xie B., Peng J., Li M., Yi C. Differential roles of human PUS10 in miRNA processing and tRNA pseudouridylation. *Nat. Chem. Biol.* 2020;16:160–169. doi: 10.1038/s41589-019-0420-5.

216. Cleynen I., González J.R., Figueroa C., Franke A., McGovern D., Bortlík M., Crusius B.J., Vecchi M., Artieda M., Szczypiorska M., et al. Genetic factors conferring an increased susceptibility to develop Crohn's disease also influence disease phenotype: Results from the IBDchip European Project. *Gut.* 2013;62:1556–1565. doi: 10.1136/gutjnl-2011-300777.

217. Bataille F., Klebl F., Rümmele P., Schroeder J., Farkas S., Wild P.J., Fürst A., Hofstädter F., Schölmerich J., Herfarth H., et al. Morphological characterisation of Crohn's disease fistulae. *Gut.* 2004;53:1314–1321. doi: 10.1136/gut.2003.038208.

218. Bruckner R.S., Spalinger M.R., Barnhoorn M.C., Feakins R., Fuerst A., Jehle E.C., Rickenbacher A., Turina M., Niechcial A., Lang S., et al. Contribution of CD3+CD8- and CD3+CD8+ T Cells to TNF-α Overexpression in Crohn Disease-Associated Perianal Fistulas and Induction of Epithelial-Mesenchymal Transition in HT-29 Cells. *Inflamm. Bowel Dis.* 2021;27:538–549. doi: 10.1093/ibd/izaa240.

219. Maggi L., Capone M., Giudici F., Santarlasci V., Querci V., Liotta F., Ficari F., Maggi E., Tonelli F., Annunziato F., et al. CD4+CD161+ T lymphocytes infiltrate Crohn's disease-associated perianal fistulas and are reduced by anti-TNF-α local therapy. *Int. Arch. Allergy Immunol.* 2013;161:81–86. doi: 10.1159/000343467.

220. van Unen V., Li N., Molendijk I., Temurhan M., Höllt T., van der Meulen-de Jong A.E., Verspaget H.W., Mearin M.L., Mulder C.J., van Bergen J., et al. Mass Cytometry of the Human Mucosal Immune System Identifies Tissue- and Disease-Associated Immune Subsets. *Immunity.* 2016;44:1227–1239. doi: 10.1016/j.immuni.2016.04.014.

221. Kotze P.G., Shen B., Lightner A., Yamamoto T., Spinelli A., Ghosh S., Panaccione R. Modern management of perianal fistulas in Crohn's disease: Future directions. *Gut.* 2018;67:1181–1194. doi: 10.1136/gutjnl-2017-314918.

222. García-Olmo D., García-Arranz M., Herreros D., Pascual I., Peiro C., Rodríguez-Montes J.A. A phase I clinical trial of the treatment of Crohn's fistula by adipose mesenchymal stem cell transplantation. *Dis. Colon Rectum.* 2005;48:1416–1423. doi: 10.1007/s10350-005-0052-6.

223. Garcia-Olmo D., Herreros D., Pascual I., Pascual J.A., Del-Valle E., Zorrilla J., De-La-Quintana P., Garcia-Arranz M., Pascual M. Expanded adipose-derived stem cells for the treatment of complex perianal fistula: A phase II clinical trial. *Dis. Colon Rectum.* 2009;52:79–86. doi: 10.1007/DCR.0b013e3181973487.

224. Cao Y., Su Q., Zhang B., Shen F., Li S. Efficacy of stem cells therapy for Crohn's fistula: A meta-analysis and systematic review. *Stem Cell Res. Ther.* 2021;12:32. doi: 10.1186/s13287-020-02095-7.

225. Kou M., Huang L., Yang J., Chiang Z., Chen S., Liu J., Guo L., Zhang X., Zhou X., Xu X., et al. Mesenchymal stem cell-derived extracellular vesicles for immunomodulation and regeneration: A next generation therapeutic tool? *Cell Death Dis.* 2022;13:580. doi: 10.1038/s41419-022-05034-x.

226. Guillamat-Prats R. The Role of MSC in Wound Healing, Scarring and Regeneration. *Cells.* 2021;10:1729. doi: 10.3390/cells10071729.

227. Carvello M., Lightner A., Yamamoto T., Kotze P.G., Spinelli A. Mesenchymal Stem Cells for Perianal Crohn's Disease. *Cells.* 2019;8:764. doi: 10.3390/cells8070764.

228. Li N., Hua J. Interactions between mesenchymal stem cells and the immune system. *Cell. Mol. Life Sci.* 2017;74:2345–2360. doi: 10.1007/s00018-017-2473-5.

229. Lightner A.L., Faubion W.A. Mesenchymal Stem Cell Injections for the Treatment of Perianal Crohn's Disease: What We Have Accomplished and What We Still Need to Do. *J. Crohn's Colitis.* 2017;11:1267–1276. doi: 10.1093/ecco-jcc/jjx046.

230. Hanna J., Hubel A. Preservation of stem cells. *Organogenesis.* 2009;5:134–137. doi: 10.4161/org.5.3.9585.

231. Dadgar N., Altemus J., Li Y., Lightner A.L. Effect of Crohn's disease mesenteric mesenchymal stem cells and their extracellular vesicles on T-cell immunosuppressive capacity. *J. Cell. Mol. Med.* 2022;26:4924–4939. doi: 10.1111/jcmm.17483.

232. Galleu A., Riffo-Vasquez Y., Trento C., Lomas C., Dolcetti L., Cheung T.S., von Bonin M., Barbieri L., Halai K., Ward S., et al. Apoptosis in mesenchymal stromal cells induces in vivo recipient-mediated immunomodulation. *Sci. Transl. Med.* 2017;9:eaam7828. doi: 10.1126/scitranslmed.aam7828.

233. Iqbal N., Constable L., Tozer P., Lung P., Hart A., Powell N. P336 Can Mesenchymal Stem Cell (MSC) apoptosis be used as a biomarker for treatment success in perianal fistulising Crohn's Disease (pCD)? Findings from a prospective pilot study. *J. Crohn's Colitis.* 2022;16((Supp. 1)):i353. doi: 10.1093/ecco-jcc/jjab232.463.

234. Altemus J., Dadgar N., Li Y., Lightner A.L. Adipose tissue-derived mesenchymal stem cells' acellular product extracellular vesicles as a potential therapy for Crohn's disease. *J. Cell Physiol.* 2022;237:3001–3011. doi: 10.1002/jcp.30756.

235. Yang E., Panaccione N., Whitmire N., Dulai P.S., Vande Casteele N., Singh S., Boland B.S., Collins A., Sandborn W.J., Panaccione R., et al. Efficacy and safety of simultaneous treatment with two biologic medications in refractory Crohn's disease. *Aliment. Pharmacol. Ther.* 2020;51:1031–1038. doi: 10.1111/apt.15719.

236. Adegbola S.O., Dibley L., Sahnan K., Wade T., Verjee A., Sawyer R., Mannick S., McCluskey D., Yassin N., Phillips R.K.S., et al. Burden of disease and adaptation to life in patients with Crohn's perianal fistula: A qualitative exploration. *Health Qual Life Outcomes.* 2020;18:370. doi: 10.1186/s12955-020-01622-7.

237. Mahadev S., Young J.M., Selby W., Solomon M.J. Self-reported depressive symptoms and suicidal feelings in perianal Crohn's disease. *Color. Dis.* 2012;14:331–335. doi: 10.1111/j.1463-1318.2011.02613.x.

238. Boudiaf R., Bouchard D., Rivière P., Brochard C., Laharie D., Abramowitz L., Pigot F., GREP members (Groupe de Recherche en Proctologie) Assessment of sexual dysfunction in patients with perianal Crohn's disease. *Color. Dis.* 2021;23:114–122. doi: 10.1111/codi.15375.

239. Schwartz D.A., Loftus E.V., Tremaine W.J., Panaccione R., Harmsen W.S., Zinsmeister A.R., Sandborn W.J. The Natural History of Fistulizing Crohn's Disease in Olmsted County, Minnesota. *Gastroenterology.* 2002;122:875–880. doi: 10.1053/gast.2002.32362.

240. Thia K.T., Sandborn W.J., Harmsen W.S., Zinsmeister A.R., Loftus E.V. Risk Factors Associated With Progression to Intestinal Complications of Crohn's Disease in a Population-Based Cohort. *Gastroenterology.* 2010;139:1147–1155. doi: 10.1053/j.gastro.2010.06.070.

241. Brochard C., Rabilloud M.-L., Hamonic S., Bajeux E., Pagenault M., Dabadie A., Gerfaud A., Viel J.-F., Tron I., Robaszkiewicz M., et al. Natural History of Perianal Crohn's Disease: Long-Term Follow-up of a Population-Based Cohort. *Clin. Gastroenterol. Hepatol.* 2022;20:e102–e110. doi: 10.1016/j.cgh.2020.12.024.

242. Tjandra D., Garg M., Behrenbruch C., McCormick J., Simkin P., Prentice R., Trinh A., Al-Ani A., Vaughan R., Macrae F., et al. Review Article: Investigation and Management of Internal Fistulae in Crohn's Disease. *Aliment. Pharmacol. Ther.* 2021;53:1064–1079. doi: 10.1111/apt.16326.

243. Tsai L., McCurdy J.D., Ma C., Jairath V., Singh S. Epidemiology and Natural History of Perianal Crohn's Disease: A Systematic Review and Meta-Analysis of Population-Based Cohorts. *Inflamm. Bowel Dis.* 2021;18:izab287. doi: 10.1093/ibd/izab287.

244. Schwartz D.A., Ghazi L.J., Regueiro M., Fichera A., Zoccali M., Ong E.M.W., Mortelé K.J. Guidelines for the Multidisciplinary Management of Crohn's Perianal Fistulas: Summary Statement. *Inflamm. Bowel Dis.* 2015;21:723–730. doi: 10.1097/MIB.0000000000000315.

245. Adegbola S.O., Dibley L., Sahnan K., Wade T., Verjee A., Sawyer R., Mannick S., McCluskey D., Yassin N., Phillips R.K.S., et al. Burden of Disease and Adaptation to Life in Patients with Crohn's Perianal Fistula: A Qualitative Exploration. *Health Qual. Life Outcomes.* 2020;18:370. doi: 10.1186/s12955-020-01622-7.

246. Mahadev S., Young J.M., Selby W., Solomon M.J. Quality of Life in Perianal Crohn's Disease: What Do Patients Consider Important? *Dis. Colon Rectum.* 2011;54:579–585. doi: 10.1007/DCR.0b013e3182099d9e.

247. Gklavas A., Sotirova I., Karageorgou M., Kozonis T., Poulaki A., Papaconstantinou I. Is the Quality of Life of Patients with Fistulizing Perianal Crohn' s Disease Impaired by the Presence of Chronic Loose, Non-Cutting Seton? *J. Gastrointest. Surg.* 2021;25:2686–2689. doi: 10.1007/s11605-021-04987-2.

248. Lee M.J., Brown S.R., Fearnhead N.S., Hart A., Lobo A.J. How Are We Managing Fistulating Perianal Crohn's Disease? Results of a National Survey of Consultant Gastroenterologists. *Frontline Gastroenterol.* 2018;9:16–22. doi: 10.1136/flgastro-2017-100866.

249. Lee M.J., Heywood N., Sagar P.M., Brown S.R., Fearnhead N.S., pCD Collaborators Surgical Management of Fistulating Perianal Crohn's Disease: A UK Survey. *Colorectal. Dis.* 2017;19:266–273. doi: 10.1111/codi.13462.

250. Panes J., Reinisch W., Rupniewska E., Khan S., Forns J., Khalid J.M., Bojic D., Patel H. Burden and Outcomes for Complex Perianal Fistulas in Crohn's Disease: Systematic Review. *WJG.* 2018;24:4821–4834. doi: 10.3748/wjg.v24.i42.4821.

251. Gecse K.B., Sebastian S., de Hertogh G., Yassin N.A., Kotze P.G., Reinisch W., Spinelli A., Koutroubakis I.E., Katsanos K.H., Hart A., et al. Results of the Fifth Scientific Workshop of the ECCO [II]: Clinical Aspects of Perianal Fistulising Crohn's Disease—the Unmet Needs. *J. Crohns Colitis.* 2016;10:758–765. doi: 10.1093/ecco-jcc/jjw039.

252. Torres J., Bonovas S., Doherty G., Kucharzik T., Gisbert J.P., Raine T., Adamina M., Armuzzi A., Bachmann O., Bager P., et al. ECCO Guidelines on Therapeutics in Crohn's Disease: Medical

Treatment. *J. Crohns Colitis.* 2020;14:4–22. doi: 10.1093/ecco-jcc/jjz180.

253. Feuerstein J.D., Ho E.Y., Shmidt E., Singh H., Falck-Ytter Y., Sultan S., Terdiman J.P., Sultan S., Cohen B.L., Chachu K., et al. AGA Clinical Practice Guidelines on the Medical Management of Moderate to Severe Luminal and Perianal Fistulizing Crohn's Disease. *Gastroenterology.* 2021;160:2496–2508. doi: 10.1053/j.gastro.2021.04.022.

254. Steinhart A.H., Panaccione R., Targownik L., Bressler B., Khanna R., Marshall J.K., Afif W., Bernstein C.N., Bitton A., Borgaonkar M., et al. Clinical Practice Guideline for the Medical Management of Perianal Fistulizing Crohn's Disease: The Toronto Consensus. *Inflamm. Bowel Dis.* 2019;25:1–13. doi: 10.1093/ibd/izy247.

255. Bemelman W.A., Warusavitarne J., Sampietro G.M., Serclova Z., Zmora O., Luglio G., de Buck van Overstraeten A., Burke J.P., Buskens C.J., Francesco C., et al. ECCO-ESCP Consensus on Surgery for Crohn's Disease. *J. Crohns Colitis.* 2018;12:1–16. doi: 10.1093/ecco-jcc/jjx061.

256. Gecse K.B., Bemelman W., Kamm M.A., Stoker J., Khanna R., Ng S.C., Panés J., van Assche G., Liu Z., Hart A., et al. A Global Consensus on the Classification, Diagnosis and Multidisciplinary Treatment of Perianal Fistulising Crohn's Disease. *Gut.* 2014;63:1381–1392. doi: 10.1136/gutjnl-2013-306709.

257. Lichtenstein G.R., Loftus E.V., Isaacs K.L., Regueiro M.D., Gerson L.B., Sands B.E. ACG Clinical Guideline: Management of Crohn's Disease in Adults. *Am. J. Gastroenterol.* 2018;113:481–517. doi: 10.1038/ajg.2018.27.

258. Sandborn W.J., Present D.H., Isaacs K.L., Wolf D.C., Greenberg E., Hanauer S.B., Feagan B.G., Mayer L., Johnson T., Galanko J., et al. Tacrolimus for the Treatment of Fistulas in Patients with Crohn's Disease: A Randomized, Placebo-Controlled Trial. *Gastroenterology.* 2003;125:380–388. doi: 10.1016/S0016-5085(03)00877-1.

259. Present D.H., Mayer L., Braakman T. Infliximab for the Treatment of Fistulas in Patients with Crohn's Disease. *N. Engl. J. Med.* 1999;340:1398–1405. doi: 10.1056/NEJM199905063401804.

260. Sands B.E., Anderson F.H., Bernstein C.N., Chey W.Y., Feagan B.G., Fedorak R.N., Kamm M.A., Korzenik J.R., Lashner B.A., Onken J.E., et al. Infliximab Maintenance Therapy for Fistulizing Crohn's Disease. *N. Engl. J. Med.* 2004;350:876–885. doi: 10.1056/NEJMoa030815.

261. West R.L., van der Woude C.J., Hansen B.E., Felt-Bersma R.J.F., van Tilburg A.J.P., Drapers J.A.G., Kuipers E.J. Clinical and Endosonographic Effect of Ciprofloxacin on the Treatment of Perianal Fistulae in Crohn's Disease with Infliximab: A Double-Blind Placebo-Controlled Study: Ciprofloxacin Plus Infliximab in Perianal Fistulae. *Aliment. Pharmacol. Ther.* 2004;20:1329–1336. doi: 10.1111/j.1365-2036.2004.02247.x.

262. Bouguen G., Siproudhis L., Gizard E., Wallenhorst T., Billioud V., Bretagne J., Bigard M., Peyrin–Biroulet L. Long-Term Outcome of Perianal Fistulizing Crohn's Disease Treated With Infliximab. *Clin. Gastroenterol. Hepatol.* 2013;11:975–981.e4. doi: 10.1016/j.cgh.2012.12.042.

263. Zhu M., Xu X., Feng Q., Cui Z., Wang T., Yan Y., Ran Z. Effectiveness of Infliximab on Deep Radiological Remission in Chinese Patients with Perianal Fistulizing Crohn's Disease. *Dig. Dis. Sci.* 2021;66:1658–1668. doi: 10.1007/s10620-020-06398-w.

264. Lee M.J., Parker C.E., Taylor S.R., Guizzetti L., Feagan B.G., Lobo A.J., Jairath V. Efficacy of Medical Therapies for Fistulizing Crohn's Disease: Systematic Review and Meta-Analysis. *Clin. Gastroenterol. Hepatol.* 2018;16:1879–1892. doi: 10.1016/j.cgh.2018.01.030.

265. Hanauer S.B., Sandborn W.J., Rutgeerts P., Fedorak R.N., Lukas M., MacIntosh D., Panaccione R., Wolf D., Pollack P. Human Anti–Tumor Necrosis Factor Monoclonal Antibody (Adalimumab) in Crohn's Disease: The CLASSIC-I Trial. *Gastroenterology.* 2006;130:323–333. doi: 10.1053/j.gastro.2005.11.030.

266. Sandborn W.J., Rutgeerts P., Enns R., Hanauer S.B., Panaccione R., D'Haens G., Li J., Rosenfeld M.R., Kent J.D., Pollack P.F. Adalimumab Induction Therapy for Crohn Disease Previously Treated with Infliximab. *Ann. Intern. Med.* 2007;146:829–838. doi: 10.7326/0003-4819-146-12-200706190-00159.

267. Colombel J., Sandborn W.J., Rutgeerts P., Enns R., Hanauer S.B., Panaccione R., Schreiber S., Byczkowski D., Li J., Kent J.D., et al. Adalimumab for Maintenance of Clinical Response and Remission in Patients With Crohn's Disease: The CHARM Trial. *Gastroenterology.* 2007;132:52–65. doi: 10.1053/j.gastro.2006.11.041.

268. Colombel J.-F., Schwartz D.A., Sandborn W.J., Kamm M.A., D'Haens G., Rutgeerts P., Enns R., Panaccione R., Schreiber S., Li J., et al. Adalimumab for the Treatment of Fistulas in Patients with Crohn's Disease. *Gut.* 2009;58:940–948. doi: 10.1136/gut.2008.159251.

269. Dewint P., Hansen B.E., Verhey E., Oldenburg B., Hommes D.W., Pierik M., Ponsioen C.I.J., van Dullemen H.M., Russel M., van Bodegraven A.A., et al. Adalimumab Combined with Ciprofloxacin Is Superior to Adalimumab Monotherapy in Perianal Fistula Closure in Crohn's Disease: A Randomised, Double-Blind, Placebo Controlled Trial (ADAFI) *Gut.* 2014;63:292–299. doi: 10.1136/gutjnl-2013-304488.

270. Lichtiger S., Binion D.G., Wolf D.C., Present D.H., Bensimon A.G., Wu E., Yu A.P., Cardoso A.T., Chao J., Mulani P.M., et al. The CHOICE Trial: Adalimumab Demonstrates Safety, Fistula Healing, Improved Quality of Life and Increased Work Productivity in Patients with Crohn's Disease Who Failed Prior Infliximab Therapy: Adalimumab Safety and Outcomes in Crohn's Patients Who Failed Infliximab. *Aliment. Pharmacol. Ther.* 2010;32:1228–1239. doi: 10.1111/j.1365-2036.2010.04466.x.

271. Castaño-Milla C., Chaparro M., Saro C., Barreiro-de Acosta M., García-Albert A.M., Bujanda L., Martín-Arranz M.D., Carpio D., Muñoz F., Manceñido N., et al. Effectiveness of Adalimumab in Perianal Fistulas in Crohn's Disease Patients Naive to Anti-TNF Therapy. *J. Clin. Gastroenterol.* 2015;49:34–40. doi: 10.1097/MCG.0000000000000169.

272. Ji C.-C., Takano S. Clinical Efficacy of Adalimumab versus Infliximab and the Factors Associated with Recurrence or Aggravation during Treatment of Anal Fistulas in Crohn's Disease. *Intest. Res.* 2017;15:182. doi: 10.5217/ir.2017.15.2.182.

273. Sands B.E., Gasink C., Jacobstein D., Gao L.-L., Johanns J., Colombel J.F., de Villiers W.J., Sandborn W.J. Fistula Healing in Pivotal Studies of Ustekinumab in Crohn's Disease. *Gastroenterology.* 2017;152:S185. doi: 10.1016/S0016-5085(17)30930-7.

274. Chapuis-Biron C., Kirchgesner J., Pariente B., Bouhnik Y., Amiot A., Viennot S., Serrero M., Fumery M., Allez M., Siproudhis L., et al. Ustekinumab for Perianal Crohn's Disease: The BioLAP Multicenter Study From the GETAID. *Am. J. Gastroenterol.* 2020;115:1812–1820. doi: 10.14309/ajg.0000000000000810.

275. Ma C., Fedorak R.N., Kaplan G.G., Dieleman L.A., Devlin S.M., Stern N., Kroeker K.I., Seow C.H., Leung Y., Novak K.L., et al. Clinical, Endoscopic and Radiographic Outcomes with Ustekinumab in Medically-Refractory Crohn's Disease: Real World Experience from a Multicentre

Cohort. *Aliment. Pharmacol. Ther.* 2017;45:1232–1243. doi: 10.1111/apt.14016.

276. Biemans V.B.C., van der Meulen-de Jong A.E., van der Woude C.J., Löwenberg M., Dijkstra G., Oldenburg B., de Boer N.K.H., van der Marel S., Bodelier A.G.L., Jansen J.M., et al. Ustekinumab for Crohn's Disease: Results of the ICC Registry, a Nationwide Prospective Observational Cohort Study. *J. Crohns Colitis.* 2020;14:33–45. doi: 10.1093/ecco-jcc/jjz119.
277. Attauabi M., Burisch J., Seidelin J.B. Efficacy of Ustekinumab for Active Perianal Fistulizing Crohn's Disease: A Systematic Review and Meta-Analysis of the Current Literature. *Scand. J. Gastroenterol.* 2021;56:53–58. doi: 10.1080/00365521.2020.1854848.
278. Godoy Brewer G.M., Salem G., Afzal M.A., Limketkai B.N., Haq Z., Tajamal M., Melia J., Lazarev M., Selaru F.M., Parian A.M. Ustekinumab Is Effective for Perianal Fistulising Crohn's Disease: A Real-World Experience and Systematic Review with Meta-Analysis. *BMJ Open Gastroenterol.* 2021;8:e000702. doi: 10.1136/bmjgast-2021-000702.
279. Feagan B.G., Schwartz D., Danese S., Rubin D.T., Lissoos T.W., Xu J., Lasch K. Efficacy of Vedolizumab in Fistulising Crohn's Disease: Exploratory Analyses of Data from GEMINI 2. *J. Crohns Colitis.* 2018;12:621–626. doi: 10.1093/ecco-jcc/jjy019.
280. Chapuis-Biron C., Bourrier A., Nachury M., Nancey S., Bouhnik Y., Serrero M., Armengol-Debeir L., Buisson A., Tran-Minh M.-L., Zallot C., et al. Vedolizumab for Perianal Crohn's Disease: A Multicentre Cohort Study in 151 Patients. *Aliment. Pharmacol. Ther.* 2020;51:719–727. doi: 10.1111/apt.15665.
281. Ayoub F., Odenwald M., Micic D., Dalal S.R., Pekow J., Cohen R.D., Rubin D.T., Sakuraba A. Vedolizumab for Perianal Fistulizing Crohn's Disease: Systematic Review and Meta-Analysis. *Intest. Res.* 2022;20:240–250. doi: 10.5217/ir.2021.00091.
282. Reinisch W., Colombel J.F., D'Haens G.R., Rimola J., DeHaas-Amatsaleh A., McKevitt M., Ren X., Serone A., Schwartz D.A., Gecse K.B. OP18 Efficacy and Safety of Filgotinib for the Treatment of Perianal Fistulizing Crohn's Disease: Results from the Phase 2 DIVERGENCE 2 Study. *J. Crohns Colitis.* 2022;16:i019–i021. doi: 10.1093/ecco-jcc/jjab232.017.
283. Papamichael K., Vande Casteele N., Jeyarajah J., Jairath V., Osterman M.T., Cheifetz A.S. Higher Postinduction Infliximab Concentrations Are Associated With Improved Clinical Outcomes in Fistulizing Crohn's Disease: An ACCENT-II Post Hoc Analysis. *Am. J. Gastroenterol.* 2021;116:1007–1014. doi: 10.14309/ajg.0000000000001111.
284. Yarur A.J., Kanagala V., Stein D.J., Czul F., Quintero M.A., Agrawal D., Patel A., Best K., Fox C., Idstein K., et al. Higher Infliximab Trough Levels Are Associated with Perianal Fistula Healing in Patients with Crohn's Disease. *Aliment. Pharmacol. Ther.* 2017;45:933–940. doi: 10.1111/apt.13970.
285. De Gregorio M., Lee T., Krishnaprasad K., Amos G., An Y.-K., Bastian-Jordan M., Begun J., Borok N., Brown D.J.M., Cheung W., et al. Higher Anti-Tumor Necrosis Factor-α Levels Correlate With Improved Radiologic Outcomes in Crohn's Perianal Fistulas. *Clin. Gastroenterol. Hepatol.* 2021;20:1306–1314. doi: 10.1016/j.cgh.2021.07.053.
286. Malian A., Rivière P., Bouchard D., Pigot F., Eléouet-Kaplan M., Favreau-Weltzer C., Poullenot F., Laharie D. Predictors of Perianal Fistula Relapse in Crohn's Disease. *Inflamm. Bowel Dis.* 2020;26:926–931. doi: 10.1093/ibd/izz200.
287. Sandborn W.J., Honiball P.J., Bloomfield R., Schreiber S. Certolizumab Pegol for the Treatment

of Crohn's Disease. *N. Engl. J. Med.* 2007;357:228–238. doi: 10.1056/NEJMoa067594.

288. Schreiber S., Thomsen O.Ø., McColm J. Maintenance Therapy with Certolizumab Pegol for Crohn's Disease. *N. Engl. J. Med.* 2007;357:239–250. doi: 10.1056/NEJMoa062897.

289. Ford A.C., Luthra P., Hanauer S.B., Travis S.P., Harris M.S., Reinisch W. Placebo Response Rate in Clinical Trials of Fistulizing Crohn's Disease: Systematic Review and Meta-Analysis. *Clin. Gastroenterol. Hepatol.* 2014;12:1981–1990. doi: 10.1016/j.cgh.2014.08.038.

290. Gonczi L., Gecse K.B., Vegh Z., Kurti Z., Rutka M., Farkas K., Golovics P.A., Lovasz B.D., Banai J., Bene L., et al. Long-Term Efficacy, Safety, and Immunogenicity of Biosimilar Infliximab After One Year in a Prospective Nationwide Cohort. *Inflamm. Bowel Dis.* 2017;23:1908–1915. doi: 10.1097/MIB.0000000000001237.

291. Gionchetti P., Dignass A., Danese S., Magro Dias F.J., Rogler G., Lakatos P.L., Adamina M., Ardizzone S., Buskens C.J., Sebastian S., et al. 3rd European Evidence-Based Consensus on the Diagnosis and Management of Crohn's Disease 2016: Part 2: Surgical Management and Special Situations. *ECCOJC.* 2017;11:135–149. doi: 10.1093/ecco-jcc/jjw169.

292. Singh S., Murad M.H., Fumery M., Sedano R., Jairath V., Panaccione R., Sandborn W.J., Ma C. Comparative Efficacy and Safety of Biologic Therapies for Moderate-to-Severe Crohn's Disease: A Systematic Review and Network Meta-Analysis. *Lancet Gastroenterol. Hepatol.* 2021;6:1002–1014. doi: 10.1016/S2468-1253(21)00312-5.

293. Lee M.J., Freer C., Adegbola S., Elkady S., Parkes M., Hart A., Fearnhead N.S., Lobo A.J., Brown S.R. Patients with Perianal Crohn's Fistulas Experience Delays in Accessing Anti-TNF Therapy Due to Slow Recognition, Diagnosis and Integration of Specialist Services: Lessons Learned from Three Referral Centres. *Colorectal. Dis.* 2018;20:797–803. doi: 10.1111/codi.14102.

294. Jeon M., Song K., Koo J., Kim S. Evaluation of a Seton Procedure Combined With Infliximab Therapy (Early vs. Late) in Perianal Fistula With Crohn Disease. *Ann. Coloproctol.* 2019;35:249–253. doi: 10.3393/ac.2018.11.23.1.

295. Zhu P., Sun J., Gu Y., Chen H., Xu M., Li Y., Yang B. Combined Therapy with Early Initiation of Infliximab Following Drainage of Perianal Fistulising Crohn's Disease: A Retrospective Cohort Study. *BMC Gastroenterol.* 2022;22:15. doi: 10.1186/s12876-021-02078-9.

296. Tandon P., Rhee G.G., Schwartz D., McCurdy J.D. Strategies to Optimize Anti-Tumor Necrosis Factor Therapy for Perianal Fistulizing Crohn's Disease: A Systematic Review. *Dig. Dis. Sci.* 2019;64:3066–3077. doi: 10.1007/s10620-019-05635-1.

297. Mak J.W.Y., Tang W., Yip T.C.F., Ran Z.H., Wei S.C., Ahuja V., Kumar S., Leung W.K., Hilmi I., Limsrivilai J., et al. Stopping Anti-Tumour Necrosis Factor Therapy in Patients with Perianal Crohn's Disease. *Aliment. Pharmacol. Ther.* 2019;50:1195–1203. doi: 10.1111/apt.15547.

298. Legué C., Brochard C., Bessi G., Wallenhorst T., Dewitte M., Siproudhis L., Bouguen G. Outcomes of Perianal Fistulising Crohn's Disease Following Anti-TNFα Treatment Discontinuation. *Inflamm. Bowel Dis.* 2018;24:1107–1113. doi: 10.1093/ibd/izy008.

299. Schwartz D.A., Peyrin-Biroulet L., Lasch K., Adsul S., Danese S. Efficacy and Safety of 2 Vedolizumab Intravenous Regimens for Perianal Fistulizing Crohn's Disease: Enterprise Study. *Clin. Gastroenterol. Hepatol.* 2021;20:1059–1067.e9. doi: 10.1016/j.cgh.2021.09.028.

300. Sandborn W.J., D'Haens G.R., Reinisch W., Panés J., Chan D., Gonzalez S., Weisel K., Germinaro M., Frustaci M.E., Yang Z., et al. Guselkumab for the Treatment of Crohn's Disease: Induction Results

from the Phase 2 GALAXI-1 Study. *Gastroenterology.* 2022;162:1650–1664.e8. doi: 10.1053/j.gastro.2022.01.047.

301. Ford A.C., Sandborn W.J., Khan K.J., Hanauer S.B., Talley N.J., Moayyedi P. Efficacy of Biological Therapies in Inflammatory Bowel Disease: Systematic Review and Meta-Analysis. *Am. J. Gastroenterol.* 2011;106:644–659. doi: 10.1038/ajg.2011.73.
302. Dejaco C., Harrer M., Waldhoer T., Miehsler W., Vogelsang H., Reinisch W. Antibiotics and Azathioprine for the Treatment of Perianal Fistulas in Crohn's Disease: Treatment for Perianal crohn's Disease. *Aliment. Pharmacol. Ther.* 2003;18:1113–1120. doi: 10.1046/j.1365-2036.2003.01793.x.
303. Hu A., Kotze P.G., Burgevin A., Tan W., Jess A., Li P.-S., Kroeker K., Halloran B., Panaccione R., Peyrin-Biroulet L., et al. Combination Therapy Does Not Improve Rate of Clinical or Endoscopic Remission in Patients with Inflammatory Bowel Diseases Treated With Vedolizumab or Ustekinumab. *Clin. Gastroenterol. Hepatol.* 2021;19:1366–1376.e2. doi: 10.1016/j.cgh.2020.07.012.
304. Yzet C., Diouf M., Singh S., Brazier F., Turpin J., Nguyen-Khac E., Meynier J., Fumery M. No Benefit of Concomitant Immunomodulator Therapy on Efficacy of Biologics That Are Not Tumor Necrosis Factor Antagonists in Patients With Inflammatory Bowel Diseases: A Meta-Analysis. *Clin. Gastroenterol. Hepatol.* 2021;19:668–679.e8. doi: 10.1016/j.cgh.2020.06.071.
305. Rasul I., Wilson S.R., MacRae H., Irwin S., Greenberg G.R. Clinical and Radiological Responses after Infliximab Treatment for Perianal Fistulizing Crohn's Disease. *Am. J. Gastroenterol.* 2004;99:82–88. doi: 10.1046/j.1572-0241.2003.04009.x.
306. Fefferman D.S., Lodhavia P.J., Alsahli M., Falchuk K.R., Peppercorn M.A., Shah S.A., Farrell R.J. Smoking and Immunomodulators Do Not Influence the Response or Duration of Response to Infliximab in Crohn's Disease. *Inflamm. Bowel Dis.* 2004;10:346–351. doi: 10.1097/00054725-200407000-00004.
307. Jones J.L., Kaplan G.G., Peyrin-Biroulet L., Baidoo L., Devlin S., Melmed G.Y., Tanyingoh D., Raffals L., Irving P., Kozuch P., et al. Effects of Concomitant Immunomodulator Therapy on Efficacy and Safety of Anti–Tumor Necrosis Factor Therapy for Crohn's Disease: A Meta-Analysis of Placebo-Controlled Trials. *Clin. Gastroenterol. Hepatol.* 2015;13:2233–2240.e2. doi: 10.1016/j.cgh.2015.06.034.
308. Privitera G., Onali S., Pugliese D., Renna S., Savarino E., Viola A., Ribaldone D.G., Buda A., Bezzio C., Fiorino G., et al. Dual Targeted Therapy: A Possible Option for the Management of Refractory Inflammatory Bowel Disease. *J. Crohns Colitis.* 2021;15:335–339. doi: 10.1093/ecco-jcc/jjaa149.
309. Goessens L., Colombel J., Outtier A., Ferrante M., Sabino J., Judge C., Saeidi R., Rabbitt L., Armuzzi A., Domenech E., et al. Safety and Efficacy of Combining Biologics or Small Molecules for Inflammatory Bowel Disease or Immune-mediated Inflammatory Diseases: A European Retrospective Observational Study. *UEG J.* 2021;9:1136–1147. doi: 10.1002/ueg2.12170.
310. Ribaldone D.G., Pellicano R., Vernero M., Caviglia G.P., Saracco G.M., Morino M., Astegiano M. Dual Biological Therapy with Anti-TNF, Vedolizumab or Ustekinumab in Inflammatory Bowel Disease: A Systematic Review with Pool Analysis. *Scand. J. Gastroenterol.* 2019;54:407–413. doi: 10.1080/00365521.2019.1597159.
311. Ahmed W., Galati J., Kumar A., Christos P.J., Longman R., Lukin D.J., Scherl E., Battat R.

Dual Biologic or Small Molecule Therapy for Treatment of Inflammatory Bowel Disease: A Systematic Review and Meta-Analysis. *Clin. Gastroenterol. Hepatol.* 2021;20:e361–e379.e3. doi: 10.1016/j.cgh.2021.03.034.

312. Yang E., Panaccione N., Whitmire N., Dulai P.S., Vande Casteele N., Singh S., Boland B.S., Collins A., Sandborn W.J., Panaccione R., et al. Efficacy and Safety of Simultaneous Treatment with Two Biologic Medications in Refractory Crohn's Disease. *Aliment. Pharmacol. Ther.* 2020;51:1031–1038. doi: 10.1111/apt.15719.

313. Schwartz D.A., Tagarro I., Carmen Díez M., Sandborn W.J. Prevalence of Fistulizing Crohn's Disease in the United States: Estimate From a Systematic Literature Review Attempt and Population-Based Database Analysis. *Inflamm. Bowel Dis.* 2019;25:1773–1779. doi: 10.1093/ibd/izz056.

314. Vuyyuru S.K., Sahu P., Kedia S., Kante B., Kumar P., Ranjan M.K., Sharma R., Makharia G., Gupta S.D., Sahni P., et al. Long-Term Outcomes in Perianal Fistulizing Crohn's Disease in a Resource-Limited Setting: A Cohort Analysis. *Indian J. Gastroenterol.* 2020;39:435–444. doi: 10.1007/s12664-020-01054-7.

315. Singh S., Facciorusso A., Dulai P.S., Jairath V., Sandborn W.J. Comparative Risk of Serious Infections With Biologic and/or Immunosuppressive Therapy in Patients With Inflammatory Bowel Diseases: A Systematic Review and Meta-Analysis. *Clin. Gastroenterol. Hepatol.* 2020;18:69–81.e3. doi: 10.1016/j.cgh.2019.02.044.

316. Wu G., Yang Y., Liu M., Wang Y., Guo Q. Systematic Review and Network Meta-Analysis: Comparative Efficacy and Safety of Biosimilars, Biologics and JAK1 Inhibitors for Active Crohn Disease. *Front. Pharmacol.* 2021;12:655865. doi: 10.3389/fphar.2021.655865.

317. Ruemmele F.M., Rosh J., Faubion W.A., Dubinsky M.C., Turner D., Lazar A., Eichner S., Maa J.-F., Alperovich G., Robinson A.M., et al. Efficacy of Adalimumab for Treatment of Perianal Fistula in Children with Moderately to Severely Active Crohn's Disease: Results from IMAgINE 1 and IMAgINE 2. *J. Crohns Colitis.* 2018;12:1249–1254. doi: 10.1093/ecco-jcc/jjy087.

318. Davidov Y., Ungar B., Bar-Yoseph H., Carter D., Haj-Natour O., Yavzori M., Chowers Y., Eliakim R., Ben-Horin S., Kopylov U. Association of Induction Infliximab Levels With Clinical Response in Perianal Crohn's Disease. *ECCOJC.* 2016;11:549–555. doi: 10.1093/ecco-jcc/jjw182.

319. El-Matary W., Walters T.D., Huynh H.Q., deBruyn J., Mack D.R., Jacobson K., Sherlock M.E., Church P., Wine E., Carroll M.W., et al. Higher Postinduction Infliximab Serum Trough Levels Are Associated With Healing of Fistulizing Perianal Crohn's Disease in Children. *Inflamm. Bowel Dis.* 2019;25:150–155. doi: 10.1093/ibd/izy217.

320. Papamichael K., Cheifetz A.S. Defining and Predicting Deep Remission in Patients with Perianal Fistulizing Crohn's Disease on Anti-Tumor Necrosis Factor Therapy. *WJG.* 2017;23:6197. doi: 10.3748/wjg.v23.i34.6197.

321. Strik A.S., Löwenberg M., Buskens C.J., Gecse K.B., Ponsioen C.I., Bemelman W.A., D'Haens G.R. Higher Anti-TNF Serum Levels Are Associated with Perianal Fistula Closure in Crohn's Disease Patients. *Scand. J. Gastroenterol.* 2019;54:453–458. doi: 10.1080/00365521.2019.1600014.

322. Plevris N., Jenkinson P.W., Arnott I.D., Jones G.R., Lees C.W. Higher Anti-Tumor Necrosis Factor Levels Are Associated with Perianal Fistula Healing and Fistula Closure in Crohn's Disease. *Eur. J. Gastroenterol. Hepatol.* 2020;32:32–37. doi: 10.1097/MEG.0000000000001561.

323. de Groof E.J., Sahami S., Lucas C., Ponsioen C.Y., Bemelman W.A., Buskens C.J. Treatment of Perianal Fistula in Crohn's Disease: A Systematic Review and Meta-Analysis Comparing Seton Drainage and Anti-Tumour Necrosis Factor Treatment. *Colorectal. Dis.* 2016;18:667–675. doi: 10.1111/codi.13311.

324. Regueiro M., Mardini H. Treatment of Perianal Fistulizing Crohn's Disease with Infliximab Alone or as an Adjunct to Exam Under Anesthesia with Seton Placement. *Inflamm. Bowel Dis.* 2003;9:98–103. doi: 10.1097/00054725-200303000-00003.

325. Gaertner W.B., Decanini A., Mellgren A., Lowry A.C., Goldberg S.M., Madoff R.D., Spencer M.P. Does Infliximab Infusion Impact Results of Operative Treatment for Crohn's Perianal Fistulas? *Dis. Colon Rectum.* 2007;50:1754–1760. doi: 10.1007/s10350-007-9077-3.

326. Kotze P.G., de Albuquerque I.C., da Luz Moreira A., Tonini W.B., Olandoski M., Coy C.S.R. Perianal Complete Remission with Combined Therapy (Seton Placement and Anti-Tnf agents) in Crohn's Disease: A Brazilian Multicenter Observational Study. *Arq. Gastroenterol.* 2014;51:284–289. doi: 10.1590/S0004-28032014000400004.

327. Adamina M., Bonovas S., Raine T., Spinelli A., Warusavitarne J., Armuzzi A., Bachmann O., Bager P., Biancone L., Bokemeyer B., et al. ECCO Guidelines on Therapeutics in Crohn's Disease: Surgical Treatment. *J. Crohns Colitis.* 2020;14:155–168. doi: 10.1093/ecco-jcc/jjz187.

328. Tanaka S., Matsuo K., Sasaki T., Nakano M., Sakai K., Beppu R., Yamashita Y., Maeda K., Aoyagi K. Clinical Advantages of Combined Seton Placement and Infliximab Maintenance Therapy for Perianal Fistulizing Crohn's Disease: When and How Were the Seton Drains Removed? *Hepatogastroenterology.* 2010;57:3–7.

329. Wasmann K.A., de Groof E.J., Stellingwerf M.E., D'Haens G.R., Ponsioen C.Y., Gecse K.B., Dijkgraaf M.G.W., Gerhards M.F., Jansen J.M., Pronk A., et al. Treatment of Perianal Fistulas in Crohn's Disease, Seton Versus Anti-TNF Versus Surgical Closure Following Anti-TNF [PISA]: A Randomised Controlled Trial. *J. Crohns Colitis.* 2020;14:1049–1056. doi: 10.1093/ecco-jcc/jjaa004.

330. Bouchard D., Abramowitz L., Bouguen G., Brochard C., Dabadie A., de Parades V., Eléouet-Kaplan M., Fathallah N., Faucheron J.-L., Maggiori L., et al. Anoperineal Lesions in Crohn's Disease: French Recommendations for Clinical Practice. *Tech. Coloproctol.* 2017;21:683–691. doi: 10.1007/s10151-017-1684-y.

331. Hirten R.P., Shah S., Sachar D.B., Colombel J.-F. The Management of Intestinal Penetrating Crohn's Disease. *Inflamm. Bowel Dis.* 2018;24:752–765. doi: 10.1093/ibd/izx108.

332. Gervais D.A., Hahn P.F., O'Neill M.J., Mueller P.R. Percutaneous Abscess Drainage in Crohn Disease: Technical Success and Short- and Long-Term Outcomes during 14 Years. *Radiology.* 2002;222:645–651. doi: 10.1148/radiol.2223010554.

333. Matsui T., Sakurai T., Yamaguchi A., Ueki T., Nakabayashi S., Yao T., Futami K., Arima S., Ono H. The Clinical Characteristics and Outcome of Intraabdominal Abscess in Crohn?S Disease. *J. Gastroenterol.* 2004;39:441–448. doi: 10.1007/s00535-003-1317-2.

334. Clancy C., Boland T., Deasy J., McNamara D., Burke J.P. A Meta-Analysis of Percutaneous Drainage Versus Surgery as the Initial Treatment of Crohn's Disease-Related Intra-Abdominal Abscess. *ECCOJC.* 2016;10:202–208. doi: 10.1093/ecco-jcc/jjv198.

335. Yang Q., Gao X., Chen H., Li M., Wu X., Zhi M., Lan P., Hu P. Efficacy of Exclusive Enteral

Nutrition in Complicated Crohn's Disease. *Scand. J. Gastroenterol.* 2017;92:995–1001. doi: 10.1080/00365521.2017.1335770.

336. Adamji M., Day A.S. An Overview of the Role of Exclusive Enteral Nutrition for Complicated Crohn's Disease. *Intest. Res.* 2019;17:171–176. doi: 10.5217/ir.2018.00079.

337. Li G., Ren J., Wang G., Hu D., Gu G., Liu S., Ren H., Wu X., Li J. Preoperative Exclusive Enteral Nutrition Reduces the Postoperative Septic Complications of Fistulizing Crohn's Disease. *Eur. J. Clin. Nutr.* 2014;68:441–446. doi: 10.1038/ejcn.2014.16.

338. Gomollón F., Dignass A., Annese V., Tilg H., Van Assche G., Lindsay J.O., Peyrin-Biroulet L., Cullen G.J., Daperno M., Kucharzik T., et al. 3rd European Evidence-Based Consensus on the Diagnosis and Management of Crohn's Disease 2016: Part 1: Diagnosis and Medical Management. *ECCOJC.* 2017;11:3–25. doi: 10.1093/ecco-jcc/jjw168.

339. Bouguen G., Huguet A., Amiot A., Viennot S., Cholet F., Nachury M., Flamant M., Reimund J.-M., Desfourneaux V., Boureille A., et al. Efficacy and Safety of Tumor Necrosis Factor Antagonists in Treatment of Internal Fistulizing Crohn's Disease. *Clin. Gastroenterol. Hepatol.* 2020;18:628–636. doi: 10.1016/j.cgh.2019.05.027.

340. Kobayashi T., Hishida A., Tanaka H., Nuki Y., Bamba S., Yamada A., Fujii T., Shinzaki S., Yokoyama Y., Yoshida A., et al. Real-World Experience of Anti–Tumor Necrosis Factor Therapy for Internal Fistulas in Crohn's Disease: A Retrospective Multicenter Cohort Study. *Inflamm. Bowel Dis.* 2017;23:2245–2251. doi: 10.1097/MIB.0000000000001276.

341. Taxonera C., Barreiro-de-Acosta M., Bastida G., Martinez-Gonzalez J., Merino O., García-Sánchez V., Gisbert J.P., Marín-Jiménez I., López-Serrano P., Gómez-García M., et al. Outcomes of Medical and Surgical Therapy for Entero-Urinary Fistulas in Crohn's Disease. *ECCOJC.* 2016;10:657–662. doi: 10.1093/ecco-jcc/jjw016.

342. Kaimakliotis P., Simillis C., Harbord M., Kontovounisios C., Rasheed S., Tekkis P.P. A Systematic Review Assessing Medical Treatment for Rectovaginal and Enterovesical Fistulae in Crohn's Disease. *J. Clin. Gastroenterol.* 2016;50:714–721. doi: 10.1097/MCG.0000000000000607.

343. Le Baut G., Peyrin-Biroulet L., Bouguen G., Gornet J.-M., Stefanescu C., Amiot A., Laharie D., Altwegg R., Fumery M., Trang C., et al. Anti-TNF Therapy for Genital Fistulas in Female Patients with Crohn's Disease: A Nationwide Study from the Groupe d'Etude Thérapeutique Des Affections Inflammatoires Du Tube Digestif (GETAID) *Aliment. Pharmacol. Ther.* 2018;48:831–838. doi: 10.1111/apt.14946.

344. Amiot A., Setakhr V., Seksik P., Allez M., Treton X., De Vos M., Laharie D., Colombel J.-F., Abitbol V., Reimund J.M., et al. Long-Term Outcome of Enterocutaneous Fistula in Patients With Crohn's Disease Treated With Anti-TNF Therapy: A Cohort Study from the GETAID. *Am. J. Gastroenterol.* 2014;109:1443–1449. doi: 10.1038/ajg.2014.183.

345. Parsi M.A., Lashner B.A., Achkar J.-P., Connor J.T., Brzezinski A. Type of Fistula Determines Response to Infliximab in Patients with Fistulous Crohn's Disease. *Am. J. Gastroenterol.* 2004;99:445–449. doi: 10.1111/j.1572-0241.2004.04083.x.

346. Saclarides T.J. Rectovaginal Fistula. *Surg. Clin. North Am.* 2002;82:1261–1272. doi: 10.1016/S0039-6109(02)00055-5.

347. Howard G., Weiner D., Bar-or I., Levine A. Dual Biologic Therapy with Vedolizumab and Ustekinumab for Refractory Crohn's Disease in Children. *Eur. J. Gastroenterol. Hepatol.* 2022;34:372–374. doi: 10.1097/MEG.0000000000002203.

348. Present D.H., Korelitz B.I., Wisch N., Glass J.L., Sachar D.B., Pasternack B.S. Treatment of Crohn's Disease with 6-Mercaptopurine. *N. Engl. J. Med.* 1980;302:981–987. doi: 10.1056/NEJM198005013021801.

349. O'Brien J.J., Bayless T.M., Bayless J.A. Use of Azathioprine or 6-Mercaptopurine in the Treatment of Crohn's Disease. *Gastroenterology.* 1991;101:39–46. doi: 10.1016/0016-5085(91)90457-V.

350. Hanauer S.B., Smith M.B. Rapid Closure of Crohn's Disease Fistulas with Continuous Intravenous Cyclosporin A. *Am. J. Gastroenterol.* 1993;88:646–649.

351. González-Lama Y., Abreu L., Vera M.I., Pastrana M., Tabernero S., Revilla J., Durán J.G., Escartin P. Long-Term Oral Tacrolimus Therapy in Refractory to Infliximab Fistulizing Crohn's Disease: A Pilot Study. *Inflamm. Bowel Dis.* 2005;11:8–15. doi: 10.1097/00054725-200501000-00002.

352. Tracanelli L., Mathieu N., Trilling B., Vergniol J., Pigot F., Faucheron J.-L. Rectovaginal Fistula in Crohn's Disease Treatment: A Low Long-Term Success Rate and a High Definitive Stoma Risk after a Conservative Surgical Approach. *Tech. Coloproctol.* 2021;25:1143–1149. doi: 10.1007/s10151-021-02506-8.

353. Iesalnieks I., Kilger A., Gla H., Obermeier F., Agha A., Schlitt H.J. Perforating Crohn's Ileitis: Delay of Surgery Is Associated with Inferior Postoperative Outcome. *Inflamm. Bowel Dis.* 2010;16:2125–2130. doi: 10.1002/ibd.21303.

354. Panés J., García-Olmo D., Van Assche G., Colombel J.F., Reinisch W., Baumgart D.C., Dignass A., Nachury M., Ferrante M., Kazemi-Shirazi L., et al. Expanded Allogeneic Adipose-Derived Mesenchymal Stem Cells (Cx601) for Complex Perianal Fistulas in Crohn's Disease: A Phase 3 Randomised, Double-Blind Controlled Trial. *Lancet.* 2016;388:1281–1290. doi: 10.1016/S0140-6736(16)31203-X.

355. Garcia-Olmo D., Gilaberte I., Binek M., D'Hoore A.J., Lindner D., Selvaggi F., Spinelli A., Panés J. Follow-up Study to Evaluate the Long-Term Safety and Efficacy of Darvadstrocel (Mesenchymal Stem Cell Treatment) in Patients with Perianal Fistulizing Crohn's Disease: ADMIRE-CD Phase 3 Randomized Controlled Trial. *Dis. Colon Rectum.* 2021. *publish ahead of print* . [PubMed] [CrossRef]

356. Panés J., Bouma G., Ferrante M., Kucharzik T., Nachury M., de la Portilla de Juan F., Reinisch W., Selvaggi F., Tschmelitsch J., Brett N.R., et al. INSPECT: A Retrospective Study to Evaluate Long-Term Effectiveness and Safety of Darvadstrocel in Patients With Perianal Fistulizing Crohn's Disease Treated in the ADMIRE-CD Trial. *Inflamm. Bowel Dis.* 2022:izab361. doi: 10.1093/ibd/izab361.

357. Abramowitz L., Brochard C., Pigot F., Roumeguere P., Pillant H., Vinson Bonnet B., Faucheron J.L., Senéjoux A., Bonnaud G., Meurette G., et al. Surgical Closure, Mainly with Glue Injection and Anti-tumour Necrosis Factor α, in Fistulizing Perianal Crohn's Disease: A Multicentre Randomized Controlled Trial. *Colorectal Dis.* 2021;24:210–219. doi: 10.1111/codi.15947.

358. Yassin N.A., Askari A., Warusavitarne J., Faiz O.D., Athanasiou T., Phillips R.K.S., Hart A.L. Systematic Review: The Combined Surgical and Medical Treatment of Fistulising Perianal Crohn's Disease. *Aliment. Pharmacol. Ther.* 2014;40:741–749. doi: 10.1111/apt.12906.

359. Haennig A., Staumont G., Lepage B., Faure P., Alric L., Buscail L., Bournet B., Moreau J. The Results of Seton Drainage Combined with Anti-TNFα Therapy for Anal Fistula in Crohn's Disease. *Colorectal Dis.* 2015;17:311–319. doi: 10.1111/codi.12851.

360. Ritchie R.D., Sackier J.M., Hodde J.P. Incontinence Rates after Cutting Seton Treatment for Anal Fistula. *Colorectal Dis.* 2009;11:564–571. doi: 10.1111/j.1463-1318.2008.01713.x.

361. Van Tets W.F., Kuijpers J.H.C. Seton Treatment of Perianal Fistula with High Anal or Rectal Opening. *Br. J. Surg.* 2005;82:895–897. doi: 10.1002/bjs.1800820711.

362. Lee M.J., Heywood N., Adegbola S., Tozer P., Sahnan K., Fearnhead N.S., Brown S.R. ENiGMA Collaborators Systematic Review of Surgical Interventions for Crohn's Anal Fistula: Surgical Interventions for Crohn's Anal Fistula. *BJS Open.* 2017;1:55–66. doi: 10.1002/bjs5.13.

363. Thornton M., Solomon M.J. Long-Term Indwelling Seton for Complex Anal Fistulas in Crohn's Disease. *Dis. Colon Rectum.* 2005;48:459–463. doi: 10.1007/s10350-004-0830-6.

364. Scott H.J., Northover J.M. Evaluation of Surgery for Perianal Crohn's Fistulas. *Dis. Colon Rectum.* 1996;39:1039–1043. doi: 10.1007/BF02054696.

365. Halme L., Sainio A.P. Factors Related to Frequency, Type, and Outcome of Anal Fistulas in Crohn's Disease. *Dis. Colon Rectum.* 1995;38:55–59. doi: 10.1007/BF02053858.

366. van Koperen P.J., Safiruddin F., Bemelman W.A., Slors J.F.M. Outcome of Surgical Treatment for Fistula *in Ano* in Crohn's Disease. *Br. J. Surg.* 2009;96:675–679. doi: 10.1002/bjs.6608.

367. van Onkelen R.S., Gosselink M.P., Schouten W.R. Ligation of the Intersphincteric Fistula Tract in Low Transsphincteric Fistulae: A New Technique to Avoid Fistulotomy: LIFT in Low Transsphincteric Fistulae. *Colorectal. Dis.* 2013;15:587–591. doi: 10.1111/codi.12030.

368. Kamiński J.P., Zaghiyan K., Fleshner P. Increasing Experience of Ligation of the Intersphincteric Fistula Tract for Patients with Crohn's Disease: What Have We Learned? *Colorectal. Dis.* 2017;19:750–755. doi: 10.1111/codi.13668.

369. Soltani A., Kaiser A.M. Endorectal Advancement Flap for Cryptoglandular or Crohn's Fistula-in-Ano. *Dis. Colon Rectum.* 2010;53:486–495. doi: 10.1007/DCR.0b013e3181ce8b01.

370. Chung W., Ko D., Sun C., Raval M.J., Brown C.J., Phang P.T. Outcomes of Anal Fistula Surgery in Patients with Inflammatory Bowel Disease. *Am. J. Surg.* 2010;199:609–613. doi: 10.1016/j.amjsurg.2010.01.007.

371. Ellis C.N., Rostas J.W., Greiner F.G. Long-Term Outcomes With the Use of Bioprosthetic Plugs for the Management of Complex Anal Fistulas. *Dis. Colon Rectum.* 2010;53:798–802. doi: 10.1007/DCR.0b013e3181d43b7d.

372. O'Connor L., Champagne B.J., Ferguson M.A., Orangio G.R., Schertzer M.E., Armstrong D.N. Efficacy of Anal Fistula Plug in Closure of Crohn's Anorectal Fistulas. *Dis. Colon Rectum.* 2006;49:1569–1573. doi: 10.1007/s10350-006-0695-y.

373. O'Riordan J.M., Datta I., Johnston C., Baxter N.N. A Systematic Review of the Anal Fistula Plug for Patients With Crohn's and Non-Crohn's Related Fistula-in-Ano. *Dis. Colon Rectum.* 2012;55:351–358. doi: 10.1097/DCR.0b013e318239d1e4.

374. Grimaud J., Munoz–Bongrand N., Siproudhis L., Abramowitz L., Sénéjoux A., Vitton V., Gambiez L., Flourié B., Hébuterne X., Louis E., et al. Fibrin Glue Is Effective Healing Perianal Fistulas in Patients with Crohn's Disease. *Gastroenterology.* 2010;138:2275–2281.e1. doi: 10.1053/j.gastro.2010.02.013.

375. Gaertner W.B., Madoff R.D., Spencer M.P., Mellgren A., Goldberg S.M., Lowry A.C. Results of Combined Medical and Surgical Treatment of Recto-Vaginal Fistula in Crohn's Disease:

Crohn's Recto-Vaginal Fistulas. *Colorectal Dis.* 2011;13:678–683. doi: 10.1111/j.1463-1318.2010.02234.x.

376. Abel M.E., Volpe P.A. Autologous Fibrin Glue in the Treatment of Rectovaginal and Complex Fistulas. *Dis. Colon Rectum.* 1993;36:447–449. doi: 10.1007/BF02050009.
377. Loungnarath R., Dietz D.W., Mutch M.G., Birnbaum E.H., Kodner I.J., Fleshman J.W. Fibrin Glue Treatment of Complex Anal Fistulas Has Low Success Rate. *Dis. Colon Rectum.* 2004;47:432–436. doi: 10.1007/s10350-003-0076-8.
378. Lindsey I., Smilgin-Humphreys M.M., Cunningham C., Mortensen N.J.M., George B.D. A Randomized, Controlled Trial of Fibrin Glue vs. Conventional Treatment for Anal Fistula. *Dis. Colon Rectum.* 2002;45:1608–1615. doi: 10.1007/s10350-004-7247-0.
379. Singer M., Cintron J., Nelson R., Orsay C., Bastawrous A., Pearl R., Sone J., Abcarian H. Treatment of Fistulas-in-Ano With Fibrin Sealant in Combination With Intra-Adhesive Antibiotics and/or Surgical Closure of the Internal Fistula Opening. *Dis. Colon Rectum.* 2005;48:799–808. doi: 10.1007/s10350-004-0898-z.
380. Singh S., Ding N.S., Mathis K.L., Dulai P.S., Farrell A.M., Pemberton J.H., Hart A.L., Sandborn W.J., Loftus E.V. Systematic Review with Meta-Analysis: Faecal Diversion for Management of Perianal Crohn's Disease. *Aliment. Pharmacol. Ther.* 2015;42:783–792. doi: 10.1111/apt.13356.
381. Kasparek M.S., Glatzle J., Temeltcheva T., Mueller M.H., Koenigsrainer A., Kreis M.E. Long-Term Quality of Life in Patients with Crohn's Disease and Perianal Fistulas: Influence of Fecal Diversion. *Dis. Colon Rectum.* 2007;50:2067–2074. doi: 10.1007/s10350-007-9006-5.
382. Lightner A.L., Ashburn J.H., Brar M.S., Carvello M., Chandrasinghe P., de Buck van Overstraeten A., Fleshner P.R., Gallo G., Kotze P.G., Holubar S.D., et al. Fistulizing Crohn's Disease. *Curr. Probl. Surg.* 2020;57:100808. doi: 10.1016/j.cpsurg.2020.100808.
383. Sandborn W.J., Fazio V.W., Feagan B.G., Hanauer S.B. American Gastroenterological Association Clinical Practice Committee AGA Technical Review on Perianal Crohn's Disease. *Gastroenterology.* 2003;125:1508–1530. doi: 10.1016/j.gastro.2003.08.025.
384. Cohen J.L., Stricker J.W., Schoetz D.J., Coller J.A., Veidenheimer M.C. Rectovaginal Fistula in Crohn's Disease. *Dis. Colon Rectum.* 1989;32:825–828. doi: 10.1007/BF02554548.
385. Yamamoto T., Bain I.M., Allan R.N., Keighley M.R. Persistent Perineal Sinus after Proctocolectomy for Crohn's Disease. *Dis. Colon Rectum.* 1999;42:96–101. doi: 10.1007/BF02235190.
386. Rius J., Nessim A., Nogueras J.J., Wexner S.D. Gracilis Transposition in Complicated Perianal Fistula and Unhealed Perineal Wounds in Crohn's Disease. *Eur. J. Surg.* 2000;166:218–222. doi: 10.1080/110241500750009311.
387. Garcia-Olmo D., Herreros D., Pascual I., Pascual J.A., Del-Valle E., Zorrilla J., De-La-Quintana P., Garcia-Arranz M., Pascual M. Expanded Adipose-Derived Stem Cells for the Treatment of Complex Perianal Fistula: A Phase II Clinical Trial. *Dis. Colon Rectum.* 2009;52:79–86. doi: 10.1007/DCR.0b013e3181973487.
388. García-Olmo D., García-Arranz M., Herreros D., Pascual I., Peiro C., Rodríguez-Montes J.A. A Phase I Clinical Trial of the Treatment of Crohn's Fistula by Adipose Mesenchymal Stem Cell Transplantation. *Dis. Colon Rectum.* 2005;48:1416–1423. doi: 10.1007/s10350-005-0052-6.
389. Scott L.J. Darvadstrocel: A Review in Treatment-Refractory Complex Perianal Fistulas in Crohn's Disease. *BioDrugs.* 2018;32:627–634. doi: 10.1007/s40259-018-0311-4.

390. Park M.Y., Yoon Y.S., Lee J.L., Park S.H., Ye B.D., Yang S.-K., Yu C.S. Comparative Perianal Fistula Closure Rates Following Autologous Adipose Tissue-Derived Stem Cell Transplantation or Treatment with Anti-Tumor Necrosis Factor Agents after Seton Placement in Patients with Crohn's Disease: A Retrospective Observational Study. *Stem Cell Res. Ther.* 2021;12:401. doi: 10.1186/s13287-021-02484-6.

391. Cao Y., Su Q., Zhang B., Shen F., Li S. Efficacy of Stem Cells Therapy for Crohn's Fistula: A Meta-Analysis and Systematic Review. *Stem Cell Res. Ther.* 2021;12:32. doi: 10.1186/s13287-020-02095-7.

392. Zabot G.P., Cassol O., Saad-Hossne R., Bemelman W. Modern Surgical Strategies for Perianal Crohn's Disease. *WJG.* 2020;26:6572–6581. doi: 10.3748/wjg.v26.i42.6572.

393. Lopez N., Ramamoorthy S., Sandborn W.J. Recent Advances in the Management of Perianal Fistulizing Crohn's Disease: Lessons for the Clinic. *Expert Rev. Gastroenterol. Hepatol.* 2019;13:563–577. doi: 10.1080/17474124.2019.1608818.

394. Sulz M.C., Burri E., Michetti P., Rogler G., Peyrin-Biroulet L., Seibold F. Treatment Algorithms for Crohn's Disease. *Digestion.* 2020;101:43–57. doi: 10.1159/000506364.

395. Adegbola S.O., Sahnan K., Twum-Barima C., Iqbal N., Reza L., Lung P., Warusavitarne J., Tozer P., Hart A. Current Review of the Management of Fistulising Perianal Crohn's Disease. *Frontline Gastroenterol.* 2021;12:515–523. doi: 10.1136/flgastro-2020-101489.

Chapter 5

THE PELVIS AND PERINEUM

Contents

Introduction

The pelvis and perineum are crucial regions in clinical anatomy, playing vital roles in supporting the body's weight, facilitating movement, and housing essential organs related to the urinary, reproductive, and digestive systems. Their complex anatomy and proximity to various vital structures make understanding these areas fundamental for healthcare professionals.

The pelvis is a bony ring formed by the sacrum, coccyx, and a pair of hip bones (ilium, ischium, and pubis). It serves as a sturdy support for the spinal column and a protective basin for the pelvic organs. The pelvic cavity is divided into the false pelvis (above the pelvic brim) and the true pelvis (below the pelvic brim). Key organs within the pelvis include the bladder, rectum, and, in females, the uterus and ovaries. The pelvic floor muscles, including the levator ani and coccygeus, form a diaphragm that supports these organs and maintains continence. The perineum is the region between the pubic symphysis and the coccyx, bordered laterally by the ischial tuberosities. It is divided into the urogenital triangle (anteriorly) and the anal triangle (posteriorly). The urogenital triangle contains the external genitalia and the openings of the urethra and vagina in females, and the base of the penis and scrotum in males. The anal triangle houses the anus and surrounding tissues. The perineum's muscles, fasciae, and ligaments provide support and play a role in functions such as urination, defecation, and sexual activity.

Understanding the anatomy of the pelvis and perineum is essential for diagnosing and treating various conditions. In obstetrics, the pelvis's shape and size are critical for childbirth. Gynecologists and urologists focus on pelvic organ health, addressing issues like pelvic organ prolapse, incontinence, and cancers. Surgeons operating in these regions must navigate the intricate anatomy to avoid complications.

Orientation and Directional Terms

Term	Definition	Illustration
Hip bones	It is comprised of two bones: the thigh bone or femur and the pelvis which is made up of three bones called ilium, ischium, and pubis.	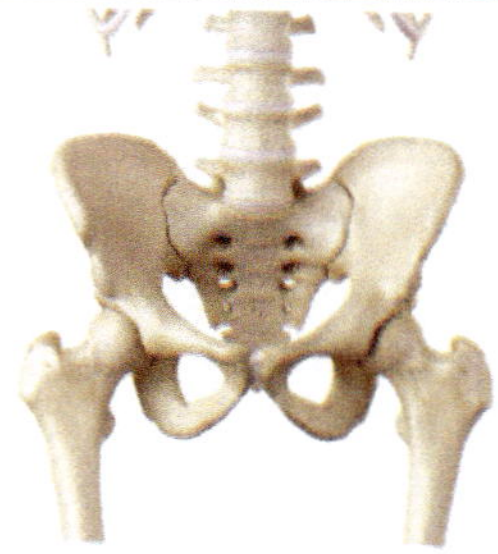
Gynecologists	A gynaecologist is a specialist doctor who manages conditions that affect the female reproductive system — which includes the vulva, vagina, uterus (womb) and ovaries.	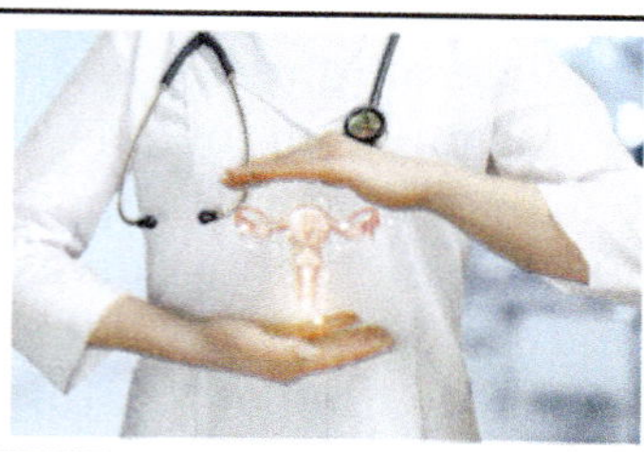
Sacrococcygeal Joint	The sacrococcygeal joint is an amphiarthrodial joint, formed between the oval surface at the apex of the sacrum, and the base of the coccyx. It is homologous with the joints between the bodies of the vertebræ, and is connected by similar ligaments: The Anterior sacrococcygeal ligament.	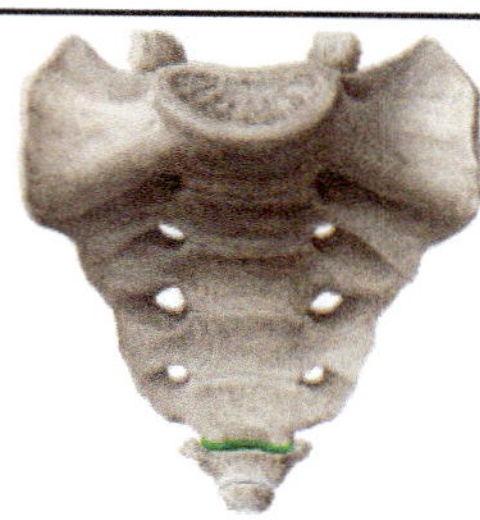
Pelvis	The pelvis is a basin-shaped structure that supports the spinal column and protects the abdominal organs. It contains the following: Sacrum. A spade-shaped bone that is formed by the fusion of 5 originally separate sacral vertebrae.	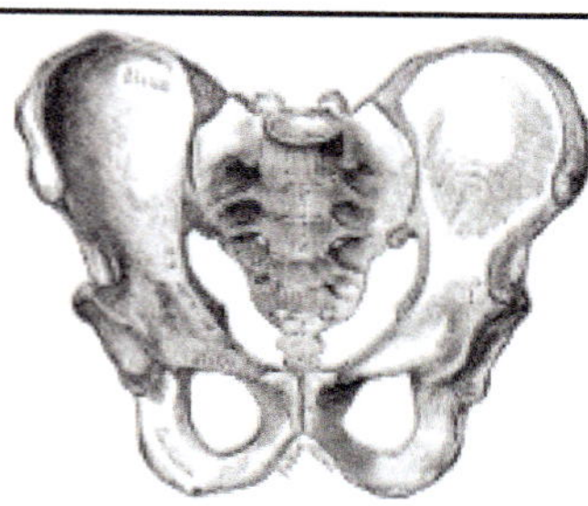
Anococcygeal body	The anococcygeal body (anococcygeal ligament or anococcygeal raphe) is a fibrous median raphe in the floor of the pelvis, which extends between the coccyx and the margin of the anus.	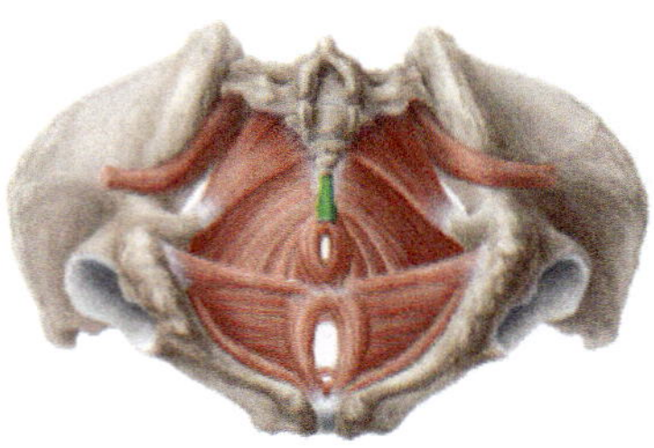

5.1. The Hip (Innominate) Bone

The ischium beneath, the pubis in front, and the ilium above make up this big, asymmetrical bone. They unite in the child's acetabulum, a laterally positioned cup-shaped fossa where the femoral head articulates, as a Y-shaped epiphyseal cartilage. By late puberty, the epiphyses close. The ilium forms the upper two-fifths of the acetabulum and expands superiorly into a flattened plate, the ala, which has lateral (gluteal) and medial (pelvic) surfaces surmounted by the iliac crest and separated by anterior and posterior borders. The ilium expands upwards as a fan-shaped bone, and below it, the pubis and ischium join to enclose the obturator foramen and form the anterolateral walls of the true pelvis. From anterior to posterior, the glutei, gluteus minimus, gluteus medius, and gluteus maximus attach to the gluteal surface. The anterior iliac fossa, from which the iliacus muscle arises, and the posterior auricular surface, which articulates with the sacrum, make up the medial surface. The roughened iliac tuberosity supporting the sacroiliac ligaments is located on its posterior side. Two small projections are present on the short anterior border: the anterior inferior iliac spine, which is the origin of the rectus femoris, and the subcutaneous anterior superior iliac spine, to which the inguinal ligament is attached. The posterior superior and posterior inferior iliac spines are two projections of the posterior border that provide attachment to the sacro tuberous ligament. The anterior to posterior superior iliac spines are separated by the curved, palpably located iliac crest. It is thick and provides attachment points for the gluteus maximus posteriorly and the tensor fascia lata anteriorly, which are the muscles of the lateral and posterior abdominal walls.

The level of the preferred lumbar puncture site is indicated by the highest points of the two iliac crests (intercristal plane), which are located at the level of the fourth lumbar vertebra (the L4/L5 intervertebral space is wide and allows access to the subarachnoid space below the termination of the spinal cord). Using the posterior superior spine as a landmark—which is located beneath the skin dimple known as the "dimple of Venus"—to the medial side of the upper buttock, the iliac crest is frequently the site of bone biopsies. It is located at the S2 level and is more pronounced in females.

An L-shaped bone with a body and ramus is called an ischium. The body expands inferiorly to form the ischial tuberosity, which provides attachment to the sacro tuberous ligament and the hamstring muscles, and forms two-fifths of the acetabulum. The obturator externus muscle is attached to the body's femoral surface. The sciatic nerve, which runs above the conical ischial spine that divides the greater sciatic notch above from the lesser sciatic notch below, crosses the body above the tuberosity. The sacrospinous ligament and levator ani are attached to the spine. The obturator internus muscle is attached to the pelvic surface of the body, while the levator ani and coccygeus muscles are attached to the medial surface of the spine.

The obturator foramen is encircled by the superior and inferior pubic rami of the ischium, which unite with the body of the pubis. The adductor muscles are attached to the body's exterior, while the levator ani muscle is attached to the body's interior, which is connected to the bladder. Hyaline cartilage covers the oval symphyseal surface, which is connected to its fellow by ligaments and a fibrocartilaginous disc (Figures 5.1 and 5.2).

Its palpable pubic crest, which forms its superior border, provides attachment to the conjoint tendon, external oblique aponeurosis, and rectus abdominis. The inguinal ligament is attached to the palpable pubic tubercle, which is located at the lateral end of the crest. A portion of the inguinal ligament is attached to the superior ramus via the pectineal line, which also bears a ridge that diverges from the pubic tubercle. The pubic arch is formed by the pubic bones articulating in the midline. There are five fused sacral vertebrae that make up the sacrum. Its shape is triangular, with two lateral surfaces, a dorsal, a pelvic, and an inferior base and apex. It is separated into a median section, which corresponds to the fused vertebral bodies, and two lateral masses, which are made up of the transverse processes, by four paired rows of sacral foramina. The sacral segmental nerves are conveyed by the pelvic and dorsal sacral foramina, which are in communication with the central sacral canal.

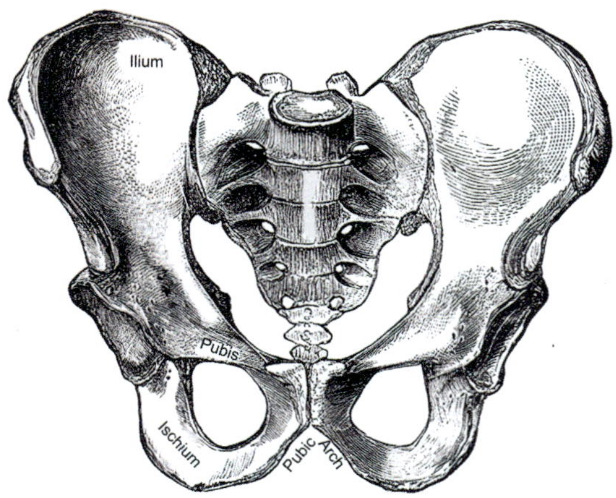

Figure 5.1. *Male pelvis.*

Source: By Henry Vandyke Carter – Henry Gray, (1918). Anatomy of the human body (see "Book" section below) Bartleby.com: Gray's Anatomy, Plate 241, Public Domain; https://commons.wikimedia.org/w/index.php?curid=323668.

The promontory is the projecting anterior margin of the base, which faces both upward and forward. It has two projecting superior articular processes on either side of the articular facet for the fifth lumbar vertebra, which is located anterior to the sacral canal opening. The coccyx and apex articulate.

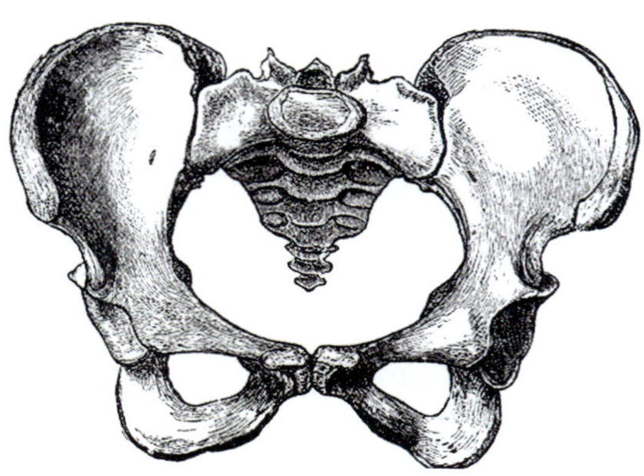

Figure 5.2. *Female pelvis.*

Source: By Henry Vandyke Carter – Henry Gray, (1918). Anatomy of the human body (see "Book" section below) Bartleby.com: Gray's Anatomy, Plate 242, Public Domain; https://commons.wikimedia.org/w/index.php?curid=323669.

The alae provide attachment to the piriformis, and the pelvic surface is concave. The rectum and the peritoneum are in contact with the lower and upper portions of the surface, respectively. The thoracolumbar fascia, gluteus maximus, and erector spinae are attached to the convex and irregular dorsal surface. It has a median sacral crest in the midline. Between paired sacral cornua, the posterior wall of the sacral canal is inferior, creating the sacral hiatus, which is sealed with fibrous tissue. The sacral canal houses the external vertebral venous plexus and spinal nerves extradurally, as well as the end of the cauda equina and cerebrospinal fluid within the meninges. The lateral surface has a pitted area for the attachment of the strong interosseous ligaments and a roughened auricular surface for articulation with the ilium (Figure 5.3).

The coccyx is small, triangular, and formed by the fusion of four coccygeal vertebrae. It articulates with the apex of the sacrum and is the remnant of a human tail.

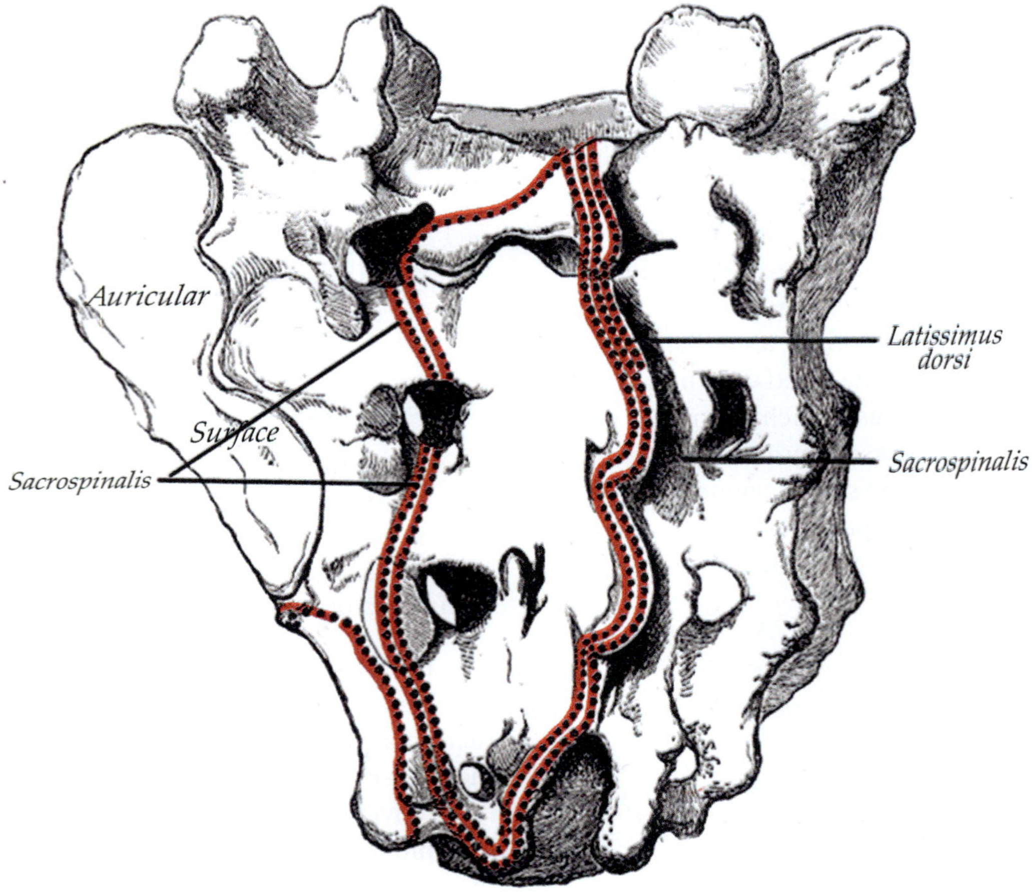

Figure 5.3. *Sacrum.*

Source: By Henry Vandyke Carter – Henry Gray, (1918). Anatomy of the human body (see "Book" section below) Bartleby.com: Gray's Anatomy, Plate 96, Public Domain; https://commons.wikimedia.org/w/index.php?curid=792303.

5.2. Joints and Ligaments of the Pelvic Girdle

5.2.1. Sacroiliac Joint

The sacroiliac joint, which connects the uneven auricular surfaces of the sacrum and ilium, is a plane synovial joint that can fuse or become partially fibrous in older individuals.

5.2.1.1. Ligaments

- Capsular ligaments are attached to the articular margins with capsular thickenings, including the very strong ventral and dorsal sacroiliac ligaments.
- Extracapsular ligaments include the interosseous sacroiliac ligament, which is also

very strong and unites the auricular surfaces of both bones.

- Accessory ligaments include:
  - o the sacrotuberous ligament, a strong thick band from the ischial tuberosity to the coccyx, the lateral crest of the sacrum, and posterior iliac spines;
  - o the sacrospinous ligament, which is triangular, converging from the lateral margin of the sacrum and coccyx to the ischial spine;
  - o the iliolumbar ligament, which attaches the 5th lumbar transverse process to the posterior iliac crest.

5.2.1.2. Functional Aspects

The irregularities in the joint limit movement to a small amount of gliding and rotation; ligaments provide stability. The sacrospinous and sacrotuberous ligaments resist the sacrum's tendency to rotate forward as a result of body weight being transmitted through the vertebral column. Using the sacral hiatus, anesthetic solutions are injected into the sacral canal and the sacral nerve roots are blocked (caudal epidural block). This allows for the anesthesia of the birth canal, pelvic floor, and perineum while sparing the lower limbs. To stop the pain of an episiotomy during labor, a pudendal nerve block is frequently used. The hormones that come with being pregnant cause these ligaments to stretch and the joint to move a little more. Together, these factors cause the female pelvis' transverse diameter to increase by 10% during the latter stages of pregnancy, which facilitates the fetus's passage.

5.2.2. Sacrococcygeal Joint

The fibrocartilaginous intervertebral disc and the capsular ligament provide stability to the sacrococcygeal joint, which is a secondary cartilaginous joint. Late pregnancy causes the ligaments to become more pliable and increases the range of motion, which increases the risk of injury during delivery.

5.2.3. Symphysis Pubis

The secondary cartilaginous joint that connects the two pubic bones is called the symphysis pubis. A fibrocartilage disc connects its articular surfaces. In late pregnancy, there is little movement other than a slight separation of the pubic bones. Sometimes symphysiotomy—splitting of this joint—is done to widen the birth canal in preparation for delivery.

5.3. The Articulated Pelvis

The pelvis lies obliquely in the erect posture, with the pubic symphysis and anterior superior iliac spines in the same vertical plane. The pelvic brim, which extends between the sacrum's promontory and the arcuate lines, divides the pelvis into greater and lesser parts. The lesser (true) pelvis is below the brim and forms the birth canal, making it a region of great obstetric significance. The greater (false) pelvis is above the brim and borders the lower abdominal cavity. It has a cavity, an outlet, and an inlet. The pelvic brim is the inlet; the female has an oval or round shape, while the male has a heart-shaped one. Its transverse diameter (13 cm) is typically larger than its anteroposterior diameter (11 cm). The cavity has a posterior wall that is three times longer than the anterior wall and is a short, curved canal. It is enclosed by the sacrum, the sacrospinous and sacrotuberous ligaments, and the true pelvic surfaces of the hip bones. The lower border of the pubic symphysis and ischiopubic rami, the sacrotuberous ligaments, and the coccyx encircle the diamond-shaped outlet. At 13 cm, the anterior diameter (conjugate) of the female is greater than the transverse diameter.

Transverse pelvic inlet and anteroposterior pelvic outlet have maximum diameters in females. As a result, in a typical labor, the head partially rotates during descent, with its greater diameter, known as the anteroposterior, normally lying along the wider diameter of the pelvic region that contains it. Comparing the pelvis to other bones, sexual differences are more noticeable. The male pelvis is thicker, rougher, and heavier than the female pelvis; the brim is heart-shaped rather than round or oval; the cavity is longer and the outlet narrower; the acetabulum is larger; the ischiopubic ramus is everted along the attachment of the penis's crura; and the subpubic angle is less than 90°, frequently as acute as 60°, while the female pelvis can reach greater than 90° (Figure 5.4).

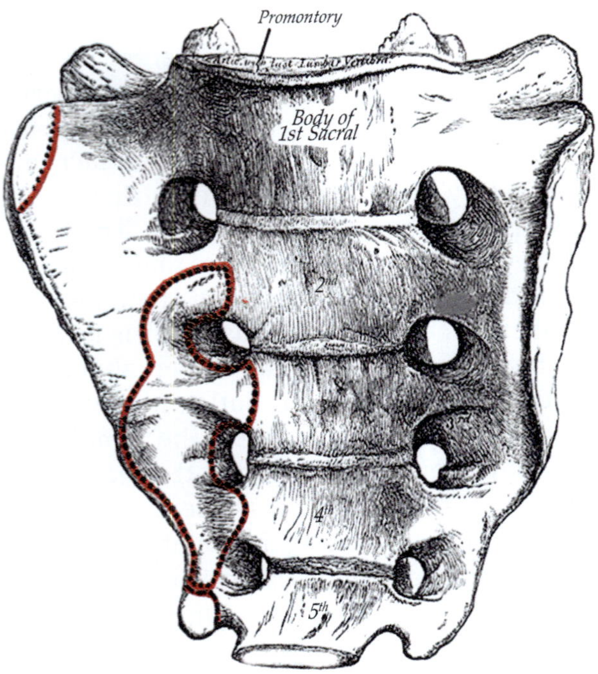

Figure 5.4. *Sacrum-pelvis.*

Source: By Henry Vandyke Carter – Henry Gray, (1918). Anatomy of the human body (see "Book" section below) Bartleby.com: Gray's Anatomy, Plate 95, Public Domain; https://commons.wikimedia.org/w/index.php?curid=792305.

5.3.1. Pelvimetry

Measuring the pregnant woman's pelvis is necessary for obstetricians to determine whether delivery-related complications are likely. What was once accomplished by X-ray is now accomplished ultrasonically. Crush injuries are a common cause of pelvic fractures, and they often result in injuries to related soft tissues, i.e., pubis fractures are linked to bladder and urethral trauma, and sacroiliac fractures and dislocations are linked to major vascular trauma (internal and common iliac).

5.4. Muscles and Fasciae of the Pelvis

Pelvic fascia covers the iliacus, obturator internus, piriformis, and other muscles that line the walls of the pelvis. Where it crosses the obturator internus, it provides attachment for the levator ani.

5.4.1. Iliacus

- **Attachments:** Pelvic – upper two-thirds of the iliac fossa and sacroiliac ligament; distal – the lesser trochanter of the femur.
- **Nerve Supply:** The femoral nerve.
- **Function:** Flexion of the trunk on the thigh; flexion and medial rotation of the femur on the trunk.

5.4.2. Obturator Internus

- **Attachments:** Pelvic – pelvic surface of the obturator membrane and adjacent bone. It is covered with the strong obturator internus fascia; femoral – the fibers converge on the lesser sciatic foramen and turn laterally to its attachment on the greater trochanter of the femur.
- **Nerve Supply:** Nerve to obturator

internus, a branch of the sacral plexus.

- **Function:** Lateral rotation of the femur.

5.4.3. Piriformis

- **Attachments:** Sacral – the lateral part of the pelvic surface of the sacrum; femoral – it passes laterally through the greater sciatic foramen to the greater trochanter of the femur.
- **Nerve Supply:** Direct branches from the sacral plexus.
- **Function:** Lateral rotation of the femur, but it is also an important landmark of the gluteal region.

5.5. The Pelvic Floor

This fibromuscular diaphragm is formed by the two-levator ani and coccygeal muscles and divides the pelvic cavity from the perineum and ischioanal fossae below. There are visceral and parietal sections of the pelvic fascia. The floor and walls of the pelvic cavity are covered by the parietal region. Along with the iliacus and transversalis fascia, it is continuous superiorly and thick over the obturator internus, where the levator ani is attached. Levator ani is covered. Spinal nerves are located outside of the pelvis, while its vessels are located inside. The rectum, uterus, and bladder are all covered by the visceral fascia. Over these viscera's lower portions, it thickens, creating ligaments that attach and suspend them from the pelvic walls (Figure 5.5).

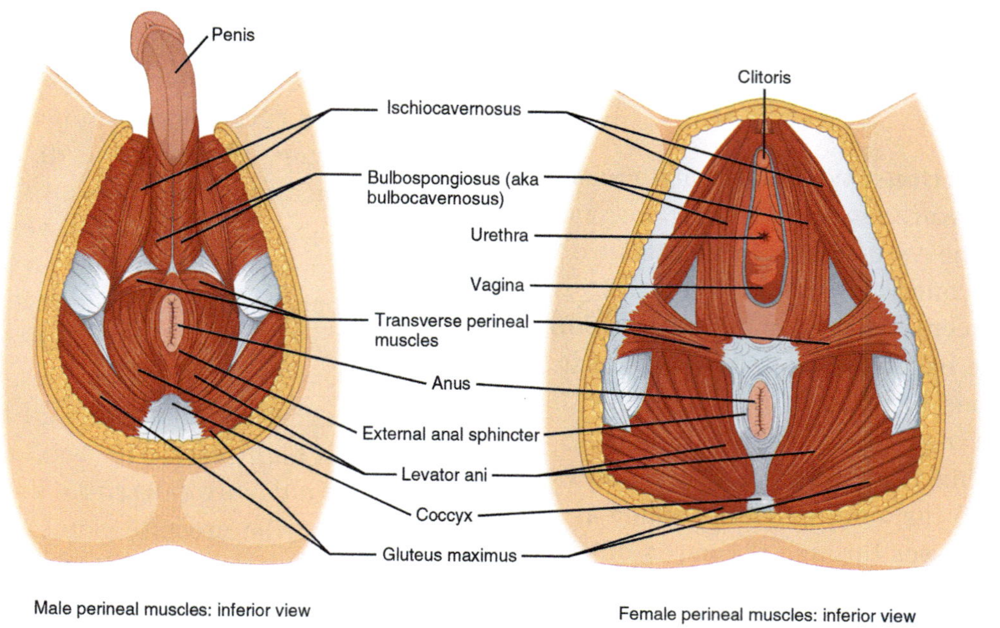

Figure 5.5. *Muscles of the pelvis.*

Source: By OpenStax – https://cnx.org/contents/FPtK1zmh@8.25:fEI3C8Ot@10/Preface, CC BY 4.0; https://commons.wikimedia.org/w/index.php?curid=30131691.

5.5.1. Levator Ani

This is a broad, flat, thin muscle.

5.5.1.1. Attachments

Lateral – in a continuous line from the back of the body of the pubis, the ischial spine, and fascia over obturator internus between the pubis and ischium. Medial – the muscle descends to the midline and there meets its fellow in the midline anococcygeal raphe.

The middle fibers travel down and backward around the puborectalis, or rectum, to the fibrous anococcygeal body; the anterior fibers travel around the prostate or vagina to the fibrous perineal body or central tendon of the perineum. Certain fibers merge with the anal sphincter. The midline raphe behind the rectum, between it and the anococcygeal body, is where the posterior fibers terminate.

5.5.2. Coccygeus

This triangular muscle passes from the ischial spine to the sides of the lower sacrum and coccyx.

- **Functions:** When intra-abdominal pressure increases during coughing or heavy lifting, both muscles work in concert to support the pelvic viscera. Defecation and micturition are expulsive processes that cause them to relax. Additionally, they strengthen the urethral and anal sphincters. The fetal head rotates into the anteroposterior plane as it passes through the pelvis during birth thanks to the gutter-like arrangement.
- **Nerve Supply:** Both are supplied by the pudendal nerve and direct branches from S3 and S4.

5.6. The Rectum and Anal Canal

The rectum connects the anal canal to the sigmoid colon. It starts in front of the third sacral segment, extends to the posterior pelvis, and curves forward with a loop to the left, ending at the tip of the coccyx. Its length is approximately 12 cm. It widens inferiorly, forming the rectal ampulla. Its lower third is extra peritoneally embedded in pelvic fascia, while its upper third is covered by the peritoneum on its front and sides. It lacks a mesentery.

- **Relations:** Its lower portion is connected to the levator ani and coccygeus, while its upper portion is in lateral contact with the small intestine's coils. It is posteriorly separated from the lower sacrum and coccyx by the superior rectal artery, the third, fourth, and fifth sacral nerves, the sympathetic plexus, and the sacral vessels. The upper two-thirds form a peritoneal pouch, known as the rectouterine (pouch of Douglas) in females and the rectovesical in males, which forms the posterior wall anteriorly in both sexes. The seminal vesicles, the ductus deferentia, the bladder, and the prostate gland are located below the pouch in males and anterior to the rectum in females (Figures 5.6 and 5.7).

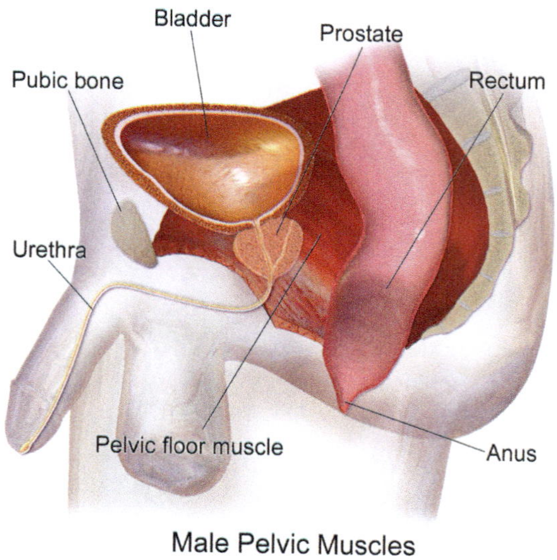

Figure 5.6. *Mid-sagittal section of the male pelvis showing peritoneal relationships.*

Source: By BruceBlaus - Own work, CC BY-SA 4.0; https://commons.wikimedia.org/w/index.php?curid=60834709.

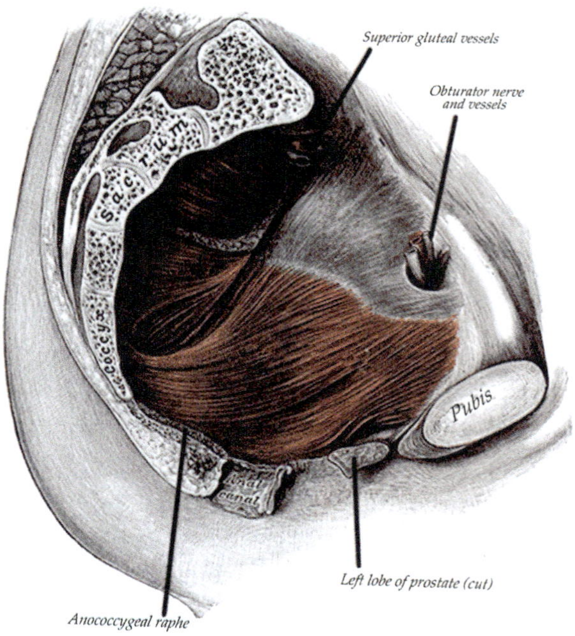

Figure 5.7. *The pelvis.*

Source: By Henry Vandyke Carter - Henry Gray, (1918). Anatomy of the human body (see "Book" section below) Bartleby.com: Gray's Anatomy, Plate 404, Public Domain; https://commons.wikimedia.org/w/index.php?curid=158672.

The lowest portion of the peritoneal cavity is made up of the rectovesical and rectouterine pouches, which can be felt in both sexes during a rectal examination. When an appendix tears, for instance, the peritoneum becomes inflamed (peritonitis), which can lead to an abscess forming in the pouch. A tender swelling located anterior to the rectal wall will be palpable. A "knitting needle" or "backstreet" abortion, in which there has been an inadvertent puncture of the uterus or posterior vaginal fornix, can potentially introduce infection into the pouch.

5.6.1. The Anal Canal

The alimentary tract's terminal segment is 2–4 cm long. Except for the sporadic passage of flatus and feces, it is kept closed by internal and external sphincters. It descends and makes a 90° turn to the rectum through the pelvic floor before opening externally at the anus. The anococcygeal body is located posteriorly; the levator ani separates it from the ischioanal fossae laterally, and the perineal body separates it from the lower vagina in females and the penis and prostate bulb in males anteriorly. Encircling its upper two-thirds is the involuntary internal sphincter, which is a continuation of the rectum's circular muscle. The voluntary external sphincter encircles the lower two-thirds of the anal canal and is arranged in deep, superficial, and subcutaneous parts:

- The deep part surrounds the middle anal canal and is reinforced by fibers of the levator ani. Damage to this part of the muscle results in fecal incontinence.
- The superficial part surrounds the lower anal canal, attached to the anococcygeal body posteriorly and the perineal body anteriorly.

- The subcutaneous part is a thick ring of muscle surrounding the anal orifice.

The anal columns are connected at their distal ends at the pectinate line by ridges or anal valves, into which the anal glands open, and the mucous membrane of the upper anal canal displays 8 to 10 longitudinal ridges. Underneath the anal mucosa are three anal cushions made of dilated venous and connective tissue, two on the right and one on the left. They help keep the anal canal closed and maintain continence. Skin lines the anal canal's lowest few centimeters.

5.6.1.1. Embryology

The pectinate or dentate line, which divides these two sections, marks the point at which the anal glands enter the tiny cavities known as the anal sinuses. The rectum and upper two-thirds of the anal canal originate from the cloaca, and the lower third from the wall of an ectodermal pouch, the proctodeum. Although it degrades before birth, the membrane dividing the cloaca and proctodeum may still exist as an imperforate anus. The variations in these two parts' blood supply, lymph drainage, and nerve supply are explained by this dual development.

5.6.1.2. Blood Supply

The superior, middle, and inferior rectal arteries are used for this. The veins create submucous plexuses that empty into the internal iliac vein via the middle and inferior rectal veins and the portal system via the superior rectal vein (Figures 5.8 and 5.9).

Congestion of the anal cushions, typically from straining during defecation, is the cause of hemorrhoids. They cause the anal mucosa to prolapse and become congested, which can sometimes cause strangulation and bleeding. The best tool for evaluating hemorrhoids is a proctoscope.

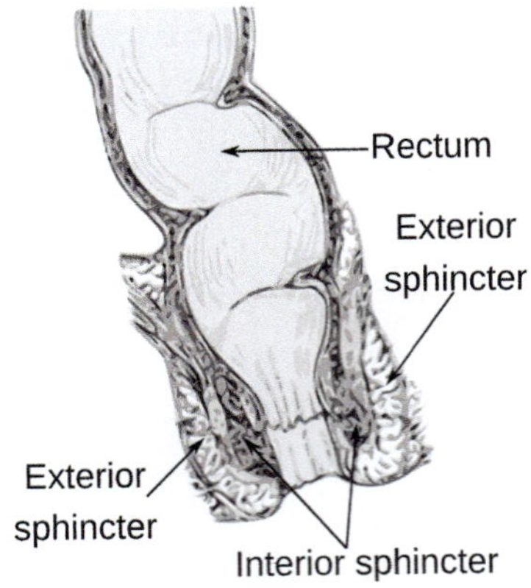

Figure 5.8. *Anal sphincter.*

Source: By Waterced, CC BY-SA 4.0; https://commons.wikimedia.org/w/index.php?curid=70161072.

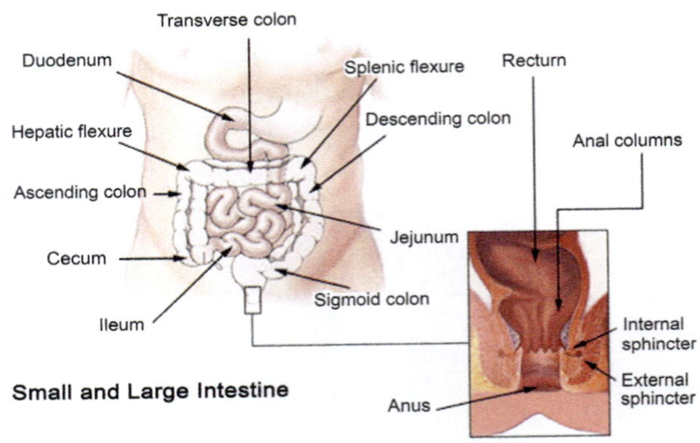

Figure 5.9. *The anus.*

Source: Public Domain; https://commons.wikimedia.org/w/index.php?curid=1354043.

The anal glands that emerge in the anal valves are the source of perianal abscesses. Subcutaneous abscesses in the perineum or ischioanal space (clinically known as ischiorectal abscesses) may develop from them as they spread. Anal fistulae, which are caused by abscesses rupturing through the skin, are typically surgically excised. Anal fissures, or tears in the anal mucosa, are common, with the posterior midline being the most common location.

5.6.2. Lymphatic Drainage

The para-aortic nodes and the preaortic nodes receive the drainage from the rectum and upper anal canal through the inferior mesenteric nodes. The lymphatics of the rectum drain upward through the upper anal canal, while the superficial inguinal nodes receive the lower anal canal's drainage. Since rectum cancer spreads through the lymphatic vessels, surgical attempts to treat the disease must also remove these nodes. The cut end of the sigmoid colon is brought out and sutured to the anterior abdominal wall to form an artificial anus (colostomy) if the entire rectum and anal canal are removed. One sign of anal cancer is an enlarged lymph gland in the groin area. The superficial inguinal lymph nodes must be removed during surgery, and the groin nodes must be included in the radiation treatment field because anal cancer typically responds to this type of treatment.

5.6.2.1. Nerve Supply

In the rectum and upper anal canal, parasympathetic nerves from the pelvic splanchnic nerves (S2, 3, 4) relax the internal sphincter while sympathetic nerves from the pelvic plexuses contract the circular muscle of the sphincter. The inferior rectal nerves and the perineal branch of the fourth sacral nerve supply the lower anal canal and the external sphincter, which are both voluntarily controlled.

5.6.3. Defecation

The urge to defecate is triggered by feces entering the rectum. Massive peristaltic waves that travel through the colon and push more feces into the rectum signal the start of defecation. Then, the anal canal relaxes and the rectum contracts, allowing the feces to pass out. This expulsion is aided by the anterior abdominal wall and diaphragm contracting simultaneously. Levator ani pulls forward the anorectal angle, squeezing the lumen flat and emptying the anal canal at the same time that the voluntary external sphincter relaxes. These sphincter muscles keep continence intact by keeping the anal canal open only when passing gas or feces.

Comprehending the intricate mechanisms that sustain fecal continence is a challenge. It involves the internal and external anal sphincters, but the puborectalis fibers of the levator ani may play the most significant role in maintaining the anorectal angle. This is typically around 90° but if it is raised to more than 100° incontinence is probably going to occur. When in good functioning, the puborectalis can be felt rectally as a firm edge situated just posteriorly above the prostate, or the anorectal ring.

The posterior tip of the sacrum and coccyx is felt during a digital examination of the rectum. In the male, the ducta deferentia and seminal vesicles, as well as the prostate, can be palpable if they are diseased; in the female, the cervix is palpable through the vaginal and rectal walls. Midwives make use of this information when evaluating cervical dilatation during labor through a rectal examination. A sigmoidoscope is needed to examine the entire rectum and lower sigmoid colon, but a proctoscope is the best tool for looking at the anal canal and lower rectum. Each provides a chance for biopsies to be performed.

5.7. The Bladder

The lower portion of the hollow, muscular bladder, which is extra peritoneally located in the anterior pelvis, is encircled by fibrous tissue. Transitional epithelium lines the smooth muscle that makes up its wall. Its dimensions and form change according to the volume of urine inside; when empty, it has a pyramidal shape with a posterior base, a superior surface, two lateral surfaces, and an apex located behind the pubic symphysis. When full, it is ovoid and distends up behind the anterior abdominal wall. The median umbilical ligament, which is a remnant of the urachus, ascends to the umbilicus from the apex. The bladder sphincter surrounds the urethra as it exits inferiorly at the narrow neck, where the ureters enter the posterolateral angles of the base.

The peritoneum covers the superior surface of the uterus and moves backward over the organ in females. The bladder base is encircled by thickened pelvic fascia, which forms ligaments that attach to the lateral walls of the pelvis (lateral ligaments of the bladder), the rectum (posterior ligament), and the back of the pubis (pubovesical and puboprostatic ligaments). The bladder's mucosa is divided into numerous folds, or trabeculations, with the exception of the trigone, a smooth triangle that lies between the two ureters and the internal urethral orifice on the inferior side.

5.7.1. Relations

The superior surface is in contact with the small intestine and, in the case of a female, the uterus; the inferolateral surfaces are separated from the pubic bones, levator ani, and obturator internus by a fat-filled retropubic space. The base is located in front of the rectum; in females, the vagina separates it from the base, whereas in males, the seminal vesicles and ducta deferentia do so. The base lies inferiorly over the urogenital diaphragm in women and the prostate in men.

5.7.2. Blood Supply

This is accomplished by the internal iliac arteries' superior and inferior vesical branches. The internal iliac veins receive venous drainage through the vesical venous plexus.

5.7.3. Lymphatic Drainage

This is to the internal and external iliac nodes.

5.7.4. Nerve Supply

These are sympathetic fibers that originate from the first and second lumbar segments via the pelvic plexuses. They are motor to the vesical sphincter and inhibitory to the bladder wall. The pelvic splanchnic nerves S2, 3 and 4 source parasympathetic fibers, which are inhibitory to the sphincter and motor to the bladder wall. The parasympathetic fibers transmit the sensation of the bladder.

5.7.5. Embryology

The trigone develops from the mesonephric (Wolffian) ducts, while the bladder primarily develops from the urogenital sinus of the cloaca. Urine may drain through the umbilicus after birth if the median umbilical ligament, a remnant of the urachus, sporadically continues to exist from the bladder to the umbilicus.

5.8. Micturition

An adult's urge to micturate is typically triggered by a bladder volume greater than approximately 300 mL. When the vesical sphincter slightly relaxes during micturition, some urine can pass through and enter the urethra, or upper urethra in females. This starts the vesical and urethral sphincter muscles relaxing and the reflex contraction of the detrusor muscle, which is located in the bladder wall. One can consciously suppress the reflexes that lead to the urge to micturate by contracting the urethral sphincter, tightening the vesical sphincter, and relaxing the detrusor. However, micturition is unavoidable once urine seeps into the urethra. It is an easy and safe procedure to introduce a needle or catheter in the midline suprapubically, without entering the peritoneum, because the enlarged obstructed bladder, as it distends into the abdomen, strips off its peritoneal covering (suprapubic catheterization). When the pubic and ischial rami are fractured, the bladder is vulnerable to harm. Urine may leak intra- or extra peritoneally if the bladder bursts when this happens if it is swollen. Cystoscopy enables bladder inspection, mucosal biopsy, and certain small cancer treatments. Bladder cancer that has progressed requires surgical removal.

5.9. The Female Internal Genital Organs

These include the ovaries, the vagina, and the uterus and uterine tubes. All of these have a connection to the broad ligament of the uterus, which is a double layer of peritoneum that extends from the lateral pelvic wall to the lateral margin of the uterus on both sides and contains fibrous tissue. The uterine tubes are located in the medial two-thirds of the ligament's free upper border, while the ovary's suspensory ligament, which forms in the lateral third, contains the ovarian vessels. The ovarian ligament, which is continuous with the uterine round ligament, is contained in the mesovarium, a peritoneal fold that connects the ovary to the posterior surface of the ligament. Ligaments that connect the uterus to pelvic structures are found in the parametrium, which is located at the base of the broad ligament fibrous tissue. The uterine artery passes lateral to the cervix over the ureter (Figure 5.10).

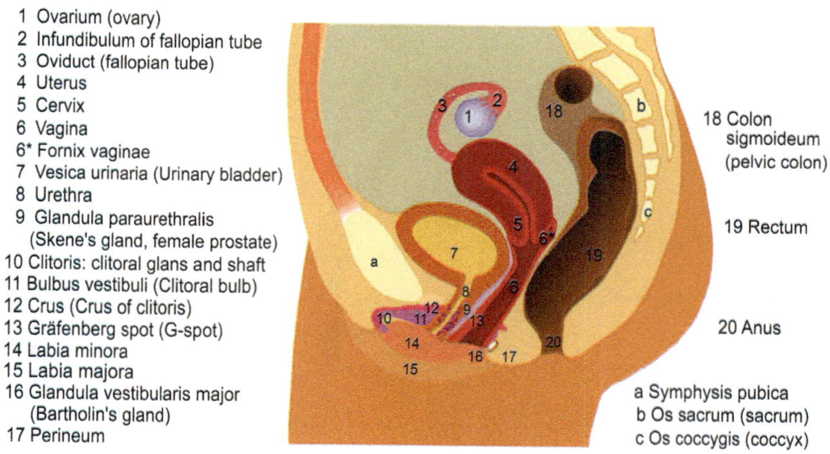

Figure 5.10. *Laparoscopic view of female pelvis: (1) bladder; (2) uterovesical pouch of peritoneum; (3) fundus of uterus; (4) uterine tube (fallopian); (5) rectouterine pouch (Douglas); (6) ligament of ovary; (7) ovary; (8) round ligament of uterus; (9) infundibulum of uterine tube; and (10) suspensory ligament of ovary.*

Source: https://bpb-us-w2.wpmucdn.com/blog.nus.edu.sg/dist/7/881/files/2022/03/Pelvis-perieum.pdf.

5.9.1. The Uterus

The uterus is a pear-shaped, hollow, muscular organ with thick walls that is located between the bladder and the rectum. Its dimensions are approximately 8 cm long, 5 cm wide, and 3 cm thick. It offers the fetus both protection and nourishment. The fetus passes through the birth canal when its muscular walls contract. Its long axis is typically oriented forward at a right angle to the vagina, causing it to open into the vagina below (anteverted). The cervix, which faces forward (anteflexion) and hangs over the bladder, meets the upper two-thirds of the body at a slight angle.

The body's upper lateral angle is where the uterine tubes connect. The fundus is the region of the body that is above the tubes.

The most fixed part of the uterus is the cylindrical cervix due to its attachments. The opening of the cervical canal is located at the apex of the cervix, and it protrudes into the upper anterior vaginal wall, encircled by the vaginal fornix, a sulcus. The parametrium and its ligamentous thickenings encircle the larger supravaginal portion of the cervix. Much of the uterus' posterior wall is covered by the peritoneum. It extends anteriorly over the fundus and body and then moves on to the superior surface of the bladder. It covers the fundus, body, supravaginal cervix, and the posterior wall (fornix) of the vagina. The peritoneum extends laterally as a broad ligament from the anterior and posterior surfaces to the lateral pelvic wall (Figure 5.11).

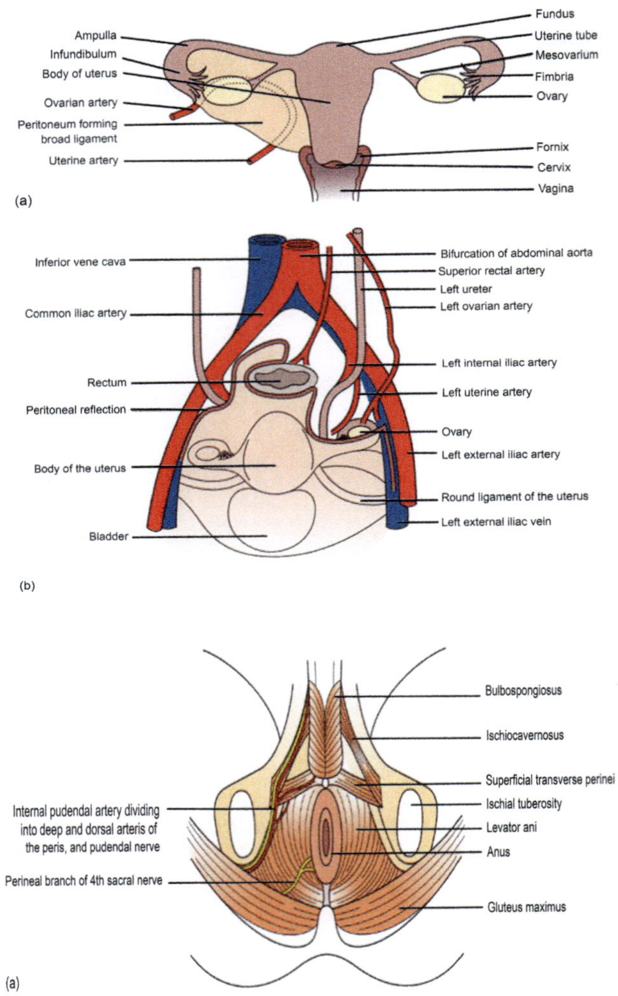

Figure 5.11. *Female reproductive system.*

Source: By The old versions were from Tsaitgaist. This new image is reworked, changed, and improved by Sciencia58 so that there is no problem any more. File: Male and female anatomy.svg, CC BY-SA 4.0; https://commons.wikimedia.org/w/index.php?curid=140544867.

An intrauterine contraceptive device (IUCD) is a tiny plastic device that is placed inside the uterine cavity to decrease the chance of conception. It is frequently covered in copper. In order to diagnose irregular menstrual bleeding, dilatation, and curettage (D&C) is commonly used. This procedure involves dilation of the cervix's neck and the removal of uterine mucosa scrapings for microscopic examination. Cervical cancer is common and can be detected early with a vaginal examination that includes a gentle scrape of the cervix to obtain a specimen of its superficial cells and a microscopically inspected stained specimen (Papanicolaou smear). This forms the cornerstone of the cervical cancer screening program.

5.9.1.1. Ligaments of the Uterus

The round ligament is a band of fibromuscular tissue that extends from the uterus's upper lateral angle, via the broad ligament, the deep inguinal ring, the inguinal canal, and the labium majus. It is a piece of the gubernaculum ovarii that connects the superficial inguinal lymph nodes to the uterus through lymph vessels.

The parametrium surrounds the supravaginal cervix. It is thickened to form three paired ligaments on the pelvic surface of levator ani:

- **The Uterosacral Ligaments** – pass posteriorly around the rectum to the sacrum.
- **The Lateral Cervical (Cardinal) Ligaments** – pass to the lateral pelvic wall.
- **The Pubocervical Ligaments** – pass forwards to the body of the pubis.

These ligaments provide stability and support for the uterus. The anteverted position might be preserved with the aid of the round ligaments. Levator ani provides significant assistance as well. The urethral sphincter is then unable to stop the unintentional loss of urine from the bladder (known as stress incontinence) when the intra-abdominal pressure is raised, for example, because the levator ani may have been torn or stretched during a difficult childbirth, making it incapable of supporting and lifting the base of the bladder when chuckling or coughing.

5.9.1.2. Relations

The uterus and the rectum are divided posteriorly by the coils of the small intestine and sigmoid colon; the bladder is located anteroinferiorly, and the broad ligaments are located on either side. The vaginal cervix is situated between the rectum posteriorly and the ureter and uterine artery laterally. It is encircled by the fornix and vaginal walls. Because of its close proximity to the uterine artery and cervix, the ureter is vulnerable to damage in the event that the artery is clamped during a hysterectomy. It also explains why advanced cervix or uterine cancer frequently results in ureteric obstruction.

5.9.1.3. Blood Supply

This originates from the internal iliac branch, or uterine artery. The veins empty into the uterine and internal iliac veins through the uterine plexus located in the lower broad ligament.

5.9.1.4. Lymphatic Drainage

Drainage is mainly to the external and common iliac nodes, but some drain along the round ligament to the superficial inguinal nodes in the groin.

5.9.1.5. Nerve Supply

There are sympathetic and parasympathetic fibers from the pelvic plexus. Pregnancy causes the uterine ligaments to stretch. In addition, if there is laxity in the vaginal wall, the bladder (cystocele) or rectum (rectocele) may protrude into the anterior vaginal wall and obstruct normal micturition and defecation. These conditions could result from the uterus failing to regain its original tension and descending into the vagina (uterine prolapse). A challenging delivery may cause a partial levator ani tear, which weakens the pelvic viscera's support and increases the risk of the uterus descending (prolapse) and developing urine incontinence. Stress incontinence, or the involuntary expulsion of a small amount of urine, is the result of sudden increases in intra-abdominal pressure, which can occur, for example, after coughing.

5.9.1.6. Age Changes

The uterine body and cervix are of equal size up until puberty, at which point the body grows. The uterine body increases 30 times during pregnancy as a result of muscle hypertrophy, following menopause, the endometrium and muscles atrophy.

5.9.2. The Uterine Tubes

The uterine tubes, which are located in the upper margins of the broad ligament, are roughly 10 cm long. The superomedial angle of the uterus is where they open. Each one overlaps the ovary's lateral surface before passing laterally and opening into the peritoneal cavity. Their function is to convey ova to the uterus. They are described as having, from medial to lateral:

- A uterine part – within the wall of the uterus;
- A narrow isthmus;
- A dilated and convoluted ampulla;
- A funnel-shaped infundibulum;
- Several finger-like fimbriae, one of which is attached to the ovary.

Throughout its course, the tube is related to coils of the small intestine.

5.9.2.1. Blood Supply

The uterine arteries, which anastomose with the ovarian vessels that emerge straight from the aorta, supply the uterine tubes.

5.9.2.2. Nerve Supply

There are sympathetic fibers from the pelvic plexuses.

5.9.2.3. Lymphatic Drainage

Drainage is to para-aortic and iliac nodes. Salpingitis, or tube infection, can result from an infection that travels straight from the uterus and vagina to the uterine tubes. This can lead to infertility and occasionally cause tubal fibrosis and blockage.

Ectopic pregnancy is the result of implantation taking place outside of the uterus, usually in the peritoneum or the uterine tubes, as opposed to the uterine body. These pregnancies typically only last 6–8 weeks in the uterine tubes before the tube bursts and an intraperitoneal bleed occurs. Hysterosalpingography, a technique that involves injecting radio-opaque material into the uterine tubes, can be used to radiographically evaluate the patency of the tube. The method of birth control known as uterine tube ligation (Table 5.1).

Table 5.1. *An Overview of the Anatomy*

Components of the Male Reproductive System		
Structure	**Location and Description**	**Function**
Bulborethral glands (2)	Pea sized organs posterior to the prostate on either side of the urethra.	Secretion of gelatinous seminal fluid called pre-ejaculate. This fluid helps to lubricate the urethra for spermatozoa to pass through, and to help flush out any residual urine or foreign matter (< 1% of semen).
Epididymis	Tightly coiled duct lying just outside each testis connecting efferent ducts to vas deferens.	Storage and maturation of sperm.
Penis	Three columns of erectile tissue: two corpora cavernosa and one corpus spongiosum. Urethra passes through penis.	Male reproductive organ and also male organ of urination.
Prostate gland	Surrounds the urethra just below the urinary bladder and can be felt during a rectal exam.	Stores and secretes a clear, slightly alkaline fluid constituting up to one-third of the volume of semen. Raise vaginal pH (25–30% of semen).
Seminal vesicles (2)	Convoluted structure attached to vas deferens near the base of the urinary bladder.	About 65–75% of the seminal fluid in humans originates from the seminal vesicles. Contain proteins, enzymes, fructose, mucus, vitamin C, flavins, phosphorylcholine, and prostaglandins. High fructose concentrations provide nutrient energy for the spermatozoa as they travel through the female reproductive system.
Testes	Inside scrotum, outside of body.	Gonads that produce sperm and male sex hormones. Production of testosterone by cells of Leydig in the testicles.
Urethra	Connects bladder to outside body, about 8 inches long.	Tubular structure that receives urine from bladder and carries it to outside of the body. Also passage for sperm.

Vas deferens	Muscular tubes connecting the left and right epididymis to the ejaculatory ducts to move sperm. Each tube is about 30 cm long.	During ejaculation the smooth muscle in the vas deferens wall contracts, propelling sperm forward. Sperm are transferred from the vas deferens into the urethra, collecting fluids from accessory sex glands en route
Components of the Female Reproductive System		
Ovaries (2)	Ovoid structures on either side of the uterus in the pelvic cavity.	Primary sex organs of female; contain ovarian follicles that contain the oocytes. Oocytes are released during the ovulation stage of the menstrual cycle.
Fallopian tubes (2)	Extend from lateral areas of the uterus to near the ovaries.	Transport oocyte to uterus after fertilization and are the sites where fertilization by sperm actually occurs.
Uterus	Pear shaped structure divided into the fundus and the cervix.	Site of fetal development during gestation.
Vagina	Located between rectum and urethra; smooth muscle lined with an epithelial mucous membrane.	Path for menstrual blood and tissue to leave the body, as well as the fetus during childbirth. Produces a variety of secretions for lubrication and receives secretions that facilitate fertilization.
Vulva	Externally located: labia majora and minora, mons pubis, clitoris, vestibule, greater and lesser vestibular glands.	Sexual function: heavily innervated and provide pleasure when properly stimulated.
Perineum	Area between vagina and anus	Helps form the muscular floor of pelvis; can be torn during vaginal childbirth.
Mammary glands	Superficial to pectoral muscles	Provide nourishment to the baby through milk secretions.

Indifferent	Male	Female
Gonad	Testis	Ovary
Müllerian duct	Appendix testis	Fallopian tubes
Müllerian duct	Prostatic utricle	Uterus, proximal vagina
Wolffian duct	Rete testis	Rete ovarii
Mesonephric tubules	Efferent ducts	Epoophoron

Wolffian duct	Epididymis	Gartner's duct
Wolffian duct	Vas deferens	–
Wolffian duct	Seminal vesicle	–
Wolffian duct	Prostate	Skene's glands
Urogenital sinus	Bladder, urethra	Bladder, urethra, distal vagina
Urogenital sinus	Bulborethral gland	Bartholin's gland
Genital swelling	Scrotum	Labia majora
Urogenital folds	Distal urethra	Labia minora
Genital tubercle	Penis	Clitoris
Prepuce	Foreskin	Clitoral hood
–	Bulb of penis	Vestibular bulbs
–	Glans penis	Clitoral glans
–	Crus of penis	Clitoral crura

Source: https://courses.lumenlearning.com/wm-biology2/chapter/reproductive-system/#:~:text=Female%20Reproductive%20System,-Produces%20eggs%20(ova&text=Primary%20sex%20organs%20of%20female,stage%20of%20the%20menstrual%20cycle.&text=Path%20for%20menstrual%20blood%20and,as%20the%20fetus%20during%20childbirth.

5.9.3. The Ovary

The ovary is a 3 cm long, almond-shaped organ. It moves and changes positions frequently, and during pregnancy, it becomes significantly displaced. It is situated behind the broad ligament and is joined by the mesovarium, a double peritoneal fold that encloses the ovary.

5.9.3.1. Relations

The ovarian fossa is occupied by the lateral surface, which is next to the pelvic wall. This is bordered anteriorly by the obliterated umbilical artery, superiorly by the internal iliac artery, and posteriorly by the ureter. The medial surface of the ovary is in close proximity to the broad ligament, and it is laterally clasped by the infundibulum and the fimbriae of the tube. One of the ovary's fimbriae and the suspensory ligament, which transports the ovarian vessels, connect the tubal end to the tube.

5.9.3.2. Blood Supply

This is accomplished through the ovarian artery and uterine artery branches. The ovarian vein, which on the left drains to the left renal vein and typically on the right directly into the inferior vena cava, receives venous drainage through the ovarian pampiniform plexus.

5.9.3.3. Lymphatic Drainage

Drainage is to para-aortic nodes.

5.9.3.4. Nerve Supply

There are sympathetic fibers from the 10th thoracic segment via the aortic plexuses.

5.9.3.5. Embryology

The mesothelium on the posterior abdominal wall, next to the paramesonephric ridge, gives rise to the ovary. As with the testis, it descends after a gubernaculum that continues as the round ligament of the ovary and the uterus. The ovary can occasionally undergo malignant transformation in addition to cyst formation. Excision of the ovary and related lymph nodes is necessary for surgical treatment of the latter. Certain women experience pain in the paraumbilical region during their ovulation (T10). The German term mittelschmerz refers to this, which happens approximately halfway through the menstrual cycle.

5.10. The Male Internal Genital Organs

5.10.1. The Prostate

The prostate is a glandular tissue-containing fibromuscular organ located on the urogenital diaphragm beneath the bladder. It has a base above, an apex below, and anterior, posterior, and two lateral surfaces. It resembles a truncated cone and has a diameter of about 3 cm. The urethra and the two ejaculatory ducts in its upper half pass through it posteriorly. It is divided into two lateral lobes and a median lobe by fibrous septae and the urethra and ejaculatory ducts; the lateral lobes are located below and lateral to these. The prostatic sheath, or pelvic fascia, covers the seminal vesicles and surrounds the organ as well as the venous plexus. Rectovesical fascia, which divides the prostate from the rectum, is continuous with the fascia that surrounds the bladder neck.

5.10.1.1. Relations

The bladder neck is located superiorly, the urethral sphincter inferiorly, the levator ani anterolaterally, and the rectum and seminal vesicles posteriorly.

5.10.1.2. Blood Supply

This is through the internal iliac artery's middle rectal and inferior vesical branches. The internal iliac veins and the vertebral venous plexus are reached by venous drainage through the prostatic plexuses.

5.10.1.3. Lymphatic Drainage

This is to the internal iliac nodes.

5.10.1.4. Nerve Supply

The pelvic plexus contains sympathetic fibers (L1, 2), while the pelvic splanchnic (S2, 3, 4) contain parasympathetic fibers. Rectal examination makes it easy to palpate the prostate; a normal gland is felt beneath the anterior rectal mucosa as a firm, smooth mass with a vertical sulcus. The glandular tissue frequently enlarges and projects upward in middle age, particularly the median lobe. This disrupts the function of the vesical sphincter and makes micturition challenging and insufficient. Even though pharmacological techniques to shrink prostate size are becoming more popular, surgical treatment is still frequently utilized. Using an operating cystoscope, transurethral resection of the prostate (TURP) allows the median lobe to be "coring out." Because of the prostate's highly coiled duct system, prostate infections, or prostatitis, are extremely difficult to treat. It is characterized by nebulous pain in the perineum, and a tender, swollen prostate may be felt rectally. Prostate cancer typically begins in the lateral lobes and can be identified by a hard, irregular mass found during a rectal examination. Because the cancer cells are transported there by the vertebral venous plexus, secondary cancer spread frequently affects the vertebral column.

5.10.2. Ductus (Vas) Deferens

Each ductus is a 45 cm long, slender muscular tube that continues the epididymis canal. It travels from the epididymis tail to the ejaculatory duct via the scrotum, inguinal canal, and pelvis.

5.10.2.1. Relations

It is located within the spermatic cord in the inguinal canal and is palpable as a firm 4-mm-diameter cord in the scrotum. It enters the pelvis at the deep inguinal ring, lateral to the inferior epigastric vessels. From there, it passes over the ureter and external iliac vessels on the lateral pelvic wall, which is covered in peritoneum. It descends medially to the seminal vesicles at the ischial spine, behind the bladder. It is dilated and referred to as the ampulla here. The common ejaculatory duct is formed by connecting it to the seminal vesicle duct at its terminus.

5.10.3. Seminal Vesicles

Each ductus deferens is a sacculated diverticulum, coiled and approximately 5 cm long, situated behind the base of the bladder and obliquely above the prostate. Above and below, the rectovesical pouch of peritoneum and the rectovesical fascia divide it from the rectum. When doing a rectal examination, the narrow lower end is rarely palpable unless it is diseased. For male sterilization, a vasectomy is frequently done: the vas is separated from the spermatic cord in the upper region of the scrotum, a 1–2 cm section is removed, and the divided ends are tied together. The sperm kept in the seminal vesicles prevents the patient from becoming sterile for three to six months. A vasectomy is a common procedure used to sterilize males. It involves separating the vas from the spermatic cord in the upper part of the scrotum, removing a 1–2 cm section, and tying the divided ends together. The sperm kept in the seminal vesicles prevents the patient from becoming sterile for three to six months.

5.10.4. Common Ejaculatory Ducts

The duct of the seminal vesicle and the terminal portion of the ductus deferens unite to form each about a 2 cm long structure behind the bladder's neck. It then passes through the upper prostate and opens into the prostatic urethra directly lateral to the posterior swelling seminal colliculus (verumontanum).

5.10.4.1. Blood Supply

The inferior vesical and middle rectal arteries supply all of these structures, and the internal iliac vein receives their venous drainage through the vesical venous plexus.

5.10.4.2. Lymphatic Drainage

Drainage is to the internal iliac nodes.

5.10.4.3. Nerve Supply

The muscles in the seminal vesicles and the walls of the ducta contract as a result of sympathetic fibers from the pelvic plexuses, also referred to as "nervi erigentes." Impotence ensues if the nervi erigentes are divided, which can happen after rectum excision. This prevents erection and ejaculation.

5.11. The Perineum

Beneath the pelvic diaphragm (coccygeus and levator ani) is the perineum. Between the pubic symphysis and the coccyx, it is a diamond-shaped area that is bordered laterally by the ischial tuberosities, posterolaterally by the sacrotuberous ligaments, and anterolaterally by the ischiopubic rami. The area is divided into an anterior urogenital triangle and a posterior anal triangle by a line connecting the ischial tuberosities.

5.11.1. The Anal Triangle

The two ischioanal fossae laterally and the anal canal in the midline make up the anal triangle. The base of the wedge-shaped ischioanal fossa is located inferiorly between the ischium and the anal canal. It is bordered superomedially by the fascia over the obturator internus, laterally by the perineal skin, and inferiorly by the levator ani's attachment to the obturator fascia above and its junction with the external anal sphincter below. It extends deep below the levator ani, all the way to the urogenital diaphragm, and extends posteriorly between the sacrotuberous and sacrospinous ligaments to the gluteus maximus. Both sexes have the same contents. The anal canal, the perineal body, and the anococcygeal body divide the two fossae, but they communicate behind the anal canal. The pudendal nerve and vessels are located on the lateral wall of each fossa, in a sheath of fascia that covers the obturator internus, or pudendal canal, which is located approximately 3 cm above the ischial tuberosity. Each fossa is composed of lobulated fat. The perineal nerve, inferior rectal nerve, and branches from the coccygeal plexus supply the perianal skin (S3, 4 and 5). Large abscesses are often the result of infection of the anal canal glands spreading through the anal wall into the ischioanal fossa (which is still referred to as the ischiorectal fossa by clinicians). If these leak through the skin, the anal canal and skin could become permanently fistulated (fistula in ano).

5.11.2. The Urogenital Triangle

The inferior layer of the urogenital diaphragm, or the perineal membrane, separates the urogenital triangle into superior and inferior compartments, or pouches. The triangular double layer of fascia, known as the urogenital diaphragm, is stronger in males than in females and spans the pubic arch between the ischiopubic rami. The perineal body, a central subcutaneous fibrous mass, is connected to its free posterior border. The female vagina and the male urethra both puncture the diaphragm. The perineal membrane, which is its inferior fascial layer, provides attachment to the bulb and crura of the penis or clitoris. Between the two levatores ani, its superior (deep) layer and the pelvic fascia meet to form the viscera. The deep layer and the posterior border of the perineal membrane fuse posteriorly to form the deep perineal pouch, a fascially bound envelope. Male and female perineal pouches differ significantly in terms of depth and superficiality.

5.11.3. The Male Urogenital Triangle

The urogenital diaphragm and the superficial fascia's membranous layer are separated by the superficial perineal pouch. The superficial fascia is continuous with the anterior abdominal wall's superficial fascia over the pubic symphysis, attached to the diaphragm's posterior border, and attached laterally to the ischiopubic rami. It offers a fascial sheath that encloses the superficial perineal muscles as well as the root and body of the penis. This fascial space, referred to as the superficial perineal pouch, contains the penis, testes, and other scrotal contents.

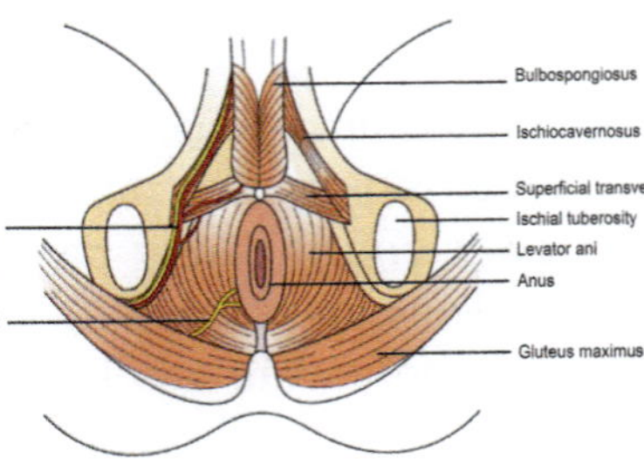

(a)

5.11.3.1. The Penis

The penis is made up of three longitudinal cylinders of erectile tissue: the two lateral corpora cavernosa, which are covered in fascia and skin, and the central corpus spongiosum, which houses the urethra. It has a root that connects it to the perineal membrane, as well as a body. The bulb of the penis posteriorly and the glans penis anteriorly are formed by the expansion of the ventral corpus spongiosum. The bulb is joined to the perineal membrane by the bulbospongiosus muscle. The urethra passes through the corpus and emerges at the top of the glans. The two cavernosa corpora unite dorsally and are inserted anteriorly into the glans. They diverge posteriorly, below the symphysis, to form the two penis crura, which are protected by the ischiocavernosus muscles. The deep fascia of the penis encloses the tunica albuginea, a tough fibrous sheath that covers the corpus spongiosum and corpora cavernosa. The suspensory ligament connecting the penis to the symphysis pubis attaches this dorsally. The prepuce, also known as the foreskin, is the fold of skin that forms over the glans and is connected to the glans by a tiny skinfold called the frenulum.

5.11.3.1.1. Blood Supply

This is accomplished by branches of the internal pudendal; the bulb, corpus spongiosum, and glans are supplied by the artery to the bulb; the corpora cavernosa is supplied by the deep artery of the penis; and the skin is supplied by the dorsal artery of the penis. During circumcision, extra care must be taken to ligate the small frenular artery to prevent significant blood loss (Figure 5.12).

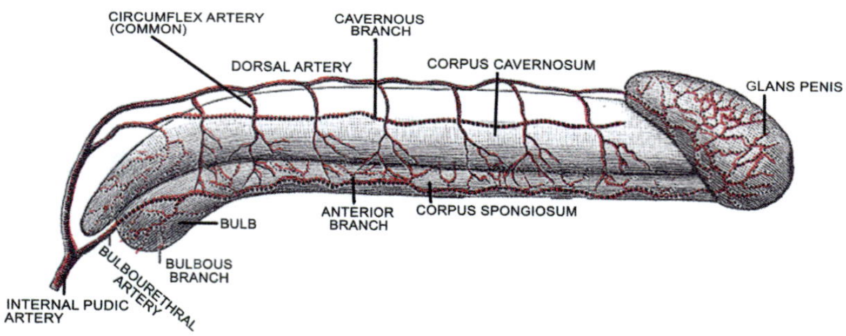

Figure 5.12. *Anatomy of the penis.*

Source: Public Domain; https://en.wikipedia.org/w/index.php?curid=62444575.

Venous drainage flows to the prostatic plexus through the deep dorsal vein of the penis and the internal pudendal vein. Engorgement of the cavernous spaces results in erection. The coiled penile arteries dilate as a result of the pelvic parasympathetic fibers. The venous drainage from the cavernous spaces is compressed by the bulbospongiosus and ischiocavernosus muscles. Somatic contractions of the bulbospongiosus muscles and closure of the bladder neck and sphincter urethrae are the mechanisms through which ejaculation is mediated by sympathetic fibers.

5.11.3.1.2. Lymphatic Drainage

This is to the superficial inguinal and iliac nodes.

5.11.3.1.3. Nerve Supply

Somatic supply is by the ilioinguinal nerve and the dorsal nerve of the penis. Parasympathetic vasodilator fibers from the pelvic splanchnic (S2, 3, 4) supply the erectile tissue.

5.11.3.1.4. The Scrotum

The scrotum is a pouch of thin, rugose skin enclosing the two testes and spermatic cords, separated by a midline raphe and septum. Its walls contain smooth muscle fibers, the dartos muscle.

5.11.3.2. The Superficial Perineal Pouch

The superficial perineal pouch houses the bulbospongiosus and ischiocavernosus muscles, which constrict the corpora and aid in ejaculation and erection. It also contains the superficial muscles of the perineum. Additionally, there are the paired superficial transverse perineal muscles located at the perineal membrane's posterior edge. All are supplied by branches of the pudendal nerve's perineal branch. The pouch contains the penile urethra and penis. Urine seeps into the superficial perineal pouch due to a ruptured penile urethra, an injury that typically results from direct trauma to the perineum or from a fractured pelvis. Its dissemination is limited by the perineal fascia's attachments; at first, it spreads into the scrotum and penis's subfascial tissues before climbing the anterior abdominal wall all the way to its superficial fascia. The attachments of the perineal fascia to the fascia lata prevent it from spreading into the thigh.

5.11.3.3. The Deep Perineal Pouch

The urogenital diaphragm's two layers are separated by a closed area known as the deep perineal pouch. It includes the sphincter urethrae muscle, which encircles the urethra, and the membranous urethra. The pudendal nerves S2, S3, and S4 supply this voluntary muscle, which is supplied by the ischiopubic ramus on both sides.

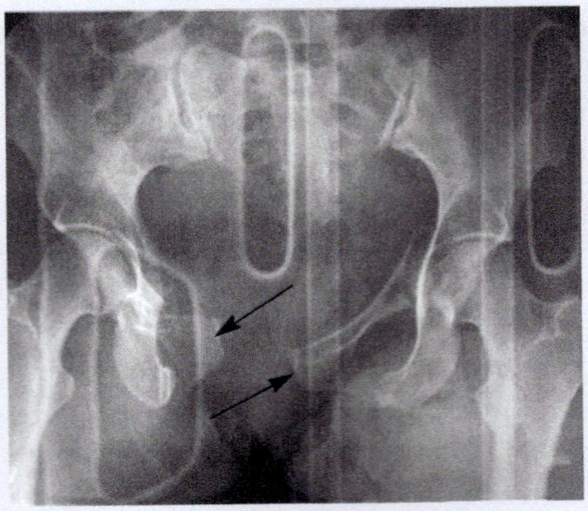

5.11.3.4. The Urethra

The male urethra is around 20 cm long and extends from the bladder's internal urethral orifice to the external urethral orifice via the prostate, deep perineal pouch, and corpus spongiosum. It is divided into prostatic, membranous, and spongy parts:

- The widest section descends through the gland and is called the prostatic urethra. It is about 3 cm long. The prostatic utricle, a small pit on top of the urethral crest (verumontanum), is where the common ejaculatory ducts and numerous prostatic ducts open. This elevation is found on the posterior wall of the body.
- The 1 cm long membranous urethra is slender. It passes through the bulbourethral glands (Cowper's) and the sphincter urethrae muscle, which encircle the deep perineal pouch.
- The entire corpus spongiosum is traversed by the spongy urethra, which is around 16 centimeters long. Its lumen, which resembles a slit, is narrowest at the external urethral meatus and dilated posteriorly in the urethral bulb.

5.11.3.4.1. Blood Supply

This is by the inferior vesical and branches of the internal pudendal artery. The veins drain to the prostatic venous plexus and internal pudendal vein.

5.11.3.4.2. Nerve Supply

The pudendal nerve.

5.11.3.4.3. Lymphatic Drainage

The spongy portion drains to the superficial inguinal nodes, while the prostatic and membranous parts drain to the internal iliac nodes. In order to relieve urinary obstruction in men, urethral catheterization is frequently necessary. The membranous urethra, which has thin walls and is narrow, is most susceptible to injury during this process. Male urethral strictures and infections are common. The passage of finely graduated urethral sounds causes dilatation.

5.11.4. The Female Urogenital Triangle

The vaginal passage passes through the superficial and deep pouches of the triangle, dividing them almost entirely. The clitoris crura, the vestibule bulb, the greater vestibular glands, the superficial perineal muscles, and the terminal portions of the vagina and urethra are all located in the superficial pouch. The sphincter urethrae, deep perineal muscles, pudendal nerve, and internal pudendal vessels are all located in the deep pouch, which is crossed by the vagina and membranous urethra. The urethra of a female is roughly 3 cm long. It descends from the neck of the bladder through the deep perineal pouch, which is encircled by the muscle known as the sphincter urethrae, and opens into the vestibule behind the clitoris. The bilateral vestibular bulbs are located in the superficial pouch next to the vagina. They are situated on the membrane that is protected by the muscles of the bulbospongiosus. The larger vestibular glands (Bartholin's) drain into this region (Wu et al., 2018).

A Bartholin's abscess near the side of the vaginal vestibule is often the result of infection of the larger vestibular glands. It is most convenient to examine the perineum in a supine position with the hips flexed and abducted, or in the "lithotomy" position. In order to avoid harming the anal sphincter or rectal wall, an episiotomy may be carried out with the aid of a pudendal nerve block if labor is prolonged and a perineal laceration appears likely. A three-centimeter mediolateral incision is made, piercing the skin, posterior vaginal wall, and bulbospongiosus muscle. Following birth, it is sutured. Bartholin's abscess at the side of the vaginal vestibule is often the result of infection of the larger vestibular glands. The most convenient way to examine the perineum is with the patient in the "lithotomy" position, i.e., lying supine with the hips abducted and flexed. Using a needle inserted into the vaginal wall and directed towards the ischial spine (palpable per vaginum), a local anesthetic is infused into the pudendal nerve, which is located 3 cm deep to the ischial tuberosity, to achieve a pudendal nerve block. The posterior vulva will become anesthetized with a pudendal block. To achieve anesthesia throughout the entire vulva, local infiltration of the lateral walls—which are supplied by the ilioinguinal nerve—is necessary.

5.11.4.1. The Female External Genitalia

The vestibule, clitoris, labia majora and minora, and mons pubis make up the female external genitalia. The pile of hairy skin and subcutaneous fat in front of the pubis is called the mons pubis. The lateral limits of the vagina are formed by the fatty, hairy folds of skin known as the labia majora. The clitoris, a tiny, sensitive mass of erectile tissue connected to the ischiopubic rami that is similar to the penis, is where the labia minora, which are thin cutaneous folds within the labia majora, unite anteriorly. It has a small glans and two small corpora cavernosae. The external urethral meatus and the vaginal entrance are located in the vestibule, which is surrounded by the labia minora.

5.11.4.1.1. The Vagina

The uterus and the pudendal cleft are connected by the vagina, an 8 cm canal. It is sustained by the fascia that surrounds it and by its connections to the perineal body. Its axis forms a 90° angle with the uterus, and it is positioned in front of the rectum, behind the bladder and urethra. Normally, its anterior and posterior walls are in contact, but at the top, the cervix projects and is encircled by a sulcus, known as the fornix. The hymen, a perforated membrane, partially occludes the lower end at birth.

5.11.4.1.2. Relations

The uterus, bladder, and urethra are located anteriorly; the anal canal, perineal body, and levator ani are located posteriorly; above is the peritoneum of the rectouterine pouch (Douglas), which divides the vagina and rectum. The perineum is where the vagina is at its lowest point.

5.11.4.1.3. Blood Supply

This is by internal iliac and uterine arteries. Venous drainage is via lateral plexuses to the internal iliac veins.

5.11.4.1.4. Lymphatic Drainage

The lower third drains to superficial inguinal nodes, and the upper two-thirds to internal and external iliac nodes. The patient lies on her back with her hips flexed in the lithotomy position during a bimanual digital vaginal examination. Combining this with a hand on the lower abdomen wall enables bimanual examination of the ovaries, uterus, and cervix. While 20% of healthy women have a retroflexed or retroverted uterus, the uterus is typically felt to be in an anteverted and anteflexed position. The cervix is soft in pregnancy, firm in non-pregnancy. The uterus's size can be determined and the ovaries can be felt in the vagina's lateral fornices.

5.11.5. Blood Supply of the Pelvic Floor and Perineum

5.11.5.1. Common Iliac Arteries

At the aortic bifurcation, which is located in front of the fourth lumbar vertebra and slightly to the left of the midline, the common iliac arteries originate. Each ends by splitting into the internal and external iliac arteries after descending laterally to the front of the corresponding sacroiliac joint.

5.11.5.1.1. Relations

Every artery has the peritoneum covering it, lymph nodes, sympathetic nerves, and plexuses surrounding it. The ureter crosses it at its bifurcation, and the root of the sigmoid colon crosses it on the left. It crosses over the psoas muscle and the lumbosacral trunk posteriorly, where it rests on the bodies of the fourth and fifth lumbar vertebrae. The arteries are preceded by the common iliac veins (Wu et al., 2018).

5.11.5.2. Internal Iliac Artery

A terminal branch of the common iliac artery is the internal iliac artery. It rises anterior to the sacroiliac joint and descends to the greater sciatic notch on the posterior pelvic wall, where it splits into the visceral and parietal branches.

5.11.5.2.1. Relations

The ureter crosses its origin, the peritoneum covers it, and lymph nodes surround it. Laterally, the obturator nerve and external iliac vein are located, and posteriorly, the lumbosacral trunk and the sacroiliac joint are located.

5.11.5.2.2. Visceral Branches

The bladder is supplied by the superior vesical artery, which emerges from the partially severed patent remnant of the umbilical artery. The uterine artery enters the broad ligament, where it anastomoses with the ovarian artery, after passing medially over the ureter and the vaginal lateral fornix. It provides blood to the uterus, uterine tubes, and vagina. The prostate, lower rectum, and seminal vesicles are supplied by the middle rectal artery. The vagina (vas deferens and seminal vesicles), bladder, and ureter are supplied by the vaginal artery (inferior vesical artery in men).

5.11.5.2.3. Parietal Branches

The umbilical artery is severed shortly after birth, but the medial umbilical ligament is still formed by the fibrous cord that lies between the pelvic wall and umbilicus. The obturator artery travels forward along the obturator internus, emerging from the pelvis by passing above the obturator membrane to supply the hip joint, which is significant in both adults and children, as well as nearby muscles. Through the larger sciatic foramen, the internal pudendal artery returns to the pelvis. It gives branches to the anal canal, scrotum (labia), and penis as it enters the pudendal canal on the obturator internus. The greater sciatic foramen, located below the piriformis, is where the inferior gluteal artery exits the pelvis to supply the hip joint, the sciatic nerve, and the gluteal muscles. Above the piriformis, the superior gluteal artery exits the pelvis through the greater sciatic foramen, supplying the hip joint and gluteal muscles. The sacral canal's contents are supplied by the lateral sacral artery. The posterior abdominal wall muscles are supplied by the iliolumbar artery, which ascends on the sacrum.

5.11.5.3. The External Iliac Artery

Starting above the sacroiliac joint, the external iliac artery is a terminal branch of the common iliac artery that wraps around the pelvic brim before continuing forward. It becomes the femoral artery as it enters the thigh below the midinguinal point.

5.11.5.3.1. Relations

It is located extra peritoneally, lateral to the external iliac vein, and encircled by lymph nodes on the psoas. The ductus deferens and the testicular vessels in the male and the ovarian vessels and the round ligament in the female cross it anteriorly.

5.11.5.3.2. Branches (Which Both Arise Just Above the Inguinal Ligament)

The posterior rectus sheath, whose contents it supplies, is reached by the inferior epigastric artery ascending medially to the deep inguinal ring behind the anterior abdominal wall. The abdominal wall is likewise supplied by the deep circumflex iliac artery.

5.11.5.4. Veins

These drain primarily to the internal iliac vein through branches that line up with its artery's branches. The prostatic, vesical, uterine, vaginal, and rectal plexuses intercommunicate with the vertebral venous plexuses, and the viscera drain through the venous plexuses that surround them.

This explains the frequency with which certain cancers affecting the pelvic organs—

particularly the prostate—spread to the skull's bones and vertebrae. The common iliac vein is formed by the union of the internal and external iliac veins. It lies posterior to the accompanying arteries and anterior to the sacroiliac joint. The inferior vena cava is formed by the common iliac vein ascending obliquely and joining its fellow just right of the midline on the fifth lumbar vertebra. With the right common iliac artery crossing it, the left vein is longer than the right. The gonadal veins, which form pampiniform plexuses and empty into the left renal vein and the right inferior vena cava, drain the ovaries and testes.

5.11.6. Lymphatic Drainage of the Pelvis and Perineum

5.11.6.1. Pelvis and Perineum

The entire pelvic viscera, including the gluteal region and the entire perineum, are drained by the internal iliac nodes, with the exception of the ovary and testis. The para-aortic nodes surrounding the renal vessels receive lymph that drains directly from the gonads. The lower limb, the lower abdominal wall, the bladder, the prostate, the uterus, and the cervix all supply vessels to the external iliac nodes. The superficial inguinal nodes receive lymph drainage from the perineum, lower anal canal, vagina, and perineal skin. The para-aortic and common iliac nodes receive efferent vessels from the iliac nodes.

5.11.6.2. Abdomen

The axillary, anterior mediastinal, and superficial inguinal nodes are reached by the lymph vessels of the anterior abdominal wall. The posterior abdominal wall and the abdominal viscera drain to the para-aortic nodes. Para-aortic nodes are located next to the aorta around the paired lateral arteries. They drain the kidneys, suprarenals, gonads, posterior abdominal wall, pelvic viscera, and lower limbs through the common iliac nodes. The left and right lumbar lymph trunks are formed by the union of their efferents.

Preaortic nodes drain the intestinal tract supplied by the three arteries that supply the alimentary tract—the coeliac, superior, and inferior mesenteric arteries. The intestinal lymph trunk, which enters the cisterna chyli, is formed when their efferents combine. The cisterna chyli is a 5–7 centimeter long sac with thin walls located in front of the upper two lumbar vertebrae, between the aorta and the right crus of the diaphragm. It receives the intestinal lymph trunk, the right and left lumbar lymph trunks, and it goes straight to the thoracic duct.

5.11.7. Nerves of the Posterior Abdominal Wall and Pelvis

These include the abdominal autonomic nervous system and the lumbar and sacral plexuses. The ventral primary rami of L1–L4 on the psoas surface form the lumbar plexus. The femoral and obturator nerves are its main branches; these also give rise to the quadriceps, sartorius, and pectineus muscles in the thigh and leg, as well as the medial and intermediate cutaneous nerves in the thigh and the saphenous nerve. The obturator nerve descends near the psoas' medial border, deep into the internal iliac vessels, and then uses the obturator foramen to enter the thigh. It supplies the obturator internus, the thigh's adductor muscles, cutaneous branches, and the thigh joints to the medial thigh (Figure 5.13).

The ventral primary rami of L4–5 and S1–4 form the sacral plexus, which is located on the surface of the piriformis in the pelvis. It should be noted that L4 contributes to both plexuses and that a branch that joins the L5 ramus to form the lumbosacral trunk contributes to the sacral plexus. The sciatic nerve and the pudendal nerve are the plexus's two main branches, though it also supplies the hip and pelvic muscles and the buttock and thigh through cutaneous branches.

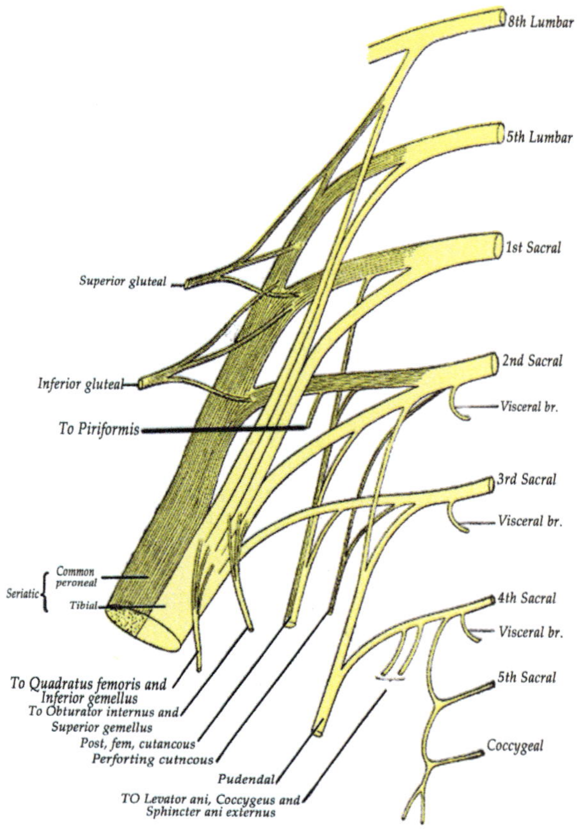

Figure 5.13. *Sacral plexus.*

Source: By Henry Vandyke Carter – Henry Gray, (1918). Anatomy of the human body (see "Book" section below) Bartleby.com: Gray's Anatomy, Plate 828, Public Domain; https://commons.wikimedia.org/w/index.php?curid=541685.

This one originates from the pelvis below the piriformis, travels through the ischial spine, and enters the perineum. It is located in the pudendal canal on the lateral wall of the ischioanal fossa, where it gives branches to the penis (clitoris), the external anal sphincter, the superficial perineal muscles, and the scrotal (vulval) skin (Figure 5.14).

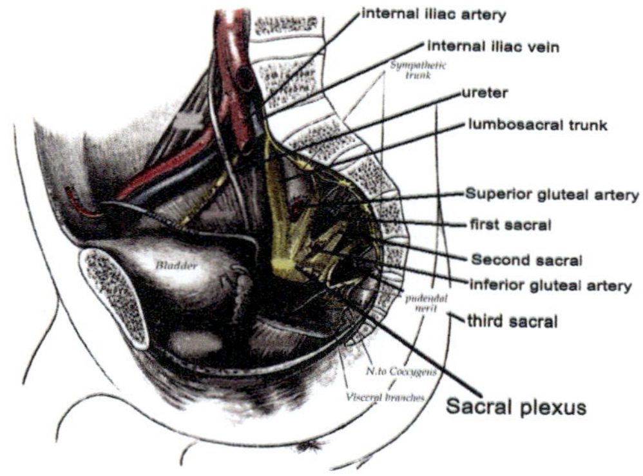

Figure 5.14. *Details of the sacral plexus.*

Source: By Mikael Häggström. When using this image in external works, it may be cited as: Häggström, M., (2014). "Medical gallery of Mikael Häggström, 2014." Wiki Journal of Medicine, 1(2). doi: 10.15347/wjm/2014.008. ISSN: 2002-4436. Public Domain. Orby Mikael Häggström, used with permission. Image:Gray829.png, Public Domain; https://commons.wikimedia.org/w/index.php?curid=2902774.

5.11.8. The Autonomic Nervous System of the Abdomen and Pelvis

The parasympathetic component, the vagus and the pelvic splanchnic nerves, as well as the lumbar sympathetic trunk, celiac, aortic, hypogastric, and pelvic plexuses, make up the autonomic nervous system of the abdomen and pelvis (S2, 3, 4). The lumbar sympathetic trunk descends on both sides of the lumbar vertebral bodies, behind the inferior vena cava and the aorta, starting deep to the medial arcuate ligament of the diaphragm as a continuation of the thoracic trunk. As the sacral trunk on the anterior sacrum, it continues distally, deep to the iliac vessels. There are typically four ganglia in the lumbar trunk, and they all send visceral branches to the aortic plexus, which is located in front of the abdominal aorta, and the hypogastric plexus on the common iliac arteries, as well as gray rami communicantes to their spinal nerves. The pelvic plexuses on the internal iliac arteries carry branches from the sacral plexus that travel to the spinal nerves and the pelvic viscera.

In some cases, lumbar sympathectomy, which involves surgically removing the lower lumbar ganglia, is used to decrease excessive sweating in individuals with hyperhidrosis and may also be used to improve blood flow to the skin in cases of arterial disease.

Two communicating celiac ganglia that are located near the celiac artery's origin make up the celiac plexus. From the thoracic sympathetic trunk, each ganglion receives greater, lesser, and occasionally the least splanchnic nerves. Each ganglion also produces branches that travel down the aorta to the aortic plexuses. Fibers travel from both plexuses to the upper digestive tract and its offshoots, including the pancreas, liver, kidneys, and gonads. The medulla of the suprarenal glands and the celiac plexus are highly communicative.

The celiac plexus and the sympathetic trunk send branches to the aortic plexus, which is located in the lower aorta. Postsynaptic fibers from it travel through the inferior mesenteric artery to the lower gastrointestinal tract, where they branch out into the hypogastric plexus. This area is situated directly beneath the aortic bifurcation, which is made up of the aortic plexus's previously mentioned branches and the sympathetic trunk. The pelvic viscera are supplied by its postsynaptic fibers.

5.11.8.1. Parasympathetic

5.11.8.1.1. Anterior and Posterior Vagal Trunks

These get contributions from the left and right vagi, travel to the coeliac plexus, and then follow the aortic branches to the alimentary tract, extending as far distally as the splenic flexure.

5.11.8.1.2. Pelvic Splanchnic Nerves

The parasympathetic nerve fibers, known as the pelvic splanchnic, originate from the anterior primary rami of S2, S3, and occasionally S4. These fibers connect to the sympathetic fibers in the inferior hypogastric plexus, which are then distributed to the distal colon, and to the pelvic plexus, which is then distributed to the pelvic viscera and perineal structures. Functionally, they supply motor fibers to the walls of the viscus and inhibitory fibers to the internal anal and vesical sphincters, thereby "emptying" the rectum (defecation) and bladder (micturition) and facilitating erection (Wu et al., 2018) (Figure 5.15).

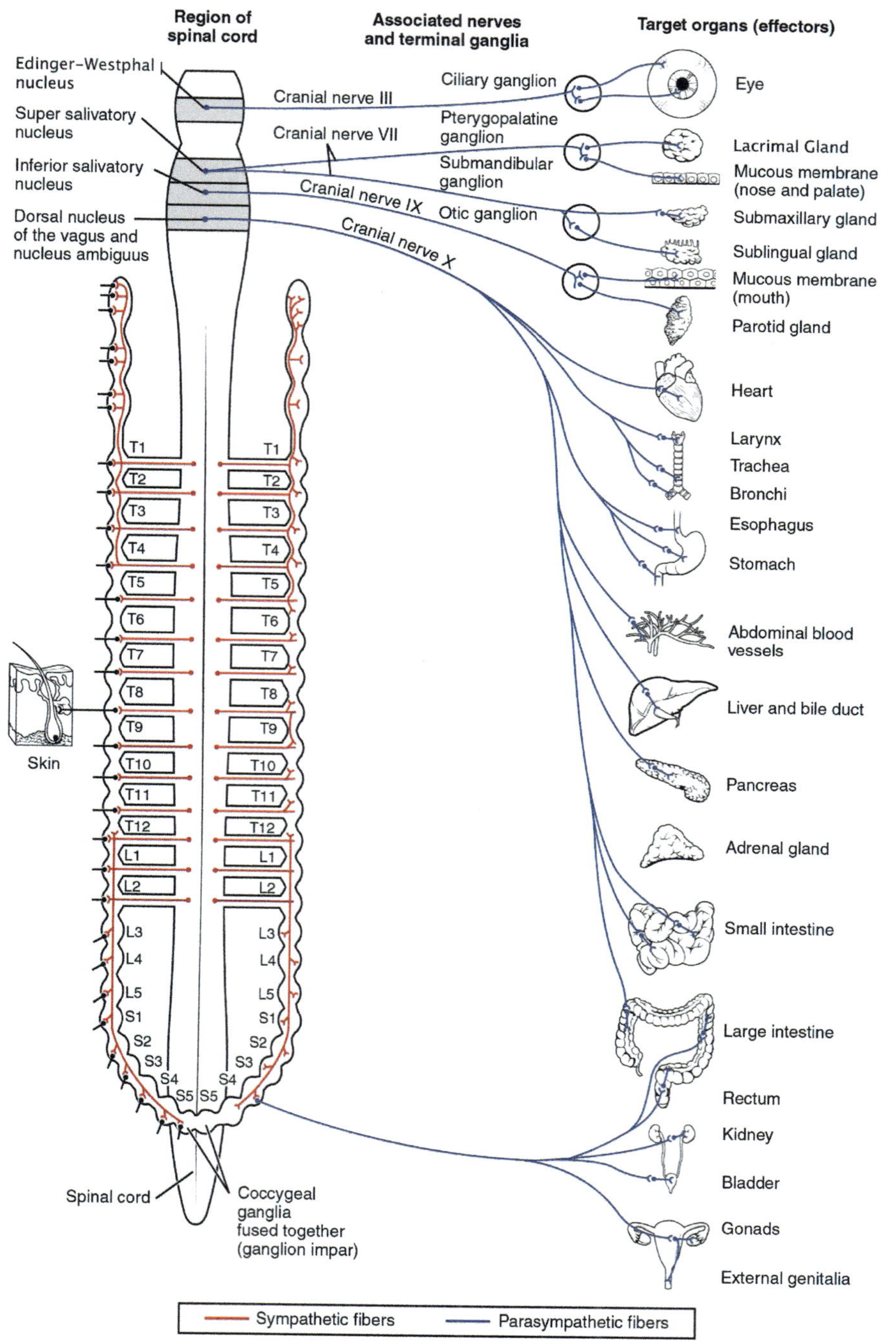

Figure 5.15. *Autonomic nerves.*

A Closer Look

Symphysis Pubis Dysfunction

Symphysis Pubis Dysfunction (SPD) is a condition characterized by discomfort and pain in the pelvic region, specifically at the symphysis pubis, a joint located at the front of the pelvis. This condition is most commonly observed in pregnant women due to the hormonal changes and physical stresses associated with pregnancy. During pregnancy, the body releases a hormone called relaxin, which relaxes the ligaments in the pelvic area to prepare for childbirth. This relaxation, coupled with the increased weight and shifting center of gravity, can lead to the misalignment or excessive movement of the symphysis pubis joint, causing pain and discomfort. The pain can vary in intensity, ranging from mild discomfort to severe, debilitating pain that can interfere with daily activities. It is often described as a sharp, shooting pain in the pelvic area, which may radiate to the lower back, hips, thighs, or groin. The pain typically worsens with activities that involve lifting one leg at a time, such as climbing stairs, getting in and out of a car, or turning over in bed.

The exact cause of SPD is not entirely understood, but it is believed to result from a combination of hormonal changes, mechanical factors, and individual anatomical differences. Certain risk factors may increase the likelihood of developing SPD, including a history of pelvic trauma, previous pelvic surgery, or a prior history of SPD in previous pregnancies. Additionally, women carrying multiple pregnancies or those with very flexible joints may be at higher risk. Diagnosis of SPD is primarily based on clinical symptoms and physical examination. Healthcare providers may perform specific tests, such as the Trendelenburg test or the modified Trendelenburg test, to assess pelvic stability and identify the presence of SPD. In some cases, imaging studies like ultrasound or MRI may be utilized to rule out other potential causes of pelvic pain and to assess the severity of the dysfunction.

Management of SPD focuses on relieving pain and improving pelvic stability. Non-pharmacological approaches are often the first line of treatment, including physical therapy, pelvic support belts, and exercises to strengthen the pelvic floor muscles and improve posture. Physical therapists may employ techniques such as manual therapy, stabilization exercises, and education on body mechanics to help manage symptoms and prevent exacerbations. In addition to physical therapy, lifestyle modifications are crucial. Pregnant women with SPD are advised to avoid activities that exacerbate pain, such as heavy lifting, standing on one leg, or prolonged sitting or standing. Applying ice or heat to the affected area, using a pillow between the knees while sleeping, and practicing good posture can also provide relief. For severe cases, pain relief medications, such as acetaminophen, may be prescribed, though the use of stronger analgesics is generally limited during pregnancy due to potential risks to the fetus.

In summary, Symphysis Pubis Dysfunction is a common condition during pregnancy that can cause significant discomfort and impact daily activities. Early diagnosis and appropriate management are essential to alleviate pain and improve the quality of life for affected women.

Through a combination of physical therapy, lifestyle modifications, and supportive measures, most women can manage their symptoms effectively and continue to engage in their usual activities. However, in some cases, symptoms may persist postpartum, necessitating continued treatment and follow-up care to ensure complete recovery. Understanding SPD and its management is crucial for healthcare providers to support and care for pregnant women experiencing this condition.

Summary

- The pelvis is the area of transition between the trunk and the lower limbs. The bony pelvis serves as the foundation for the pelvic region and provides strong support for the vertebral column and the lower limbs.
- The perineal body, also called the central tendon of the perineum, is an irregularly shaped fibromuscular structure located at the central point of the perineum, midway between the ischial tuberosities.
- As the urinary bladder fills, the peritoneal reflection is elevated above the level of the pubis and is raised from the anterior abdominal wall. A filled urinary bladder can be approached with a needle just superior to the pubis without entering the peritoneal cavity.
- In the pelvic cavity, make a midline cut, beginning posterior to the pubic symphysis. Carry this midline cut through the superior surface of the urinary bladder. Open the urinary bladder and sponge the interior, if necessary.
- The urinary bladder is a reservoir for urine. When empty, it is located within the pelvic cavity. When filled, it extends into the abdominal cavity. The urinary bladder is a subperitoneal organ that is surrounded by endopelvic fascia.
- The uterus is a pear-shaped, thick-walled, hollow muscular organ about 8 cm long, 5 cm wide, and 3 cm thick, lying between the bladder and rectum. It provides protection and nourishment for the fetus.
- The round ligament is a fibromuscular band passing from the upper lateral angle of the uterus through the broad ligament to the deep inguinal ring, and then through the inguinal canal to end in the labium majus.
- The ovary is an almond-shaped organ about 3 cm long. Its position and mobility vary, and it is displaced considerably during pregnancy.
- The superficial perineal pouch lies between the membranous layer of the superficial fascia and the urogenital diaphragm. The superficial fascia is attached to the posterior border of the diaphragm, laterally to the ischiopubic rami, and anteriorly is continuous with the superficial fascia of the anterior abdominal wall over the pubic symphysis.
- The penis comprises three longitudinal cylinders of erectile tissue: the central corpus spongiosum containing the urethra, and the two lateral corpora cavernosa covered by fascia and skin. It has a body and a root, and the root attaches it to the perineal membrane.
- The deep perineal pouch is a closed space sandwiched between the two layers of the urogenital diaphragm. It contains the membranous urethra and the sphincter urethrae muscle, which surrounds the urethra.

References

1. Abe, H., Hayashi, S., Kim, J. H., Murakami, G., Rodríguez-Vázquez, J. F., & Jin, Z. W. (2021). Fetal development of the thoracolumbar fascia with special reference to the fascial connection with the transversus abdominis, latissimus dorsi, and serratus posterior inferior muscles. *Surgical and Radiologic Anatomy, 43*(6), 917–928.
2. Ashton-Miller, J. A., Howard, D., & DeLancey, J. O. (2001). The functional anatomy of the female pelvic floor and stress continence control system. *Scandinavian Journal of Urology and Nephrology. Supplementum, 207*, 1–7; discussion 106–125.
3. Asil, K., & Yaldiz, M. (2018). Conus medullaris levels on ultrasonography in term newborns: Normal levels and dermatological findings. *Journal of Korean Neurosurgical Society, 61*(6), 731–736.
4. B, S. N., & Rodenbaugh, D. W. (2008). Modeling the anatomy and function of the pelvic diaphragm and perineal body using a "string model". *Advances in Physiology Education, 32*(2), 169–170.
5. Bayot, M. L., Nassereddin, A., & Varacallo, M. (2023). Anatomy, shoulder and upper limb, brachial plexus. In *StatPearls*. StatPearls Publishing.
6. Bley, T. A., Duffek, C. C., François, C. J., Schiebler, M. L., Acher, C. W., Mell, M., Grist, T. M., & Reeder, S. B. (2010). Presurgical localization of the artery of Adamkiewicz with time-resolved 3.0-T MR angiography. *Radiology, 255*(3), 873–881.
7. Bogduk, N., Wilson, A. S., & Tynan, W. (1982). The human lumbar dorsal rami. *Journal of Anatomy, 134*(Pt 2), 383–397.
8. Chevalier, F., Fernandez-Lao, C., & Cuesta-Vargas, A. I. (2014). Normal reference values of strength in pelvic floor muscle of women: A descriptive and inferential study. *BMC Women's Health, 14*, 143.
9. Choi, S., Trieu, J., & Ridley, L. (2010). Radiological review of intercostal artery: Anatomical considerations when performing procedures via intercostal space. *Journal of Medical Imaging and Radiation Oncology, 54*(4), 302–306.
10. Dewhurst, C., O'Neill, S., O'Regan, K., & Maher, M. (2012). Demonstration of the course of the posterior intercostal artery on CT angiography: Relevance to interventional radiology procedures in the chest. *Diagnostic and Interventional Radiology, 18*(2), 221–224.
11. Evans, L., O'Donohoe, T., Morokoff, A., & Drummond, K. (2023). The role of spinal surgery in the treatment of low back pain. *Medical Journal of Australia, 218*(1), 40–45.
12. Farrell, C., & Kiel, J. (2023). Anatomy, back, rhomboid muscles. In *StatPearls*. StatPearls Publishing.
13. Gailloud, P. (2019). Spinal vascular anatomy. *Neuroimaging Clinics of North America, 29*(4), 615–633.
14. Gole, R. A., Meshram, P. M., & Hattangdi, S. S. (2014). Anencephaly and its associated malformations. *Journal of Clinical and Diagnostic Research, 8*(9), AC07-9.
15. Gong, Z., Li, D., Zou, F., Liu, S., Wang, H., & Ma, X. (2022). Low lumbar multifidus muscle status and bone mineral density are important risk factors for adjacent segment disease after lumbar fusion: A case-control study. *Journal of Orthopedic Surgery and Research, 17*(1), 490.

16. Hall, B. K. (2018). Germ layers, the neural crest and emergent organization in development and evolution. *Genesis, 56*(6–7), e23103.
17. Hall, M. I., Rodriguez-Sosa, J. R., & Plochocki, J. H. (2017). Reorganization of mammalian body wall patterning with cloacal septation. *Scientific Reports, 7*(1), 9182.
18. Henson, B., Kadiyala, B., & Edens, M. A. (2023). Anatomy, back, muscles. In *StatPearls*. StatPearls Publishing.
19. Hinata, N., Hieda, K., Sasaki, H., Kurokawa, T., Miyake, H., Fujisawa, M., Murakami, G., & Fujimiya, M. (2014). Nerves and fasciae in and around the paracolpium or paravaginal tissue: An immunohistochemical study using elderly donated cadavers. *Anatomy & Cell Biology, 47*(1), 44–54.
20. Hodges, P. W., Sapsford, R., & Pengel, L. H. (2007). Postural and respiratory functions of the pelvic floor muscles. *Neurourology and Urodynamics, 26*(3), 362–371.
21. Hsieh, P. C., Lee, S. T., & Chen, J. F. (2014). Lower thoracic degenerative spondylithesis with concomitant lumbar spondylosis. *Clinical Neurology and Neurosurgery, 118*, 21–25.
22. Jing, D., Ashton-Miller, J. A., & DeLancey, J. O. (2012). A subject-specific anisotropic visco-hyperelastic finite element model of female pelvic floor stress and strain during the second stage of labor. *Journal of Biomechanics, 45*(3), 455–460.
23. Kaiser, J. T., Reddy, V., & Lugo-Pico, J. G. (2023). Anatomy, back, spinal cord arteries. In *StatPearls*. StatPearls Publishing.
24. Kiecker, C., Bates, T., & Bell, E. (2016). Molecular specification of germ layers in vertebrate embryos. *Cellular and Molecular Life Sciences, 73*(5), 923–947.
25. Knezevic, N. N., Candido, K. D., Vlaeyen, J. W. S., Van Zundert, J., & Cohen, S. P. (2021). Low back pain. *The Lancet, 398*(10294), 78–92.
26. Kocbek, L., & Rakuša, M. (2018). Common trunk of the posterior intercostal arteries from the thoracic aorta: Anatomical variation, frequency, and importance in individuals. *Surgical and Radiologic Anatomy, 40*(4), 465–470.
27. Kraima, A. C., West, N. P., Treanor, D., Magee, D., Roberts, N., van de Velde, C. J., DeRuiter, M. C., Quirke, P., & Rutten, H. J. (2016). The anatomy of the perineal body in relation to abdominoperineal excision for low rectal cancer. *Colorectal Disease, 18*(7), 688–695.
28. Larson, K. A., Yousuf, A., Lewicky-Gaupp, C., Fenner, D. E., & DeLancey, J. O. (2010). Perineal body anatomy in living women: 3-dimensional analysis using thin-slice magnetic resonance imaging. *American Journal of Obstetrics and Gynecology, 203*(5), 494.e15–21.
29. Lee, J. M., & Kim, N. K. (2018). Essential anatomy of the anorectum for colorectal surgeons focused on the gross anatomy and histologic findings. *Annals of Coloproctology, 34*(2), 59–71.
30. Malik, N., Tedder, B. L., Fakoya, A. O., & Zemaitis, M. R. (2023). Anatomy, thorax, triangle of auscultation. In *StatPearls*. StatPearls Publishing.
31. Mense, S. (2019). Innervation of the thoracolumbar fascia. *European Journal of Translational Myology, 29*(3), 8297.
32. Mitchell, B., Imonugo, O., & Tripp, J. E. (2023). Anatomy, back, extrinsic muscles. In *StatPearls*. StatPearls Publishing.
33. Mühl-Benninghaus, R. (2018). [Spina bifida]. *Der Radiologe, 58*(7), 659–663.

34. Nyangoh Timoh, K., Moszkowicz, D., Zaitouna, M., Lebacle, C., Martinovic, J., Diallo, D., Creze, M., Lavoue, V., Darai, E., Benoit, G., & Bessede, T. (2018). Detailed muscular structure and neural control anatomy of the levator ani muscle: A study based on female human fetuses. *American Journal of Obstetrics and Gynecology, 218*(1), 121.e1–121.e12.

35. Petersen, E. A., Schatman, M. E., Sayed, D., & Deer, T. (2021). Persistent spinal pain syndrome: New terminology for a new era. *Journal of Pain Research, 14*, 1627–1630.

36. Prakash, S., Kalra, P., Khan, Y., & Dhal, A. (2020). Ventral scapular osteochondroma excision through 'triangle of auscultation': A case series. *Journal of Orthopedic Surgery (Hong Kong), 28*(1), 2309499019892848.

37. Ranade, A. V., Rai, R., Rai, A. R., Dass, P. M., Pai, M. M., & Vadgaonkar, R. (2018). Variants of latissimus dorsi with a perspective on tendon transfer surgery: An anatomic study. *Journal of Shoulder and Elbow Surgery, 27*(1), 167–171.

38. Rider, L. S., & Marra, E. M. (2023). Cauda equina and conus medullaris syndromes. In *StatPearls*. StatPearls Publishing.

39. Robinson, W. A., Nassr, A. N., & Sebastian, A. S. (2019). Thoracic disc herniation, avoidance, and management of the surgical complications. *International Orthopaedics, 43*(4), 817–823.

40. Sahni, M., Alsaleem, M., & Ohri, A. (2023). Meningomyelocele. In *StatPearls*. StatPearls Publishing.

41. Sato, T., Koizumi, M., Kim, J. H., Kim, J. H., Wang, B. J., Murakami, G., & Cho, B. H. (2011). Fetal development of deep back muscles in the human thoracic region with a focus on transvers spinalis muscles and the medial branch of the spinal nerve posterior ramus. *Journal of Anatomy, 219*(6), 756–765.

42. Shafik, A., Sibai, O. E., Shafik, A. A., & Shafik, I. A. (2007). A novel concept for the surgical anatomy of the perineal body. *Diseases of the Colon & Rectum, 50*(12), 2120–2125.

43. Sinhorim, L., Amorim, M. D. S., Ortiz, M. E., Bittencourt, E. B., Bianco, G., da Silva, F. C., Horewicz, V. V., Reed, W. R., Mazzardo-Martins, L., & Martins, D. F. (2021). Potential nociceptive role of the thoracolumbar fascia: A scope review involving in vivo and ex vivo studies. *Journal of Clinical Medicine, 10*(19), 2595.

44. Sugiura, K., Morimoto, M., Higashino, K., Takeuchi, M., Manabe, A., Takao, S., Maeda, T., & Sairyo, K. (2021). Transitional vertebrae and numerical variants of the spine: Prevalence and relationship to low back pain or degenerative spondylolisthesis. *Bone & Joint Journal, 103-B* (7), 1301–1308.

45. Uçar, İ., Karartı, C., Cüce, İ., Veziroğlu, E., Özüdoğru, A., Koçak, F. A., & Dadalı, Y. (2021). The relationship between muscle size, obesity, body fat ratio, pain and disability in individuals with and without nonspecific low back pain. *Clinical Anatomy, 34*(8), 1201–1207.

46. Wagenlehner, F. M., Del Amo, E., Santoro, G. A., & Petros, P. (2013). Live anatomy of the perineal body in patients with third-degree rectocele. *Colorectal Disease, 15*(11), 1416–1422.

47. Waxenbaum, J. A., & Lu, M. (2022). Physiology, muscle energy. In *StatPearls*. StatPearls Publishing.

48. Wilke, J., Schleip, R., Klingler, W., & Stecco, C. (2017). The lumbodorsal fascia as a potential source of low back pain: A narrative review. *BioMed Research International, 2017*, 5349620.

49. Willard, F. H., Vleeming, A., Schuenke, M. D., Danneels, L., & Schleip, R. (2012). The

thoracolumbar fascia: Anatomy, function and clinical considerations. *Journal of Anatomy, 221*(6), 507–536.

50. Wu, Y., Dabhoiwala, N. F., Hagoort, J., Hikspoors, J. P. J. M., Tan, L. W., Mommen, G., Hu, X., Zhang, S. X., & Lamers, W. H. (2018). Architecture of structures in the urogenital triangle of young adult males; comparison with females. *Journal of Anatomy, 233*(4), 447–459.

51. Wu, Y., Dabhoiwala, N. F., Hagoort, J., Shan, J. L., Tan, L. W., Fang, B. J., Zhang, S. X., & Lamers, W. H. (2015). 3D topography of the young adult anal sphincter complex reconstructed from undeformed serial anatomical sections. *PLOS ONE, 10*(8), e0132226.

Chapter

THE BACK

6

Contents

Introduction

The back, a crucial area in clinical anatomy, encompasses the posterior aspect of the trunk, extending from the base of the skull to the coccyx. It plays a vital role in providing structural support, enabling movement, and protecting the spinal cord and other neural elements. The anatomy of the back can be divided into several key components: the vertebral column, muscles, nerves, and blood vessels.

The vertebral column, or spine, is the central structural element of the back. It consists of 33 vertebrae, divided into five regions: cervical, thoracic, lumbar, sacral, and coccygeal. These vertebrae are separated by intervertebral discs, which act as shock absorbers and allow flexibility. The spine not only supports the body's weight but also houses the spinal cord, a critical component of the central nervous system that transmits neural signals between the brain and the rest of the body.

Muscles of the back are categorized into superficial, intermediate, and deep layers. The superficial muscles, such as the trapezius and latissimus dorsi, are primarily responsible for movements of the shoulder and upper limb. Intermediate muscles, including the serratus posterior, aid in respiratory functions. The deep muscles, like the erector spinae and multifidus, are crucial for maintaining posture and enabling complex movements of the spine.

The back's innervation is primarily provided by the dorsal rami of the spinal nerves, which supply the muscles and skin. Proper functioning of these nerves is essential for sensory perception and motor control. Additionally, the blood supply to the back muscles and spine is ensured by branches of the major arteries, such as the vertebral and lumbar arteries.

Clinically, the back is a common site of musculoskeletal disorders, including herniated discs, spinal stenosis, and muscle strains, which can lead to pain and impaired mobility. Diagnostic techniques like MRI and CT scans, along with physical examination, are crucial in identifying the underlying causes of back pain. Treatment approaches vary from conservative methods, such as physical therapy and medications, to surgical interventions in severe cases.

The back is a complex anatomical region integral to movement, support, and neural function. Understanding its anatomy is essential for diagnosing and managing clinical conditions that affect the back, thereby enhancing patient care and outcomes.

Orientation and Directional Terms

Term	Definition	Illustration
Lumbar spine	Lumbar spine is the lower back region of your spinal column or backbone. It consists of five bones (L1-L5). Other structures in or around your lumbar spine are your intervertebral disks, spinal cord and nerves, muscles, tendons and ligaments.	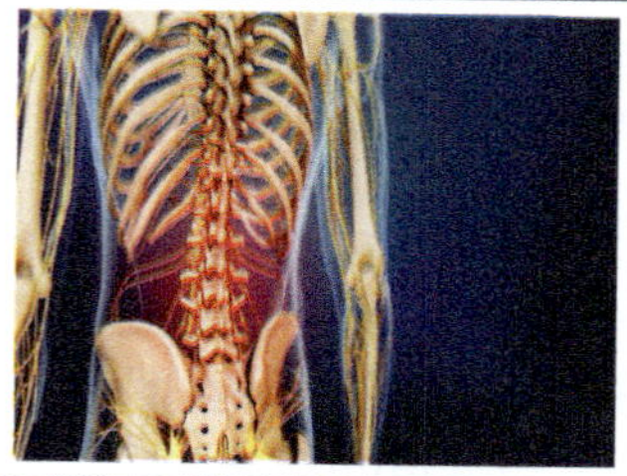
Thoracolumbar fascia (TLF)	The TLF is a critical part of a myofascial girdle that surrounds the lower portion of the torso, playing an important role in posture, load transfer and respiration. The fascial system is a "fibrous collagenous tissue which is part of a body-wide tensional force transmission system".	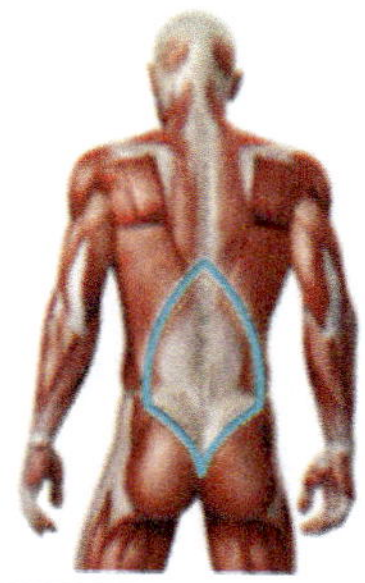
Axial skeleton	Axial skeleton is made up of the 80 bones within the central core of your body. This includes bones in your head, neck, back and chest. Your axial skeleton protects and cushions your brain, spinal cord and organs.	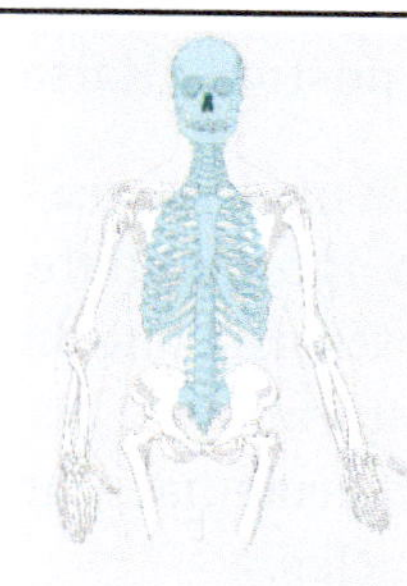
Spina bifida	Spina bifida is a birth defect in which an area of the spinal column doesn't form properly, leaving a section of the spinal cord and spinal nerves exposed through an opening in the back. Spina bifida occurs in 1 per 2,000 live births in the United States and is the most common central nervous system birth defect.	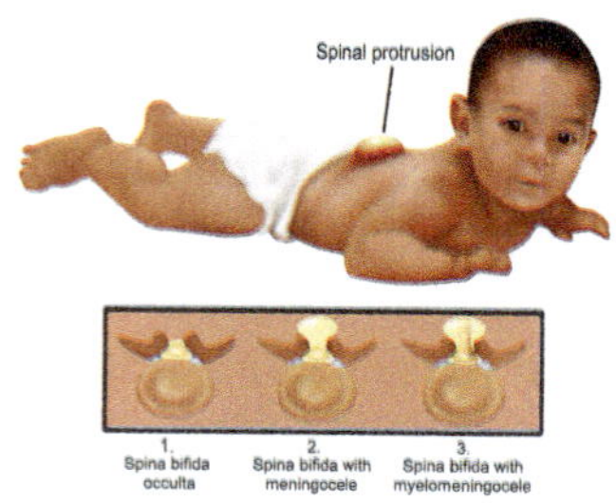
Vertebral canal	Vertebral canal is an elongated body cavity enclosed within the dorsal bony arches of the vertebral column, which contains the spinal cord, spinal roots and dorsal root ganglia.	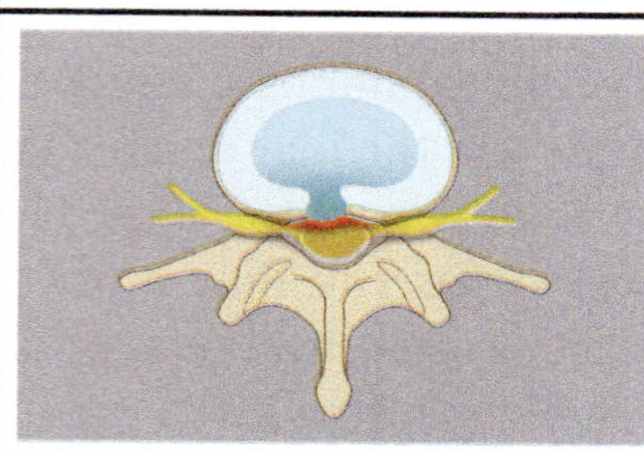

6.1. Back Anatomy

One of the body's most important topographical regions, the back is vital to posture, movement, and the movement of the upper and lower limbs (Kaiser et al., 2023). The body is divided into uneven anterior and posterior segments by the spine, which is positioned in the midline. The back region is the part of the body that lies between the neck and gluteal regions in the posterior segment. It is located inferiorly in the pelvis and superiorly in the neck. The back is made up of muscle groups, nerves, vessels, presacral vertebrae, scapulae, skin, and fascia covering the spine. The three main movements of the back are trunk rotation, flexion/extension, and lateral bending. While some back muscles are involved in upper extremity movement, others attach to the lateral and posterior processes of the vertebrae to support the spine in an erect posture (Kaiser et al., 2023).

The back muscles are categorized into three layers: deep, intermediate, and superficial, also known as extrinsic and intrinsic back muscles in certain literature. This section will explore the deep, intermediate, and superficial groups of back muscles.

6.1.1. Structure and Function

The deep and superficial fascia cover the back. The outermost layer of fascia serves as a robust and dense layer (Waxenbaum et al., 2022). It consists of adipose or areolar connective tissue located immediately deep under the back's skin. This fascia runs parallel to the upper limb, gluteal, and cervical superficial fascias. Attached to the occipital bone, spinous processes of the vertebrae, and the iliac crest is the dense fibrous structure known as the deep fascia of the neck and back area. The iliac crest and the twelfth rib are separated by the thoracolumbar fascia (TLF), which is also a strong aponeurosis. The thoracolumbar fascia is made up of the upper and middle transversus muscle fibers as well as the internal oblique muscle fibers. In addition, a variety of ligaments connect the successive vertebrae and the thoracic vertebrae to the various parts of the ribs. A fibrous membrane makes up the ligamentum nuchae, one of these ligaments. It connects to the spinous process of the cervical vertebrae after beginning at the external occipital protuberance. It is solely the rudiment of a crucial ligament in humans, but in lower animals it aids in maintaining the head position.

The human back has a wide range of purposes in the body. It permits flexibility in movement and acts as the human torso's principal structural support. The spinal column runs centrally down the posterior midline (Figure 6.1).

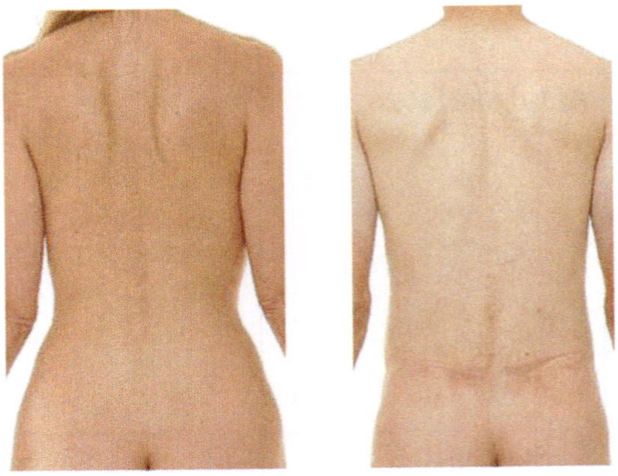

Figure 6.1. *Surface Anatomy of the Back. This illustration shows the trapezius, spine of the scapula, rhomboideus major, teres major, deltoideus, inferior angle of the scapula, sacrospinalis, iliac crest, latissimus dorsi, and glutaeus medius and maximus.*

Source: By Taken at City Studios in Stockholm (www.stockholmsfotografen.se), September 29, 2011, with assistance from KYO (The organization of life models) in Stockholm. Both models have consented to the license of the image, and its usage in Wikipedia. Images uploaded by Mikael Häggström. – File:Posterior_view_of_human_female_and_male,_without_labels.jpg, CC0; https://commons.wikimedia.org/w/index.php?curid=125344968.

The human spinal cord is housed and protected by the bony vertebrae that make up the spinal column (Kaiser et al., 2023). The column consists of five lumbar vertebrae and 12 thoracic vertebrae, which are arranged more superiorly. It is a continuation of the seven cervical vertebrae in the neck. The sacrum marks the end of the column. The 12 thoracic vertebrae are connected with the ribs. Laterally, there are two bony scapulae on either side of the spinal column (Mitchell et al., 2023). They serve as a bony attachment point for a number of muscles, including the upper limb rotator cuff muscles (Mitchell et al., 2023). The back is made up of three muscle groups in addition to the bones. The deep, superficial, and intermediate muscle groups are collectively referred to as the intrinsic muscle group (Benson et al., 2023). These groups permit flexion/extension, rotation, side bending, limb locomotion, and support for respiratory effort in addition to basic back movements (Benson et al., 2023). These muscles enable the trunk, posture, and locomotor functions of the entire body in addition to supporting respiratory function.

6.1.2. Embryology

The ectoderm, mesoderm, and endoderm are the three germ layers in human development (Kiecker et al., 2016). The paraxial mesoderm, which creates the skin's dermis, is also responsible for the development of the body's skeletal muscles and most of the axial skeleton (Kiecker et al., 2016). The ectoderm gives rise to the epidermis of the skin on the back. The neural plate is an ectodermal structure that gives rise to the spinal cord (Hall, 2018). The neural tube is formed by the bilateral development of neural folds from the neural plate that rise, converge, and fuse. By day 27, the tube fully fuses and stops communicating with the amniotic cavity. A lack of fusion in this area may cause anencephaly (Gole et al., 2016). Because the back's superficial and intermediate muscles develop embryologically from hypaxial myotomes, they are referred to as extrinsic muscles. Back intrinsic muscles originate from epaxial myotomes (Sato et al., 2011).

6.1.3. Blood Supply and Lymphatics

The dorsal branches of the posterior intercostal arteries provide the majority of the blood supply to the skin and muscles in the back. In certain variants, these arteries originate directly from the descending aorta, or they may arise from intercostal arteries.

The intercostal vein and nerve run in a groove that extends caudal to the ribs, as do the intercostal arteries. The thoracic aorta extends slightly laterally on the left side and anteriorly to the spinal column. It is also possible for the azygos and hemiazygos veins to exist anterior to the spinal cord. Depending on its location and stage of development during embryonic development, the spinal cord itself receives blood from multiple sources (Kaiser et al., 2023). The vascular supply to the spinal cord is provided by the artery of Adamkiewicz, the posterior spinal arteries, and the anterior spinal arteries. The veins in the back that supply venous blood are the anterior and posterior intercostal veins.

6.1.4. Nerves

The dorsal branches of the spinal nerves, also referred to as posterior rami, are the primary source of the nervous supply to the back. The organization of the back's sensory innervation follows a dermatomal pattern, each of which correlates to a distinct spinal nerve at various spinal nerves. The dorsal branches of the spinal nerves innervate the intrinsic muscles of the back in addition to giving sensation to the skin on the back. The extrinsic back muscles, on the other hand, are innervated by spinal nerves, in contrast to this innervation (Bayot et al., 2023).

6.1.5. Muscles

The muscles of the back are divided into three categories. The first category is the superficial back muscles; these are part of the extrinsic back muscles. These muscles are located superficially, and they assist in the movement of the upper limbs. The superficial muscles include:

- **Trapezius:**
  - Originates from the superior nuchal line, external occipital protuberance, nuchal ligament, and spinous processes of C7–T12.
  - Attach to the lateral third of the clavicle, acromion, and spine of the scapula.
  - Innervated by the accessory nerve (12th cranial nerve).
- **Latissimus Dorsi:**
  - Originates from spinous processes of T7–L5, sacrum, thoracolumbar fascia, iliac crest, and 10th through 12th rib.
  - Inserts to the intertubercular groove of the humerus.
  - Innervated by the thoracodorsal nerve.
- **Levator Scapulae:**
  - Originates from the transverse processes of the first four cervical vertebrae.
  - Inserts to the superior angle of the scapula.
  - Innervated by the dorsal scapular nerve.
- **Rhomboids*:**
  - **Minor:**
    - § Originated from the nuchal ligament and spinous processes of C7–T1.
    - § Inserts to the superior part of the medial border of the scapula (the line which is located between the superior angle and trigonum scapula.
    - § Innervated by the dorsal scapular nerve.
  - **Major:**
    - § Originated from spinous processes of T2–T5.
    - § Inserts to the inferior part of the medial border of the scapula (the line which is located between the inferior angle and trigonum scapula).

*Rhomboid major and rhomboid minor are part of the deep shoulder girdle muscle group (Farrell et al., 2023).

The second group of muscles is the intermediate group. It is part of the extrinsic back muscle. These muscles assist in human respiratory function and are intimately associated with the ribs. This muscle group consists of the following:

- **Serratus Posterior Inferior:**
  - Originated from the ligamentum nuchae and spinous processes of C7–T3 vertebrae;
  - Inserts to the superior aspect of 2nd through 5th ribs;
  - Innervated by the anterior rami of the T1–T4 spinal nerves.
- **Serratus Posterior Superior:**
  - Originated from the spinous processes of T11–L3 vertebrae;
  - Inserts to the inferior border of the 9th through 12th ribs;
  - Innervated by the T9–T12 spinal nerves.

The deep back or intrinsic muscles make up the last group of muscles. The axial skeleton moves as a result of these muscles. The intrinsic muscles are covered in a thick layer of fascia. In the lumbar and thoracic regions, the deep fascia forms a sheath called the thoracolumbar fascia. This fascia runs along the midline, connecting the skull and ligament nuchae to the medial crest of the sacrum. It affixes laterally to the ribs' angles and transverse processes. Its layers are anterior, middle, and posterior. Over the surface of the erector spinae muscles, the posterior layer is situated laterally between the lumbar and sacral spinous processes. Beginning at the lumbar transverse processes, the middle layer joins the iliac crest and the last rib. The iliac crest, the transverse processes of the lumbar vertebrae, and the quadratus lumborum muscle are attached to the anterior layer.

In the back and neck, this group is further divided into multiple categories. The splenius muscles, which are found in the lateral and posterior neck regions, make up the superficial layer. The transvers spinalis group and the erector spinae muscles are the two primary muscle groups that make up the intrinsic muscles. These muscles primarily move in three directions: rotation, side bending, and flexion/extension. The erector spinae group, which is the largest group of the intrinsic back muscles, consists of the following:

- Iliocostalis, most laterally located;
- Longissimus, the largest part of the group;
- Spinalis, most medially located.

This muscle group is responsible for maintaining posture, elongating the spine, and allowing for side bending. When activated bilaterally, it serves as the main extensor of the back. When activated unilaterally, it functions as a lateral flexor and rotator of the spine. Another set of muscles in the human back, known as the transvers spinalis muscles, are situated between the transverse processes and spinous processes of the vertebrae. These muscles are positioned beneath the erector spinae muscles. The transvers spinalis group contains:

- Semispinalis is located in the cervical and thoracic regions and has thoracic, cervicis, and capitis muscles.
- The multifidi lie deep to the semispinalis muscles, located along the entire spine, particularly in the lumbar region.
- The rotatores are the deepest part of this group, located along the entire spine, particularly in the thoracic region.

The transvers spinalis group is situated bilaterally on the vertebral column, just like the erector spinae group. When contracted bilaterally, these muscles help to bend the back posteriorly. They aid in lateral bending and rotation when unilateral contraction takes place.

6.1.6. Physiologic Variants

The latissimus dorsi muscle may be punctured by the radial nerve or a communicating branch between the radial nerve and the axillary nerve. It is also known that a connection between the latissimus dorsi muscle and the teres major muscle may exist through muscle fibers (with a frequency of 10%) (Ranade et al., 2018). It is possible to view the numerical variations of the vertebrae in the thoracolumbar region as a risk factor for the development of back clinical symptoms (Sugiura et al., 2021).

6.1.7. Surgical Considerations

Prior to any surgical procedures, the primary surgical consideration with the back is where to place the needle to administer spinal anesthesia. The spinal cord's furthest distal end is called the conus medullaris. In neonates, it ends at the L2/L3 level; in adults, it ends at the L1 level. When administering anesthesia prior to surgery, the surgeon places a needle into the dural sac between the L3/L4 levels in adults in order to avoid the conus medullaris (Lancester et al., 2023).

6.1.8. Clinical Significance

Patients frequently present with back pain, which can usually be adequately treated conservatively with physical therapy, anti-inflammatory drugs, and/or muscle relaxants. But identifying and treating the underlying cause of back pain is the most crucial aspect of this intervention. While acute low back pain frequently goes away on its own, for a significant portion of patients, it recurs often and develops into chronic low back pain (Evans et al., 2023). A common presenting symptom for patients with spinal diseases is generalized back pain. Skeletal muscle strain is the most common underlying etiology of the pain. Spinal diseases or vertebral disc herniation could be the cause. Back pain can have many different causes, and lumbar disc problems such as herniation or rupture as well as vertebral fractures should be taken into account. Furthermore, back pain can also be brought on by osteoarthritis and spondylolisthesis, a disorder in which one vertebra slips anteriorly relative to the others in the column. Recent research on spinal diseases has concentrated on the paraspinal muscles because these muscle structures are the paraspinal muscles' spinal attachment points. Because of this, there is growing evidence that the amount and caliber of paraspinal muscles play a significant role in the development of spinal cord disorders (Gong et al., 2022).

6.1.8.1. Persistent Pain Following Spine Surgery

The terminological approach, which entered the literature in the 1970s as "post-laminectomy syndrome" and "failed back surgery syndrome" (FBSS), was revised as "chronic pain after spinal surgery" (CPSS) in ICD-11 in 2019. This term describes pain that does not subside or even worsens following spine surgery (Petersen et al., 2021).

6.1.8.2. Spina Bifida

Spina bifida is a congenital condition seen on the back when there is incomplete closure of the vertebral column. There are three different subcategories of the condition:

- Spina bifida occulta results from the incomplete fusion of the vertebral arch. The patients are usually asymptomatic, and the only clinical index of suspicion may be a small tuft of hair overlying the defect.
- Spina bifida cystica with meningocele occurs when the bony vertebral arch fails to form and there is a herniation of the spinal meninges.
- Spina bifida cystica with meningomyelocele is the most severe and involves herniation of the meninges and the spinal cord (Sahni et al., 2023; Bayot, Nassereddin, & Varacallo, 2023; Mitchell, Imonugo, & Tripp, 2023).

6.2. The Vertebral Column and Spinal Cord

The flexible, curved column that makes up the skeleton's central axis bears the weight of the head, trunk, and upper limbs before sending it to the lower limbs through the pelvic girdle. The size, articulation, and strength of its ligaments and muscles, as well as the vertebrae themselves, are what give it its tremendous strength. Ligaments and cartilaginous discs, which make up approximately 25% of the vertebrae's length, connect the 33 vertebrae together. About 70 centimeters in length, the column encloses and shields the spinal cord within its canal. Cervical (7), thoracic (12), lumbar (5), sacral (5), and coccygeal (4) are the five groups of vertebrae, each with distinct properties. The vertebral foramen is enclosed by the vertebral arch, which is located behind the anterior body of a typical vertebra. A spinous process arises posteriorly and two transverse processes emerge near the junction of the laminae and pedicles, making up the arch, which is composed of paired anterior pedicles and posterior flattened laminae. Two superior and two inferior articular processes are present (Figure 6.2).

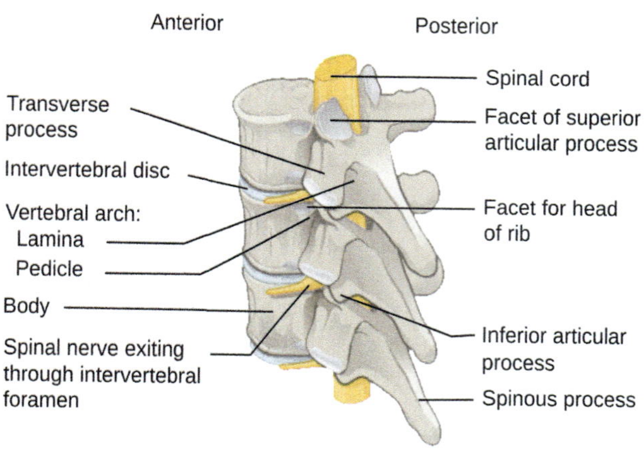

Figure 6.2. *Typical vertebra.*

Source: By Jmarchn - Own work, CC BY-SA 3.0; https://commons.wikimedia.org/w/index.php?curid=45613313.

The body has flat upper and lower articular surfaces and is short and cylindrical. The body's posterolateral region extends the short, rounded pedicles backward. Spinal nerves travel through intervertebral foramina, which are bound by adjacent pedicles. The flat laminae fuse posteriorly to form a spinous process that protrudes. Like roof tiles, adjacent laminae overlap one another. It is possible to feel the tips of the spinous process posteriorly in the midline. Near the intersection of the pedicles and laminae, superior and inferior pairs of articular processes are located. These processes have articular facets covered in hyaline cartilage that articulate in synovial joints between neighboring vertebral arches. The robust transverse processes extend laterally, providing articulation with the ribs in the thorax and attachment to muscles.

6.2.1. Regional Variations

6.2.1.1. Cervical

A comparatively large vertebral foramen and a small oval body characterize the typical cervical vertebra. Each transverse process is broad but short, and it bears anterior and posterior tubercles in addition to enclosing a foramen transversarium that houses vertebral vessels.

The superior articular facet's surface faces upward and backward, while the inferior facet faces the other way. There is a bifid spine. The cervical vertebrae ranked first, second, and seventh exhibit deviations from this pattern. To enable unrestricted head movement, the atlas (first cervical vertebrae) is adapted. It is a ring of bone that has two large articular lateral masses but no body or spine. The occipital condyles articulate with the kidney-shaped upper articular facets.

The second cervical vertebra articulates with the lower circular articular facets. The medial aspect of the lateral masses is where the transverse ligament of the atlas is attached. A facet on the posterior side of the anterior arch is present for articulation with the axis dens. The vertebral artery grooves the posterior arch superiorly on each side. Its long transverse processes have palpable tips behind the mandibular angle, and the spinal accessory nerve crosses them (Figures 6.3 and 6.4).

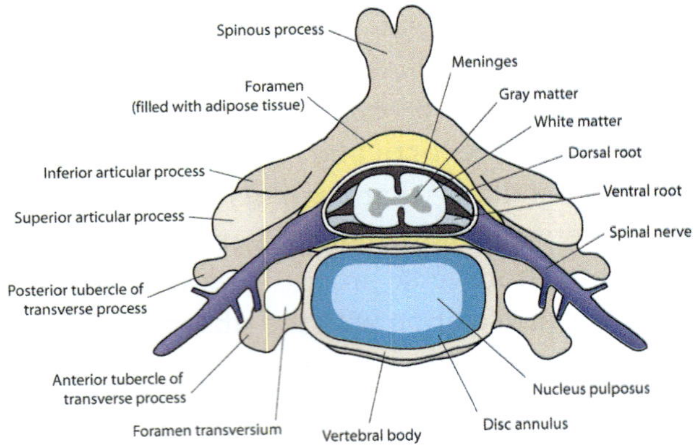

Figure 6.3. *Typical cervical vertebra.*

Source: By user: debivort – Own work, CC BY-SA 3.0; https://commons.wikimedia.org/w/index.php?curid=1675049.

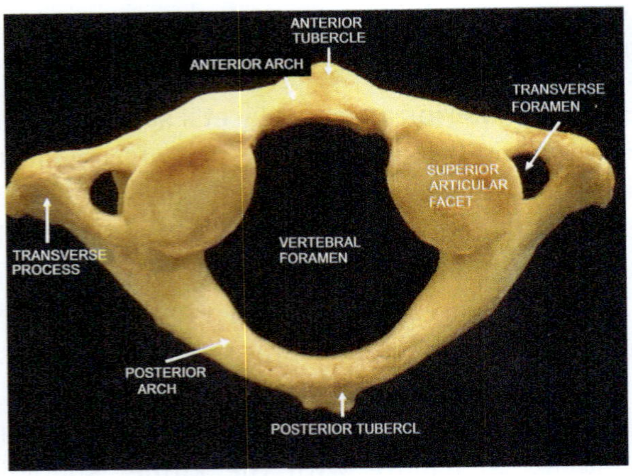

Figure 6.4. *Superior surface of the atlas vertebra.*

Source: https://en.m.wikipedia.org/wiki/File:Atlas_vertebrae.jpg.

The dens, also known as the odontoid peg, is a conical projection on the upper surface of the axis (second cervical). At the point of articulation, the transverse ligament of the atlas holds the dens in place at the rear of the anterior arch. Its apex and the occiput are joined by the alar ligaments. Facing upward, the superior articular facets are nearly horizontal. The vertebra prominens, the seventh cervical vertebra, is a long, non-bifid spine that is easily palpable and frequently visible in the midline at the level of the collarbone on the back of the neck.

6.2.1.2. Thoracic

The body of a thoracic vertebra is wedge-shaped and has a deeper posterior recess. Each body's sides articulate at the superior and inferior costal facets with paired ribs. The ends of the transverse processes, which have a facet for articulation with the tubercle of the corresponding rib, are oriented laterally and backwards. The superior facets have lateral and backward faces. The downward-projecting spines and broad laminae overlap with those below (Figures 6.5–6.7; Table 6.1).

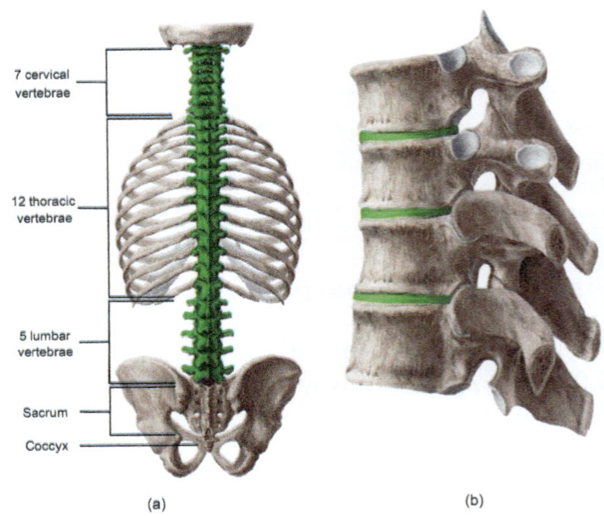

Figure 6.5. *Overview.*

Source: Frost, B. A., Camarero-Espinosa, S., & Foster, E. J., (2019). Materials for the spine: Anatomy, problems, and solutions. Materials, 12(2), 253. https://doi.org/10.3390/ma12020253.

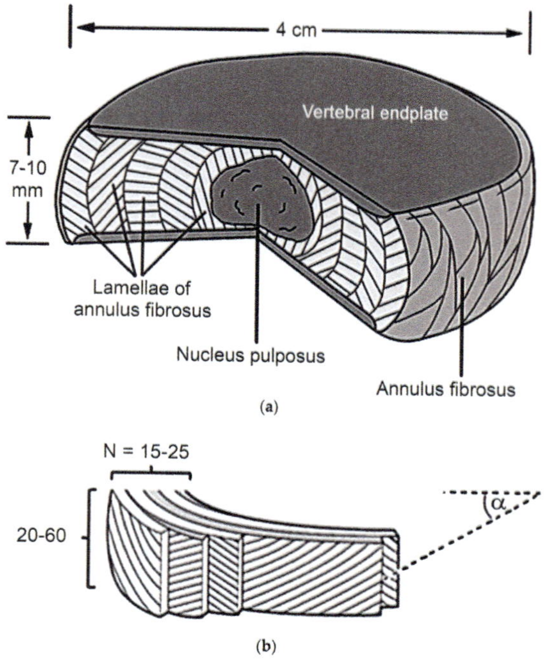

Figure 6.6. *Pictured (a) is a cut out portion of a normal disc depicting the nucleus pulposus, vertebral endplates, and annulus fibrosus. The chosen intervertebral disc is 4 cm wide and 7–10 mm thick [Raj P.P. 2008]. Depicted in the lower image (b) is a diagram showing the detailed structure of the annulus fibrosus, with its 15–25 lamellae comprised of 20–60 collagen fiber bundles. Also shown, is the angle α, which correlates to the directionality of the fibers' bundles in relation to the vertebrae.*

Source: *Frost, B. A., Camarero-Espinosa, S., & Foster, E. J., (2019). Materials for the spine: Anatomy, problems, and solutions. Materials, 12(2), 253. https://doi.org/10.3390/ma12020253.*

Table 6.1. *Average Dimensions of the Intervertebral Discs in the Cervical, Thoracic, and Lumbar Spine*

Cervical IVD Dimensions	C2/C3	C3/C4	C4/C5	C5/C6	C6/C7	C7/T1
Area (mm^2)	190 ± 10	280 ± 40	240 ± 20	300 ± 30	460 ± 5	440 ± 5
Thickness (mm)	3.51 ± 0.71	3.74 ± 0.36	4.07 ± 0.36	4.45 ± 0.21	4.11 ± 0.28	4.50 ± 0.53
Thoracic IVD dimensions	T1/T2	T2/T3	T3/T4	T4/T5	T5/T6	T6/T7
Area (mm^2)	510 ± 50	490 ± 5	485 ± 5	450 ± 40	605 ± 20	750 ± 10
Thickness (mm)	4.40 ± 0.65	3.50 ± 0.69	3.30 ± 0.50	3.20 ± 0.47	3.50 ± 0.47	4.10 ± 0.47

Thoracic IVD dimensions	T7/T8	T8/T9	T9/T10	T10/T11	T11/T12	T12/L1
Area (mm^2)	710 ± 30	900 ± 10	840 ± 30	1,080 ± 20	1,170 ± 30	1,190 ± 40
Thickness (mm)	3.90 ± 0.72	5.30 ± 0.80	4.80 ± 1.07	6.50 ± 0.97	5.40 ± 0.95	6.8 ± 0.21

Lumbar IVD dimensions	L1/L2	L2/L3	L3/L4	L4/L5	L5/S1
Area (mm^2)	1,400 ± 20	1,640 ± 50	1,690 ± 40	1,660 ± 30	1,680 ± 30
Thickness (mm)	7.65 ± 0.57	8.90 ± 0.25	9.25 ± 0.29	9.90 ± 0.49	9.35 ± 1.06

Source: Frost, B. A., Camarero-Espinosa, S., & Foster, E. J., (2019). Materials for the spine: Anatomy, problems, and solutions. Materials, 12(2), 253. https://doi.org/10.3390/ma12020253.

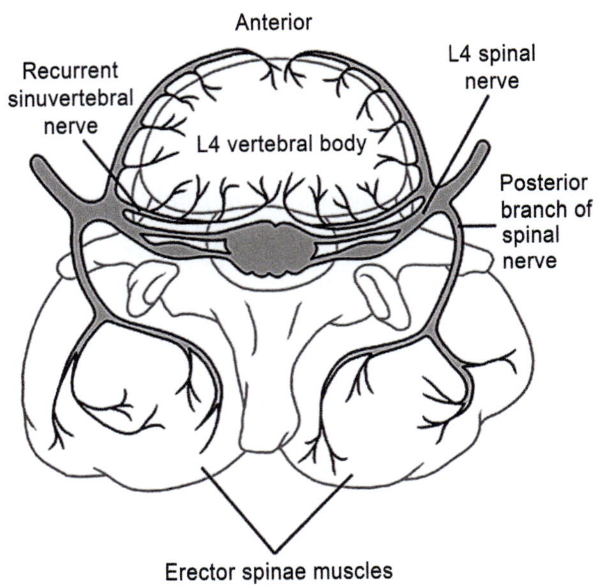

Figure 6.7. *The innervation of a healthy intervertebral disc, showing the sinuvertebral nerves and rami communicantes extending into the vertebral foramen and the outer annulus of the disc.*

Source: Frost, B. A., Camarero-Espinosa, S., & Foster, E. J., (2019). Materials for the spine: Anatomy, problems, and solutions. Materials, 12(2), 253. https://doi.org/10.3390/ma12020253.

Cervical disc thicknesses were taken from 19 Chinese cadaveric humans of unspecified age or gender. Standard deviations were estimated from graphical error bars. Thoracic disc thicknesses were taken from 15 healthy female and male cadaveric humans with average ages of 58.67 ± 10.74 years and 56.20 ± 11.65 years, respectively. Lumbar disc thicknesses were taken from 607 female and 633 male human spines with age ranges from 20 to 92 years and 20 to 87 years, respectively.

Standard deviations were estimated from graphical error bars. All of the cross-sectional areas were taken from 4 full human cadaver spines of the following demographics: Male of 73 years, female of 86 years, female of 85 years, and female of 80 years.

While the lower vertebrae have larger bodies and more horizontal spines, the upper vertebrae have smaller bodies. On the bodies of the 10th, 11th, and 12th vertebrae, the costal facets are typically single and complete.

6.2.1.3. Lumbar

The body of a lumbar vertebra is large and kidney-shaped, with wider sides. Its superior articular facets face medially and backward, and its bulky transverse processes project laterally. The wide, rectangular spinous process extends backward in a horizontal direction.

The fifth lumbar vertebra is unique in that it has a small, conical transverse process and a wedge-shaped body that is thicker anteriorly. It is prevented from sliding anteriorly over the top of the sacrum by its inferior articular facet, which faces forward.

The common congenital anomaly known as spina bifida occulta is characterized by the failure of the laminae of L5 or S1 to develop. The bony defect usually doesn't cause any issues, but on rare occasions, it can become larger, causing meninges and occasionally the spinal cord to herniate (a condition known as spina bifida cystica), which can result in neurological symptoms like lower limb paralysis. The cervical, thoracic, and lumbar vertebrae are easily identified from one another because the former have costal facets on both sides of the body and the latter do not. The lumbar vertebrae lack both costal facets and a foramen in the transverse process (Figure 6.8).

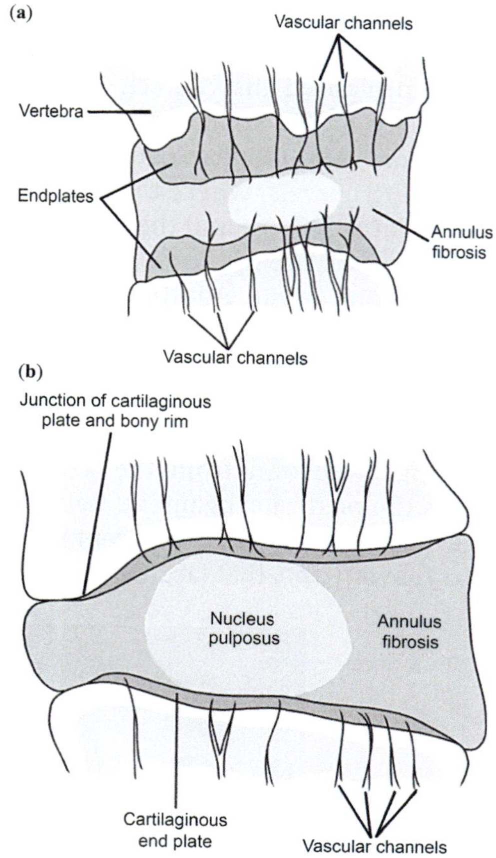

Figure 6.8. *(a) Schematic representation of the multiple longer and thicker vascular channels throughout the intervertebral disc on a 10-month-old female; while (b) represents the vascular channels throughout the disc of a 50-year-old adult, showing the retraction and thinning of the channels.*

Source: Frost, B. A., Camarero-Espinosa, S., & Foster, E. J., (2019). Materials for the spine: Anatomy, problems, and solutions. Materials, 12(2), 253.

6.2.2. Joints and Ligaments

Hyaline cartilage covers the articular surfaces of neighboring vertebrae, and a thick fibrocartilaginous intervertebral disc connects them. The nucleus pulposus, the center of the disc, is surrounded by the fibrous annulus fibrosus and has a consistency similar to toothpaste. The disc functions as a cushion. Sometimes the semisolid nucleus protrudes through a prolapsed disc defect, pressing on a spinal nerve or the spinal cord, resulting in symptoms and signs of nerve compression. The L4/L5 or L5/S1 levels, where the spinal nerve roots are relatively large and the intervertebral foramina are small, are where most symptomatic disc protrusions occur. Additionally, anterior and posterior longitudinal ligaments bind the vertebral bodies together. Each ligament, which is attached to each vertebral body and disc, extends from the occiput to the sacrum in the anterior ligament and from the axis to the sacrum in the posterior ligament. Between the paired articular processes of adjacent vertebrae are two synovial joints that facilitate articulation.

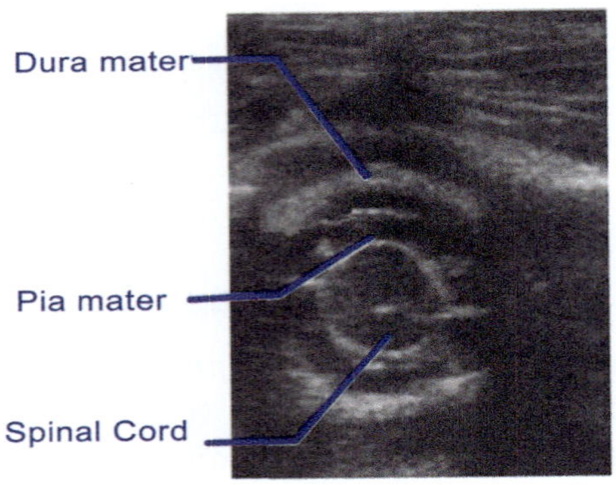

Figure 6.9. *Ultrasound of the spinal cord.*

Source: Benjdira, B., Ouni, K., Al-Rahhal, M. M., Albakr, A., Al-Habib, A., & Mahrous, E., (2020). Spinal cord segmentation in ultrasound medical imagery. Applied Sciences, 10(4), 1370. https://doi.org/10.3390/app10041370.

Additional support to the vertebral column is provided by (Figure 6.9):

- The ligamenta flava, which unite adjacent laminae. These ligaments contain a large amount of yellow elastic tissue and are strong. They maintain the curvatures of the spinal column and support it when it is flexed.
- The supraspinous, interspinous, and intertransverse ligaments, which help unite adjacent vertebrae.

6.2.2.1. Variations

The head can move freely thanks to modifications made to the atlantoaxial and atlanto-occipital joints. These joints are seen in X-rays obtained with the mouth open. The convex occipital condyles and the concave upper articular surfaces of the atlas form the condyloid synovial joints known as the atlanto-occipital joints. The anterior and posterior atlanto-occipital membranes support them. The atlantoaxial joints are made up of a midline synovial pivot between the dens and a ring formed by the anterior arch and the transverse ligament of the atlas, as well as two lateral synovial plane joints between the lateral mass of the atlas and the axis's pedicle. The membrana tectoria, accessory ligaments that join the occiput, rear of the axis, and the nearby cruciate (cruciform) ligament, strengthen the joint.

6.2.3. Functional Aspects

6.2.3.1. Curvatures and Mobility

The primary curvature of the vertebral column is flexed during fetal life. Two secondary curvatures form after birth: the lumbar region extends after adopting an erect posture, and the cervical region is extended by the muscles that raise the head. The sacral and thoracic regions still have their original curvature. The column gains some resilience and spring from these curves and the intervertebral discs. There are irregularities in the vertebral column's curvature. Lordosis, which is frequently momentarily present in late pregnancy, causes an excessive hollowness in the back and an accentuated lumbar curvature. It may be caused by weakened trunk muscles. Excessive lateral curvature, or scoliosis, is invariably accompanied by rotation of the vertebral bodies, with the spinous processes pointing in the direction of the curve's concavity. It frequently results from weak back muscles or is linked to a vertebra's failure to grow fully (hemivertebra). Osteoporosis, a generalized bone atrophy, is typically the cause of kyphosis, an exaggeration of the thoracic curvature, which results in the erosion and collapse of multiple nearby vertebrae. Localized kyphosis (kyphus) results from the collapse of a single vertebra due to a tuberculous infection or fracture.

6.2.4. Muscles

The head and spinal column are extended by the extensor muscles of the neck and back. They extend from the sacrum to the occiput and form a large composite mass that lies deep to the girdle and trapezius muscles. The erector spinae are the biggest and strongest muscles, but they are supported by smaller muscles that are connected to nearby ribs and other vertebrae. Because the center of gravity is located anterior to the vertebral column, these muscles are involved in maintaining posture and are always active when at rest. The head's flexion, rotation, and extension are produced by the muscles that are attached to the skull (Figures 6.10 and 6.11).

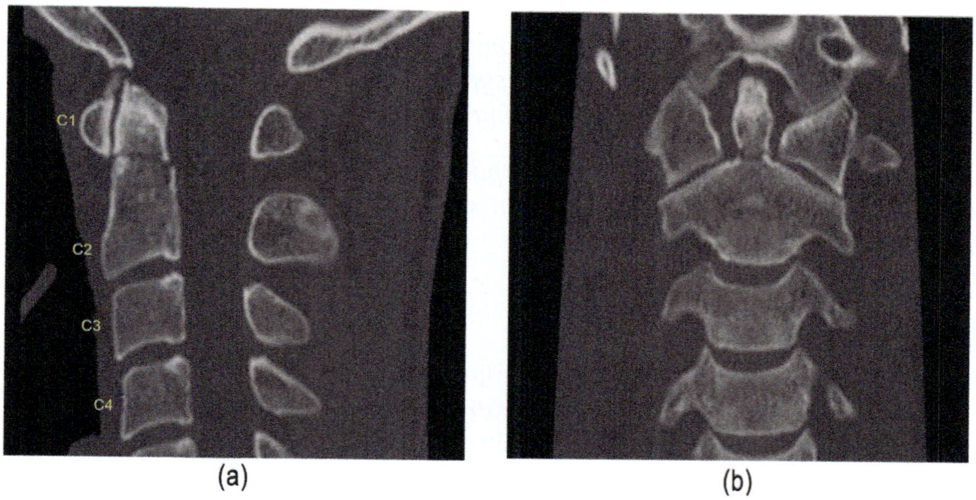

Figure 6.10. *(a) Sagittal; and (b) coronal view of CT showing type II dens fracture. "C1–C4" designate each corresponding spinal level.*

Source: *Hussain, O., Kaushal, M., Agarwal, N., Kurpad, S., & Shabani, S., (2023). The role of magnetic resonance imaging and computed tomography in spinal cord injury. Life, 13(8), 1680. https://doi.org/10.3390/life13081680.*

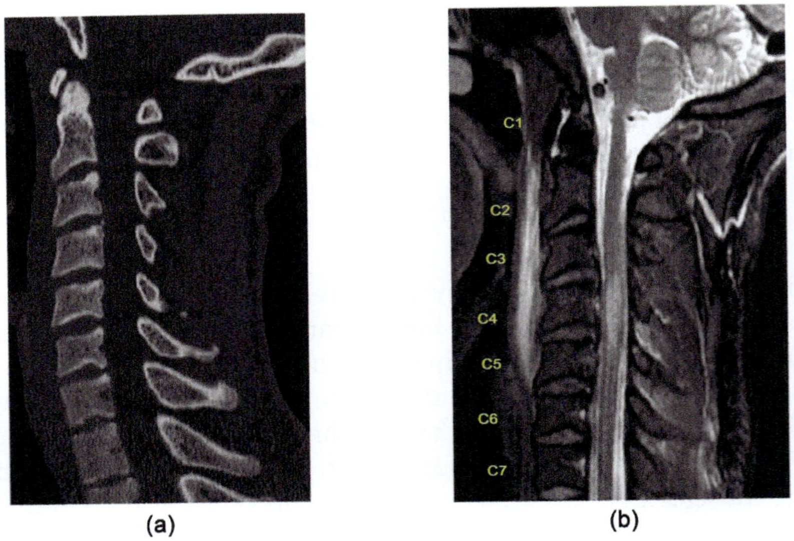

Figure 6.11. *(a) Sagittal CT demonstrating no bony injury or malalignment to a trauma patient. (b) Sagittal MRI STIR sequence demonstrating cord signal change with evidence of contusion spanning from C3–C5. "C1–C7" designate each corresponding spinal level.*

Source: Hussain, O., Kaushal, M., Agarwal, N., Kurpad, S., & Shabani, S., (2023). The role of magnetic resonance imaging and computed tomography in spinal cord injury. Life, 13(8), 1680. https://doi.org/10.3390/life13081680.

6.2.4.1. Movements

Only limited movements are possible between adjacent vertebrae, but because these can augment each other, it is possible to produce extensive movement of the whole vertebral column. Flexion is most marked in the cervical region, rotation in the thoracic, and rotation and lateral flexion in the lumbar region:

- **Flexion** – rectus abdominis and prevertebral muscles.
- **Lateral Flexion** – in the neck by sternocleidomastoid and trapezius; in the trunk by the oblique abdominal muscles and quadratus lumborum.
- **Rotation** – sternocleidomastoid and oblique abdominal muscles.
- **Extension** – erector spinae muscles of the back.

6.2.4.2. Movements of the Head

Rotation occurs at the atlantoaxial joints and all other movements, flexion, extension, and lateral flexion, at the atlanto-occipital joints:

- **Rotation** – sternocleidomastoid, trapezius.
- **Flexion** – longus capitis and the muscles depressing the fixed mandible.
- **Extension** – postvertebral muscles.

- **Lateral Flexion** – sternocleidomastoid and trapezius aided and supported by stout muscles joining the atlas and axis to each other and to the base of the skull.

6.2.4.3. Stability

The ligamenta flava and pre- and postvertebral muscles play a major role in this; neither the bones nor the ligaments by themselves could sustain the significant forces that periodically act on the vertebral column (Table 6.2).

Table 6.2. *Muscles and Actions*

Muscles	Actions	
Major muscles of upper limb	Deltoid	Shoulder abduction, flexion, and extension
	Biceps brachii	Flexes elbow
	Triceps brachii	Extends forearm
Major muscles of lower limb	Gluteus maximus	External rotation and extension of the hip joint.
	Sartorius	Lateral rotation and abduction of thigh; flexion and medial rotation of leg.
	Quadriceps group (4 muscles together)	Knee extension; hip flexion.
	Hamstrings group (3 muscles together)	Flexes knee, extends hip joint, medially rotates leg at knee.
	Tibialis anterior	Dorsiflex and invert the foot.
	Gastrocnemius	Plantar flexes foot – extension or flexion of the foot at the ankle, flexes knee.
Major muscles of trunk – anterior	Pectoralis	Control the movement of the arm, create lateral, vertical, or rotational motion.
	Rectus abdominus	Pulls the ribs and the pelvis in and curves the back (doing crunches).
	External oblique	Rotate the trunk.
Major muscles of trunk – posterior	Trapezius (upper back)	Tilt and turn the head and neck, shrug, steady the shoulders, and twist the arms. Elevates, depresses, rotates, and retracts the scapula, or shoulder blade.
	Latissimus dorsi (lower back)	When flexed, the muscle works at extending, adducting, and rotating the arm.

Agonist and Antagonist Skeletal Muscle Pairs		
Agonist	Antagonist	Movement
Biceps brachii: in the anterior compartment of the arm.	Triceps brachii: in the posterior compartment of the arm.	The biceps brachii flexes the forearm, whereas the triceps brachii extends it.
Hamstrings: group of three muscles in the posterior compartment of the thigh.	Quadriceps femoris: group of four muscles in the anterior compartment of the thigh.	The hamstrings flex the leg, whereas the quadriceps femoris extend it.

Source: https://courses.lumenlearning.com/suny-dutchess-ap1/chapter/the-muscular-system/.

Flexion-compression injuries, which most frequently occur at the thoracolumbar junction and involve T12 and/or L1, are the most common cause of vertebral fractures. These injuries result in "wedging" of the affected vertebrae. Most of these fractures do not result in vertebral column instability because the posterior longitudinal ligament is still intact. On the other hand, the ligamenta flava and interspinous ligaments are ruptured and the vertebral column becomes unstable if severe flexion is combined with forcible rotation of the vertebral column. Compression of the spinal cord and irreversible nerve damage may result from further displacement.

A cervical vertebral fracture-dislocation can result in serious consequences, particularly if the atlas transverse ligament ruptures, leading to atlantoaxial subluxation (incomplete dislocation) or complete dislocation. The injury may be fatal if the fracture impacts the spinal cord and causes quadriplegia, which is the paralysis of all four limbs. Although they can happen anywhere along the vertebral column, fractures of the vertebral bodies typically occur at the thoracolumbar junction, which connects the more mobile lumbar spine to the rigid thoracic region. These fractures are typically the result of forced flexion of the vertebral column. Spondylolisthesis, or a gap in the pars interarticularis of the lumbar vertebra pedicle, is a common genetic defect that can cause the vertebrae to slip. An oblique X-ray of the lumbar spine shows this. Compression of a nerve root is frequently the result of disc prolapse, most commonly in the posterolateral direction. The spinal cord may be compressed by the less common posterocentral protrusion. The use of MRI scans has greatly facilitated the diagnosis of disc prolapse. The fifth lumbar nerve is compressed by the prolapse of the L4/5 disc, and the first sacral nerve is compressed by the disc below.

Pain radiates down the leg and posterior thigh in either of these scenarios. Clinical confirmation of the diagnosis can be achieved through the "straight leg raising" test, which causes pain along the irritated nerve root. Although common, back pain is not well understood. Severe spinal column movements or unusual physical activity involving lifting and/or bending are often the cause of acute cases. In these cases, minor tears in the muscle or ligaments are most likely the cause. Back pain that has persisted for a long time is not uncommon; its causes include bad posture, an imbalance in the body's weight on the vertebral column, and uneven strain on the erector spinae muscles. Protective muscular spasm in the spine's extensor muscles is linked to both forms of back pain.

6.2.5. The Vertebral Canal and Spinal Cord

The ligaments that connect the vertebral foramina form the bony-ligamentous vertebral canal. It connects to the sacral canal below the sacral hiatus, where it continues from the foramen magnum. It houses the spinal cord, nerve roots, and spinal meninges. The epidural (extradural) space, which houses the internal vertebral venous plexus, fat, and emerging spinal nerves, divides the bony wall of the canal from the meninges. The second lumbar and second sacral vertebrae are where the spinal cord and dural sac end, respectively. The internal vertebral venous plexus and extradural fat separate the latter from the walls of the vertebral canal, but the ventral and dorsal nerve roots of the spinal nerves pierce it. Up to the intervertebral foramina, it envelops the nerves. The subarachnoid space of the posterior cranial fossa and the spinal subarachnoid space communicate above the foramen magnum. The cauda equina is the only structure located in the space below the spinal cord's termination at the level of L2.

A lumbar puncture involves inserting a needle just below the fourth lumbar spine in the midline. This level is located on the intercristal plane, which connects the iliac crests' highest points. The interspinous ligament is punctured by the needle, which then enters the epidural space and pierces the dura to enter the spinal canal, where cerebrospinal fluid can be extracted for analysis. Additionally, local anesthetic solution injections into the spinal canal (spinal anesthesia) or the extradural space (epidural anesthesia) are performed at this site (Table 6.3).

Table 6.3. *MRI*-Based Injury Classification Schemes*

Classification Scheme	Type	Name
Kulkarni et al. (1987) MRI patterns for prognosticating acute spinal cord injury.	Pattern 1	Cord hemorrhage
	Pattern 2	Cord edema
	Pattern 3	Mixed
Bondurant et al. (1990) classification scheme for prognostication of acute spinal cord injury.	Pattern 1	Normal MRI signal
	Pattern 2	Single level edema
	Pattern 3	Multi-level edema
	Pattern 4	Mixed hemorrhage and edema
Schaefer et al. (1992) types of MRI findings associated with acute spinal cord injury.	Type 1	Central intramedullary cord hemorrhage
	Type 2	T2 hyperintense contusion extending longitudinally greater than 1 vertebral body.
	Type 3	T2 hyperintense contusion, confined to a single vertebral body.
	Type 4	No evidence of SCI on MRI.
The brain and spinal injury center score (BASIC) for classifying acute SCIs on the basis of axial T2-weighted imaging.	Basic 0	No intramedullary cord signal abnormality.
	Basic 1	Intramedullary T2 hyperintensity confined to central gray matter.
	Basic 2	Intramedullary T2 hyperintensity involves both gray and white matter but does not cover the entire transverse extent of the spinal cord.
	Basic 3	Intramedullary T2 hyperintensity covers the entire transverse extent of the spinal cord.
	Basic 4	Intramedullary T2 hyperintensity covers the entire transverse extent of the spinal cord plus T2 hypointense foci.

Source: Hussain, O., Kaushal, M., Agarwal, N., Kurpad, S., & Shabani, S., (2023). The role of magnetic resonance imaging and computed tomography in spinal cord injury. Life, 13(8), 1680. https://doi.org/10.3390/life13081680.

6.2.5.1. Blood Supply

The tiny segmental spinal arteries supply blood to the vertebral column. The veins empty into the internal and external vertebral venous plexuses, which then empty into the internal iliac, lumbar, azygos, and basivertebral veins. These veins subsequently empty into the pelvic plexuses and the intracranial sinuses, draining the vertebrae.

Two posterior spinal arteries branch off of the posterior inferior cerebellar or vertebral arteries, and a single anterior spinal artery from both vertebral arteries provides the arterial supply. Each posterior artery descends posterior to the nerve rootlets, while the anterior artery descends in the cord's anterior median fissure. The vertebral, deep cervical, posterior intercostal, lumbar, and lateral sacral arteries all branch off into these three arteries in the lower spinal cord, providing reinforcement for them. The midline anterior and posterior spinal veins are responsible for venous drainage, leading to the vertebral venous plexus. One of the main sources of blood supply to the cord is the segmental extensions of the longitudinal arteries. Thus, spinal cord ischemia may be present in spinal trauma, fractures, and fracture-dislocations. Similarly, spinal cord ischemia, muscle weakness, and paralysis may be caused by occlusive arterial disease in these small vessels, particularly in the great radicular artery (of Adamkiewicz), a particularly significant segmental vessel that supplies blood to the lower half of the spinal cord. Spinal cord ischemia may occur during surgery if the aorta is clamped. The basivertebral veins, which remove the newly formed cells from the vertebral marrow, connect the vertebral venous plexus (also known as Batson's valveless plexus) to every vertebral body through multiple connections and up to six longitudinal channels. It acts as an easy transport system for metastases, particularly those of the prostate, ovary, and breast, to both the vertebral column and the cranial cavity. It connects the outside and inside of the spinal canal from the pelvis to the skull (Bayot, Nassereddin, & Varacallo, 2023; Mitchell, Imonugo, & Tripp, 2023).

A Closer Look

Spine

The human spine, also known as the vertebral column, is a remarkable and complex structure that plays a critical role in supporting the body's weight, protecting the spinal cord, and enabling a wide range of movements. Comprising 33 vertebrae divided into five distinct regions, the spine is both a pillar of strength and a marvel of flexibility. These regions include the cervical spine (neck), thoracic spine (upper and mid-back), lumbar spine (lower back), sacrum, and coccyx (tailbone). Each region has unique characteristics and functions, contributing to the overall integrity and mobility of the spine.

The cervical spine consists of seven vertebrae (C1–C7) and is responsible for supporting the head and enabling its movement. The first cervical vertebra, known as the atlas, and the second, the axis, are specially designed to allow for the nodding and rotation of the head. The thoracic spine, composed of 12 vertebrae (T1–T12), serves as the attachment point for the ribs, providing stability and protection for the heart and lungs. This region is less mobile than the cervical and lumbar regions due to the ribcage's presence but allows for some degree of bending and twisting.

The lumbar spine, comprising five vertebrae (L1–L5), bears the most weight and endures the greatest strain of all the spinal regions. It provides flexibility for movements such as bending and twisting while maintaining stability for the upper body's weight. The sacrum, a triangular bone formed by the fusion of five sacral vertebrae (S1–S5), connects the spine to the pelvis and supports the weight of the upper body when sitting and standing. Below the sacrum is the coccyx, or tailbone, consisting of four fused vertebrae. Although considered a vestigial structure, the coccyx provides attachment points for ligaments and muscles.

Intervertebral discs, located between each vertebra, play a crucial role in cushioning the spine and absorbing shocks. These discs are composed of a tough outer layer called the annulus fibrosus and a gel-like inner core called the nucleus pulposus. They allow the spine to flex, extend, and rotate while maintaining its structural integrity. Additionally, the spine's curvature—cervical and lumbar lordosis (inward curves) and thoracic and sacral kyphosis (outward curves)—help distribute mechanical stress during movement and at rest.

The spinal cord, a vital part of the central nervous system, runs through the vertebral foramen, a central cavity in each vertebra. Protected by the vertebrae, the spinal cord transmits nerve signals between the brain and the rest of the body. Nerve roots extend from the spinal cord through spaces between the vertebrae, known as intervertebral foramina, to innervate different body parts.

Maintaining spinal health is essential for overall well-being. Common spinal issues include herniated discs, spinal stenosis, and scoliosis. Herniated discs occur when the nucleus pulposus protrudes through a tear in the annulus fibrosus, potentially compressing nearby nerves and causing pain. Spinal stenosis involves the narrowing of the spinal canal, which can lead to nerve compression. Scoliosis, a lateral curvature of the spine, can affect posture and mobility if severe.

Prevention and management of spinal problems often involve regular exercise, proper ergonomics, and maintaining a healthy weight. Strengthening core muscles, practicing good posture, and avoiding prolonged periods of inactivity can help preserve spinal health. In cases of injury or degenerative conditions, medical interventions such as physical therapy, medication, or surgery may be necessary.

The spine's intricate structure and functions are fundamental to human movement, stability, and protection of the nervous system. Understanding the spine's anatomy and taking proactive measures to maintain its health are crucial for a pain-free and active life. Whether through daily habits, exercise, or medical care, supporting spinal health is a lifelong endeavor that significantly impacts overall quality of life.

Summary

- The back is a key topographical region of the body, with crucial importance for posture, locomotion, and upper and lower limb movements.
- The spine, located in the midline, divides the body into unequal anterior and posterior segments. In the posterior segment, the body area between the neck and gluteal regions is defined as the back region.
- The deep fascia of the neck and the back area, a dense fibrous structure, is attached to the occipital bone, spinous processes of the vertebrae, and the iliac crest. The thoracolumbar fascia (TLF), which also may be classified as a strong aponeurosis, is located between the twelfth rib and the iliac crest.
- Blood supply to the skin and muscles in the back is primarily from the dorsal branches of the posterior intercostal arteries. These arteries arise from intercostal arteries or directly from the descending aorta in some variants.
- The primary surgical considerations with the back must consider the needle placement for administering spinal anesthesia before surgical procedures. The conus medullaris is the most distal end of the spinal cord.
- The curved, flexible column that forms the central axis of the skeleton supports the weight of the head, trunk, and upper limbs and transmits it through the pelvic girdle to the lower limbs.
- The typical cervical vertebra has a small oval body and a relatively large vertebral foramen. Each short, but wide, transverse process encloses a foramen transversarium containing vertebral vessels, and bears anterior and posterior tubercles.
- A thoracic vertebra has a wedge-shaped body which is deeper posteriorly. The sides of each body articulate with paired ribs at superior and inferior costal facets. The transverse processes are directed backwards and laterally, and their ends bear a facet for articulation with the tubercle of the corresponding rib.
- A lumbar vertebra has a large kidney-shaped body, wider from side to side. Its bulky transverse processes project laterally and its superior articular facets face backwards and medially.
- The articular surfaces of the bodies of adjacent vertebrae are covered by hyaline cartilage and united by a thick fibrocartilaginous intervertebral disc. The center of the disc (nucleus pulposus) is gelatinous, with the consistency of toothpaste, and surrounded by a fibrous part, the annulus fibrosus.
- The extensor muscles of the back and neck extend the head and vertebral column. They form a large composite mass lying deep to trapezius and girdle muscles, and extend from the sacrum to the occiput.
- This depends almost entirely on the pre- and postvertebral muscles, helped by the ligamenta flava; neither the bones nor the ligaments alone could withstand the large forces that occasionally act on the vertebral column (Bayot, Nassereddin, & Varacallo, 2023; Mitchell, Imonugo, & Tripp, 2023).

References

1. Abe, H., Hayashi, S., Kim, J. H., Murakami, G., Rodríguez-Vázquez, J. F., & Jin, Z. W. (2021). Fetal development of the thoracolumbar fascia with special reference to the fascial connection with the transversus abdominis, latissimus dorsi, and serratus posterior inferior muscles. *Surgical and Radiologic Anatomy, 43*(6), 917–928.
2. Asil, K., & Yaldiz, M. (2018). Conus medullaris levels on ultrasonography in term newborns: Normal levels and dermatological findings. *Journal of Korean Neurosurgical Society, 61*(6), 731–736.
3. Bayot, M. L., Nassereddin, A., & Varacallo, M. (2023). Anatomy, shoulder and upper limb, brachial plexus. In *StatPearls*. StatPearls Publishing.
4. Bley, T. A., Duffek, C. C., François, C. J., Schiebler, M. L., Acher, C. W., Mell, M., & Reeder, S. B. (2010). Presurgical localization of the artery of Adamkiewicz with time-resolved 3.0-T MR angiography. *Radiology, 255*(3), 873–881.
5. Bogduk, N., Wilson, A. S., & Tynan, W. (1982). The human lumbar dorsal rami. *Journal of Anatomy, 134*(Pt 2), 383–397.
6. Choi, S., Trieu, J., & Ridley, L. (2010). Radiological review of intercostal artery: Anatomical considerations when performing procedures via intercostal space. *Journal of Medical Imaging and Radiation Oncology, 54*(4), 302–306.
7. Dewhurst, C., O'Neill, S., O'Regan, K., & Maher, M. (2012). Demonstration of the course of the posterior intercostal artery on CT angiography: Relevance to interventional radiology procedures in the chest. *Diagnostic and Interventional Radiology, 18*(2), 221–224.
8. Evans, L., O'Donohoe, T., Morokoff, A., & Drummond, K. (2023). The role of spinal surgery in the treatment of low back pain. *Medical Journal of Australia, 218*(1), 40–45.
9. Farrell, C., & Kiel, J. (2023). Anatomy, back, rhomboid muscles. In *StatPearls*. StatPearls Publishing.
10. Gailloud, P. (2019). Spinal vascular anatomy. *Neuroimaging Clinics of North America, 29*(4), 615–633.
11. Gole, R. A., Meshram, P. M., & Hattangdi, S. S. (2014). Anencephaly and its associated malformations. *Journal of Clinical and Diagnostic Research, 8*(9), AC07–AC09.
12. Gong, Z., Li, D., Zou, F., Liu, S., Wang, H., & Ma, X. (2022). Low lumbar multifidus muscle status and bone mineral density are important risk factors for adjacent segment disease after lumbar fusion: A case-control study. *Journal of Orthopedic Surgery and Research, 17*(1), 490.
13. Hall, B. K. (2018). Germ layers, the neural crest and emergent organization in development and evolution. *Genesis, 56*(6–7), e23103.
14. Henson, B., Kadiyala, B., & Edens, M. A. (2023). Anatomy, back, muscles. In *StatPearls*. StatPearls Publishing.
15. Hsieh, P. C., Lee, S. T., & Chen, J. F. (2014). Lower thoracic degenerative spondylithesis with concomitant lumbar spondylosis. *Clinical Neurology and Neurosurgery, 118*, 21–25.
16. Kaiser, J. T., Reddy, V., & Lugo-Pico, J. G. (2023). Anatomy, back, spinal cord arteries. In *StatPearls*. StatPearls Publishing.

17. Kiecker, C., Bates, T., & Bell, E. (2016). Molecular specification of germ layers in vertebrate embryos. *Cellular and Molecular Life Sciences, 73*(5), 923–947.

18. Knezevic, N. N., Candido, K. D., Vlaeyen, J. W. S., Van Zundert, J., & Cohen, S. P. (2021). Low back pain. *The Lancet, 398*(10294), 78–92.

19. Kocbek, L., & Rakuša, M. (2018). Common trunk of the posterior intercostal arteries from the thoracic aorta: Anatomical variation, frequency, and importance in individuals. *Surgical and Radiologic Anatomy, 40*(4), 465–470.

20. Malik, N., Tedder, B. L., Fakoya, A. O., & Zemaitis, M. R. (2023). Anatomy, thorax, triangle of auscultation. In *StatPearls*. StatPearls Publishing.

21. Mense, S. (2019). Innervation of the thoracolumbar fascia. *European Journal of Translational Myology, 29*(3), 8297.

22. Mitchell, B., Imonugo, O., & Tripp, J. E. (2023). Anatomy, back, extrinsic muscles. In *StatPearls*. StatPearls Publishing.

23. Mühl-Benninghaus, R. (2018). Spina bifida. *Der Radiologe, 58*(7), 659–663.

24. Petersen, E. A., Schatman, M. E., Sayed, D., & Deer, T. (2021). Persistent spinal pain syndrome: New terminology for a new era. *Journal of Pain Research, 14*, 1627–1630.

25. Prakash, S., Kalra, P., Khan, Y., & Dhal, A. (2020). Ventral scapular osteochondroma excision through 'triangle of auscultation': A case series. *Journal of Orthopaedic Surgery (Hong Kong), 28*(1), 2309499019892848.

26. Ranade, A. V., Rai, R., Rai, A. R., Dass, P. M., Pai, M. M., & Vadgaonkar, R. (2018). Variants of latissimus dorsi with a perspective on tendon transfer surgery: An anatomic study. *Journal of Shoulder and Elbow Surgery, 27*(1), 167–171.

27. Rider, L. S., & Marra, E. M. (2023). Cauda equina and conus medullaris syndromes. In *StatPearls*. StatPearls Publishing.

28. Robinson, W. A., Nassr, A. N., & Sebastian, A. S. (2019). Thoracic disc herniation, avoidance, and management of the surgical complications. *International Orthopedics, 43*(4), 817–823.

29. Sahni, M., Alsaleem, M., & Ohri, A. (2023). Meningomyelocele. In *StatPearls*. StatPearls Publishing.

30. Sato, T., Koizumi, M., Kim, J. H., Kim, J. H., Wang, B. J., Murakami, G., & Cho, B. H. (2011). Fetal development of deep back muscles in the human thoracic region with a focus on transvers spinalis muscles and the medial branch of the spinal nerve posterior ramus. *Journal of Anatomy, 219*(6), 756–765.

31. Sinhorim, L., Amorim, M. D. S., Ortiz, M. E., Bittencourt, E. B., Bianco, G., da Silva, F. C., & Martins, D. F. (2021). Potential nociceptive role of the thoracolumbar fascia: A scope review involving in vivo and ex vivo studies. *Journal of Clinical Medicine, 10*(19), 4342.

32. Sugiura, K., Morimoto, M., Higashino, K., Takeuchi, M., Manabe, A., Takao, S., & Sairyo, K. (2021). Transitional vertebrae and numerical variants of the spine: Prevalence and relationship to low back pain or degenerative spondylolisthesis. *The Bone & Joint Journal, 103-B* (7), 1301–1308.

33. Uçar, İ., Karartı, C., Cüce, İ., Veziroğlu, E., Özüdoğru, A., Koçak, F. A., & Dadalı, Y. (2021). The relationship between muscle size, obesity, body fat ratio, pain and disability in individuals with and without nonspecific low back pain. *Clinical Anatomy, 34*(8), 1201–1207.

34. Waxenbaum, J. A., & Lu, M. (2022). Physiology, muscle energy. In *StatPearls*. StatPearls Publishing.

35. Wilke, J., Schleip, R., Klingler, W., & Stecco, C. (2017). The lumbodorsal fascia as a potential source of low back pain: A narrative review. *BioMed Research International, 2017*, 5349620.

36. Willard, F. H., Vleeming, A., Schuenke, M. D., Danneels, L., & Schleip, R. (2012). The thoracolumbar fascia: Anatomy, function and clinical considerations. *Journal of Anatomy, 221*(6), 507–536.

37. van Den Hauwe L.S.P., Flanders A.E. Spinal Trauma and Spinal Cord Injury (SCI) In: Hodler J., Kubik-Huch R.A., von Schulthess G.K., editors. *Diseases of the Brain, Head and Neck, Spine 2020–2023: Diagnostic Imaging [Internet]* Springer; Cham, Germany: 2020. [(accessed on 15 February 2020)]. Chapter 19. Available online: https://www.ncbi.nlm.nih.gov/books/NBK554330/

38. Shabani S., Kaushal M., Soliman H.M., Nguyen H.S., Aarabi B., Fehlings M.G., Kotter M., Kwon B.K., Harrop J.S., Kurpad S.N. AOSpine Global Survey: International Trends in Utilization of Magnetic Resonance Imaging/Computed Tomography for Spinal Trauma and Spinal Cord Injury across AO Regions. *J. Neurotrauma.* 2019;36:3323–3331. doi: 10.1089/neu.2019.6464.

39. Goldman L.W. Principles of CT and CT Technology. *J. Nucl. Med. Technol.* 2007;35:115–128. doi: 10.2967/jnmt.107.042978. quiz 129–130.

40. Goldberg A.L., Kershah S.M. Advances in Imaging of Vertebral and Spinal Cord Injury. *J. Spinal Cord Med.* 2010;33:105–116. doi: 10.1080/10790268.2010.11689685.

41. Riedel C.H., Zoubie J., Ulmer S., Gierthmuehlen J., Jansen O. Thin-slice reconstructions of nonenhanced CT images allow for detection of thrombus in acute stroke. *Stroke.* 2012;43:2319–2323. doi: 10.1161/STROKEAHA.112.649921.

42. Daffner R.H., Hackney D.B. ACR Appropriateness Criteria® on Suspected Spine Trauma. *J. Am. Coll. Radiol.* 2007;4:762–775. doi: 10.1016/j.jacr.2007.08.006.

43. Platzer P., Jaindl M., Thalhammer G., Dittrich S., Wieland T., Vecsei V., Gaebler C. Clearing the cervical spine in critically injured patients: A comprehensive C-spine protocol to avoid unnecessary delays in diagnosis. *Eur. Spine J.* 2006;15:1801–1810. doi: 10.1007/s00586-006-0084-1.

44. Wintermark M., Mouhsine E., Theumann N., Mordasini P., van Melle G., Leyvraz P.F., Schnyder P. Thoracolumbar Spine Fractures in Patients Who Have Sustained Severe Trauma: Depiction with Multi–Detector Row CT. *Radiology.* 2003;227:681–689. doi: 10.1148/radiol.2273020592.

45. Glover G.H. Overview of Functional Magnetic Resonance Imaging. *Neurosurg. Clin. N. Am.* 2011;22:133–139. doi: 10.1016/j.nec.2010.11.001.

46. Shah N.G., Keraliya A., Nunez D.B., Schoenfeld A., Harris M.B., Bono C.M., Khurana B. Injuries to the Rigid Spine: What the Spine Surgeon Wants to Know. *RadioGraphics.* 2019;39:449–466. doi: 10.1148/rg.2019180125.

47. Girão M.M.V., Miyahara L.K., Dwan V.S.Y., Baptista E., Taneja A.K., Gotfryd A., Castro A.D.A. Imaging features of the postoperative spine: A guide to basic understanding of spine surgical procedures. *Insights Imaging.* 2023;14:103. doi: 10.1186/s13244-023-01447-0.

48. Pomerantz S.R. Myelography: Modern technique and indications. *Handb. Clin. Neurol.* 2016;135:193–208.

49. Esquivel A., Ferrero A., Mileto A., Baffour F., Horst K., Rajiah P.S., Inoue A., Leng S., McCollough

C., Fletcher J.G. Photon-Counting Detector CT: Key Points Radiologists Should Know. *Korean J. Radiol.* 2022;23:854–865. doi: 10.3348/kjr.2022.0377.

50. Rajiah P., Sundaram M., Subhas N. Dual-Energy CT in Musculoskeletal Imaging: What Is the Role Beyond Gout? *Am. J. Roentgenol.* 2019;213:493–505. doi: 10.2214/AJR.19.21095.
51. Cicero G., Ascenti G., Albrecht M.H., Blandino A., Cavallaro M., D'angelo T., Carerj M.L., Vogl T.J., Mazziotti S. Extra-abdominal dual-energy CT applications: A comprehensive overview. *La Radiol. Medica.* 2020;125:384–397.
52. Foti G., Serra G., Iacono V., Zorzi C. Identification of Traumatic Bone Marrow Oedema: The Pearls and Pitfalls of Dual-Energy CT (DECT) *Tomography.* 2021;7:387–396. doi: 10.3390/tomography7030037.
53. Bäcker H.C., Wu C.H., Perka C., Panics G. Dual-Energy Computed Tomography in Spine Fractures: A Systematic Review and Meta-Analysis. *Int. J. Spine Surg.* 2021;15:525–535. doi: 10.14444/8074.
54. Cavallaro M., D'Angelo T., Albrecht M.H., Yel I., Martin S.S., Wichmann J.L., Lenga L., Mazziotti S., Blandino A., Ascenti G., et al. Comprehensive comparison of dual-energy computed tomography and magnetic resonance imaging for the assessment of bone marrow edema and fracture lines in acute vertebral fractures. *Eur. Radiol.* 2022;32:561–571. doi: 10.1007/s00330-021-08081-8.
55. Edward Boas D.F. CT artifacts: Cases and reduction techniques. *Imaging Med.* 2012;4:229–240. doi: 10.2217/iim.12.13.
56. Fehlings M.G., Rao S.C., Tator C.H., Skaf G., Arnold P., Benzel E., Dickman C., Cuddy B., Green B., Hitchon P., et al. The optimal radiologic method for assessing spinal canal compromise and cord compression in patients with cervi-cal spinal cord injury. Part II: Results of a multicenter study. *Spine.* 1999;24:605–613. doi: 10.1097/00007632-199903150-00023.
57. Magu S., Singh D., Yadav R.K., Bala M. Evaluation of Traumatic Spine by Magnetic Resonance Imaging and Correlation with Neurological Recovery. *Asian Spine J.* 2015;9:748–756. doi: 10.4184/asj.2015.9.5.748.
58. Maynard F.M., Jr., Bracken M.B., Creasey G., Ditunno J.F., Jr., Donovan W.H., Ducker T.B., Garber S.L., Marino R.J., Stover S.L., Tator C.H., et al. International Standards for Neurological and Functional Classification of Spinal Cord Injury. *Spinal Cord.* 1997;35:266–274. doi: 10.1038/sj.sc.3100432.
59. Bondurant F.J., Cotler H.B., Kulkarni M.V., McArdle C.B., Harris J.H. Acute spinal cord injury. A study using physical examination and magnetic resonance imaging. *Spine.* 1990;15:161–168. doi: 10.1097/00007632-199003000-00002.
60. Marciello M.A., Flanders A.E., Herbison G.J., Schaefer D.M., Friedman D.P., Lane J.I. Magnetic resonance imaging related to neurologic outcome in cervical spinal cord injury. *Arch. Phys. Med. Rehabil.* 1993;74:940–946.
61. Yamashita Y., Takahashi M., Matsuno Y., Kojima R., Sakamoto Y., Oguni T., Sakae T., Kim E.E. Acute spinal cord injury: Magnetic resonance imaging correlated with myelopathy. *Br. J. Radiol.* 1991;64:201–209. doi: 10.1259/0007-1285-64-759-201.
62. Sliker C.W., Mirvis S.E., Shanmuganathan K. Assessing Cervical Spine Stability in Obtunded Blunt Trauma Patients: Review of Medical Literature. *Radiology.* 2005;234:733–739. doi: 10.1148/radiol.2343031768.

63. Ghaffari-Rafi A., Peterson C., Leon-Rojas J.E., Tadokoro N., Lange S.F., Kaushal M., Tetreault L., Fehlings M.G., Martin A.R. The Role of Magnetic Resonance Imaging to Inform Clinical Decision-Making in Acute Spinal Cord Injury: A Systematic Review and Meta-Analysis. *J. Clin. Med.* 2021;10:4948. doi: 10.3390/jcm10214948.

64. Bozzo A., Marcoux J., Radhakrishna M., Pelletier J., Goulet B., Malomo T., Brown A.A., Bale K., Yung A., Kozlowski P., et al. The Role of Magnetic Resonance Imaging in the Management of Acute Spinal Cord Injury. *J. Neurotrauma.* 2011;28:1401–1411. doi: 10.1089/neu.2009.1236.

65. Haefeli J., Mabray M., Whetstone W., Dhall S., Pan J., Upadhyayula P., Manley G., Bresnahan J., Beattie M., Ferguson A., et al. Multivariate Analysis of MRI Biomarkers for Predicting Neurologic Impairment in Cervical Spinal Cord Injury. *Am. J. Neuroradiol.* 2017;38:648–655. doi: 10.3174/ajnr.A5021.

66. Kumar Y., Hayashi D. Role of magnetic resonance imaging in acute spinal trauma: A pictorial review. *BMC Musculoskelet. Disord.* 2016;17:310. doi: 10.1186/s12891-016-1169-6.

67. Flanders A.E., Spettell C.M., Tartaglino L.M., Friedman D.P., Herbison G.J. Forecasting motor recovery after cervical spinal cord injury: Value of MR imaging. *Radiology.* 1996;201:649–655. doi: 10.1148/radiology.201.3.8939210.

68. Hackney D.B., Asato R., Joseph P.M., Carvlin M.J., McGrath J.T., Grossman R.I., Kassab E.A., DeSimone D. Hemorrhage and edema in acute spinal cord compression: Demonstration by MR imaging. *Radiology.* 1986;161:387–390. doi: 10.1148/radiology.161.2.3763906.

69. Wang M., Dai Y., Han Y., Haacke E.M., Dai J., Shi D. Susceptibility weighted imaging in detecting hemorrhage in acute cervical spinal cord injury. *Magn. Reson. Imaging.* 2011;29:365–373. doi: 10.1016/j.mri.2010.10.016.

70. Kulkarni M.V., McArdle C.B., Kopanicky D., Miner M., Cotler H.B., Lee K.F., Harris J.H. Acute spinal cord injury: MR imaging at 1.5 T. *Radiology.* 1987;164:837–843. doi: 10.1148/radiology.164.3.3615885.

71. Mabray M.C., Talbott J.F., Whetstone W.D., Dhall S.S., Phillips D.B., Pan J.Z., Manley G.T., Bresnahan J.C., Beattie M.S., Haefeli J., et al. Multidimensional Analysis of Magnetic Resonance Imaging Predicts Early Impairment in Thoracic and Thoracol-umbar Spinal Cord Injury. *J. Neurotrauma.* 2016;33:954–962. doi: 10.1089/neu.2015.4093.

72. Talbott J.F., Whetstone W.D., Readdy W.J., Ferguson A.R., Bresnahan J.C., Saigal R., Hawryluk G.W.J., Beattie M.S., Mabray M.C., Pan J.Z., et al. The Brain and Spinal Injury Center score: A novel, simple, and reproducible method for assessing the severity of acute cervical spinal cord injury with axial T2-weighted MRI findings. *J. Neurosurg. Spine.* 2015;23:495–504. doi: 10.3171/2015.1.SPINE141033.

73. Schaefer D.M., Flanders A.E., Osterholm J.L., Northrup B.E. Prognostic significance of magnetic resonance imaging in the acute phase of cervical spine injury. *J. Neurosurg.* 1992;76:218–223. doi: 10.3171/jns.1992.76.2.0218.

74. Flanders A.E., Spettell C.M., Friedman D.P., Marino R.J., Herbison G.J. The Relationship between the Functional Abilities of Patients with Cervical Spinal Cord Injury and the Severity of Damage Revealed by MR Imaging. *Am. J. Neuroradiol.* 1999;20:926–934.

75. Boldin C., Raith J., Fankhauser F., Haunschmid C., Schwantzer G., Schweighofer F. Predicting Neurologic Recovery in Cervical Spinal Cord Injury with Postoperative MR

Imaging. *Spine.* 2006;31:554–559. doi: 10.1097/01.brs.0000201274.59427.a4.

76. Ramón S., Domínguez R., Ramírez L., Paraira M., Olona M., Castelló T., Fernández L.G. Clinical and magnetic resonance imaging correlation in acute spinal cord injury. *Spinal Cord.* 1997;35:664–673. doi: 10.1038/sj.sc.3100490.

77. Kaushal M., Shabani S., Budde M.D., Kurpad S.N. Diffusion Tensor Imaging in Acute Spinal Cord Injury: A Review of Animal and Human Studies. *J. Neurotrauma.* 2019;36:2279–2286. doi: 10.1089/neu.2019.6379.

78. Cheran S., Shanmuganathan K., Zhuo J., Mirvis S.E., Aarabi B., Alexander M.T., Gullapalli R.P. Correlation of MR Diffusion Tensor Imaging Parameters with ASIA Motor Scores in Hemorrhagic and Nonhemorrhagic Acute Spinal Cord Injury. *J. Neurotrauma.* 2011;28:1881–1892. doi: 10.1089/neu.2010.1741.

79. Shanmuganathan K., Zhuo J., Chen H.H., Aarabi B., Adams J., Miller C., Menakar J., Gullapalli R.P., Mirvis S.E. Diffusion Tensor Imaging Parameter Obtained during Acute Blunt Cervical Spinal Cord Injury in Pre-dicting Long-Term Outcome. *J. Neurotrauma.* 2017;34:2964–2971. doi: 10.1089/neu.2016.4901.

80. Shabani S., Kaushal M., Budde M., Kurpad S.N. Correlation of magnetic resonance diffusion tensor imaging parameters with American Spinal Injury Association score for prognostication and long-term outcomes. *Neurosurg. Focus.* 2019;46:E2. doi: 10.3171/2018.12.FOCUS18595.

81. Poplawski M.M., Alizadeh M., Oleson C.V., Fisher J., Marino R.J., Gorniak R.J., Leiby B.E., Flanders A.E. Application of Diffusion Tensor Imaging in Forecasting Neurological Injury and Recovery after Human Cervi-cal Spinal Cord Injury. *J. Neurotrauma.* 2019;36:3051–3061. doi: 10.1089/neu.2018.6092.

82. Farzaneh F., Riederer S.J., Pelc N.J. Analysis of T2 limitations and off-resonance effects on spatial resolution and artifacts in echo-planar imaging. *Magn. Reson. Med.* 1990;14:123–139. doi: 10.1002/mrm.1910140112.

83. Jezzard P., Barnett A.S., Pierpaoli C. Characterization of and correction for eddy current artifacts in echo planar diffusion imaging. *Magn. Reason. Med.* 1998;39:801–812. doi: 10.1002/mrm.1910390518.

84. Skinner N.P., Kurpad S.N., Schmit B.D., Muftuler L.T., Budde M.D. Rapid in vivo detection of rat spinal cord injury with double-diffusion-encoded magnetic resonance spectroscopy. *Magn. Reson. Med.* 2017;77:1639–1649. doi: 10.1002/mrm.26243.

85. Skinner N.P., Lee S.-Y., Kurpad S.N., Schmit B.D., Muftuler L.T., Budde M.D. Filter-probe diffusion imaging improves spinal cord injury outcome prediction. *Ann. Neurol.* 2018;84:37–50. doi: 10.1002/ana.25260.

86. Krzyżak A.T., Olejniczak Z. Improving the accuracy of PGSE DTI experiments using the spatial distribution of b matrix. *Magn. Reson. Imaging.* 2015;33:286–295. doi: 10.1016/j.mri.2014.10.007.

87. Freund P., Seif M., Weiskopf N., Friston K., Fehlings M.G., Thompson A.J., Curt A. MRI in traumatic spinal cord injury: From clinical assessment to neuroimaging biomarkers. *Lancet Neurol.* 2019;18:1123–1135. doi: 10.1016/S1474-4422(19)30138-3.

88. Landelle C., Lungu O., Vahdat S., Kavounoudias A., Marchand-Pauvert V., De Leener B., Doyon J. Investigating the human spinal sensorimotor pathways through functional magnetic resonance

imaging. *Neuroimage.* 2021;245:118684. doi: 10.1016/j.neuroimage.2021.118684.

89. Martin A.R., Aleksanderek I., Cohen-Adad J., Tarmohamed Z., Tetreault L., Smith N., Cadotte D.W., Crawley A., Ginsberg H., Mikulis D.J., et al. Translating state-of-the-art spinal cord MRI techniques to clinical use: A systematic review of clinical studies uti-lizing DTI, MT, MWF, MRS, and fMRI. *NeuroImage: Clin.* 2016;10:192–238. doi: 10.1016/j.nicl.2015.11.019.

90. Petrella J.R., Provenzale J.M. MR Perfusion Imaging of the Brain. *Am. J. Roentgenol.* 2000;175:207–219. doi: 10.2214/ajr.175.1.1750207.

91. Meyer B.P., Hirschler L., Lee S., Kurpad S.N., Warnking J.M., Barbier E.L., Budde M.D. Optimized cervical spinal cord perfusion MRI after traumatic injury in the rat. *J. Cereb. Blood Flow Metab.* 2021;41:2010–2025. doi: 10.1177/0271678X20982396.

92. Meyer B.P., Lee S.-Y., Kurpad S.N., Budde M.D. Differential Trajectory of Diffusion and Perfusion Magnetic Resonance Imaging of Rat Spinal Cord Injury. *J. Neurotrauma.* 2022;40:918–930. doi: 10.1089/neu.2022.0283.

93. Lee S., Wilkins N., Schmit B.D., Kurpad S.N., Budde M.D. Relationships between spinal cord blood flow measured with flow-sensitive alternating inversion recovery (FAIR) and neurobehavioral outcomes in rat spinal cord injury. *Magn. Reson. Imaging.* 2021;78:42–51. doi: 10.1016/j.mri.2021.02.004.

Chapter 7

THE UPPER LIMB

Contents

Introduction

The upper limb is recognized for its range of motion and its capacity to grasp, strike, and perform tasks involving fine motor skills (manipulation). The hand is a very useful tool for identifying these characteristics. How well the hand can carry out its tasks depends in part on its ability to position it in the proper way using movements at the radio-ulnar, scapulothoracic, elbow, wrist, and glenohumeral joints. The elbow, shoulder, wrist, and hand are the four sections that make up the upper limb, and each section is further divided into regions (Marciniak, 2011). Shoulder: includes the lateral portion of the cervical region as well as the scapular, pectoral, and deltoid muscles. The pectoral (shoulder) girdle is incomplete at the posterior end and has a bony border formed by the scapulae and clavicles. The anterior ring is completed by the sternum's manubrium (Maciejasz et al., 2014). The arm (*L. brachium*), centered on the humeral bone, is located between the elbow and the shoulder. The front and back of the arm are included in its composition. The forearm, also known as the antebrachium in Latin, is located between the wrist and the elbow and houses both the ulna and the radius (Cordella et al., 2016).

The hand, also known as the manus in Latin, is located distal to the forearm and is made up of the carpus, the metacarpus, and the phalanges. Equipped with the sensitive sensory nerve endings for the receptors of pain, temperature, and touch, the hand is composed of the palm, wrist, dorsum, and digits (which include the thumb along with four fingers) (Al-Qattan et al., 2009).

Orientation and Directional Terms

Term	Definition	Illustration
Upper limb	The upper limb is divided into three regions. These consist of the arm, located between the shoulder and elbow joints; the forearm, which is between the elbow and wrist joints; and the hand, which is located distal to the wrist. There are 30 bones in each upper limb	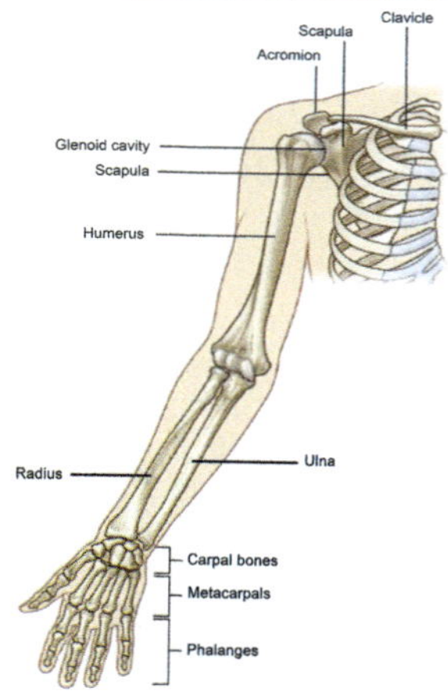
Shoulder joint	The shoulder joint (glenohumeral joint) is an articulation between the scapula and the humerus. It is a ball and socket-type synovial joint, and one of the most mobile joints in the human body.	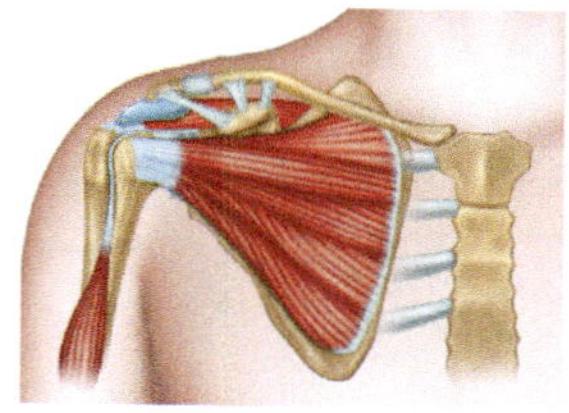
Humeral head	The humerus bone is located in the upper arm, between the shoulder joint and the elbow joint. The shoulder joint, also known as the glenohumeral joint, is a ball and socket joint. The ball is the humeral head, and the socket is the glenoid fossa of the scapula.	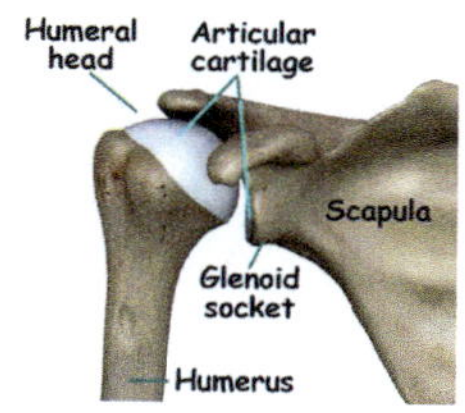
Elbow Joint	The elbow is the joint that connects your upper arm to your forearm. Like all your joints, your elbows are part of your skeletal system. Your elbows also contain cartilage, muscles, ligaments, nerves and blood vessels.	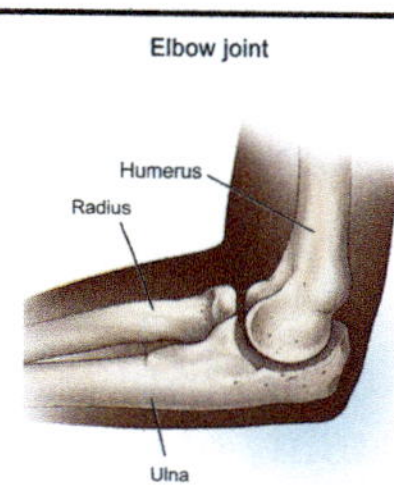
Wrist Joint	The wrist joint also referred to as the radiocarpal joint is a condyloid synovial joint of the distal upper limb that connects and serves as a transition point between the forearm and hand. A condyloid joint is a modified ball and socket joint that allows for flexion, extension, abduction, and adduction movements.	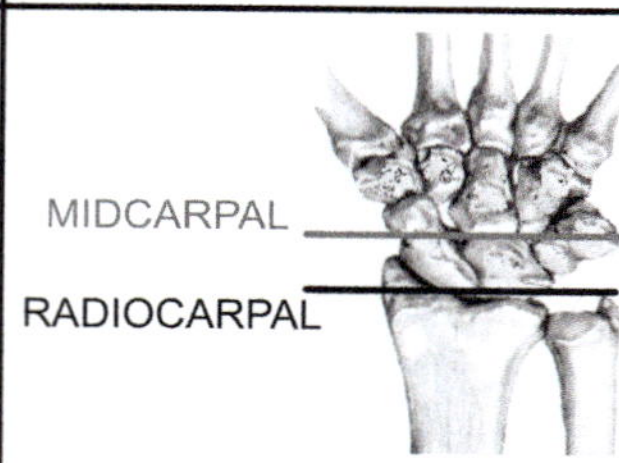

7.1. Surface Anatomy of Upper Limb

Studying surface anatomy is a convenient topic. A friend with an appropriate body mass index or oneself can be used to study the anatomy of the limb (Azer, 2012) (Figure 7.1).

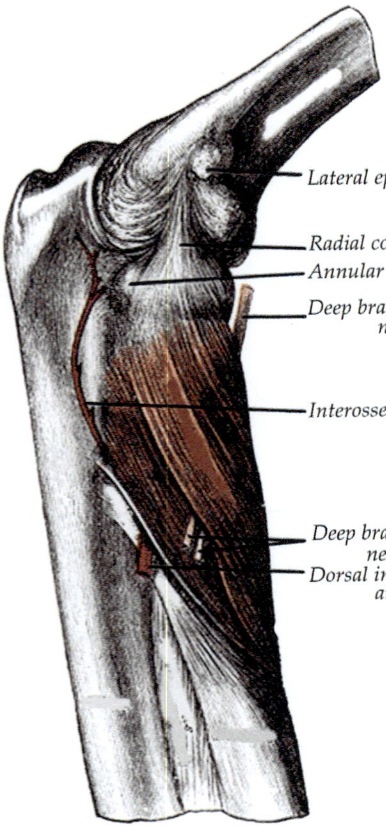

Figure 7.1. *The epicondyles.*

Source: By Henry Vandyke Carter – Henry Gray, (1918). Anatomy of the human body (see "Book" section below) Bartleby.com: Gray's anatomy, Plate 420, Public Domain; https://commons.wikimedia.org/w/index.php?curid=552307.

7.1.1. Joints and Bones

The subcutaneous border is palpable along the entire length of the clavicle; in rare cases, the supraclavicular nerves that traverse the surface of the clavicle can be felt against the underlying bone. The prominent bony border on the side of the scapular spine is known as the acromion process. It is situated directly above the smooth bulge of the deltoid muscle, which encloses the larger humeral tubercle (Brook, 2008). The medial border of the scapula is palpable. However, abduction of the arm is a difficult movement that includes abduction at the shoulder joint, sternoclavicular joint depression, and scapular rotation. Self-palpation is a simple method of verifying the latter two (Watts & Lifeso, 1996). When the shoulder is abducted, you can feel the humerus head close to the top of the axilla; observe how it moves as the arm rotates. The olecranon process and epicondyles are two elbow bone markers (Jaffe, 1959).

Pronation and supination cause the head of the radius to rotate, resting on the depression in the posterolateral region of the extended elbow. The ulna's posterior border can be surgically exposed from beginning to end without risk because it is completely subcutaneous and not crossed by any known arteries or nerves. The radial styloid is located on the bottom of the anatomical snuffbox, whereas the ulnar styloid is situated on the dorsal side of the ulna's head. Lister's dorsal tubercle is situated posteriorly on the distal extremity of the radius. You can feel the pisiform at the hypothenar eminence in your hand. The hamate's hook can be felt with deep palpation slightly distoradial to the pisiform. There is typical soreness inside the anatomical snuffbox and near the base of the thenar eminence when this bone breaks. When the wrist is stretched, the scaphoid and pisiform tubercles in a thin person may be seen as bulges (Scotece et al., 2014).

7.1.2. Tendons and the Muscles

The teres major and latissimus dorsi form the posterior fold of the axilla, whereas the pectoralis major forms the anterior fold. The deltoid muscle in the upper arm forms the curve of the shoulder. The brachialis and biceps make up the anterior side of the arm, and the triceps make up the posterior side. The biceps tendon is visible and palpable when the elbow is extended to a right angle. Just medially to this, you can check the pulse of the brachial artery. As the median nerve is touched, applying firm pressure directly medially to this location will cause hand paresthesia (Alexander, 2002) (Figure 7.2).

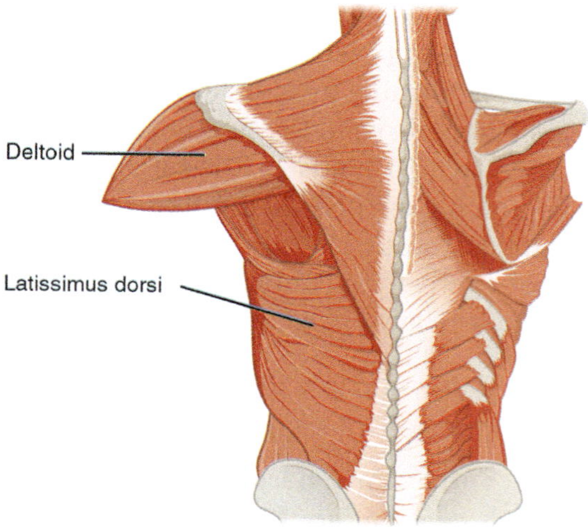

Figure 7.2. *Latissimus dorsi.*

Source: By OpenStax College – https://cnx.org/contents/FPtK1zmh@8.108:y9_gDy74@5, CC BY 3.0; https://commons.wikimedia.org/w/index.php?curid=64291142.

The brachioradialis muscle is easily seen along the radial border when the forearm is moved. To locate the radial pulse at the wrist, start at the most convenient point. Moving from there, you will first encounter the flexor carpi radialis tendon, followed by the palmaris longus (which may be absent), and finally, the cluster of tendons from the flexor digitorum superficialis. When checking for the ulnar pulse at the wrist, it is only detectable on the radial side of the pisiform bone, where the flexor carpi ulnaris tendon enters from the palm (Kjaer, 2004).

In the anatomical snuffbox, the flexor pollicis longus tendon marks the ulnar boundary as it originates from the end of the thumb. Additionally, the tendons of the extensor digitorum can be observed running down behind the phalanges of the fingers when the hand is extended (Kjaer et al., 2006) (Figure 7.3).

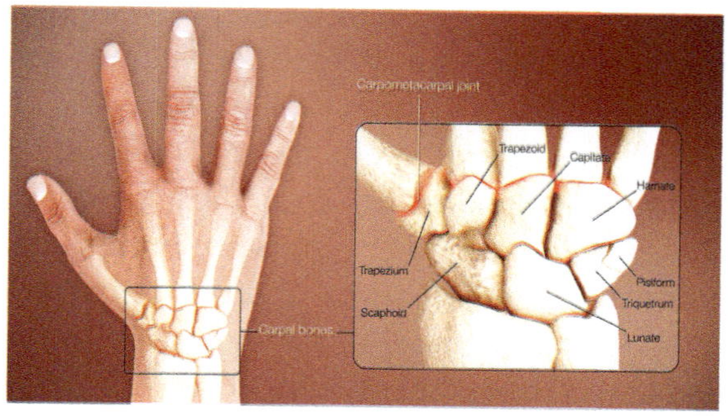

Figure 7.3. *The anatomical features of the back of the right wrist.*

Source: By https://www.scientificanimations.com – https://www.scientificanimations.com/wiki-images/, CC BY-SA 4.0; https://commons.wikimedia.org/w/index.php?curid=92031630.

7.1.3. Vessels

The brachial artery on the humerus, the radial artery at the first knuckle, the ulnar arteries at the wrist, the subclavian artery against the first rib, and the radial artery in the anatomical snuffbox (Mitchell & Schoen, 2010) (Figure 7.4).

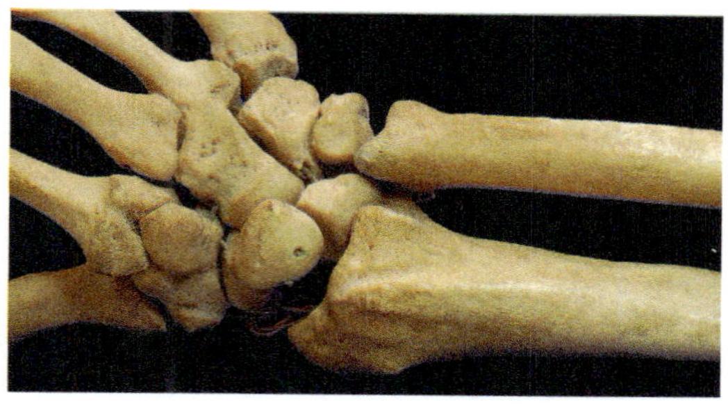

Figure 7.4. *The region is situated directly above the wrist articulation.*

Source: By Brian C. Goss – Own work, Public Domain; https://commons.wikimedia.org/w/index.php?curid=982489.

The brachial artery divides into radial and ulnar branches at the level of the radius's neck, and the radial artery corresponds to the small hole seen along the tightened brachioradialis (Cormack & Lamberty, 1984). The deeper, more superficial deep venae comitantes that connect the primary arteries are smaller and less useful clinically than the superficial veins, which are larger and utilized for venipuncture and transfusion. The medial basilic vein and the lateral cephalic vein on the palm of the hand receive the drainage from these superficial veins. Even if a cephalic vein is not immediately visible, it is safe to sever it there because its origin is usually found in the superficial fascia, just behind the radial styloid. It passes through the anterior forearm, into a depression, and then into the space between the pectoralis major and the deltoid after entering the deep fascia (Sherman, 1981). It eventually penetrates both the clavipectoral fascia and the axillary vein. The basilic vein travels along the anterior and posteromedial sides of the forearm before entering the deep fascia of the upper arm. The venae comitantes of the brachial artery unite to form the axillary vein in the posterior axillary fold (Lewis, 1926).

Slightly distal to the front of the elbow, the median cubital vein joins the basilic and cephalic veins. It is the body's most noticeable superficial vein and is visible even when other veins are obscured by fat or swollen from shock. As it ascends and moves medially from the cephalic vein to the basilic vein, the median forearm vein joins it. This forms the letter "H." The median forearm vein can occasionally divide somewhat distal to the fossa, with one branch flowing to the basilic vein and the other to the cephalic vein. This results in a pattern that resembles an 'M' and serves as a substitute for the median cubital vein. You'll get used to the next two looks very quickly because venipuncture happens here a lot. Currently, this vein is avoided for the intravenous injection of barbiturates and other irritating medications due to the risk of accessing the brachial artery and damaging the ulnar artery in rare situations of high brachial artery bifurcation (Louveau et al., 2015).

7.1.4. Nerves

Many of the nerves in the upper limbs can be palpated, particularly in a thin individual. The median nerve usually makes a superficial crossing of the brachial artery in the mid-upper arm, but in a few uncommon instances, it makes a deeper crossing. Nelson's arm was amputated above the elbow due to an inadvertent inclusion of his median nerve in the ligation surrounding the artery, which holds historical significance. It is commonly acknowledged that Lord Nelson (Viscount) Horatio Nelson (1758–1805) was the most captivating commander in the history of the Royal Navy (Zahalka & Frenette, 2020).

The following is a list of useful surface markers of other intangible nerves:

1. The axillary nerve is located about 5 centimeters (2 inches) below the acromion process, close to the humerus.
2. At the midpoint of the humeral shaft, the radial nerve travels behind the bone.
3. In Henry's approach, the radial nerve's posterior bony branch is identified as it loops around the radius. You can feel the radial head rotate with pronation by placing your middle finger on the radial head and your ring finger over the nerve at the end of the radius (Dibona, 1982).
4. Because the median nerve in the forearm is located in the plane of the median meridian, local anesthesia fed in the midline of the

wrist blocks the nerve's distribution in hand.

5. Located in between the ulnar pulse at the wrist, the ulnar nerve is an important sensory and motor nerve. After traveling down the pisiform's radial region, it rests on the hamate's hook in hand. Touching the area between the pisiform bone and the ulnar two fingers with a fingernail causes tingling (Müller et al., 2003).

7.2. The Skeletal Structures of the Upper Limb

7.2.1. The Scapula

The glenoid depression on the outside edge, the spine on the outer edge, and the coracoid on the inner edge constitute the three main components of the scapula, a triangular bone of the upper limb (Ben Kibler, 1998). The muscles surrounding the scapula provide strong protection, and only very severe trauma can result in a fracture (Nikander et al., 2006) (Figure 7.5).

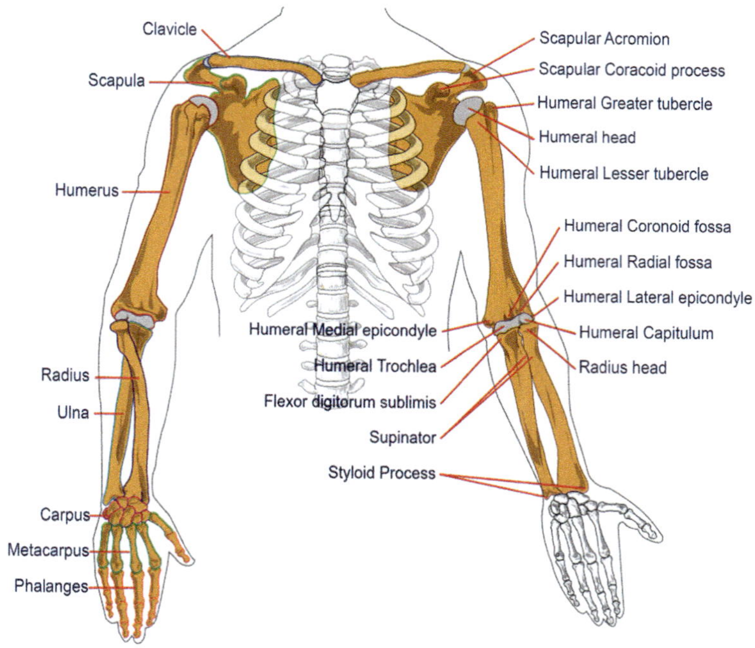

Figure 7.5. *The skeleton of the upper limb.*

Source: https://upload.wikimedia.org/wikipedia/commons/4/49/Human_arm_bones_diagram.svg.

7.2.2. The Clavicle

The clavicle, also known as the collarbone, is a long, thin, S-shaped bone that connects the shoulder blade to the breastbone. It is approximately 15 cm long. There are two clavicles in the human body since there is one on each side of the chest. Together with the shoulder blade, it forms the shoulder girdle. It is a bone that is easily felt, and in those with less fat in this area, the position of the bone can be recognized as a protrusion through the skin. Because the bone spins like a key along its axis when the shoulder is abducted, the term "clavicula," which means small key, is derived from it (Khan et al., 2009). The clavicle is the bone that breaks the most frequently. Impacts to the shoulder, such as those resulting from falling on outstretched arms or from direct contact, are frequently the cause of shoulder fractures (Abbott & Lucas, 1954).

This lengthy bone has several interesting characteristics:

- There is no medullary cavity;
- It is the earliest fetal organ to harden (5th–6th week);
- It grows in the membrane;
- It is the body's usually shattered lengthy bone (Nordqvist & Petersson, 1994).

The clavicle is separated into two sections: the lateral one-third is flattened in section and convex posteriorly, and the medial two-thirds are circular in section and convex anteriorly. The manubrium forms an articulation with the sternoclavicular joint, which is distinguished by a cartilaginous disc. This is a ball-and-socket joint that revolves around the costoclavicular ligament, which acts as its fulcrum, in lockstep with the shoulder joint.

The acromioclavicular joint is located in the middle of the clavicle. The third portion of the subclavian vessels and the trunks of the brachial plexus are only isolated from the middle third of the shaft of the clavicle by the thin subclavius muscle, which is the only muscle of its sort. Although clavicle fractures are common, injury to the underlying subclavian arteries is relatively rare due to the protection provided by this muscle slip. These vessels are torn by clavicle pieces; Sir Robert Peel, who served as Prime Minister of the United Kingdom, died as a result of this fracture after falling off his horse (Gardner, 1968).

The brachiocephalic artery bifurcation, which is situated behind the sternoclavicular joints, and the carotid artery are closely related to the clavicle's end that is close to the breastbone. The internal jugular vein is situated somewhat laterally on either side. These veins are kept apart from the bone by the strap muscles, the sternohyoid and sternothyroid (Post, 1989).

The clavicle transmits force from the upper limb to the axial skeleton, acts as a strut to keep the arm hanging freely from the trunk, and is where muscles attach to the body. The clavicle is most likely to break at the junction of the inner and outer thirds. The majority of fractures are caused by indirect forces greater than the strength of the bone at the impact site, which is typically the hand or shoulder, and which are then transferred to the axial skeleton. A person with a fractured collarbone will typically be seen supporting his limp upper arm with the other arm because the trapezius muscle is less able to support the weight of the arm.

7.2.3. The Humerus

A long bone consists of two ends (articular and lateral surfaces) and a shaft (diaphysis) (epiphysis). It is the longest bone in the upper body. The malformed hemisphere that comprises the upper extremity's proximal articular surface is referred to as the head of the humerus (Zlotolow et al., 2006).

- The term "anatomical neck" refers to the region of the body that is situated between the head and the tuberosities.
- The term "surgical neck" refers to the region that can be found between the tuberosities and the shaft.
- The portion of the bigger tuberosity that is closest to the head can be found at its proximal end. The lesser

tuberosity is very discernible and can be felt; it is located on the front of the humerus, directly behind the head, and it is very prominent (Jupiter et al., 1985).

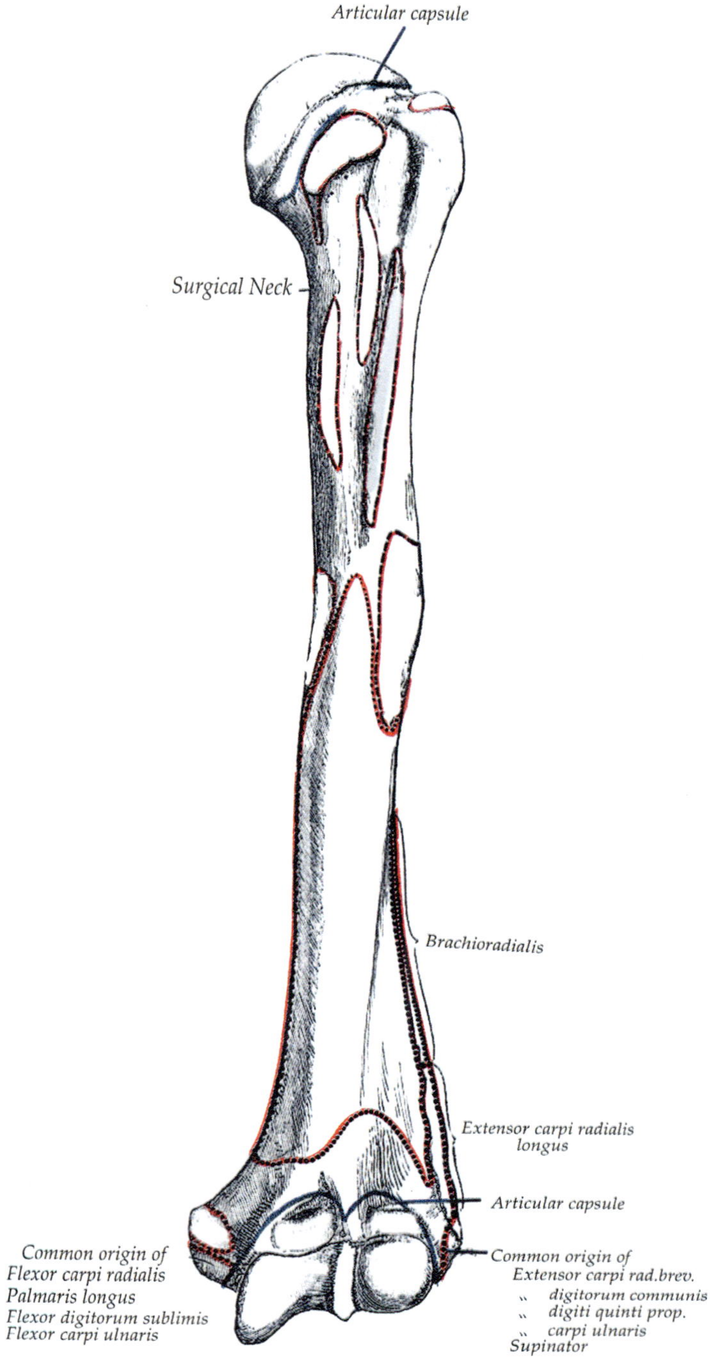

Figure 7.6. *The humerus.*

Source: By Henry Vandyke Carter – Henry Gray, (1918). Anatomy of the human body (see "Book" section below) Bartleby.com: Gray's Anatomy, Plate 207, Public Domain; https://commons.wikimedia.org/w/index.php?curid=327856.

The bicipital groove is a depression that lies between the two tuberosities. The long head of the tendon that joins the biceps muscle is located here. Three borders make up the humeral body, i.e., three surfaces, namely the lateral, anterior, and medial ones, posterior, lateral, and antero-medial surfaces (Volgas et al., 2004) (Figure 7.6).

Due to their close proximity to the humerus, the radial, ulnar, and axillary nerves may sustain damage when the humeral neck, midshaft, and lower end are destroyed. The distal end is angled forward at a 45° angle on the shaft, and this must be considered. A lateral radiograph of the elbow, which shows that the capitulum is divided by a vertical line that runs along the front of the shaft, makes this easily verifiable. A reduction in this angulation is a clear indication of a supracondylar fracture because it indicates that the distal end of the humerus has moved posteriorly (Horak & Nilsson, 1975).

7.2.4. The Radius and Ulna

The forearm is made up of the radius and ulna, which run from the elbow to the wrist. The ulna is located in the medial forearm, whereas the radius is found in the lateral forearm (Evans, 1951). The head, neck, shaft, and distal end comprise the radius. The ulna is composed of the olecranon, coronoid process, trochlear fossa, small distal head, and shaft. It connects to the inferior radioulnar joint on the medial side of the radius's distal end. The radius's shaft wraps around the relatively stationary ulnar shaft during supination and pronation, the radius's head spins against the ulna's radial notch, and the radius's proximal end spins against the ulna's head. An interosseous ligament made of fibrous tissue connects the two bones. According to Davis et al., this rotating axis runs from the radial head to the distal ulnar head (1995) (Figures 7.7–7.9).

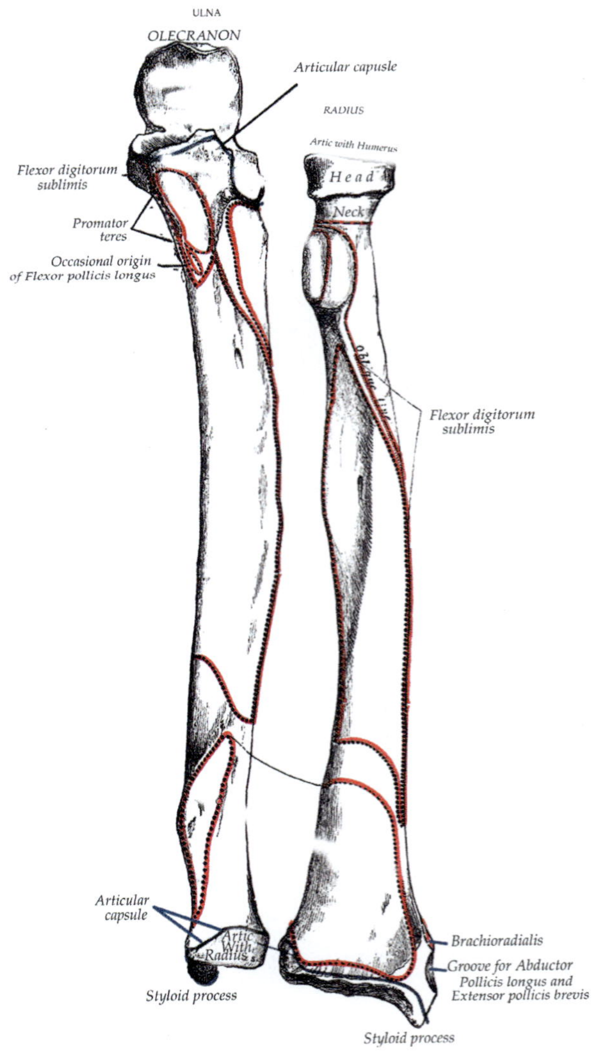

Figure 7.7. *The anterior view of the radius and ulna.*

Source: By Henry Vandyke Carter – Henry Gray, (1918). Anatomy of the human body (see "Book" section below) Bartleby.com: Gray's Anatomy, Plate 213, Public Domain; https://commons.wikimedia.org/w/index.php?curid=303960.

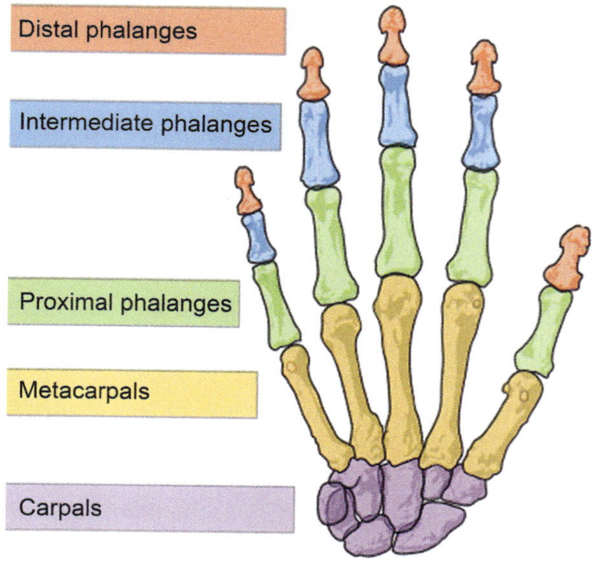

Figure 7.8. *The anterior view of the right carpus, metacarpus, and phalanges.*

Source: By Mariana Ruiz Villarreal (lady of hats); retouches by Nyks – Own work. Image renamed from image: Human hand bones simple-edit1-2.svg, Public Domain; https://commons.wikimedia.org/w/index.php?curid=3949051.

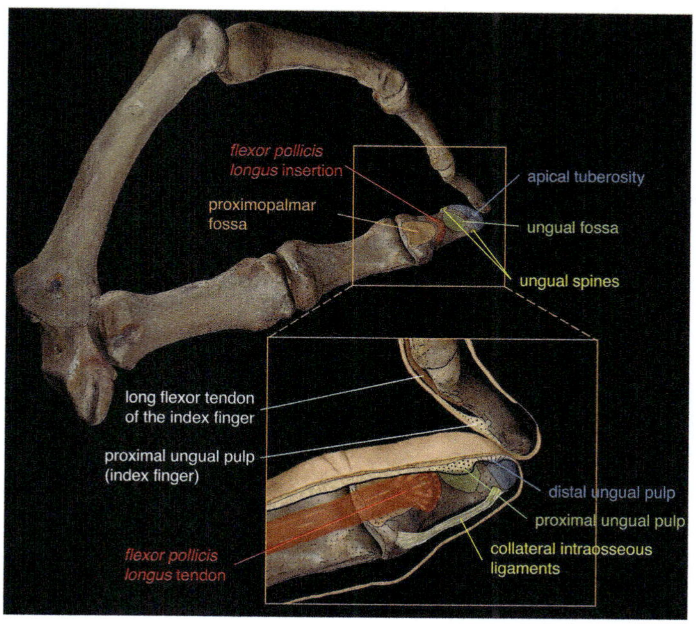

Figure 7.9. *Gripping.*

Source: By Almécija, S., Moyà-Solà, S., & Alba, D. M., (2010). Early origin for human-like precision grasping: A comparative study of pollical distal phalanges in fossil hominins. PLoS One, 5(7), e11727. doi: 10.1371/journal.pone.0011727, CC BY 3.0; https://commons.wikimedia.org/w/index.php?curid=12463663.

7.2.5. The Shoulder Joint

The humerus and scapula are joined at the shoulder joint, which is a ball and socket joint. The most important joint in the human body, the shoulder joint connects the upper limb to the trunk. Although it is one of the most mobile joints in the human body, joint stability is sacrificed in the process. Although the cartilaginous ring of the labrum glenoidale significantly improves the glenoid fossa, the glenoid fossa is situated between the relatively large head of the humerus and the relatively short and shallow glenoid fossa. The intercondylar space is the name given to this gap. The joint capsule is attached to the epiphyseal lines of both the glenoid and the humeral head, not to either of these bones. The shoulder contains the joint capsule (Inman et al., 1944). Situated between the relatively large head of the humerus and the relatively small and shallow glenoid fossa, the shoulder joint is a ball-and-socket synovial joint. According to Lucas (1973), the joint capsule is loose and attached all the way around the glenoid's epiphyseal lines and the humerus' head (Figures 7.10 and 7.11).

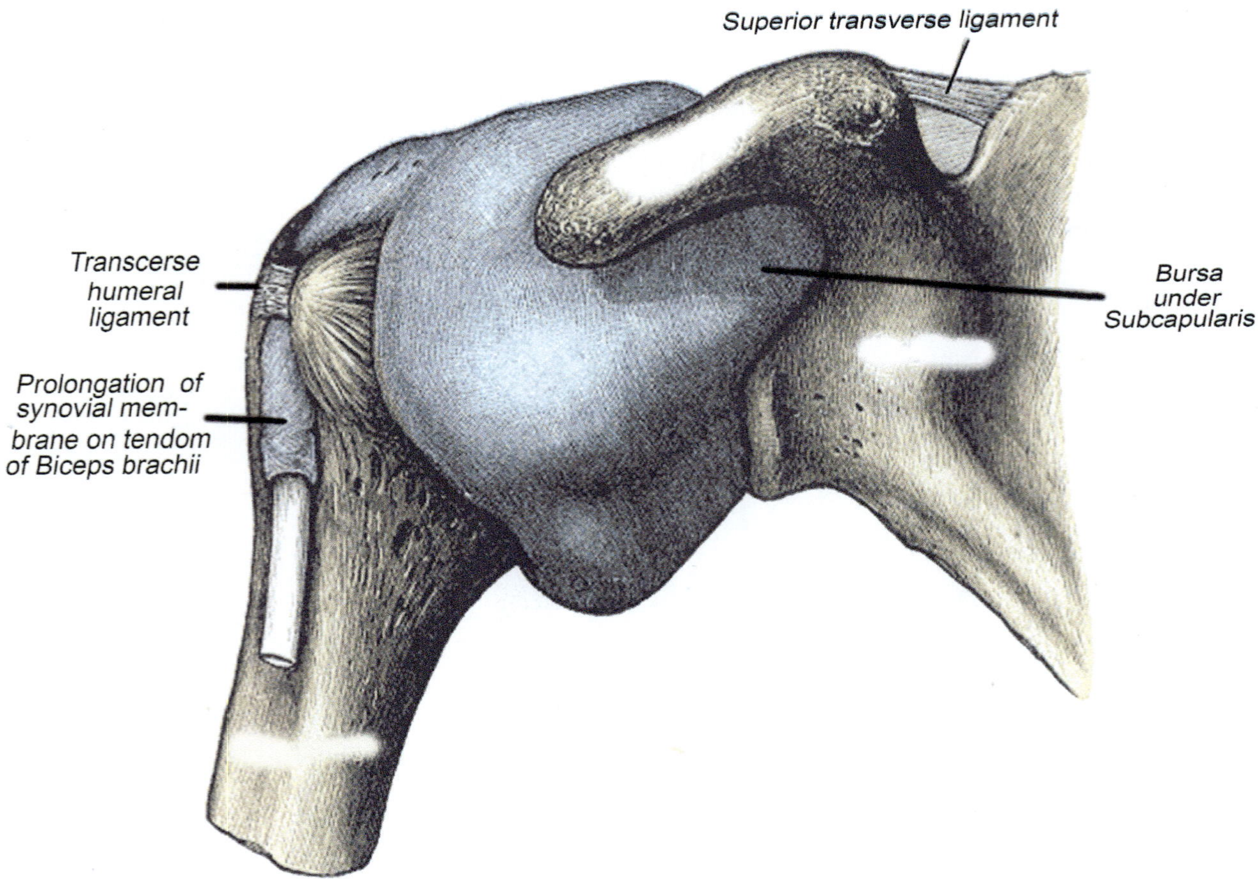

Figure 7.10. *The shoulder joint.*

Source: By Henry Vandyke Carter – Henry Gray, (1918). Anatomy of the human body (see "Book" section below) Bartleby.com: Gray's anatomy, Plate 327, Public Domain; https://commons.wikimedia.org/w/index.php?curid=108237.

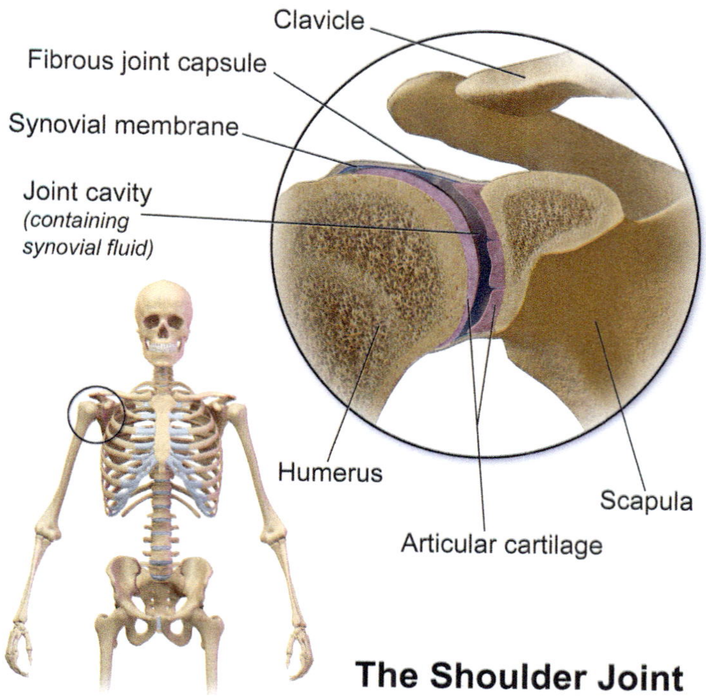

Figure 7.11. *The shoulder joint.*

Source: By BruceBlaus. When using this image in external sources it can be cited as: Blausen.com staff (2014). "Medical gallery of Blausen Medical, (2014)." Wiki Journal of Medicine, 1(2). doi: 10.15347/wjm/2014.010. ISSN: 2002-4436. Own work, CC BY 3.0; https://commons.wikimedia.org/w/index.php?curid=27796970.

Osteomyelitis of the humeral shaft, however, may directly connect the joint as it descends to the diaphysis on the humeral neck (Rowe & Yee, 1944). As the tendon of the head of the biceps muscle passes through the joint, the synovial membrane, which lines the inside of the capsule, enlarges to encircle it. The entire interior of the capsule is covered by this membrane. Furthermore, a link is established between the subscapular bursa, situated just below the subscapularis tendon, and the synovium (Inman & Abbott, 1996).

The strength of this joint is dependent on the solidity of the accompanying muscles, which can be classified as (Figure 7.12):

- The rotator cuff's connected short muscles;
- The long head of the biceps muscle, which emerges from the supraglenoid tubercle and then crosses over the head of the humerus, hence residing within the joint while being enclosed in a synovium tube;
- The more distantly related long shoulder muscles: the deltoid, long triceps head, teres major, latissimus dorsi, and pectoralis major (Prescher, 2000).

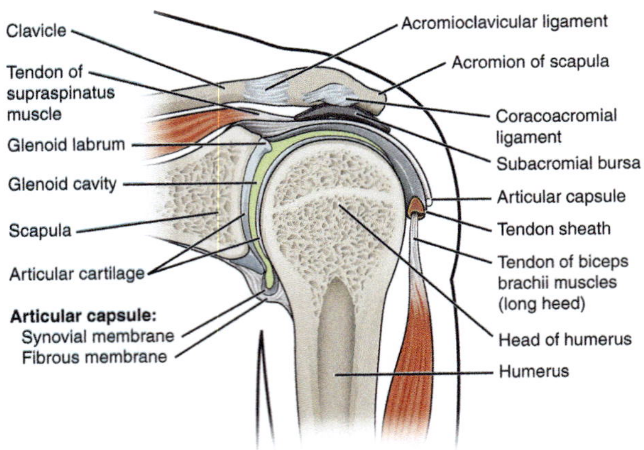

Figure 7.12. *The muscles.*

Source: https://commons.wikimedia.org/wiki/File:914_Shoulder_Joint.jpg.

Shoulder girdle movements: A great deal of mobility is present in the shoulder girdle. The movement of the shoulder girdle is principally made possible by the scapulothoracic joint. Scapular mobility is very important because it allows the shoulder blades to move freely, which is necessary for the proper positioning of the shoulder girdle in space. The following is a description of how scapular movements are mirrored in the shoulder girdle:

- **Scapular Protraction:** The shoulders are shifted anteriorly and inwards by sliding the scapula laterally aside from the spine (Ovesen & Nielsen, 1985).
- **Scapular Retraction:** This is the movement that is involved in medially sliding the scapula towards the spine. This happens because of a continuous backward and inwards movement of the shoulders.
- **Scapular Elevation:** It lets the shoulder girdle raise or move upward (O'Connell et al., 1990).
- **Scapular Depression:** Unlike the latter, this action permits the shoulder girdle and scapula to descend lower.
- **Scapular Upward Rotation:** The shoulder girdle rotates upwards and inwards by turning the lower scapula laterally and upwards (Högfors et al., 1991).
- **Downward Scapular Rotation:** The scapula is slid towards the spinal column because of this movement. As a consequence of this, the shoulder girdle is moved downwards.

The deltoid can abduct to a 90° angle after the supraspinatus initiates the abduction of the shoulder. The scapula is rotated upward by the serratus anterior and trapezius, moving it to an elevation of 180°. The movements of the shoulder and shoulder girdle come together into one seamless motion. To test this, find your own or a colleague's lower pole of the scapula. This should sway outwards when shoulder abduction is started. In addition to the scapular movements, the reciprocal movement also takes place at the sternoclavicular joint. The tendon layers from the shoulder muscles that encircle and integrate with the joint are referred to as the rotator cuff. The muscles are the subscapularis, which enters from below, and the infraspinatus, teres minor, and supraspinatus, which enter from above the humeral tubercle. The base of everything is the scapula (Bankart, 1923).

When it comes to its functional significance, the supraspinatus is the most significant muscle. As it passes over the shoulder's peak, the subacromial bursa divides it from the acromion process and the coracoacromial ligament. This sac, which forms the largest bursa in the body, continues beneath the deltoid. In the event that damage results in injury to the supraspinatus tendon, abduction cannot begin properly, and the patient must learn to tilt his torso to the affected side (Bureau et al., 1996). Shoulder Impingement Syndrome, also referred to as supraspinatus tendonitis, is a common shoulder ailment. Symptoms of supraspinatus may develop gradually over time without apparent cause, or they may occur rapidly following an injury. The pain associated with supraspinatus tendonitis appears as an arc when the arm is moved between 60 and 120° of abduction because the tendon becomes compressed against the bone at those angles. Regarding its symptoms, they typically manifest in middle age (Eckmann et al., 2017).

7.2.6. The Elbow Joint

Elbow joint is present between the forearm and the arm. Three bones constitute this synovial joint: the radius, ulna, and humerus.

This joint is made up of three different articulations (Fornalski et al., 2003):

1. **Humeroulnar:** A hinge joint between the humerus and ulna trochlea.
2. **Superior Radioulnar:** The link between the head of the radius and the ulna's radial notch, with the head held in position by the annular ligament.
3. **Humeroradial:** The ball-and-socket joint between the capitulum and radial head.

Hyaline cartilage acts as a separating layer between the articular surfaces of the bones in synovial joints, which are movable joints. Viscous synovial fluid lubricates these joints to allow for easy mobility. The fibrous capsule of the joint is lined with the synovial membrane (An et al., 1981) (Figures 7.13 and 7.14).

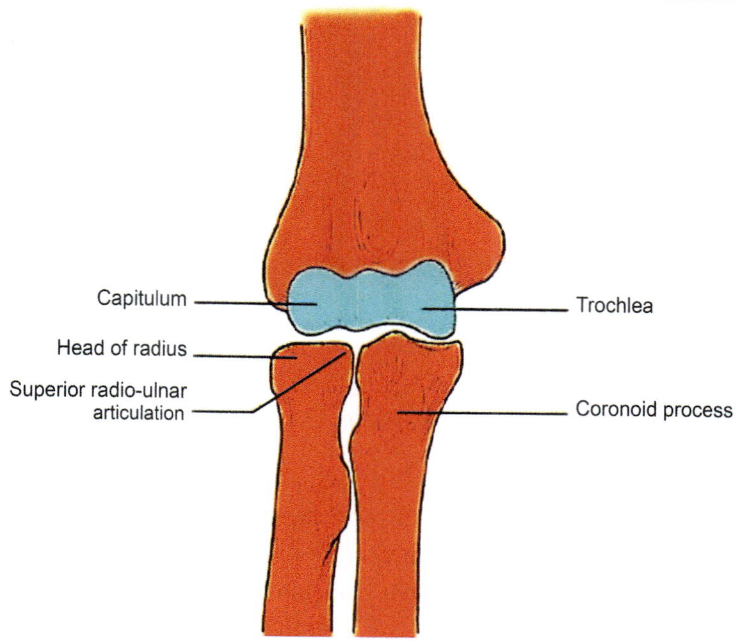

Figure 7.13. *Elbow skeleton parts (right side) take note of the three groups of articular surfaces.*

Source: https://encrypted-tbn3.gstatic.com/images?q=tbn:ANd9GcQd7QASrzjN4XNm9gd8iH6pvzOaM_BXmxjHRwf4m5QkInH293Lq.

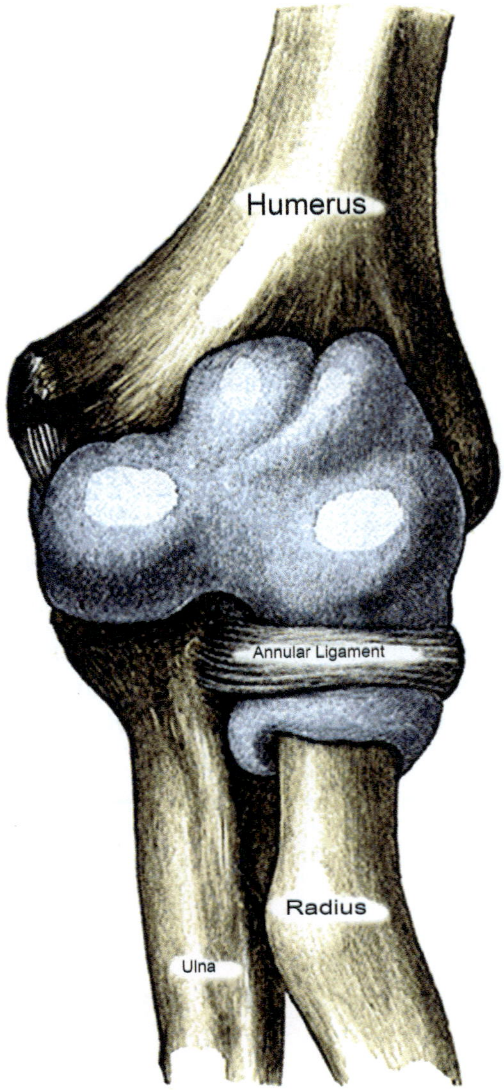

Figure 7.14. *The view of the joint capsule of the elbow.*

Source: By Henry Vandyke Carter – Henry Gray, (1918). Anatomy of the human body (see "Book" section below) Bartleby.com: Gray's anatomy, Plate 331, Public Domain; https://commons.wikimedia.org/w/index.php?curid=792116.

The extracapsular location of the lateral and medial epicondyles indicates that they are not articulated into the elbow joint. While the lateral and medial ligaments thicken and strengthen the sides, the anterior and posterior capsules are thin and loose to permit flexion and extension. The lateral ligament's distal attachment point is the annular ligament of the radial head. The synovium slides into the radius to allow the annular ligament to be accessed, facilitating the rotation of the radius (Regan et al., 1991). The proximal radioulnar and ulnar collateral joints pronate and supinate, along with concurrent distal radio-ulnar and ulnar collateral joint movements, whereas the humeroulnar and humeroradial joints bend and extend (Halls & Travill, 1964).

7.2.7. The Wrist Joint

The wrist joint, which joins the hand and forearm, is a synovial joint. It consists of the articular disc, the distal end of the radius, and the proximal row of carpal bones, also known as the distal row (Hagert, 2010). The distal radioulnar joint, which is located just above the wrist, is where the ulna and radius articulate, in contrast to the radius. The articular disc, a fibrocartilaginous ligament covering the ulna's superior surface, prevents the ulna in humans from articulating with the carpal bones (Ryu et al., 1991). The concave surface of the radius and articular disc articulate with the convex surface of the carpal bones (Figure 7.15).

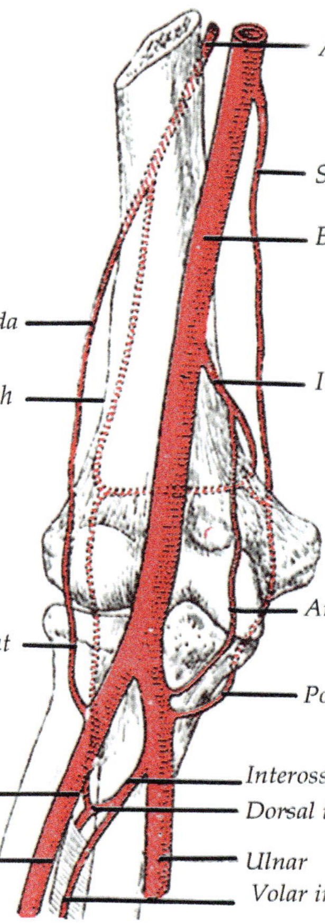

Figure 7.15. *The arteries of the hand.*

Source: By Henry Vandyke Carter – Henry Gray, (1918). Anatomy of the human body (see "Book" section below) Bartleby.com: Gray's anatomy, Plate 526, Public Domain; https://commons.wikimedia.org/w/index.php?curid=559534s.

The ellipsoidal synovial joint that makes up the wrist allows for movement in two directions. This demonstrates that flexion, extension, adduction, and abduction are among the ranges of motion it can display (Lewis et al., 1970). The forearm muscles must be used in order to move the wrist. Flexion is produced by the flexor carpi ulnaris and radialis with assistance from the flexor digitorum superficialis. Together with the extensor carpi ulnaris, the extensor carpi radialis longus and brevis are primarily responsible for the extension. The extensor digitorum aids in the extension as well. Adduction is produced by the flexor and extensor carpi ulnaris working in tandem. Contracting the abductor pollicis longus, flexor carpi radialis, and extensor carpi radialis longus and brevis is how abduction is performed (Bawa et al., 2000).

7.2.8. The Articulations in the Hand

Gliding motions are produced by joints that are located in between the carpal bones. Thumb flexion and extension, abduction and adduction, and opposition—where the thumb crosses over and makes contact with the fifth finger—are all possible at the carpometacarpal joint, which resembles a saddle (Wu et al., 2001). This joint's range is very large in comparison to the limited motions of the carpometacarpal joints, which only allow the second and third metacarpals to glide in a few degrees and the fourth and fifth metacarpals to flex and extend in a narrow range. According to Choi et al. (2017), its range permits complete range of motion in the flexion, extension, and gliding planes of motion.

At the metacarpophalangeal joints, the situation is completely different. The thumb's metacarpophalangeal joint can only flex and extend 60°, while the other four metacarpophalangeal joints can flex and extend 90° in addition to abduction, adduction, and circumduction. Be aware that when the metacarpophalangeal joints are flexed, the finger cannot move in either direction and cannot be abducted or adducted. This is due to the fact that each metacarpal head is straight at the front and circular at the distal end (Oikonomidis et al., 2011).

Once a firm grasp is established, strong deep transverse ligaments connect the metacarpophalangeal joints of the fingers but not the thumb joint. The thumb joint is not affected by this. These ligaments tighten when one grasps something, preventing the palm from extending in any direction. Because each interphalangeal joint has opposing surfaces that resemble pulleys, all interphalangeal joints are hinge joints that can only move in two directions: flexion and extension. Every metacarpophalangeal and interphalangeal joint has the same ligament configuration (Panchal-Kildare & Malone, 2013).

1. When viewed from the back, the joint capsule is substituted by the extension of the extensor tendon of the digit under examination.
2. In the front of the capsule, fibrocartilage serves as the structure's foundation. The friction caused by the neighboring flexor tendons has resulted in the formation of this palmar ligament.
3. The collateral ligaments provide additional support to the joint. These ligaments are loose when the joint is extended, but they become taut when the joint is flexed (Oikonomidis et al., 2014).

7.3. Important Upper Limb Zones

7.3.1. The Axilla

The axilla is the area of the human body that is directly beneath the shoulder joint. It includes the axillary space, which is a region inside the shoulder girdle that lies between the thoracic cage and the arm. The imaginary plane created by the superior margins of the clavicle, scapula, and first rib defines it anteriorly (Guéro, 2018). On the medial side, it is bordered by the thoracolumbar fascia and the serratus anterior muscle. The lateral portions of the upper four intercostal spaces make up the medial wall of the axilla (Ikeda et al., 2001), and the lateral wall is the medial aspect of the upper arm segment. These are covered by serratus anterior digitations. The back axilla is surrounded by the latissimus dorsi, teres major, and subscapularis muscles (Evans & Guyton, 1995). The base of the axillary pyramid is the deep fascia, which emerges from the rear of the chest and extends to the arm's medial region. The latissimus dorsi and the pectoralis major are connected by the axillary fascia (Ikeda et al., 2000).

7.3.2. The Cubital Fossa

It is a triangular curve on the front of the elbow joint, acting as a transition zone between the forearm and the arm. The cubital fossa consists of three borders, a floor, and a roof (Loewenthal et al., 2002):

- The brachioradialis muscle has a medial border and a lateral border.
- The pronator teres muscle has a lateral border and a medial border.
- A line between the epicondyles of the humerus is the superior boundary (Yammine & Erić, 2017).
- Roof fascia, subcutaneous fat, skin, and bicipital aponeurosis. Several superficial veins can also be found on the cubital fossa's roof. A typical location for venipuncture is the median cubital vein, which joins the basilic and cephalic veins and is easily accessible.
- Floor proximally brachialis and supinator (distally) (Singh et al., 1982).

Its contents are:

- **The Radial Nerve:** It runs along the lateral border of the cubital fossa, splitting into branches. It performs motor and sensory functions in the forearm and hand's posterior region.
- **The Biceps Tendon:** It grows centrally through the cubital fossa and connects to the radial tuberosity.
- **The Brachial Artery:** The brachial artery splits into the radial and ulnar arteries at the apex of the cubital fossa.
- **The Median Nerve:** It goes via the cubital fossa, exiting between the two heads of the pronator teres. It performs motor and sensory functions in the forearm and hand (Yamada et al., 2008) (Figure 7.16).

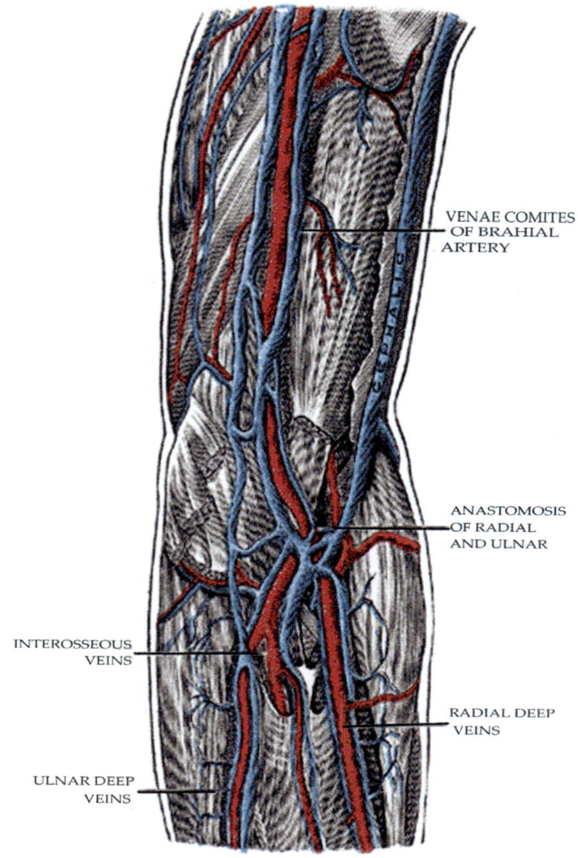

Figure 7.16. *Anterior slicing of the forearm to reveal the veins.*

Source: By Henry Vandyke Carter – Henry Gray, (1918). Anatomy of the human body (see "Book" section below) Bartleby.com: Gray's Anatomy, Plate 575, Public Domain; https://commons.wikimedia.org/w/index.php?curid=538691.

7.3.3. The Carpal Tunnel

It is a very small wrist canal. It is where the median nerve and numerous tendons enter the palm. The carpal tunnel is made up of the flexor retinaculum and the carpal arch. The concave surface of the deep carpal arch becomes a tunnel due to the overlaying flexor retinaculum. The tunnel's sides and bottom are formed by the concave carpal arch on the palmar side (Werner & Andary, 2002). The scaphoid and trapezium bones' tubercles help it develop laterally. It is formed by the hook of the pisiform bone and is situated in the center of the hamate bone. In humans, the ceiling of the carpal tunnel is made of dense connective tissue called the flexor retinaculum. The carpal arch becomes the carpal tunnel when the space between the medial and lateral sections of the arch is connected (Atroshi et al., 1999). You can tell where the carpal tunnel begins by looking at your distal wrist crease, which is located in line with the tunnel's entrance.

Given below is the list of tendons that make up the carpal tunnel:

- Flexor pollicis longus tendon;
- Four flexor digitorum profundus tendons;
- Four flexor digitorum superficialis tendons (Gelberman et al., 1981).

A synovial sheath surrounds the eight tendons of the flexor digitorum and the flexor digitorum profundus superficialis. The tendon of the flexor pollicis longus is encased in synovial fluid. These sheaths allow the tendons to move freely. Though it is actually located in the flexor retinaculum rather than the carpal tunnel, the flexor carpi radialis tendon is sometimes said to be located in the carpal tunnel (Viera, 2003). The median nerve splits into the recurrent branch and the palmar digital nerves after going through the carpal tunnel. The dorsal nail beds and palmar skin of the lateral three-and-a-half digits receive sensory information from the palmar digital nerves. Additionally, they provide motor nerve innervation to the lateral two lumbricals. The cyclic branch supplies the thenar muscle group. CTS (Carpal tunnel syndrome) is a serious syndrome linked to carpal tunnel malfunction. The compression of the median nerve within the carpal tunnel is the cause of it. Enlarged ligaments and tendon sheaths are the cause of the most common kind of mononeuropathy. Thermal muscle atrophy and weakening may result from CTS if treatment is not received (Phalen, 1972).

7.4. The Upper Limb's Arteries

7.4.1. The Axillary Artery

One of the main blood vessels in the human anatomy, the axillary artery carries oxygenated blood to the thorax, axilla, and upper limb. It starts at the subclavian artery, which is located close to the edge of the first rib. It passes through the bottom edge of the teres major and changes into the brachial artery (Rodríguez-Niedenführ et al., 2001).

The axillary artery is commonly divided into three sections:

- The first section is the portion of the artery superior to the pectoralis minor;
- The second section is the portion of the artery posterior to the pectoralis minor; and
- The third section is the artery below the pectoralis minor (Çavdar et al., 2000).

The axillary artery is divided into multiple smaller branches, and the genesis of these branches varies greatly (Schachner et al., 2005).

- **The First Section:** Superior thoracic artery (supreme thoracic artery).

- **The Second Section:** Thoracoacromial artery and lateral thoracic artery. It is likely to branch from one of the following arteries if it does not come from the axillary artery: (i) thoracoacromial artery; (ii) third axillary artery; (iii) suprascapular artery; or (iv) subscapular artery (Sabik et al., 2004).
- **The Third Section:** The anterior humeral circumflex artery, the posterior humeral circumflex artery, and the subscapular artery. According to Natsis et al., the brachial artery continues past the teres major's inferior border (2006).

7.4.2. The Brachial Artery

The axillary artery extends past the teres major muscle to become the brachial artery. It moves to the cubital fossa at the elbow by traveling along the ventral surface of the arm. After that, the radial and ulnar arteries split off and proceed down the forearm. The ulnar and radial arteries run through the upper arm, and in some individuals, the bifurcation occurs much earlier (Bots et al., 2005). There is a close relationship between the brachial artery and the median nerve. The median nerve crosses the medial side of the brachial artery just in front of the elbow joint. The following branches emerge from the brachial artery (Sorensen et al., 1997):

- Profunda brachii artery;
- Superior ulnar collateral artery;
- Inferior ulnar collateral artery;
- Radial artery;
- Ulnar artery;
- Nutrient branches to the humerus (Faulx et al., 2003).

7.4.3. The Radial Artery

The radial artery starts at the biceps tendon at the level of the radial neck. It is accompanied in its upper half by the brachioradialis, which is a tightened muscle that displays the artery's surface marking on the medial side. In the proximal region of the forearm, between the tendons of the brachioradialis and flexor carpi radialis, is where the artery is felt at the wrist. The radial nerve passes through the middle third of the forearm on the lateral side of the artery (Acar et al., 1992). To help form the superficial palmar arch, the artery branches distal to the radial pulse. It then penetrates the first dorsal interosseous muscle and the abductor pollicis between the first and second metacarpals, enters the anatomical snuffbox through the tendons of the abductor pollicis longus and extensor pollicis brevis, structures the palmar arch with the ulnar artery's branch, and exits the body (Slogoff et al., 1983).

7.4.4. The Ulnar Artery

The ulnar artery travels from its starting point to its ending, passing beneath the muscles that originate from the flexor, resting on the flexor digitorum profundus, and being covered by the flexor carpi ulnaris. The head of the pronator teres, a small muscle, is the only structure that lies between the ulnar artery and the median nerve as they pass each other superficially (Hazlett, 1949). The ulnar nerve tracks the artery on the medial side of its course, along the distal two-thirds of its path through the forearm and over the flexor retinaculum (Lovie et al., 1984).

Note: Around every major joint, there is a dense network of arteries that have been connected.

7.5. The Brachial Plexus

The muscles and skin of the upper limb are supplied with nerve fibers by the brachial plexus. It passes through the axilla and all of the upper extremities, starting at the base of the neck (Thompson & Rorie, 1983).

The plexus is created in the following manner (Figure 7.17):

- Five roots from the anterior major rami of C5, C6, C7, C8, and T1 connect to form:
- Three trunks created by the junction of C5 and C6; C7 alone; and C8 and T1; which separate into (Foad et al., 2008):
- Six segregations are formed by the division of each trunk into an anterior and a posterior division, which then recombine to form:
- Three cords, lateral, medial, and posterior (Winnie, 1970).

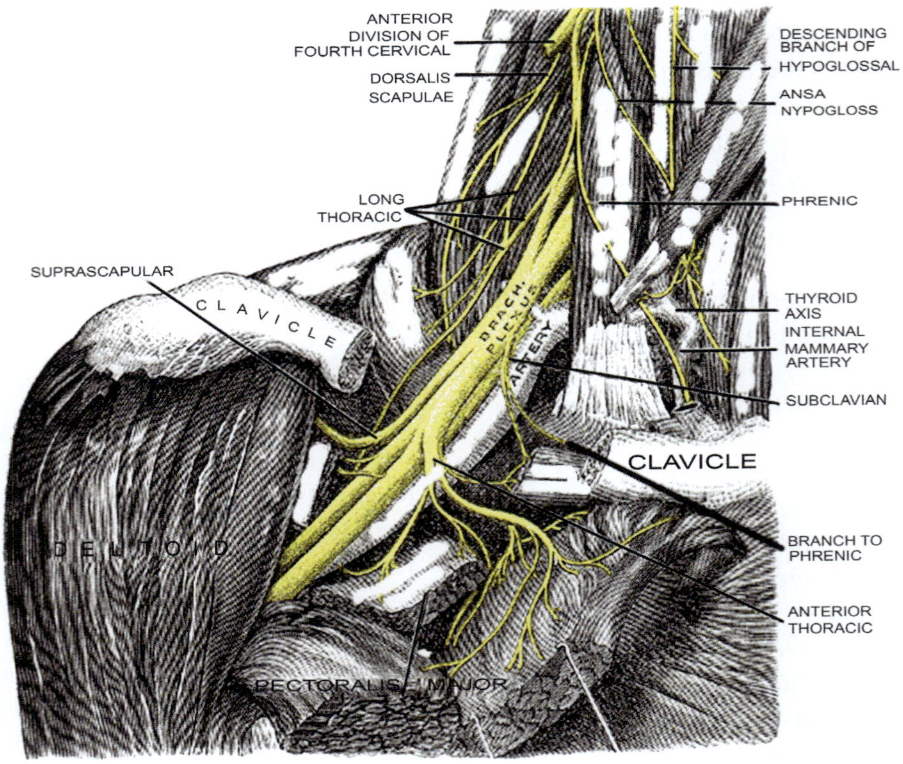

Figure 7.17. *Scheme of the brachial plexus.*

Source: By Henry Vandyke Carter – Henry Gray, (1918). Anatomy of the human body (see "Book" section below) Bartleby.com: Gray's anatomy, Plate 808, Public Domain; https://commons.wikimedia.org/w/index.php?curid=541664.

The space between the anterior and middle scalene muscles is where the roots are situated. The posterior triangle of the neck's fascial floor contains the trunks at a considerable depth. The axilla, which is located posterior to the collarbone, displays both the partitions and the cords. Following their continuation distally, the cords give rise to the primary nerve trunks of the upper limb, which include (Narakas, 1985) (Figure 7.18):

- The lateral cord;
- The medial cord; and
- The posterior cord (radial nerve and the axillary nerve) (Narakas & Hentz, 1988);
- The median nerve is formed through communication between the medial and lateral cords.

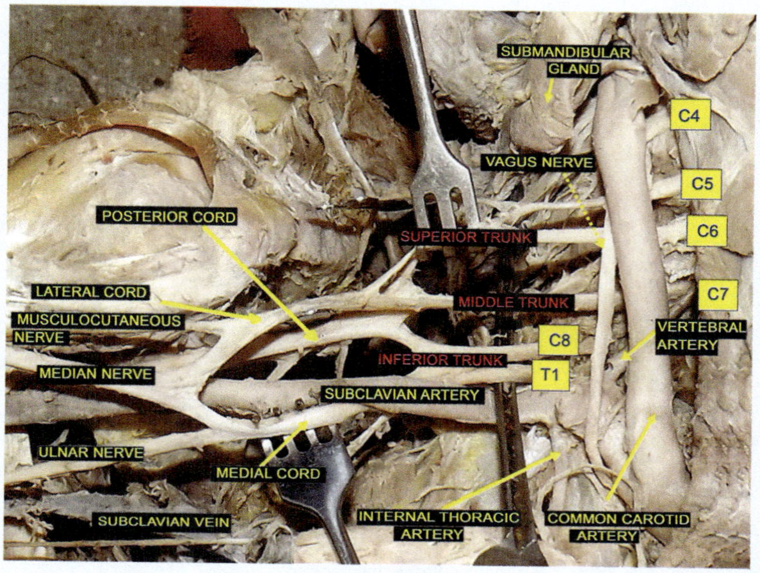

Figure 7.18. *The branches extend out from the brachial plexus.*

Source: By Anatomist90 – Own work, CC BY-SA 3.0; https://commons.wikimedia.org/w/index.php?curid=18940042.

The descendants of the various brachial plexus parts are listed below:

1. **From the Roots:** Nerve to rhomboids, serratus anterior, and subclavius.
2. **From the Trunk:** Suprascapular nerve – from the upper trunk (Lusk et al., 1987).
3. **From the Lateral Cord:** Musculocutaneous, lateral pectoral, and the lateral root of the median nerve.
4. **From the Medial Cord:** Medial cutaneous nerves medial, pectoral nerve, the medial root of the median nerve, and the ulnar nerve (Van Es, 2001).
5. **From the Posterior Cord:** Nerve to latissimus dorsi, subscapular nerves, axillary, and radial nerve.

It is important to remember that the anteriorly positioned medial and lateral cords supply the tissues of the anterior compartment, while the posterior cord supplies the muscles and skin of the posterior portion of the limb (Vargas et al., 2010) (Figure 7.19).

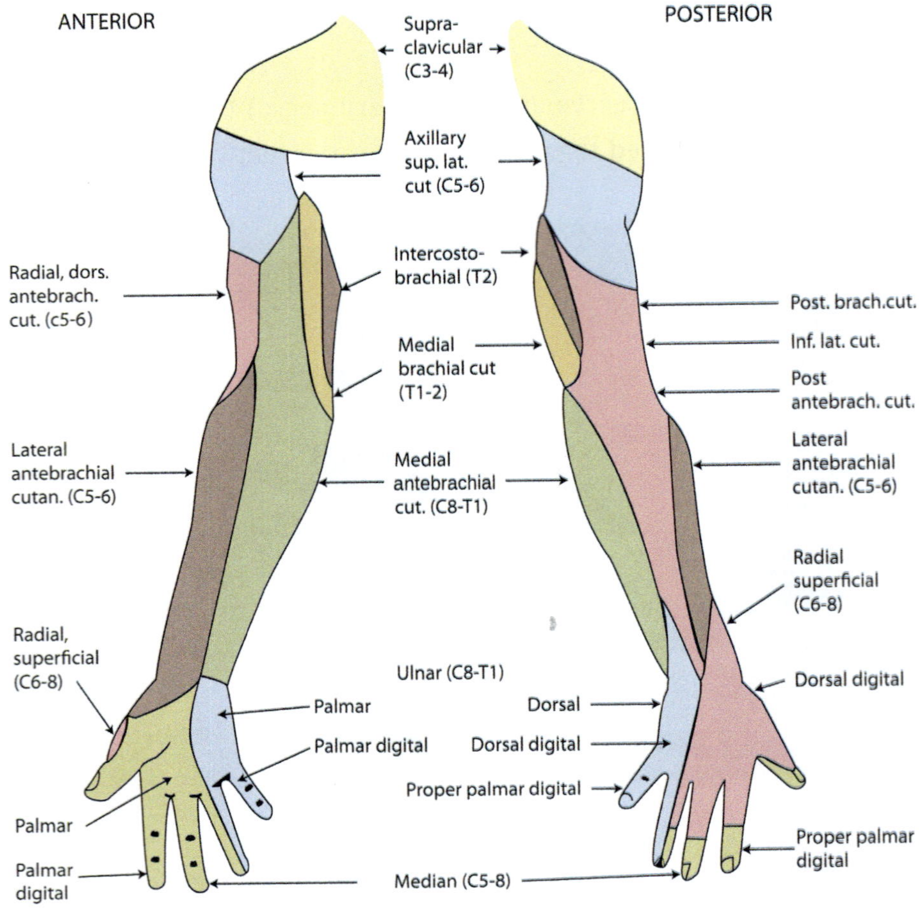

Figure 7.19. *The segmental cutaneous innervation.*

Source: By Henry Vandyke Carter – Henry Gray, (1918). Anatomy of the human body (see "Book" section below) Bartleby.com: Gray's Anatomy, Plate 812. This is a retouched picture, which means that it has been digitally altered from its original version. Modifications: Vectorized. The original can be viewed here: Gray812 an d814.PNG. Modifications made by Fred the Oyster., Public Domain; https://commons.wikimedia.org/w/index.php?curid=9821685.

A Closer Look

Upper Limb Analysis

Upper limb analysis is a critical area of study within biomechanics, physical therapy, and sports science, focusing on the complex movements and functions of the human arm. This analysis encompasses the shoulder, elbow, wrist, and hand, examining their individual roles and the intricate coordination required for various activities. Understanding the mechanics of these joints and their interactions is essential for diagnosing and treating injuries, enhancing athletic performance, and designing prosthetics and rehabilitation protocols.

The shoulder complex, comprising the glenohumeral joint, acromioclavicular joint, sternoclavicular joint, and the scapulothoracic articulation, is highly mobile, allowing for a wide range of movements. These movements include flexion, extension, abduction, adduction, internal and external rotation, and circumduction. The stability of the shoulder is maintained by a combination of muscles, tendons, and ligaments, with the rotator cuff playing a pivotal role. Upper limb analysis often involves evaluating the function and coordination of these components to understand their contribution to movement and identify any dysfunctions.

The elbow joint, a hinge joint formed by the humerus, radius, and ulna, allows for flexion and extension of the forearm, as well as supination and pronation. The integrity and function of the elbow are crucial for tasks that require lifting, throwing, and precision. Analyzing the elbow involves assessing the strength and coordination of the muscles involved, such as the biceps brachii, triceps brachii, and the muscles of the forearm, as well as the stability provided by the ligaments.

The wrist is a complex joint composed of the distal ends of the radius and ulna, and the carpal bones. It permits a wide range of motions, including flexion, extension, radial and ulnar deviation, and circumduction. The intricate arrangement of bones, ligaments, and tendons in the wrist requires detailed analysis to understand its role in fine motor skills and load-bearing activities. Disorders such as carpal tunnel syndrome, tendinitis, and fractures necessitate thorough evaluation and targeted interventions.

Hand analysis delves into the fine motor skills and dexterity essential for various tasks, from typing and writing to gripping and manipulating objects. The hand comprises numerous bones, joints, muscles, and tendons, working in unison to perform precise movements. Each finger and the thumb have unique roles, with the thumb's opposition providing a significant functional advantage. Analyzing hand function involves examining grip strength, range of motion, coordination, and the integrity of structures such as the flexor and extensor tendons.

Upper limb analysis employs various techniques, including kinematic and kinetic assessments, electromyography (EMG), and motion capture systems. Kinematic analysis focuses on the movement patterns and joint angles, while kinetic analysis examines the forces involved in these movements. EMG measures the electrical activity of muscles to assess their activation patterns and coordination.

Motion capture systems provide detailed, real-time data on limb movements, aiding in the accurate assessment of upper limb function.

This comprehensive analysis is crucial in clinical settings for diagnosing and treating musculoskeletal disorders, planning surgical interventions, and designing rehabilitation programs. In sports science, upper limb analysis helps optimize performance, prevent injuries, and enhance recovery strategies for athletes. In the field of prosthetics, it informs the design of advanced prosthetic limbs that mimic natural movements. Overall, upper limb analysis is a vital tool in understanding the complexities of arm function, leading to improved health outcomes and performance in various activities.

Summary

- The upper limb is known for its movement and its potential to grab, strike, and engage in activities requiring fine motor abilities (manipulation). The hand is a particularly good indicator of these traits.
- Along the entire length of the clavicle, the subcutaneous border can be detected; on rare occasions, the underlying bone can be felt against the supraclavicular nerves that cross the clavicle's surface.
- The pectoralis major creates the front of the axilla, while the teres major and latissimus dorsi make the posterior fold. The shoulder curve is created by the deltoid muscle in the upper arm.
- The subclavian artery is situated against the first rib, the radial artery in the anatomical snuffbox, the brachial artery on the humerus, the radial artery at the first knuckle, and the ulnar arteries at the wrist.
- The superficial veins, which are used for venipuncture and transfusion, are greater in size and have a stronger clinical value due to their use than the smaller and more superficial deep venae comitantes, which join the primary arteries.
- The scapula is a triangular bone of the upper limb and has three significant elements: the glenoid depression on its outer edge, the spine on its outer edge, and the coracoid on its inner edge.
- The clavicle (collarbone) is a long, narrow, S-shaped bone about 15 cm long that acts as a link between the breastbone and the shoulder blade. Each side of the chest has one clavicle, which means there are two clavicles in the human body.
- The radius and ulna constitute the forearm while extending from the elbow to the wrist. The radius is present in the lateral forearm, while the ulna is placed in the medial forearm.
- The shoulder joint is a ball and socket joint that links the humerus to the scapula. Linking the upper limb to the trunk, the shoulder joint serves as the most significant joint of the human body.
- The lateral and medial epicondyles, which are not part of the elbow joint's articulation, are located in extracapsular fashion. The anterior and posterior capsules are thin and loose to allow for flexion and extension, while the lateral and medial ligaments thicken and strengthen the sides.
- The wrist joint is a synovial joint that connects the forearm to the hand. It is made up of the proximal row of carpal bones, which is referred to as the distal row, and the radius's distal end, and the articular disc.
- The region of the human body located right under the shoulder joint is referred to as the axilla. It contains the axillary space, which is a space between the thoracic cage and the arm, within the shoulder girdle.
- It is a tiny channel inside the wrist. It is the entry point for many tendons and the median nerve into the palm. A carpal arch and a flexor retinaculum make up the carpal tunnel.

References

1. Abbott, L. C., & Lucas, D. B. (1954). The function of the clavicle: Its surgical significance. *Annals of Surgery, 140*(4), 583.
2. Acar, C., Jebara, V. A., Portoghese, M., Beyssen, B., Pagny, J. Y., Grare, P., & Carpentier, A. F. (1992). Revival of the radial artery for coronary artery bypass grafting. *The Annals of Thoracic Surgery, 54*(4), 652–660.
3. Alexander, R. M. (2002). Tendon elasticity and muscle function. *Comparative Biochemistry and Physiology Part A: Molecular & Integrative Physiology, 133*(4), 1001–1011.
4. Al-Qattan, M. M., Yang, Y., & Kozin, S. H. (2009). Embryology of the upper limb. *The Journal of Hand Surgery, 34*(7), 1340–1350.
5. An, K. N., Hui, F. C., Morrey, B. F., Linscheid, R. L., & Chao, E. Y. (1981). Muscles across the elbow joint: A biomechanical analysis. *Journal of Biomechanics, 14*(10), 659–669.
6. Atroshi, I., Gummesson, C., Johnsson, R., Ornstein, E., Ranstam, J., & Rosén, I. (1999). Prevalence of carpal tunnel syndrome in a general population. *JAMA, 282*(2), 153–158.
7. Azer, S. A. (2012). Can "YouTube" help students in learning surface anatomy? *Surgical and Radiologic Anatomy, 34*(5), 465–468.
8. Bankart, A. B. (1923). Recurrent or habitual dislocation of the shoulder-joint. *British Medical Journal, 2*(3285), 1132.
9. Bawa, P., Chalmers, G. R., Jones, K. E., Søgaard, K., & Walsh, M. L. (2000). Control of the wrist joint in humans. *European Journal of Applied Physiology, 83*(2), 116–127.
10. Ben Kibler, W. (1998). The role of the scapula in athletic shoulder function. *The American Journal of Sports Medicine, 26*(2), 325–337.
11. Bots, M. L., Westerink, J., Rabelink, T. J., & de Koning, E. J. (2005). Assessment of flow-mediated vasodilatation (FMD) of the brachial artery: Effects of technical aspects of the FMD measurement on the FMD response. *European Heart Journal, 26*(4), 363–368.
12. Brook, I. (2008). Microbiology and management of joint and bone infections due to anaerobic bacteria. *Journal of Orthopedic Science, 13*(2), 160–169.
13. Bureau, N. J., Dussault, R. G., & Keats, T. E. (1996). Imaging of bursae around the shoulder joint. *Skeletal Radiology, 25*(6), 513–517.
14. Çavdar, S., Zeybek, A., & Bayramiçli, M. (2000). Rare variation of the axillary artery. *Clinical Anatomy: The Official Journal of the American Association of Clinical Anatomists and the British Association of Clinical Anatomists, 13*(1), 66–68.
15. Chakravarty, K., & Webley, M. (1993). Shoulder joint movement and its relationship to disability in the elderly. *The Journal of Rheumatology, 20*(8), 1359–1361.
16. Choi, C., Kim, S., & Ramani, K. (2017). Learning hand articulations by hallucinating heat distribution. In *Proceedings of the IEEE International Conference on Computer Vision* (pp. 3104–3113).
17. Cordella, F., Ciancio, A. L., Sacchetti, R., Davalli, A., Cutti, A. G., Guglielmelli, E., & Zollo, L. (2016). Literature review on needs of upper limb prosthesis users. *Frontiers in Neuroscience, 10*, 209.

18. Cormack, G. C., & Lamberty, B. G. H. (1984). Fasciocutaneous vessels. *Anatomia Clinica, 6*(2), 121–131.

19. Davis, A. P., Witte, D. P., Hsieh-Li, H. M., Potter, S. S., & Capecchi, M. R. (1995). Absence of radius and ulna in mice lacking hoxa-11 and hoxd-11. *Nature, 375*(6534), 791–795.

20. Dibona, G. F. (1982). The functions of the renal nerves. *Reviews of Physiology, Biochemistry and Pharmacology, 94*, 75–181.

21. Eckmann, M. S., Bickelhaupt, B., Fehl, J., Benfield, J. A., Curley, J., Rahimi, O., & Nagpal, A. S. (2017). Cadaveric study of the articular branches of the shoulder joint. *Regional Anesthesia & Pain Medicine, 42*(5), 564–570.

22. Evans, D. M., & Guyton, D. P. (1995). Carcinoma of the axillary breast. *Journal of Surgical Oncology, 59*(3), 190–195.

23. Evans, E. M. (1951). Fractures of the radius and ulna. *The Journal of Bone and Joint Surgery. British Volume, 33*(4), 548–561.

24. Faulx, M. D., Wright, A. T., & Hoit, B. D. (2003). Detection of endothelial dysfunction with brachial artery ultrasound scanning. *American Heart Journal, 145*(6), 943–951.

25. Foad, S. L., Mehlman, C. T., & Ying, J. (2008). The epidemiology of neonatal brachial plexus palsy in the United States. *JBJS, 90*(6), 1258–1264.

26. Fornalski, S., Gupta, R., & Lee, T. Q. (2003). Anatomy and biomechanics of the elbow joint. *Sports Medicine and Arthroscopy Review, 11*(1), 1-9.

27. Gardner, E. (1968). 2 The embryology of the clavicle. *Clinical Orthopedics and Related Research (1976–2007), 58*, 9–16.

28. Gelberman, R. H., Hergenroeder, P. T., Hargens, A. R., Lundborg, G. N., & Akeson, W. H. (1981). The carpal tunnel syndrome. A study of carpal canal pressures. *The Journal of Bone and Joint Surgery. American Volume, 63*(3), 380–383.

29. Guéro, S. (2018). Developmental biology of the upper limb. *Hand Surgery and Rehabilitation, 37*(5), 265–274.

30. Hagert, E. (2010). Proprioception of the wrist joint: A review of current concepts and possible implications on the rehabilitation of the wrist. *Journal of Hand Therapy, 23*(1), 2–17.

31. Halls, A. A., & Travill, A. (1964). Transmission of pressures across the elbow joint. *The Anatomical Record, 150*(3), 243–247.

32. Hazlett, J. W. (1949). The superficial ulnar artery. *Canadian Medical Association Journal, 61*(3), 289.

33. Högfors, C., Peterson, B., Sigholm, G., & Herberts, P. (1991). Biomechanical model of the human shoulder joint—II. The shoulder rhythm. *Journal of Biomechanics, 24*(8), 699–709.

34. Horak, J., & Nilsson, B. E. (1975). Epidemiology of fracture of the upper end of the humerus. *Clinical Orthopedics and Related Research, (112)*, 250–253.

35. Huber, W. P., & Putz, R. V. (1997). Periarticular fiber system of the shoulder joint. *Arthroscopy: The Journal of Arthroscopic & Related Surgery, 13*(6), 680–691.

36. Ikeda, Y., Takami, H., Niimi, M., Kan, S., Sasaki, Y., & Takayama, J. (2001). Endoscopic thyroidectomy by the axillary approach. *Surgical Endoscopy, 15*(11), 1362–1364.

37. Ikeda, Y., Takami, H., Sasaki, Y., Kan, S., & Niimi, M. (2000). Endoscopic neck surgery by the axillary approach1. *Journal of the American College of Surgeons, 191*(3), 336–340.

38. Inman, V. T., & Abbott, L. C. (1996). Observations of the function of the shoulder joint. *Clinical Orthopedics and Related Research (1976–2007), 330*, 3–12.

39. Inman, V. T., Saunders, J. D. M., & Abbott, L. C. (1944). Observations on the function of the shoulder joint. *JBJS, 26*(1), 1–30.

40. Jaffe, H. L. (1959). Tumors and tumorous conditions of the bones and joints. *Academic Medicine, 34*(1), 72.

41. Jupiter, J. B., Neff, U. R. S., Holzach, P., & Allgöwer, M. (1985). Intercondylar fractures of the humerus. An operative approach. *The Journal of Bone and Joint Surgery. American Volume, 67*(2), 226–239.

42. Khan, L. K., Bradnock, T. J., Scott, C., & Robinson, C. M. (2009). Fractures of the clavicle. *JBJS, 91*(2), 447–460.

43. Kjaer, M. (2004). Role of extracellular matrix in adaptation of tendon and skeletal muscle to mechanical loading. *Physiological Reviews, 84*(2), 649–698.

44. Kjær, M., Magnusson, P., Krogsgaard, M., Møller, J. B., Olesen, J., Heinemeier, K., & Langberg, H. (2006). Extracellular matrix adaptation of tendon and skeletal muscle to exercise. *Journal of Anatomy, 208*(4), 445–450.

45. Lewis, O. J., Hamshere, R. J., & Bucknill, T. M. (1970). The anatomy of the wrist joint. *Journal of Anatomy, 106*(Pt 3), 539.

46. Lewis, T. (1926). The blood vessels of the human skin. *British Medical Journal, 2*(3418), 61.

47. Loewenthal, M. R., Dobson, P. M., Starkey, R. E., Dagg, S. A., Petersen, A., & Boyle, M. J. (2002). The peripherally inserted central catheter (PICC): A prospective study of its natural history after cubital fossa insertion. *Anesthesia and Intensive Care, 30*(1), 21–24.

48. Louveau, A., Smirnov, I., Keyes, T. J., Eccles, J. D., Rouhani, S. J., Peske, J. D., & Kipnis, J. (2015). Structural and functional features of central nervous system lymphatic vessels. *Nature, 523*(7560), 337–341.

49. Lovie, M. J., Duncan, G. M., & Glasson, D. W. (1984). The ulnar artery forearm free flap. *British Journal of Plastic Surgery, 37*(4), 486–492.

50. Lucas, D. B. (1973). Biomechanics of the shoulder joint. *Archives of Surgery, 107*(3), 425–432.

51. Lusk, M. D., Kline, D. G., & Garcia, C. A. (1987). Tumors of the brachial plexus. *Neurosurgery, 21*(4), 439–453.

52. Maciejasz, P., Eschweiler, J., Gerlach-Hahn, K., Jansen-Troy, A., & Leonhardt, S. (2014). A survey on robotic devices for upper limb rehabilitation. *Journal of Neuroengineering and Rehabilitation, 11*(1), 1–29.

53. Marciniak, C. (2011). Poststroke hypertonicity: Upper limb assessment and treatment. *Topics in Stroke Rehabilitation, 18*(3), 179–194.

54. Mitchell, R. N., & Schoen, F. J. (2010). Blood vessels. In R. S. Cotran & V. Kumar (Eds.), *Robbins and Cotran: Pathologic Basis of Disease (8th ed., pp. 516–517)*. Saunders Elsevier.

55. Müller, L. J., Marfurt, C. F., Kruse, F., & Tervo, T. M. (2003). Corneal nerves: Structure, contents and function. *Experimental Eye Research, 76*(5), 521–542.

56. Narakas, A. O. (1985). The treatment of brachial plexus injuries. *International Orthopedics, 9*(1), 29–36.

57. Narakas, A. O., & Hentz, V. R. (1988). Neurotization in brachial plexus injuries. Indication and results. *Clinical Orthopedics and Related Research, (237)*, 43–56.

58. Natsis, K., Papadopoulou, A. L., Paraskevas, G., Totlis, T., & Tsikaras, P. (2006). High origin of a superficial ulnar artery arising from the axillary artery: Anatomy, embryology, clinical significance and a review of the literature. *Folia Morphological, 65*(4), 400–405.

59. Nikander, R., Sievänen, H., Uusi-Rasi, K., Heinonen, A., & Kannus, P. (2006). Loading modalities and bone structures at nonweight-bearing upper extremity and weight-bearing lower extremity: A pQCT study of adult female athletes. *Bone, 39*(4), 886–894.

60. Nordqvist, A. N. D. E. R. S., & Petersson, C. L. A. E. S. (1994). The incidence of fractures of the clavicle. *Clinical Orthopedics and Related Research, (300)*, 127–132.

61. O'Connell, P. W., Nuber, G. W., Mileski, R. A., & Lautenschlager, E. (1990). The contribution of the glenohumeral ligaments to anterior stability of the shoulder joint. *The American Journal of Sports Medicine, 18*(6), 579–584.

62. Oikonomidis, I., Kyriazis, N., & Argyros, A. A. (2011). Efficient model-based 3D tracking of hand articulations using Kinect. In *BmVC (Vol. 1, No. 2, p. 3)*.

63. Oikonomidis, I., Lourakis, M. I., & Argyros, A. A. (2014). Evolutionary quasi-random search for hand articulations tracking. In *Proceedings of the IEEE Conference on Computer Vision and Pattern Recognition (pp. 3422–3429)*.

64. Ovesen, J., & Nielsen, S. (1985). Stability of the shoulder joint: Cadaver study of stabilizing structures. *Acta Orthopaedical Scandinavica, 56*(2), 149–151.

65. Panchal-Kildare, S., & Malone, K. (2013). Skeletal anatomy of the hand. *Hand Clinics, 29*(4), 459–471.

66. Phalen, G. S. (1972). The Carpal-tunnel Syndrome: Clinical Evaluation of 598 Hands. *Clinical Orthopedics and Related Research (1976–2007), 83*, 29–40.

67. Post, M. E. L. V. I. N. (1989). Current concepts in the treatment of fractures of the clavicle. *Clinical Orthopedics and Related Research, (245)*, 89–101.

68. Prescher, A. (2000). Anatomical basics, variations, and degenerative changes of the shoulder joint and shoulder girdle. *European Journal of Radiology, 35*(2), 88–102.

69. Regan, W. D., Korinek, S. L., Morrey, B. F., & An, K. N. (1991). Biomechanical study of ligaments around the elbow joint. *Clinical Orthopedics and Related Research, (271)*, 170–179.

70. Rodríguez-Niedenführ, M., Vázquez, T., Nearn, L., Ferreira, B., Parkin, I., & Sanudo, J. R. (2001). Variations of the arterial pattern in the upper limb revisited: A morphological and statistical study, with a review of the literature. *The Journal of Anatomy, 199*(5), 547–566.

71. Rowe, C. R., & Yee, L. B. (1944). A posterior approach to the shoulder joint. *JBJS, 26*(3), 580–584.

72. Ryu, J., Cooney III, W. P., Askew, L. J., An, K. N., & Chao, E. Y. (1991). Functional ranges of motion of the wrist joint. *The Journal of Hand Surgery, 16*(3), 409–419.

73. Sabik, J. F., Nemeh, H., Lytle, B. W., Blackstone, E. H., Gillinov, A. M., Rajeswaran, J., & Cosgrove, D. M. (2004). Cannulation of the axillary artery with a side graft reduces morbidity. *The Annals of Thoracic Surgery, 77*(4), 1315–1320.

74. Schachner, T., Nagiller, J., Zimmer, A., Laufer, G., & Bonatti, J. (2005). Technical problems and complications of axillary artery cannulation. *European Journal of Cardio-Thoracic Surgery, 27*(4), 634–637.

75. Scotece, M., Conde, J., Vuolteenaho, K., Koskinen, A., Lopez, V., Gómez-Reino, J., & Gualillo, O. (2014). Adipokines as drug targets in joint and bone disease. *Drug Discovery Today, 19*(3), 241–258.

76. Sherman, T. F. (1981). On connecting large vessels to small. The meaning of Murray's law. *The Journal of General Physiology, 78*(4), 431–453.

77. Singh, S. P., Ekandem, G. J., & Bose, S. (1982). A study of the superficial veins of the cubital fossa in Nigerian subjects. *Cells Tissues Organs, 114*(4), 317–320.

78. Slogoff, S., Keats, A. S., & Arlund, C. (1983, July). On the safety of radial artery cannulation. *The Journal of the American Society of Anesthesiologists, 59*(1), 42–47.

79. Sorensen, K. E., Kristensen, I. B., & Celermajer, D. S. (1997). Atherosclerosis in the human brachial artery. *Journal of the American College of Cardiology, 29*(2), 318–322.

80. Thompson, G. E., & Rorie, D. K. (1983). Functional anatomy of the brachial plexus sheaths. *Anesthesiology, 59*(2), 117–122.

81. Van Es, H. W. (2001). MRI of the brachial plexus. *European Radiology, 11*(2), 325–336.

82. Vargas, M. I., Viallon, M., Nguyen, D., Beaulieu, J. Y., Delavelle, J., & Becker, M. (2010). New approaches in imaging of the brachial plexus. *European Journal of Radiology, 74*(2), 403–410.

83. Viera, A. J. (2003). Management of carpal tunnel syndrome. *American Family Physician, 68*(2), 265–272.

84. Volgas, D. A., Stannard, J. P., & Alonso, J. E. (2004). Nonunion of the humerus. *Clinical Orthopedics and Related Research (1976–2007), 419*, 46–50.

85. Watts, H. G., & Lifeso, R. M. (1996). Current concepts review-tuberculosis of bones and joints. *JBJS, 78*(2), 288–299.

86. Werner, R. A., & Andary, M. (2002). Carpal tunnel syndrome: Pathophysiology and clinical neurophysiology. *Clinical Neurophysiology, 113*(9), 1373–1381.

87. Winnie, A. P. (1970). Interscalene brachial plexus block. *Anesthesia & Analgesia, 49*(3), 455–466.

88. Wu, Y., Lin, J. Y., & Huang, T. S. (2001, July). Capturing natural hand articulation. In *Proceedings Eighth IEEE International Conference on Computer Vision. ICCV 2001 (Vol. 2, pp. 426–432)*. IEEE.

89. Yamada, K., Yamada, K., Katsuda, I., & Hida, T. (2008). Cubital fossa venipuncture sites based on anatomical variations and relationships of cutaneous veins and nerves. *Clinical Anatomy: The Official Journal of the American Association of Clinical Anatomists and the British Association of Clinical Anatomists, 21*(4), 307–313.

90. Yammine, K., & Erić, M. (2017). Patterns of the superficial veins of the cubital fossa: A meta-analysis. *Phlebology, 32*(6), 403–414.

91. Zahalka, A. H., & Frenette, P. S. (2020). Nerves in cancer. *Nature Reviews Cancer, 20*(3), 143–157.

92. Zlotolow, D. A., Catalano III, L. W., Barron, A. O., & Glickel, S. Z. (2006). Surgical exposures of the humerus. *JAAOS-Journal of the American Academy of Orthopedic Surgeons, 14*(13), 754–765.

Chapter

THE LOWER LIMB

8

Contents

Introduction

An essential component of the human anatomy, the lower limb is principally in charge of sustaining the body's weight, enabling movement, and preserving equilibrium. It is divided into the hip, thigh, knee, and foot as its four primary regions. These areas cooperate to facilitate a variety of motions, such as running, jumping, and climbing.

The hip joint, located where the lower limb meets the pelvis, is a ball-and-socket joint that allows for a wide range of motion in various directions. It provides the stability and strength necessary for weight-bearing activities. Within the thigh is the femur, the body's longest and strongest bone, which plays a key role in supporting body weight and facilitating movement. Muscles in the thigh, like the quadriceps and hamstrings, are vital for activities like walking, running, and jumping. The knee is a hinge joint created by the femur, tibia, and patella (kneecap). It enables flexion and extension, which are essential for most lower limb movements. Ligaments and muscles support the knee, providing stability and control. Injuries to the knee, such as ligament tears or meniscus damage, can significantly impact mobility and must be carefully managed. The lower leg, including the tibia and fibula, supports foot movement and muscle attachment. This area connects to the foot through the ankle joint, enabling crucial movements like dorsiflexion and plantarflexion for walking and running. The foot itself is a complex structure with various bones, joints, muscles, and ligaments that aid in shock absorption, balance, and propulsion. The arches of the foot, supported by tendons and ligaments, help distribute weight and provide stability. Overall, the lower limb is a sophisticated system designed for strength, stability, and flexibility. Its intricate anatomy allows for a wide range of functions necessary for daily activities and physical performance. Understanding this structure and function is essential for diagnosing and treating related injuries and conditions.

Orientation and Directional Terms

Term	Definition	Illustration
Triradiate cartilage	Triradiate cartilage is the Y- shaped epiphyseal plate that occurs at the junction where the ischium, ilium, and pubis meet in the skeletally immature skeleton. The vertical component of the "Y" is the meeting of the ischium and pubic bone. The anterior arm is the junction of the ilium and pubis.	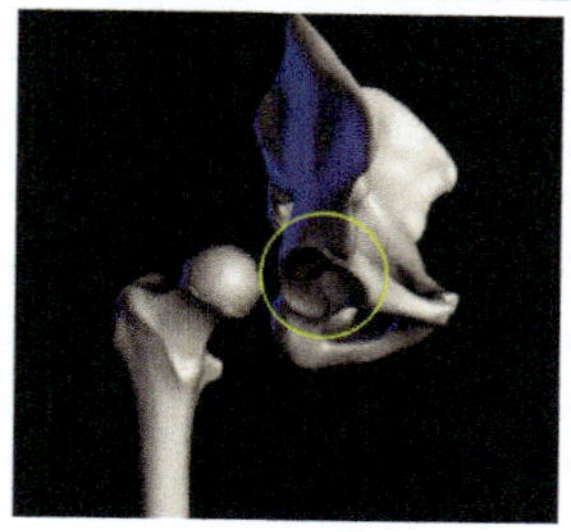
Patella	The patella is your kneecap. It's the bone at the front of your knee joint. It's the biggest bone in your body embedded in a tendon (a sesamoid bone). Your patella helps your quadriceps muscle move your leg, protects your knee joint, and supports lots of important muscles, tendons and ligaments.	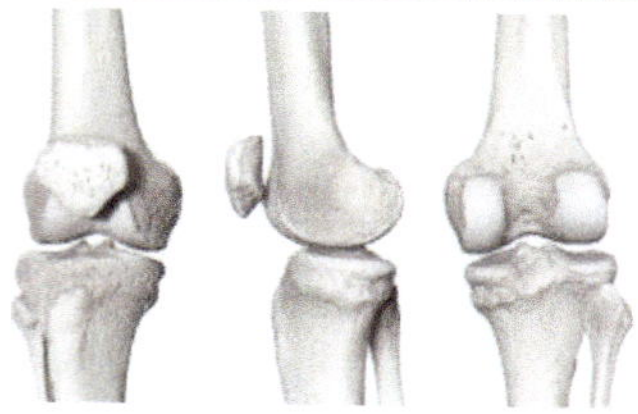
Tarsus	The tarsus consists of 7 bones which form the posterior aspect of the foot. Bones of the tarsus include the calcaneus, talus, navicular, cuboid and cuneiform (medial, intermediate and lateral) bones.	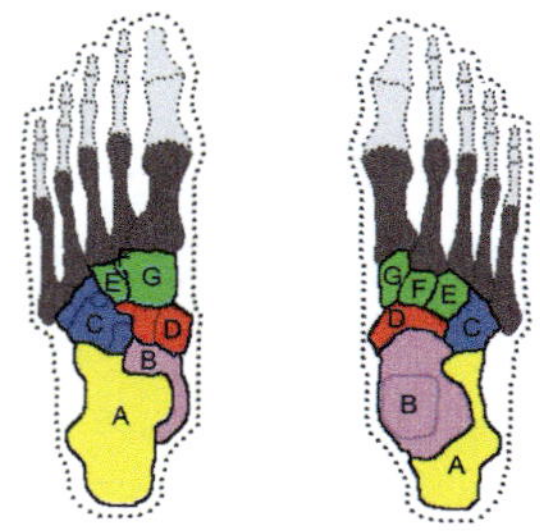
Femur nerve	The femoral nerve is one of the largest nerves in the leg. It has a motor function to help you move your hips, legs, ankles and feet. It also has a sensory function, helping you feel touch, pain and hot or cold temperatures. The femoral nerve is part of the peripheral nervous system.	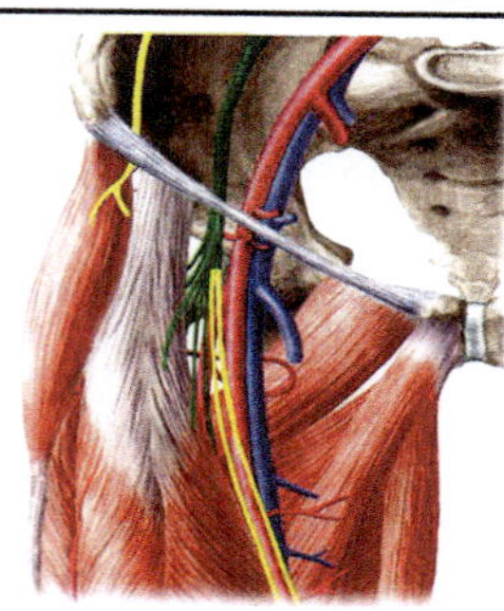
Lower limb	The lower limb is divided into three regions. These are the thigh, located between the hip and knee joints; the leg, located between the knee and ankle joints; and distal to the ankle, the foot. There are 30 bones in each lower limb.	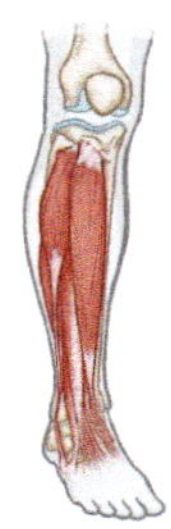

8.1. Bones of Lower Limb

Body weight is distributed through all sacroiliac joints from the vertebra to the pelvic girdle, then from the pelvic girdle to the hips and finally to the femur bone (L. feet), and lastly to the ankles and knees. After that, the tibial bone shifts the weight from the knee to the ankle. In addition to not flexing with the femur, the fibula cannot really support weight. At the ankle, the talus bears the unsteady weight. Every foot has a linear arch made up of the tarsal and metatarsal components, which when standing evenly distributes weight between the forefoot and the heels. This arch's talus serves as its cornerstone (Della Croce et al., 1999) (Figure 8.1).

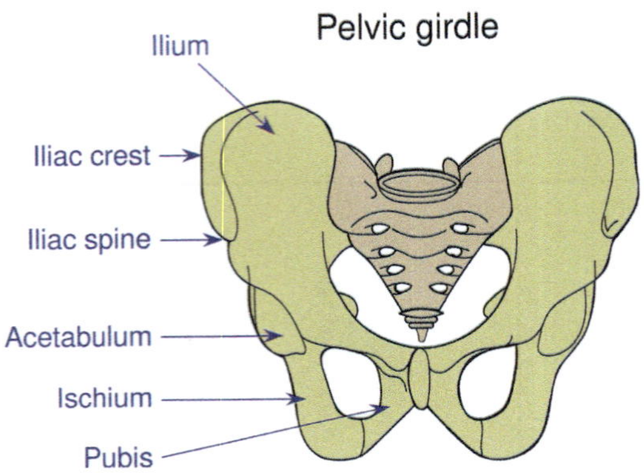

Figure 8.1. *Pelvic girdle.*

Source: https://en.wikipedia.org/wiki/File:Pelvic_girdle_illustration.svg.

The femur bone is angled downwards and towards the middle of the thigh to provide optimal support for walking upright. This positioning allows the knee to be near and directly under the body, aligning the center of mass with the vertical support of the feet and legs. Women tend to have slightly more angled thigh bones than men due to their wider pelvises (Valente et al., 2012).

8.1.1. Hip Bone

The three primary bones that come together to create the hip bone in adults are the ischium, pubis, and ilium. During adolescence, these bones are separated by a triradiate ligament. As individuals age between 15 and 17 years old, the cartilage disappears and the bones begin to fuse together. The fusion process is typically completed between the ages of 20 and 25 (Figure 8.2).

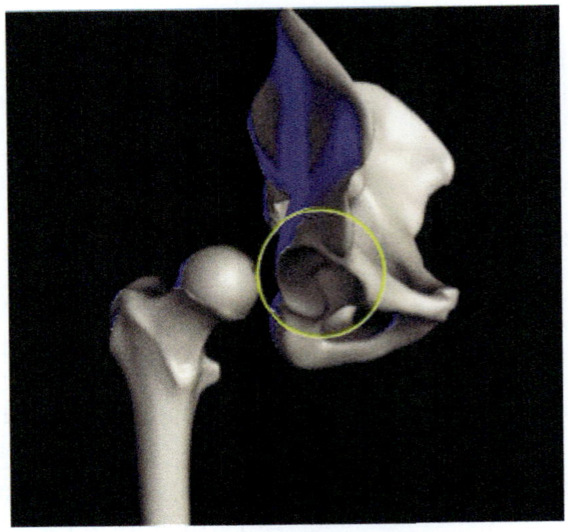

Figure 8.2. *The triradiate cartilage.*

Source: By Protohiro at the English-language Wikipedia, CC BY-SA 3.0; https://commons.wikimedia.org/w/index.php?curid=3911259.

The acetabulum, the cup-shaped chamber or hole on the lateral edge of the hip where the femoral head articulates, is composed in part of the superior portion of the hip bone, the largest and uppermost part of the hip. The ilium consists of a core that joins the pubic area and ischium to the acetabulum, and an ala (wing) that is bounded apically by the iliac crest (Shoji et al., 2013). The ischium forms the posterio-inferior portion of the acetabulum and the thigh bone. The ischium is made up of a core that joins the ilium and the superior dorsum of the pubis to form the acetabulum. When the inferior ramus of the pubis and the ischium converge, the ischiopubic ramus is formed (Schmalzried et al., 1997). The frontal and anterio-medial parts of the acetabulum are formed by the pubis, respectively. The left pubis is encased in the body of the right pubis at the symphysis pubis. It also has both superior and inferior rami (Byrne et al., 2010).

To spot the pelvic bone or skeletal pelvis in the natural position, locate it such that the following conditions are met. The anterio-superior iliac spine and anterio-superior region of the pubis should lie in a similar coronal (frontal) plane;

The pubis' symphysial area should be perpendicular and collinear to the middle plane:

- The inside of the pubis should be located superiorly.
- Inferio-laterally, the Acetabulum lies with the notch lying inferior.
- Inferio-medially to the acetabulum should lie the Obturator Foramen (Macchiarelli et al., 1999).

8.1.2. Femur

The femur is the biggest and most massive bone in the skeleton. It is primarily made up of the proximal, distal, and superior extremities. The majority of the body is smooth and round, with the exception of a prominent dual furrow known as the linea aspera that deviates inferiorly on the posterior side of the shaft (King-Heiden & Litster, 2019). The proximal end of the femur is composed of the greater and smaller trochanters, the head, and the neck. The femur's head is entirely covered in fibrocartilage, with the exception of a central dip or pit that acts as the fovea for the head ligaments. The neck of the femur is trapezoid; the head is carried by its narrower extremity, while its broad base is contiguous with the shaft (Weiner, 1996). The junction of the neck and shaft is home to the two massive, blunt peaks known as the trochanters. The smaller trochanter's rounded tip extends medially from the femur's posterior-medial neck region to the shaft juncture. The larger, laterally positioned bulk, called the greater trochanter, extends where the neck and shaft converge. The intertrochanteric line is a rough surface ridge that extends from the greater to the smaller trochanter. The intertrochanteric crest, a similar but smoother crest, connects the trochanters posteriorly (Garden, 1961) (Figure 8.3).

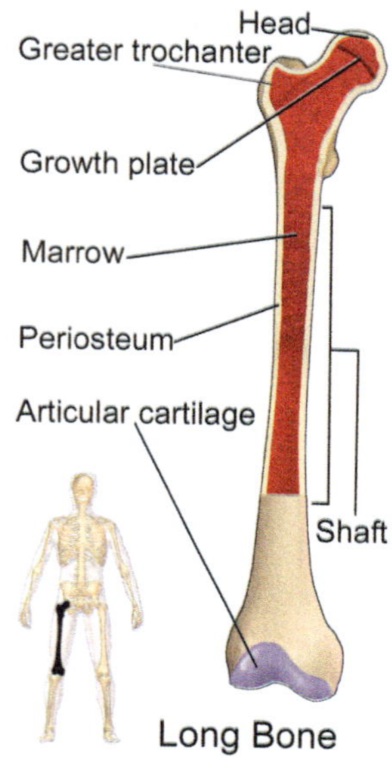

Figure 8.3. *The anterior aspect of the femur.*

Source: By BruceBlaus. When using this image in external sources it can be cited as: Blausen.com staff (2014). "Medical gallery of Blausen Medical, 2014." Wiki Journal of Medicine, 1(2). doi: 10.15347/wjm/2014.010. ISSN: 2002-4436. Own work, CC BY 3.0; https://commons.wikimedia.org/w/index.php?curid=27796927.

Two femoral condyles that curve spirally terminate the proximal end of the femur. The articulation of the femoral and tibial condyles forms the knee joint. The proximal femur's bend, which gives the femur an L-shape, allows the longer axes of the neck and head to extend superior-medially at an angle to that of the slant-placed shaft. Adults typically have a steep inclination angle between 115° and 140°. Women have a lower inclination because their acetabula are wider and the rod is more common. The femur can move more freely at the hip because the neck and head are more vertical to the acetabulum as a result of the angle of inclination. The femur's collar is heavily stressed, despite the fact that this aids in bipedal movement. An elderly person's minor stumble could result in a fracture if osteoporosis has compromised the collar (Abulhasan & Grey, 2017) (Figure 8.4).

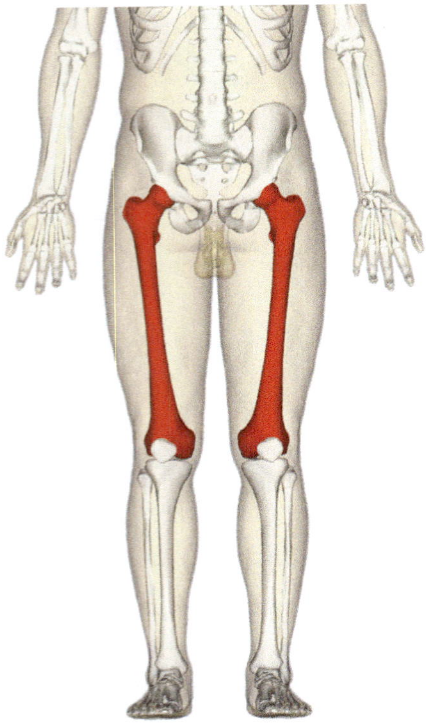

Figure 8.4. *The femur.*

Source: By Anatomography – en: Anatomography (setting page of this image), CC BY-SA 2.1 jp; https://commons.wikimedia.org/w/index.php?curid=23652071.

The neck and head planes of the femur align with the transversal axes of the femoral condyles at the femur's longer shaft axis, forming torsional angles. These angles, also known as the angle of declination, are observed when the femur is viewed from above with the proximal end overlapping the distal tip. Men typically have a torsional angle of 7°, while women have a torsional angle of 12°. This torsional angle, along with the inclination angle, allows for rotational motion of the femoral head within the acetabulum, facilitating extension, flexion, adduction, abduction, and rotary movements of the thighs (Dixon, 1910).

8.1.3. Patella

The patella, also referred to as the kneecap, is a large sesamoid bone structure that grows intravenously at birth. This triangle-shaped bone is located ahead of the femoral condyles and attaches to the patellar region of the femur.

A perpendicular ridge divides the patella's posterior layer into the medial and lateral articular outer surfaces. The posterior layer is seamless and covered in a substantial amount of articular cartilage. The two lateral boundaries congregate inferiorly to form the sharp apex, while the tough outer base (outstanding boundary) slopes infero-anteriorly. The subcutaneous frontal surface of the kneecap is curved (Fox et al., 2012).

8.1.4. Tibia

The talus at the lower border, the fibula at the lateral position, and the femoral condyles apically convey the length of the massive, load-bearing tibia (shinbone) at both its distal and proximal ends.

The far end of the tibia is shorter than the nearest end and has grooves for contact with the fibula and talus. The medial malleolus is an inferiorly oriented protrusion that arises from the distal tip of the tibia's midline. The large nutritional foramen is located in the proximal third of the tibia's nearest face.

This is the point on the tibia where the nutrition canal enters the medullary (marrow) chamber. For additional information on bony characteristics, *see* Figure 8.5 (Hwang et al., 2012).

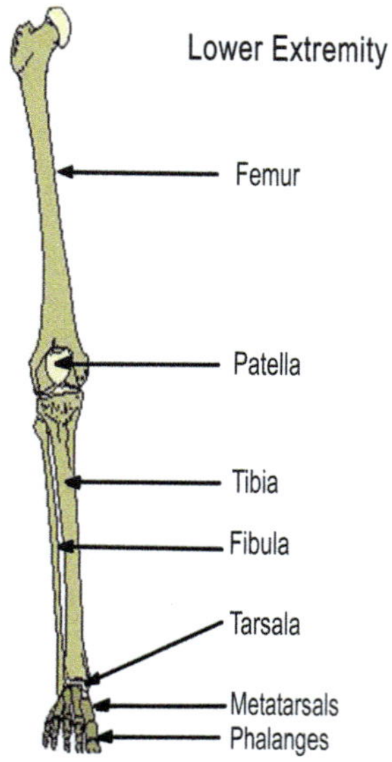

Figure 8.5. *The tibia and fibula.*

Source: Public Domain; https://commons.wikimedia.org/w/index.php?curid=789643.

8.1.5. Fibula

The thin fibula is situated posterior-laterally to the tibia and is mainly utilized for muscle attachment. At its closest end, the fibula has an expanded cap in front of a wide collar. The fibula expands at its distal tip to form the laterally positioned malleolus, which is one centimeter more distal, much more noticeable, and posteriorly situated than the medial malleolus. While not directly involved in weight-bearing activities, the sidelong malleolus of the fibula functions as the lateral portion of the sockets of the trochlea of the talus. An interosseous membrane connects the shafts of the tibia and fibula for the majority of their length (Weinert Jr et al., 1973).

8.1.6. Tarsus

The tarsus is composed of the talus, cuboid, calcaneus, navicular, and three cuneiform bones. The talus is the only bone that connects the legs. The calcaneus, or heel bone, is the largest and strongest bone in the foot. It joins the talus superiorly and the cube-shaped object anteriorly. The calcaneus is responsible for moving most of the body weight from the talus to the floor. The sustentaculum tali, which extends from the medial side of the superior boundary of the calcaneus, supports the tip of the talus. On its heel aspect, the calcaneal tuberosity (L. tuber calcanei), a prominent protrusion on the posterior aspect of the calcaneus, has both medial and lateral extensions. Further anteriorly is the calcaneal tubercle, a lesser protrusion (Tomlinson et al., 2003).

The talus's head, collar, and core (anklebone). The body mass that is transferred from the tibia is carried by the trochlea, the superior edge of the talus, which joins the two malleoli. The talus is supported by the top 2/3 of the calcaneus. There are no tendons or muscles that attach to the talus because cartilage makes up the majority of its surface. The talus's curved shape rests partially on the sustentaculum tali of the calcaneus and forms an anterior connection with the navicular (Novas, 1989).

Seen between the talar tip and the cuneiforms lies a flat, yacht-shaped bone called the navicular (L. small shape). As just the tuberosity of the navicular, the midline side of the navicular extends on the lower border. Leg pain could result from an excessively protruding tuberosity rubbing up against the medial portion of the footwear (Raes et al., 2011).

Mostly in the distal series of the tarsus, the cube-shaped (cuboid) is the bone that is most to the side. A trough for the tendons of the fibularis longus muscular structure can be found on the lateral and plantar sides of the cuboid, anterior to the tuberosity of the bone (Sammarco, 2004).

Midline (first), intermediate (second), and lateral are the 3 cuneiforms (third). Each cuneiform (*L. cuneus*, chisel-shaped) connects with the base of the corresponding metatarsal anteriorly and the navicular posteriorly. Additionally, the cuboid and the lateral cuneiform articulate (Jotoku et al., 2006).

8.2. Metatarsus

The phalanges and the tarsus are joined by the five long bones that make up the metatarsus. These are classified based on their location from the midfoot. The first metatarsal is thicker and shorter in length than the others. The second metatarsal is the largest. Each metatarsal consists of a head, a shaft, and a base that is situated proximally (distally). The bases of the metatarsals articulate with the cuneiform and cuboid bones. The bases of the first and fifth metatarsals have large tuberosities; the tuberosity of the fifth metatarsal extends well over the lateral border of the cuboid. Moreover, the heads flex when proximal phalanges are present (McCormick & Blount, 1949).

8.2.1. Phalanges

There are 14 phalanges in total. The first digit (big toe) has just two phalanges (proximal and distal), in contrast to the remaining four digits, which have three phalanges each (proximal, middle, and distal). According to Ridola & Palma (2001), each phalanx consists of a head, a shaft (rod), and a base that is adjacent to it (distally).

8.3. Fascia, Vessels, and Cutaneous Nerves of the Lower Limb

8.3.1. Subcutaneous Tissue and Fascia

The superficial fascia, sometimes referred to as subcutaneous tissue, is composed of lymphatic vessels, surface veins, lymph arteries, epidermal nerves, and loosely packed connective tissue that is located deep beneath the skin. There is a contiguous subcutaneous layer between the hips and the thighs and the lower part of the anterolateral abdomen. Within this subcutaneous tissue of both legs, fat is retained in the posterior aspect in the popliteal fossa and again far to the knees; at the knees, however, the subcutaneous tissue sheds its lateral and anterior adipose and combines with the deeper fascia (Cormack & Lamberty, 1984).

Stronger than the outer fascia, the deeper fascia envelops the leg like an elastic sock. Muscle contractions are more effective at constricting veins and directing blood toward the heart because the fascia limits the muscles' ability to expand outward. Fascia lata is the name for the deep fascia of the thighs (*L. lata*, broad). Fascia lata has (Niranjan et al., 2000):

Fascia lata is the name for the deep fascia of the thighs (*L. lata*, broad). *Fascia lata* has:

i. The inguinal ligament, pelvic arch, core of the pubis, and pubic mound are connected to and contiguous well with fascia lata on the upper side. Just beneath the inguinal ligament, the flexible covering of subcutaneous tissue (Scarpa fascia) of the inferior abdomen connects to the fascia lata as well (Haertsch, 1981).
ii. Posteriorly and laterally, the iliac crest (ridge).
iii. The ischial tuberosity, coccyx, sacrum, sacrotuberous ligaments, and the posterior aspect.
iv. The deep fascia of the legs distal and the outside portions of the knee bones.

The fascia lata is substantial because it encapsulates the major leg muscles, especially where it thickens sideways to develop the iliotibial tract. It is true that an aponeurosis of the gluteus maximus and tensor fasciae latae muscles is composed of such a broad band of fiber. The iliotibial tract extends from the iliac tubercle to the anterior-lateral tibial tubercle (also known as the Gerdy tubercle) on the lateral condyle of the tibia (O'Hare et al., 1983).

The leg muscles are divided into three superficial and deep compartments: the anterior, medial, and posterior. The external walls of these divisions are made up of the fascia lata and the three fascia lata intermuscular septa, which branch off of the fascia lata's inner edge and join the linea aspera on the femur's posterior surface. The sideways intermuscular septum is strong, but the other two septa are quite weak. The iliotibial tract and the lateral intermuscular septum are one continuous structure. The saphenous aperture is a hole or gap in the fascia lata located below the inguinal ligament's midline. Its middle gap is smoother, but its transverse, upper, and lower borders come together to form a jagged edge known as the falciform margin (O'Hare et al., 2013) (Figure 8.6).

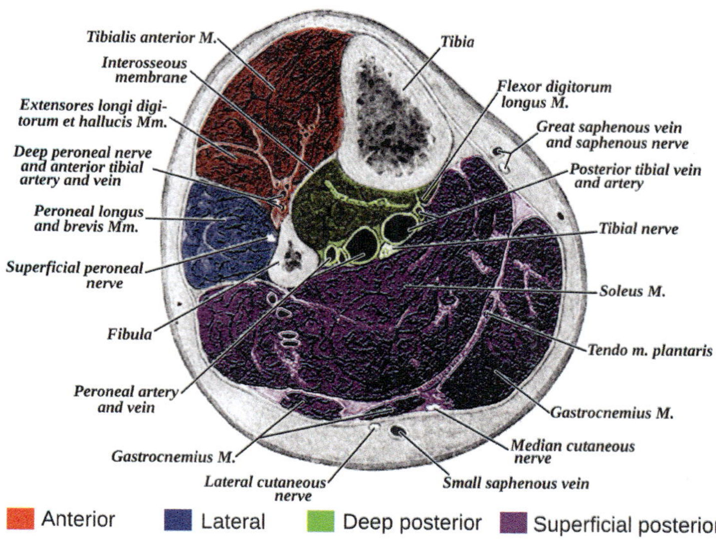

Figure 8.6. *Fascial compartments of the leg.*

Source: By Henry Vandyke Carter – Fig. 440 from Gray's Anatomy. File:Gray440.png, Public Domain; https://commons.wikimedia.org/w/index.php?curid=88465446.

The cribriform fascia, which resembles a strainer, is a local layer of subcutaneous tissue that covers the saphenous aperture (*L. cribrum*, sieve). The femoral vein and deep inguinal lymphatic system are reached by the great saphenous veins and certain lymphatic vessels, which in turn reach the saphenous aperture and cribriform fascia (Lidman et al., 1987). The deep fascia of the legs, also referred to as the crural fascia (L crus, leg), joins at the front and middle margins of the tibia. It is contiguous with the periosteum of the tibia. The basic connections of all the supporting muscles are found in the proximal part of the anterior portion of the leg, where the crural fascia is dense. In the distal part of the legs, the crural fascia is thin, but it is thicker where it generates the extensor retinacula (Rajacic et al., 1996). The anterior and posterior intermuscular septa leave the deeper layer of the crural fascia and join the corresponding fibular edges. The interosseous membrane and the intermuscular septa (plantar flexor) divide the leg's lateral (fibular), posterior, and anterior (dorsiflexor) portions. The crosswise intermuscular septum divides the plantar flexor muscle in the rear segment into deep and superficial sections (Capdevila et al., 2002).

8.3.2. Venous Drainage of Lower Limb

The lower extremities of limbs contain both fascial and deeper veins; surface veins are found in the subcutaneous tissue, whereas deeper veins run alongside the main arteries and reach the deep fascia.

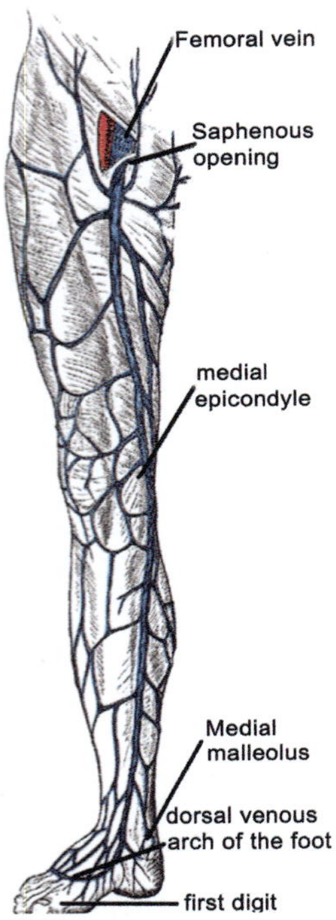

Figure 8.7. *Superficial venous and lymphatic drainage of the lower limb.*

Source: By Mikael Häggström. When using this image in external works, it may be cited as: Häggström, M., (2014). "Medical gallery of Mikael Häggström, 2014." Wiki Journal of Medicine, 1(2). doi: 10.15347/wjm/2014.008. ISSN: 2002-4436. Public Domain, or By Mikael Häggström, used with permission. Image:Gray581.png, Public Domain; https://commons.wikimedia.org/w/index.php?curid=2902242.

There are valves in both fascial and deep veins, but there are more in the deeper veins. The two main surface veins are the larger and smaller saphenous veins. The dorsal digital vein of the big toe joint, as well as the dorsal venous arch of the feet, combine to create the great saphenous vein (Chatterjee Sasanka, 2012) (Figure 8.7).

The great saphenous vein can:

i. Ascends anterior to the medial malleolus.
ii. Passes posterior to the medial condyle of the femur (about a hand's breadth posterior to the medial border of the patella).
iii. Anastomoses freely with the small saphenous vein.
iv. Traverses the saphenous opening in the fascia lata.
v. The dorsal digital vein of the fifth toe connects well with the rear venous arch to form the tiny saphenous vein, which emerges on the side of the leg. The deep fascia is penetrated by the little saphenous vein, which rises posteriorly to the sideways malleolus as a prolongation of the lateral border vein and travels all along the lateral side of the calcaneal tendon (Topham & Mortimer, 2002).
vi. The popliteal veins in the popliteal fossa are where it discharges after ascending between both ends of the gastrocnemius muscle.

Many perforating veins pierce the deep fascia and cross between the deeper and superficial veins. Their valves, or gates, only allow fluid to move from superficial veins into deeper veins. Squeezing the perforating veins prevents blood from flowing from the deep veins towards the superficial veins when the musculature tenses and stress within the deep fascia increases. Consequently, the deep fascia is punctured at sharp angles by the perforating veins. This pattern of venous blood circulation from the superficial to the deep helps muscle contractions push blood toward the heart against gravity for an effective venous return from the limb (Mortimer et al., 2019) (Figure 8.8).

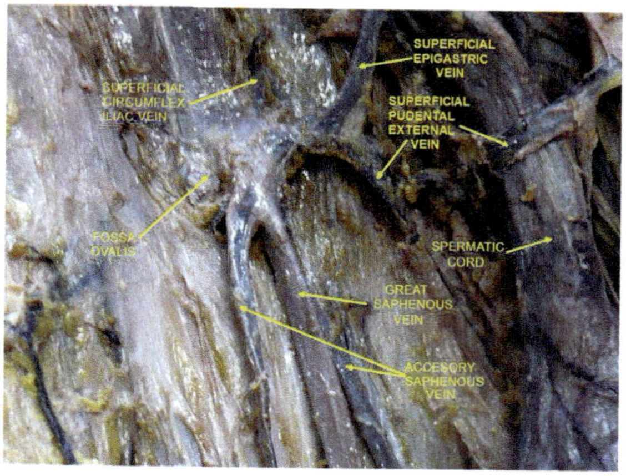

Figure 8.8. *The venous and lymphatic drainage of the lower limb.*

Source: By Anatomist90 – Own work, CC BY-SA 3.0; https://commons.wikimedia.org/w/index.php?curid=29759492.

Deep veins run alongside the main arterial system and its branches inside the lower limb. Usually occurring in pairs, the deeper veins frequently connect companion veins (*L. venae* comitantes) that encircle the arteries rather than showing up in the legs as a single vein (Nicolaides et al., 2008). They are covered in a vascular sheath along with the arteries, where pulses also help to compress and move the flow in the veins. The popliteal vein, located behind the knees, receives the veins from the deeper leg and develops into the femoral vein in the thighs. The profunda femoris vein connects to the last segment of the femoral vein. As the femoral vein deepens and enters the inguinal ligament, the iliofemoral vein forms in the hip (Uhl & Gillot, 2007) (Figure 8.9).

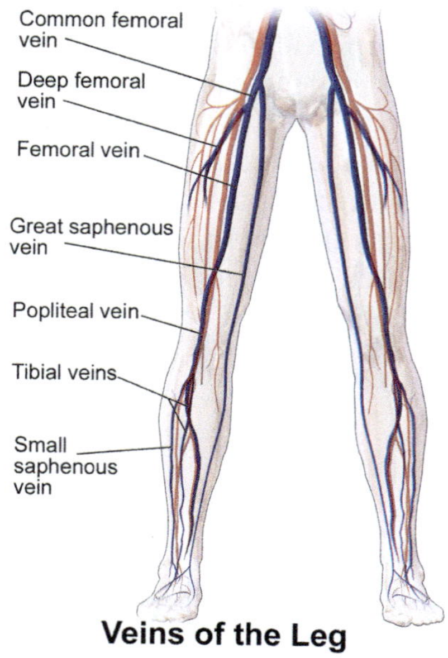

Figure 8.9. *Deep venous drainage of the lower limb.*

Source: By BruceBlaus. When using this image in external sources it can be cited as: Blausen.com staff (2014). "Medical gallery of Blausen Medical, 2014." Wiki Journal of Medicine, 1(2). doi: 10.15347/wjm/2014.010. ISSN: 2002-4436. Own work, CC BY 3.0; https://commons.wikimedia.org/w/index.php?curid=30634279.

8.3.3. Lymphatic Drainage of Lower Limb

Lower leg lymph vessels are both shallow and deeper. The superficial lymphatic capillaries cross and follow the saphenous vein and its branches. The lymph veins that trail the greater saphenous vein terminate at the superficial lymph nodes. The external iliac lymphatic vessels along the external iliac vein receive the majority of the lymph produced by these nodes, although the deep inguinal lymphatic vessels, which are located on the midline of the femoral vein, may also occasionally receive lymph from all of these nodes (Shinaoka et al., 2020). The lymph veins that follow the smaller saphenous vein enter the popliteal lymphatic nodes, which are situated in the fat surrounding the popliteal veins in the popliteal fossa. The popliteal lymph glands are reached by the leg's deeper lymphatic vessels in addition to its deep veins. Through deep lymphatic arteries, the majority of the lymph from these nodes rises to the deeper inguinal lymph nodes. According to Topham & Mortimer (2002), the deeper nodes supply fluid to the outer iliac lymph nodes.

8.3.4. Cutaneous Innervation of the Lower Limb

Cutaneous neurons in the subcutaneous tissue supply the lower extremity of the limb's epidermis. Except for a small number in the proximal part of the limbs, these neurons are extensions of the sacral and lumbar sensory nerves.

The area of the skin that gets nourishment from a specific vertebral neuron's cutaneous branching is called a dermatome. Dermatomes L1–L5 spread out as a series of strips from the hind middle of the body through into the legs, traveling sideways and inferiorly all-around limbs towards its forward and middle sides to reflect the medial rotations that occur throughout growth (Macefield et al., 1989). Dermatomes S1 and S2 descend the posterior aspect and anterior portion of the limbs, diverging around the ankles to reach the medial and lateral borders of the feet.

In addition to the axial map, even though dermatome mapping has divided them into discrete sections, the path of the union of dermatomes fed by separated spinal regions and nearby dermatomes intersects. Two separate dermatome maps are frequently used. Since Foerster's (1933) design is correlated with clinical outcomes, most people support it; however, some people support the design because it is correlated with limb growth and development (Nakajima et al., 2006).

8.4. Thigh and Gluteal Regions

The development of well-defined buttocks is closely related to the evolution of walking on two legs and standing upright. Changes in the shape of the thigh bone necessary for walking upright allow the muscles that lift the thighs to be positioned more effectively in the buttocks. This repositioning of the thigh muscles in the buttocks is made possible by the femur taking on a different shape to accommodate walking on two legs. The muscles in the legs are divided into three sections by intermuscular septa: the front (extensor), middle (adductor), and back (flexor). The nerves that control the thigh muscles, such as the obturator nerve and the tibial portion of the sciatic nerve, directly stimulate the different bands of muscle in the legs (Shaer, 1984).

8.4.1. Anterior Thigh Muscles

The large anterior portion of the thigh houses the muscles of the front thighs, hip flexors, and knee extensors. An overview of all these muscles' neural supplies, connections, and main purposes can be found in Figure 8.10 The muscles of the front thigh are (Hallock, 1984) (Figure 8.10):

- The flattened quadrangular Pectineus muscle is situated in the front of the superomedial side of the thigh. The iliacus and psoas muscles combine to produce the iliopsoas, which is the main flexor of the hips.

The larger pelvic and abdominal walls house the meaty parts of the two muscles. When these reach the thighs, they unite by passing through the inguinal ligament and attaching to the thigh's trochanter. They hold a unique ability to initiate motion and keep it going (fixate). In addition, the aforementioned muscles maintain appropriate lumbar lordosis during standing, which influences compensatory thoracic kyphosis (spinal column curvature) (Koshima et al., 2005).

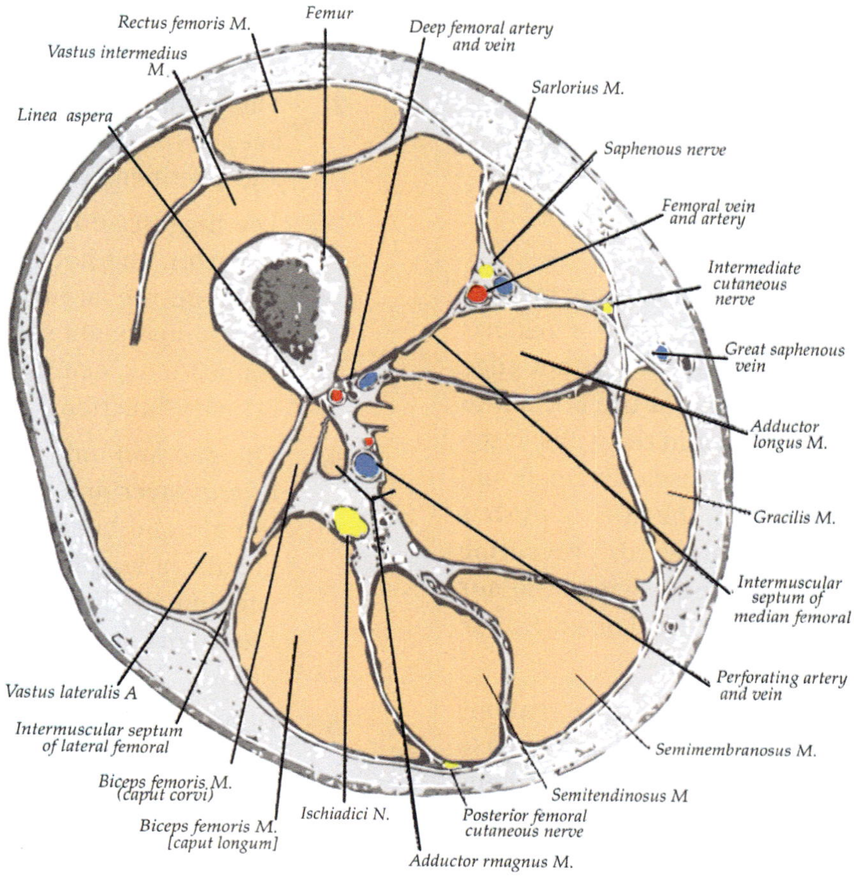

Figure 8.10. *Anterior and medial thigh muscles.*

Source: By Henry Vandyke Carter – Henry Gray, (1918). Anatomy of the human body (see "Book" section below) Bartleby.com: Gray's Anatomy, Plate 432, Public Domain; https://commons.wikimedia.org/w/index.php?curid=3450591.

Sartorius, also known as the tailor's muscle (L sart, a tailor), is a long, ribbon-like muscle that crosses the supero-anterior region of the thighs transversely (from medial to lateral). It is the front thigh's most noticeable superficial muscle. When bilaterally active, the muscle moves the knee and hip joints to position the limbs in the cross-legged sitting position. Since none of the movements are very strong, they are mainly produced by a synergist that collaborates with other leg muscles.

The Quadriceps femoris, sometimes known as the "four-headed femoral muscle," is the major knee extensor and the principal component of the front leg muscles. It almost completely encloses the femur's anterior aspect and edges. Four components make up a particular muscle:

- The "kicking muscle," or rectus femoris (*L. rectus*, direct), traverses the hip and aids in iliopsoas flexion. Hip flexion reduces its capacity to extend the knees (Mechelli et al., 2019).
- Vastus lateralis: the biggest quadriceps muscle, running the entire course of the lateral thighs.

- Vastus medialis spans the middle side of the distant 2/3 of the thigh, while vastus intermedius reaches deeper to the rectus femoris in between vastus lateralis and vastus medialis (Agyapong-Badu et al., 2014).

The branch of the vastus intermedius muscle, commonly referred to as the articularis genus, attaches at the top to the bottom edge of the front of the femur and at the bottom to the synovium of the patella and the walls of the suprapatellar bursa. This muscle is small and flat. During knee extension, the muscle pushes the synovial membranes upward, preventing them from getting caught between the femur and patella inside the knee joint (Loeb & Hoffer, 1985).

At the distal end of the leg, the tendons from each of the four quadriceps muscle groups combine to form the quadriceps tendons. Following the kneecap's insertion, the quadriceps tendons form the patellar ligament (ligamentum patellae), which is attached to the tibial tuberosity. The vastus medialis and lateralis separately attach to the kneecap along the path that leads to the anterior aspect of the tibial component. These connections form the lateral and medial patellar retinacula, which reinforce the knee capsules on either side of the kneecap. By shifting the tendon anteriorly and away from the plane of the joint, the kneecap provides the quadriceps with increased traction, enabling it to reach the tibia with a mechanical advantage (Loeb et al., 1985).

8.4.2. Medial Thigh Muscles

The middle segment of the thighs contains the adductor group of muscles, which are largely activated by the obturator nerves. The members of the adductor group are (Angrigiani et al., 2001):

1. The adductor longus, which is the most frontal.
2. The adductor brevis, which is deeper (posterior) to the adductor and pectineus longus muscles.
3. The biggest adductor muscle, adductor, and hamstrings sections make up the adductor magnus. The components vary in their connections, neural supplies, and primary functions.
4. The one and only adductor muscle to crossover and function at both the hip and knee joints is the gracilis, a lengthy, strap-like muscle running all along the midline side of the thighs and knees (Satake et al., 2014).
5. Obturator externus is a fan-shaped muscle that is firmly ingrained in the superomedial region of the thighs.

The adductor hiatus is the gap located between the tendons of the hamstrings and the distant aponeurotic connection of the adductor portion of the adductor magnus (Eom et al., 2011).

The popliteal fossa, located behind the knees, receives the femoral arteries and veins as they exit the thigh's appendicular skeleton. The main job of the muscles in the adductor family is to raise the hip joint. These are employed in the event of a side-to-side transition, to maintain posture while resting on both legs, and to counteract lateral body swaying. The adductors assist in stretching the hip when it is contracted and bending it when it is stretched during sprinting or working against resistance (Persichetti et al., 2003).

8.5. Neurovascular Structures and Relationships in Anteromedial Thigh

8.5.1. Femoral Triangle and Adductor Canal

The femoral triangle is a subfascial region located in the anterosuperior part of the thighs. When the thighs are contracted, abducted, or twisted, it appears as a triangular dip below the inguinal ligament.

- The femoral ligament, which also serves as the femoral triangle's foundation, and the adductor longus, which constitutes its middle, encircle it.
- Laterally, it is positioned by the sartorius; the peak is located where the sartorius' medial boundary intersects the adductor longus' sideways boundary (Grob et al., 2015).

The femoral triangle's muscular flooring is composed of the iliopsoas (laterally) and the pectineus (medially). The roof of the triangle is composed of the epidermis, fascia lata, subcutaneous tissue, and cribriform fascia. The trunks and abdominopelvic chamber are connected to the lower extremity of the limb by the retro-inguinal gap, which reaches deeper to the inguinal ligament. The separation is brought about by the inguinal ligament bridging the gap between the pubic tubercle and ASIS. The region is divided into two sections by the iliopsoas fascia. The laterally oriented portion acts as the muscle segment where the femoral nerves and the iliopsoas muscle pass, while the middle segment allows blood vessels, veins, and lymphatics to travel between the femoral triangle and the larger pelvis (Stewart et al., 2019).

Prominent components of the said triangle, from sideways to middle, are the following:

- The femoral nerve and its (end) branches.
- The femoral artery, along with its multiple branches.
- The femoral vein, along with its closest branches.
- The unique femoral canal.
- The lymph vessels that connect the deeper inguinal lymph nodes.

The femoral vein and artery, which run from and to the adductor canals at the summit of the triangle, are located in the femoral triangle. The adductor canal, sometimes referred to as the sub-sartorial canal or Hunter canal, extends from the tip of the triangle to the adductor hiatus in the adductor magnus tendon, where it crosses over the adductor longus at the point where another sartorius muscle bridges (Lubowitz, 2009). An intermuscular pathway leads the femoral artery and vein, saphenous nerves, and vastus medialis nervous system to the popliteal fossa, where they become popliteal arteries. The adductor longus and adductor magnus form the adductor canal's lateral and anterior borders, respectively, while the sartorius fills in the space between the aforementioned muscles to form the canal's ceiling (Jiamton & Apivatthakakul, 2015).

8.5.2. Femoral Nerve

The femoral nerve (L2–L4) is the main branch off of the lumbar plexus. From its source in the psoas major muscle in the abdomen, the nerve runs posterior-laterally into the pelvis, eventually reaching the midpoint of the inguinal ligament. After passing deeper into this ligament (within the muscle segment of the retro-inguinal area), it then reaches the femoral triangle and travels laterally to the femoral blood vessels (Vloka et al., 1999). When the femoral nerve reaches the triangle, it divides into several terminal branches that innervate the muscles of the upper leg. It also gives rise to articular branches to the hip and knee joints, as well as cutaneous branches to the anterior-medial aspect of the leg. The final cutaneous branch of the femoral nerve, the saphenous nerve, exits the triangle and courses alongside the femoral sheath where the femoral blood vessels are located. The saphenous nerve continues alongside the major vein and artery through the adductor canal when the femoral vessels pass through the adductor hiatus. It then becomes superficial by passing between the gracilis and the sartorius muscles at this point. Running antero-inferiorly, the saphenous nerve supplies the skin and fascia on the anterior-medial surfaces of the knee, foot, and leg (Ishiguro et al., 2012) (Figure 8.11).

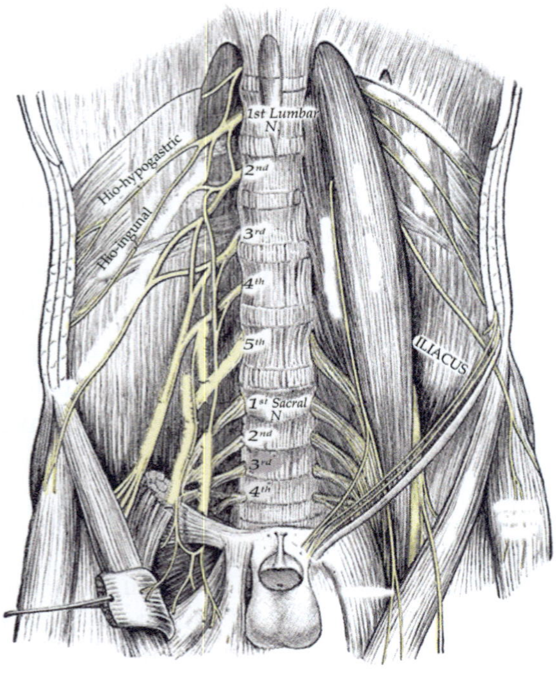

Figure 8.11. *The femoral nerve.*

Source: By Henry Vandyke Carter – Henry Gray, (1918). Anatomy of the human body (see "Book" section below) Bartleby.com: Gray's Anatomy, Plate 823, Public Domain; https://commons.wikimedia.org/w/index.php?curid=541679.

8.5.3. Femoral Sheath

The femoral sheath, a spiral fascial tube of varying length (typically three to four centimeters) that extends deep to the inguinal ligament and forms the femoral canal above it, encloses the basal portions of the femoral vessels. The sheath is created by inferiorly prolonging the transversalis and iliopsoas fascia that emerge from the abdominal region/pelvis (Salsbury, 1937). The femoral sheath does not shield the femoral nerve. The lower border of the sheath terminates at the tunica adventitia, the loose collagenous covering of the femoral vessels. The median border of a long femoral sheath is breached by the great saphenous vein and lymph vessels. The femoral sheath allows the femoral vein and artery to glide smoothly down to the inguinal ligament when the hip moves. The femoral sheath is divided into three sections by straight septa of extraperitoneal fibrous tissue that extend from the belly along the femoral arteries.

The sideways segment houses the femoral artery, the middle segment houses the femoral vein, and the lowest segment houses the femoral canal. These are the segments of the femoral sheath (Skandalakis et al., 1989).

The lowest of the three segments is the femoral canal. It is small and cone-shaped and is located between the femoral vein and the midline border of the femoral sheath. The femoral canal has the following characteristics (Lata et al., 2018):

1. The basal margin of the saphenous aperture is where the femoral canal extends beyond.
2. It includes lax connective tissue, fats, a few lymph vessels, and occasionally a deeper inguinal lymphatic node.
3. It permits the femoral vein to enlarge whenever circulatory flow

out from the lower extremity of the limb is enhanced and whenever increasing intra-abdominal stress produces a brief stagnation in the veins (Cloquet node) (Schnyder et al., 2001).

The femoral canal is formed by the basal orifice at its abdominal end, which is modest in diameter (about 1 centimeter) and functions as the femoral rings. The pectineal ligament wraps the upper ramus of the pubic area downward; the femoral septum is situated between the femoral canal and the femoral vein; the lacunar ligament is located centrally; the median half of the inguinal ligament is located apically (Nobel et al., 1980).

8.5.4. Femoral Artery

The external iliac artery branches off to form the femoral artery, which serves as the major artery to the lower limb and extends distal to the inguinal ligament. The femoral artery (Schnyder et al., 2001):

1. Joins the femoral triangle deeper to the midway of the inguinal ligament (currently halfway between both the ASIS and the pubic tubercle); buried dormant to the fascia lata; drops on the surrounding boundaries of the iliopsoas as well as pectineus;
2. Splits the femoral triangle in half and enters the adductor canal at the top, deeper to the sartorius.
3. Leaves the adductor canal by traversing the adductor gap and then changing its name to the popliteal (afferent) artery (Siddharth et al., 1985).

The profunda femoris artery is the main artery that reaches the thighs and the largest branching of the femoral artery. It begins where the artery is, at the aforementioned triangle. It is divided from the femoral vein and artery in the middle of the thigh by the adductor longus. Three to four perforating arteries emerge and wrap around the back of the thigh to supply the muscles of the hamstring, the adductor magnus, and the vastus lateralis (Grier & Hartnell, 1990). The circumflex femoral artery arises from the profunda femoris artery, though it can also develop on its own. These arteries anastomose with each other and adjacent arteries to supply the femoral muscles and the closest end of the thigh (Turi, 2008). The majority of the circulation to the neck and head of the thigh is supplied by the middle circumflex femoral artery and the rear retinacular arteries, along with their branches. It runs very deep (anterior) between the iliopsoas and pectineus at the back of the femur neck, where it meets the quadratus femoris. The lateral circumflex femoral artery crosses the joints sideways to mainly supply blood to the musculature of the thigh (Irani et al., 2009).

8.5.5. Femoral Vein

In the vicinity of the adductor gap, the popliteal veins continue into the femoral vein. As it ascends into the adductor canal, the femoral vein is only posterior-lateral after moving dorsal to the main artery. The femoral vein travels lateral to the femoral sheathing and the femoral canal. It becomes the external iliac vein as it passes behind the inguinal ligament (Warkentine et al., 2008). In the lower part of the triangle, the profunda femoris veins, the great saphenous veins, and other branches enter the femoral vein. This femoral profunda femoris, or deeper vein, joins the femoral vein below the inguinal ligament and descends to the great saphenous vein's terminus. Three to four puncturing veins combine to form it (Moore et al., 2011).

8.5.6. Obturator Artery and Nerve

The origin of the obturator arteries is usually the internal iliac artery. In approximately 20% of cases, an expanded pelvic branching of the lower epigastric artery replaces or attaches the obturator arteries (Akata et al., 1999). Following its penetration of the obturator foramen in the middle segment of the thighs, the obturator artery divides into anterior and posterior branches that cross the adductor brevis muscles.

The obturator artery supplies blood to the pectineus, obturator externus, gracilis, and adductors of thighs. The femur end is fed by an acetabular branching that arises from its posterior offshoot (Sañudo et al., 2011). Together with the obturator vein and artery, the obturator nerves (L2–L4) enter the obturator foramen to enter the thighs. It is distributed evenly across the psoas muscle's medial surface. Similar to channels, it divides into posterior and anterior branching that crosses the adductor brevis. The front stream supplies the adductor brevis, adductor longus, gracilis, and pectineus, while the rear stream supplies the adductor magnus and the obturator externus (Kendir et al., 2008).

8.6. Gluteal and Posterior Thigh Regions

The gluteal region, encompassing the hips and buttocks, is situated behind the pelvic region. Its lower boundary is marked by gluteal folds, while its upper boundary is defined by the iliac crest, greater trochanter, and ASIS. Gluteal wrinkles separate the upper leg from the lower buttock (Ramirez et al., 1984).

The intergluteal fissure divides the buttocks from one another. The skeletal pelvis is composed of the sacral and tailbone bones and joints, which are connected by the gluteal tendons. The sacrotuberous and sacrospinous ligaments form the larger and smaller sciatic foramina from the sciatic grooves in the hips. The great sciatic foramen is a passageway for tissues that enter or exit the pelvis, as opposed to the smaller sciatic foramen, which channels tissues that enter or exit the groin area. Imagine the great sciatic foramen as the gate that allows blood vessels and arteries to leave the pelvis and enter the gluteal region. Through this opening, arteries and neurons leave the pelvis (Hurwitz & Walton, 1982) (Figure 8.12).

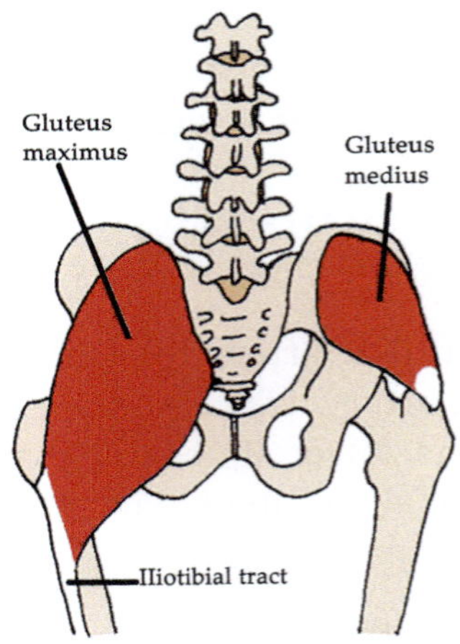

Figure 8.12. *Gluteal regions.*

Source: CC BY-SA 3.0; https://commons.wikimedia.org/w/index.php?curid=545381.

8.6.1. Gluteal Muscles

There are two layers to the gluteal muscles: the deep (not shallow) and the superficial (shallow). The external surface is composed of the tensor fasciae latae and the three glutei (medius, maximus, and minimus). The gluteus maximus primarily facilitates sideways rotations and flexion of the hip joint (Flack et al., 2012). It is most effective when transitioning from a flexed to a standing position, such as when standing up from a seated or bent position, climbing stairs, or sprinting. Beside the gluteus (maximus) is the fan-shaped gluteus medius and minimus. These are the medial abductors and provide better, more precise results from the thigh. The tensor fasciae latae is located on the side of the hip, between two layers of fascia lata. The tensor fasciae latae is an abductor of the hip and a midline spinner, but it usually doesn't work by itself (Mendieta, 2006). It produces flexion when combined with the rectus femoris and iliopsoas. The tensor fasciae latae further tenses the fascia lata and iliotibial tract, helping to stabilize the thigh on the tibia when standing (Centeno & Young, 2006). The obturator internus, piriformis, inferior and superior gemelli, as well as quadratus femoris are among the minor muscles that make up the deeper layer. The above muscles, which are sideways rotators of the thighs and are protected by the inferior part of the gluteus maximus, aid in maintaining the hip joint by supporting the femoral head in the acetabulum alongside the powerful tendons of the hip (Mendieta & Sood, 2018).

8.6.2. Gluteal Bursae

Gluteal bursae are flat membrane pouches that contain a synovial capillary layer, separating the gluteus maximus from other organs. The bursae are positioned in abrasion-prone areas, such as the space between a tendon and a skeletal protrusion, to reduce resistance and allow for unhindered mobility. The following bursae are connected to the gluteus maximus (Lequesne et al., 2008):

1. The ischial bursa connects the lower boundary of the gluteus maximus to the ischial tuberosity.
2. The trochanteric bursa divides the deeper face of the gluteus maximus from the larger trochanter of the thigh.
3. The upper portion of the basal connection of the vastus lateralis is separated from the iliotibial tract by the gluteofemoral bursa (Walsh et al., 2011).

8.6.3. Posterior Thigh Muscles

The three primary hamstring muscles that comprise the back of the thighs (the long head) are the semimembranosus, semitendinosus, and biceps femoris. The hamstrings, which originate from the ischial tuberosity and extend deeper to the gluteus maximus before inserting on the femurs, are innervated by the tibial subdivision of the sciatic nerve. They cover and have an impact on the flexion and extension of the knee and hip joints, respectively. One cannot maximize the effectiveness of both activities at the same time (Abe et al., 2016). A full range of extension knees shortens the hamstring muscles, making it impossible for them to tighten further and enlarge the hip joint. A full-extension hip also shortens these hamstrings, preventing them from affecting the knees. When the thigh and leg remain still, the hamstrings may help extend the body at the hips. They are always engaged in hip extension, such as when maintaining an upright posture, with the exception of complete knee flexion.

The fourth muscle group in the posterior segment is not the hamstrings; rather, it is the small head of the biceps femoris, which only crosses the knee joints and is innervated by the fibular subdivision of the sciatic nerve (Hupkens et al., 2013).

A Closer Look

Mortality After Lower Extremity Amputation

Mortality after lower extremity amputation is a significant concern, reflecting the complex interplay of underlying health conditions, the severity of the disease leading to amputation, and the postoperative care received. Lower extremity amputations, often necessitated by peripheral arterial disease (PAD), diabetes, or trauma, carry a high risk of morbidity and mortality, with various factors influencing patient outcomes.

The immediate postoperative period is critical. Studies indicate that the 30-day mortality rate following major lower extremity amputation can range from 5% to 15%, with higher rates observed in older patients and those with comorbid conditions such as cardiovascular disease, renal insufficiency, or severe diabetes. The risk of complications, including infections, cardiac events, and thromboembolic events, is heightened during this period, necessitating vigilant medical supervision.

Long-term mortality rates are even more striking. One-year mortality rates following major amputations, such as above-knee or below-knee amputations, can exceed 30%, with five-year mortality rates approaching 50% to 70%. These rates are comparable to those seen in some malignancies, underscoring the severe impact of the underlying health issues that necessitate amputation. Factors contributing to long-term mortality include the progression of cardiovascular disease, renal failure, recurrent infections, and the high prevalence of comorbidities in this patient population.

Diabetes is a significant factor influencing mortality after lower extremity amputation. Diabetic patients are more prone to complications such as poor wound healing and infections due to impaired immune responses and vascular complications. Additionally, the presence of diabetic nephropathy or retinopathy can further complicate the clinical picture and contribute to higher mortality rates.

Peripheral arterial disease, often coexisting with diabetes, is another critical determinant of outcomes post-amputation. The severity of PAD can lead to significant ischemia and tissue necrosis, necessitating more extensive amputations, which are associated with higher mortality rates compared to minor amputations like toe or foot amputations. Moreover, PAD patients often have widespread atherosclerosis, impacting not just the limbs but also coronary and cerebral arteries, thereby increasing the risk of fatal cardiovascular events.

Socioeconomic factors and access to healthcare also play vital roles in determining outcomes. Patients with limited access to postoperative rehabilitation and prosthetic services may experience reduced mobility and independence, leading to secondary complications such as pressure ulcers, muscle atrophy, and cardiovascular deconditioning, all of which can increase mortality risk. Psychological factors, including depression and reduced quality of life, are also critical as they can affect recovery and long-term survival. Efforts to reduce mortality after lower extremity amputation focus on comprehensive preoperative assessment and optimization of the patient's medical condition, meticulous surgical technique, and robust postoperative care. This includes managing cardiovascular risks, ensuring effective wound care, preventing infections, and facilitating rehabilitation and psychosocial support. Early involvement of a multidisciplinary team, including surgeons, internists, rehabilitation specialists, and social workers, is crucial for improving patient outcomes.

In summary, mortality after lower extremity amputation remains high, influenced by a range of medical, surgical, and socio-economic factors. Addressing these challenges requires a holistic approach, targeting both the underlying causes necessitating amputation and the multifaceted needs of patient's post-surgery. Improving preoperative optimization, enhancing surgical techniques, and providing comprehensive postoperative care can help reduce mortality rates and improve the quality of life for patients undergoing these life-altering procedures.

Summary

- The lower limb is a crucial part of the human anatomy, primarily responsible for supporting the body's weight, facilitating locomotion, and maintaining balance.
- The hip joint, where the lower limb connects to the pelvis, is a ball-and-socket joint that allows for a high degree of motion in multiple directions. It provides stability and strength needed for weight-bearing activities.
- Body weight is distributed from the vertebrae to the pelvic girdle through all the sacroiliac joints, first from the pelvic girdle towards the hips, to the femur bone (*L. femora*), and finally to the knees and ankles.
- Ischium, pubis, and ilium are the three main bones that fuse together to form every adult's hip bone. These bones still are divided by something like a triradiate ligament during adolescence.
- The acetabulum, the cup-shaped chamber (hole) on the lateral edge of the hip for articulating with the femoral head, is made up of part of the superior portion of the hip bone, which is the upper and greatest component of the hip.
- The trochanters, two massive, blunt peaks, are located where the collar and rod connect. The round tip of the cone lesser trochanter reaches medially from the posterior-medial portion of the neck of the femur and shaft juncture.
- The patella, often known as the cap of the knee, is a substantial sesamoid bony structure that develops intravenously upon birth. This triangle-shaped bone connects to the patellar region of the femur and is situated forward to the femoral condyles.
- The massive, load-bearing tibia (shinbone) conveys at its distal and proximal ends long with the femoral condyles apically, the talus at the lower border, and the fibula at the lateral position.
- The skinny fibula, which is primarily used for the attachment of muscles, is located posterior-laterally to the tibia. The fibula has a broad collar in front of an expanded cap at its closest end.
- The talus, cuboid, calcaneus, navicular, and 3 cuneiform bones make up the tarsus. The legs' bones only connect with the talus. The biggest and sturdiest bone in the feet is the calcaneus (heelbone). It connects anteriorly with the cube-shaped and superiorly with the talus.
- The epidermis of the lower extremity of the limb is supplied by cutaneous neurons in the subcutaneous tissue. These neurons are extensions of the sacral and lumbar sensory nerves, with the exception of a few in the proximal portion of the limbs.
- The formation of a prominent gluteal area is intimately linked to the adoption of bipedalism and an erect posture. The modification of the femur shape required for bipedal walking allows for superior positioning of the thigh abductors into the gluteal region.
- The major branching of the lumbar plexus is the femoral nerve (L2–L4). The inguinal ligament midway is reached by the neuron as it drops posterior-laterally into the pelvis from its source in the psoas major in the belly.

- The popliteal veins continue into the femoral vein close to the adductor gap. The femoral vein is dorsal to the main artery but then just posterior-lateral as it moves up into the adductor canal.

References

1. Abe, T., Loenneke, J. P., & Thiebaud, R. S. (2016). Ultrasound assessment of hamstring muscle size using posterior thigh muscle thickness. *Clinical Physiology and Functional Imaging, 36*(3), 206–210.
2. Abulhasan, J. F., & Grey, M. J. (2017). Anatomy and physiology of knee stability. *Journal of Functional Morphology and Kinesiology, 2*(4), 34.
3. Agyapong-Badu, S., Warner, M., Samuel, D., Narici, M., Cooper, C., & Stokes, M. (2014). Anterior thigh composition measured using ultrasound imaging to quantify relative thickness of muscle and non-contractile tissue: A potential biomarker for musculoskeletal health. *Physiological Measurement, 35*(10), 2165.
4. Akata, T., Murakami, J., & Yoshinaga, A. (1999). Life-threatening hemorrhage following obturator artery injury during transurethral bladder surgery: A sequel of an unsuccessful obturator nerve block. *Acta Anesthesiologic Scandinavica, 43*(7), 784–788.
5. Angrigiani, C., Grilli, D., & Thorne, C. H. (2001). The adductor flap: A new method for transferring posterior and medial thigh skin. *Plastic and Reconstructive Surgery, 107*(7), 1725–1731.
6. Byrne, D. P., Mulhall, K. J., & Baker, J. F. (2010). Anatomy & biomechanics of the hip. *The Open Sports Medicine Journal, 4*(1) 51-57.
7. Capdevila, X., Biboulet, P., Morau, D., Bernard, N., Deschodt, J., Lopez, S., & d'Athis, F. (2002). Continuous three-in-one block for postoperative pain after lower limb orthopedic surgery: Where do the catheters go? *Anesthesia & Analgesia, 94*(4), 1001–1006.
8. Centeno, R. F., & Young, V. L. (2006). Clinical anatomy in aesthetic gluteal body contouring surgery. *Clinics in Plastic Surgery, 33*(3), 347–358.
9. Chatterjee, S. S. (2012). Venous ulcers of the lower limb: Where do we stand? *Indian Journal of Plastic Surgery, 45*(2), 266.
10. Cormack, G. C., & Lamberty, B. G. H. (1984). Fasciocutaneous vessels. *Anatomia Clinica, 6*(2), 121–131.
11. Della Croce, U., Cappozzo, A., & Kerrigan, D. C. (1999). Pelvis and lower limb anatomical landmark calibration precision and its propagation to bone geometry and joint angles. *Medical & Biological Engineering & Computing, 37*(2), 155–161.
12. Dixon, A. F. (1910). The architecture of the cancellous tissue forming the upper end of the femur. *Journal of Anatomy and Physiology, 44*(Pt 3), 223.
13. Eom, J. S., Sun, S. H., & Hong, J. P. (2011). Use of the upper medial thigh perforator flap (gracilis perforator flap) for lower extremity reconstruction. *Plastic and Reconstructive Surgery, 127*(2), 731–737.
14. Flack, N. A. M. S., Nicholson, H. D., & Woodley, S. J. (2012). A review of the anatomy of the hip abductor muscles, gluteus medius, gluteus minimus, and tensor fascia lata. *Clinical Anatomy, 25*(6), 697–708.

15. Fox, A. J., Wanivenhaus, F., & Rodeo, S. A. (2012). The basic science of the patella: Structure, composition, and function. *The Journal of Knee Surgery, 25*(02), 127–142.

16. Garden, R. S. (1961). The structure and function of the proximal end of the femur. *The Journal of Bone and Joint Surgery. British Volume, 43*(3), 576–589.

17. Grand, T. I. (1968). The functional anatomy of the lower limb of the howler monkey (*Alouatta caraya*). *American Journal of Physical Anthropology, 28*(2), 163–181.

18. Grier, D., & Hartnell, G. (1990). Percutaneous femoral artery puncture: Practice and anatomy. *The British Journal of Radiology, 63*(752), 602–604.

19. Grob, K., Monahan, R., Gilbey, H., Yap, F., Filgueira, L., & Kuster, M. (2015). Distal extension of the direct anterior approach to the hip poses risk to neurovascular structures: An anatomical study. *JBJS, 97*(2), 126–132.

20. Haertsch, P. (1981). The blood supply to the skin of the leg: A post-mortem investigation. *British Journal of Plastic Surgery, 34*(4), 470–477.

21. Hallock, G. G. (1991). Simultaneous transposition of anterior thigh muscle and fascia flaps: An introduction to the chimera flap principle. *Annals of Plastic Surgery, 27*(2), 126–131.

22. Hupkens, P., Ozturk, E., Wittens, S., Hoevenaren, I. A., Kooloos, J. G., & Ulrich, D. J. (2013). Posterior thigh perforator flaps: An anatomical study to localize and classify posterior thigh perforators. *Microsurgery, 33*(5), 376–382.

23. Hurwitz, D. J., & Walton, R. L. (1982). Closure of chronic wounds of the perineal and sacral regions using the gluteal thigh flap. *Annals of Plastic Surgery, 8*(5), 375–386.

24. Hwang, M. D., Piefer, J. W., & Lubowitz, J. H. (2012). Anterior cruciate ligament tibial footprint anatomy: Systematic review of the 21st century literature. *Arthroscopy: The Journal of Arthroscopic & Related Surgery, 28*(5), 728–734.

25. Irani, F., Kumar, S., & Colyer Jr, W. R. (2009). Common femoral artery access techniques: A review. *Journal of Cardiovascular Medicine, 10*(7), 517–522.

26. Ishiguro, S., Yokochi, A., Yoshioka, K., Asano, N., Deguchi, A., Iwasaki, Y., & Maruyama, K. (2012). Anatomy and clinical implications of ultrasound-guided selective femoral nerve block. *Anesthesia & Analgesia, 115*(6), 1467–1470.

27. Jiamton, C., & Apivatthakakul, T. (2015). The safety and feasibility of minimally invasive plate osteosynthesis (MIPO) on the medial side of the femur: A cadaveric injection study. *Injury, 46*(11), 2170–2176.

28. Jotoku, T., Kinoshita, M., Okuda, R., & Abe, M. (2006). Anatomy of ligamentous structures in the tarsal sinus and canal. *Foot & Ankle International, 27*(7), 533–538.

29. Kachlik, D., Pechacek, V., Hnatkova, G., Hnatek, L., Musil, V., & Baca, V. (2019). The venous perforators of the lower limb–A new terminology. *Phlebology, 34*(10), 650–668.

30. Kendir, S., Akkaya, T., Comert, A., Sayin, M., Tatlisumak, E., Elhan, A., & Tekdemir, I. (2008). The location of the obturator nerve: A three-dimensional description of the obturator canal. *Surgical and Radiologic Anatomy, 30*(6), 495–501.

31. King-Heiden, T. C., & Litster, M. (2019). Using case-study based modules to promote a better understanding of evolution in an undergraduate anatomy and physiology course. *Journal of Biological Education, 53*(5), 477–491.

32. Koshima, I., Fujitsu, M., Ushio, S., Sugiyama, N., & Yamashita, S. (2005). Flow-through anterior thigh flaps with a short pedicle for reconstruction of lower leg and foot defects. *Plastic and Reconstructive Surgery, 115*(1), 155–162.

33. LaMont, J. G. (1986). Functional anatomy of the lower limb. *Clinics in Plastic Surgery, 13*(4), 571–579.

34. Lata, K., Kaki, A., Grines, C., Blank, N., Elder, M., & Schreiber, T. (2018). Pre-close technique of percutaneous closure for delayed hemostasis of large-bore femoral sheaths. *Journal of Interventional Cardiology, 31*(4), 504–510.

35. Lequesne, M., Mathieu, P., Vuillemin-Bodaghi, V., Bard, H., & Djian, P. (2008). Gluteal tendinopathy in refractory greater trochanter pain syndrome: Diagnostic value of two clinical tests. *Arthritis Care & Research, 59*(2), 241–246.

36. Lidman, D., Nettelblad, H., Berggren, A., & Rajan, S. (1987). Reconstruction of soft tissue defects including the Achilles tendon with free neurovascular tensor fascia lata flap and fascia lata: Case report. *Scandinavian Journal of Plastic and Reconstructive Surgery, 21*(2), 213–218.

37. Loeb, G. E., & Hoffer, J. A. (1985). Activity of spindle afferents from cat anterior thigh muscles. II. Effects of fusimotor blockade. *Journal of Neurophysiology, 54*(3), 565–577.

38. Loeb, G. E., Hoffer, J. A., & Marks, W. B. (1985). Activity of spindle afferents from cat anterior thigh muscles. III. Effects of external stimuli. *Journal of Neurophysiology, 54*(3), 578–591.

39. Lubowitz, J. H. (2009). Anteromedial portal technique for the anterior cruciate ligament femoral socket: Pitfalls and solutions. *Arthroscopy: The Journal of Arthroscopic & Related Surgery, 25*(1), 95–101.

40. Macchiarelli, R., Bondioli, L., Galichon, V., & Tobias, P. V. (1999). Hip bone trabecular architecture shows uniquely distinctive locomotor behavior in South African australopithecines. *Journal of Human Evolution, 36*(2), 211–232.

41. Macefield, G., Gandevia, S. C., & Burke, D. (1989). Conduction velocities of muscle and cutaneous afferents in the upper and lower limbs of human subjects. *Brain, 112*(6), 1519–1532.

42. McCormick, D. W., & Blount, W. P. (1949). Metatarsus adductovarus: Skewfoot. *Journal of the American Medical Association, 141*(7), 449–453.

43. Mechelli, F., Arendt-Nielsen, L., Stokes, M., & Agyapong-Badu, S. (2019). Validity of ultrasound imaging versus magnetic resonance imaging for measuring anterior thigh muscle, subcutaneous fat, and fascia thickness. *Methods and Protocols, 2*(3), 58.

44. Mendieta, C. G. (2006). Classification system for gluteal evaluation. *Clinics in Plastic Surgery, 33*(3), 333–346.

45. Mendieta, C. G., & Sood, A. (2018). Classification system for gluteal evaluation: Revisited. *Clinics in Plastic Surgery, 45*(2), 159–177.

46. Moore, H. M., Gohel, M., & Davies, A. H. (2011). Number and location of venous valves within the popliteal and femoral veins–A review of the literature. *Journal of Anatomy, 219*(4), 439–443.

47. Nakajima, T., Sakamoto, M., Tazoe, T., Endoh, T., & Komiyama, T. (2006). Location specificity of plantar cutaneous reflexes involving lower limb muscles in humans. *Experimental Brain Research, 175*(3), 514–525.

48. Nicolaides, A. N., Allegra, C., Bergan, J., Bradbury, A., Cairols, M., Carpentier, P., & Taft, A.

(2008). Management of chronic venous disorders of the lower limb's guidelines according to scientific evidence. *International Angiology, 27*(1), 1.

49. Niranjan, N. S., Price, R. D., & Govilkar, P. S. (2000). Fascial feeder and perforator-based VY advancement flaps in the reconstruction of lower limb defects. *British Journal of Plastic Surgery, 53*(8), 679–689.
50. Nobel, W., Marks, S. C., & Kubik, S. (1980). The anatomical basis for femoral nerve palsy following iliacus hematoma. *Journal of Neurosurgery, 52*(4), 533–540.
51. Novas, F. E. (1989). The tibia and tarsus in Herrerasauridae (Dinosauria, incertae sedis) and the origin and evolution of the dinosaurian tarsus. *Journal of Paleontology, 63*(5), 677–690.
52. O'Hare, P. M., Leonard, A. G., & Brennen, M. D. (1983). Experience with the tensor fasciae latae free flap. *British Journal of Plastic Surgery, 36*(1), 98–104.
53. Persichetti, P., Simone, P., Berloco, M., Casadei, R. M., Marangi, G. F., Cagli, B., & Di Lella, F. (2003). Vulvo-perineal reconstruction: Medial thigh septo-fascio-cutaneous island flap. *Annals of Plastic Surgery, 50*(1), 85–89.
54. Raes, E. V., Bergman, E. H., van der Veen, H., Vanderperren, K., Van der Vekens, E., & Saunders, J. H. (2011). Comparison of cross-sectional anatomy and computed tomography of the tarsus in horses. *American Journal of Veterinary Research, 72*(9), 1209–1221.
55. Rajacic, N., Darweesh, M., Jayakrishnan, K., Gang, R. K., & Kojic, S. (1996). The distally based superficial sural flap for reconstruction of the lower leg and foot. *British Journal of Plastic Surgery, 49*(6), 383–389.
56. Ramirez, O. M., Hurwitz, D. J., & Futrell, J. W. (1984). The expansive gluteus maximus flap. *Plastic and Reconstructive Surgery, 74*(6), 757–770.
57. Ridola, C., & Palma, A. (2001). Functional anatomy and imaging of the foot. *Italian Journal of Anatomy and Embryology= Archivio Italiano di Anatomia ed Embriologia, 106*(2), 85–98.
58. Salsbury, C. R. (1937). The development of the femoral sheath. *Canadian Medical Association Journal, 37*(6), 579.
59. Sammarco, V. J. (2004). The talonavicular and calcaneocuboid joints: Anatomy, biomechanics, and clinical management of the transverse tarsal joint. *Foot and Ankle Clinics, 9*(1), 127–145.
60. Sanudo, J. R., Mirapeix, R., Rodriguez-Niedenführ, M., Maranillo, E., Parkin, I. G., & Vázquez, T. (2011). Obturator artery revisited. *International Urogynecology Journal, 22*(10), 1313–1318.
61. Satake, T., Muto, M., Ko, S., Yasumura, K., Ishikawa, T., & Maegawa, J. (2014). Breast reconstruction using free posterior medial thigh perforator flaps: Intraoperative anatomical study and clinical results. *Plastic and Reconstructive Surgery, 134*(5), 880–891.
62. Schmalzried, T. P., Akizuki, K. H., Fedenko, A. N., & Mirra, J. (1997). The role of access of joint fluid to bone in periarticular osteolysis: A report of four cases. *JBJS, 79*(3), 447–452.
63. Schnyder, G., Sawhney, N., Whisenant, B., Tsimikas, S., & Turi, Z. G. (2001). Common femoral artery anatomy is influenced by demographics and comorbidity: Implications for cardiac and peripheral invasive studies. *Catheterization and Cardiovascular Interventions, 53*(3), 289–295.
64. Shaer, W. D. (1984). Gluteal and thigh reduction: Reclassification, critical review, and improved technique for primary correction. *Aesthetic Plastic Surgery, 8*(3), 165–172.
65. Shinaoka, A., Koshimune, S., Suami, H., Yamada, K., Kumagishi, K., Boyages, J., & Ohtsuka, A.

(2020). Lower-limb lymphatic drainage pathways and lymph nodes: A CT lymphangiography cadaver study. *Radiology, 294*(1), 223–229.

66. Shoji, T., Yasunaga, Y., Yamasaki, T., Mori, R., Hamanishi, M., & Ochi, M. (2013). Bony impingement depends on the bone morphology of the hip after total hip arthroplasty. *International Orthopedics, 37*(10), 1897–1903.

67. Siddharth, P., Smith, N. L., Mason, R. A., & Giron, F. (1985). Variational anatomy of the deep femoral artery. *The Anatomical Record, 212*(2), 206–209.

68. Skandalakis, J. E., Gray, S. W., Skandalakis, L. J., Colborn, G. L., & Pemberton, L. B. (1989). Surgical anatomy of the inguinal area. *World Journal of Surgery, 13*(5), 490–498.

69. Stecco, C., Tiengo, C., Stecco, A., Porzionato, A., Macchi, V., Stern, R., & De Caro, R. (2013). Fascia redefined: Anatomical features and technical relevance in fascial flap surgery. *Surgical and Radiologic Anatomy, 35*(5), 369–376.

70. Stewart, M., Brassett, C., & Abood, A. (2019). Neurovascular Anatomy at the "Box Junction": Considerations in the Anterolateral Thigh Flap. *Journal of Reconstructive Microsurgery, 35*(04), 254–262.

71. Tomlinson, J. E., Rich Redding, W., Berry, C., & Smallwood, J. E. (2003). Computed tomographic anatomy of the equine tarsus. *Veterinary Radiology & Ultrasound, 44*(2), 174–178.

72. Topham, E. J., & Mortimer, P. S. (2002). Chronic lower limb oedema. *Clinical Medicine, 2*(1), 28.

73. Turi, Z. G. (2008). An evidence-based approach to femoral arterial access and closure. *Reviews in Cardiovascular Medicine, 9*(1), 6–19.

74. Uhl, J. F., & Gillot, C. (2007). Embryology and three-dimensional anatomy of the superficial venous system of the lower limbs. *Phlebology, 22*(5), 194–206.

75. Valente, G., Martelli, S., Taddei, F., Farinella, G., & Viceconti, M. (2012). Muscle discretization affects the loading transferred to bones in lower-limb musculoskeletal models. *Proceedings of the Institution of Mechanical Engineers, Part H: Journal of Engineering in Medicine, 226*(2), 161–169.

76. Vloka, J. D., Hadzic, A., Drobnik, L., Ernest, A., Reiss, W., & Thys, D. M. (1999). Anatomical landmarks for femoral nerve block: A comparison of four needle insertion sites. *Anesthesia & Analgesia, 89*(6), 1467.

77. Walsh, M. J., Walton, J. R., & Walsh, N. A. (2011). Surgical repair of the gluteal tendons: A report of 72 cases. *The Journal of Arthroplasty, 26*(8), 1514–1519.

78. Warkentine, F. H., Pierce, M. C., Lorenz, D., & Kim, I. K. (2008). The anatomic relationship of femoral vein to femoral artery in euvolemic pediatric patients by ultrasonography: Implications for pediatric femoral central venous access. *Academic Emergency Medicine, 15*(5), 426–430.

79. Weiner, D. (1996). Pathogenesis of slipped capital femoral epiphysis: Current concepts. *Journal of Pediatric Orthopedics. Part B, 5*(2), 67–73.

80. Weinert Jr, C. R., McMaster, J. H., & Ferguson, R. J. (1973). Dynamic function of the human fibula. *American Journal of Anatomy, 138*(2), 145–149.

Chapter 9

THE HEAD AND NECK

Contents

Introduction

The human head and neck region contain a multitude of structures that are necessary for many different functions, including sensory perception, communication, and basic physiological processes. It is an intricate and vital region of the body. This area contains the neck, which connects the head to the rest of the body and supports important structures like the trachea and esophagus, as well as the skull, which forms the structure of the face and protects the brain. The brain, which is the main component of the central nervous system, and the sense organs that are in charge of sight, hearing, smell, and taste—the eyes, ears, nose, and mouth—are all included in the head. The face is made up of complex muscles that allow for various expressions and eating and speaking functions. Important anatomical components of the neck include the cervical spine, which supports and moves the head, large blood vessels like the jugular veins and carotid arteries, and important nerves like the accessory and vagus nerves. The parathyroid and thyroid glands, which control calcium homeostasis and metabolism, are also housed there. The head is made up of the ears, the face, the brain, and its coverings. The cranium, or skull, is the skeleton of the head. Understanding the features of the skull offers a fundamental foundation for comprehending the head region (Holland et al., 1998).

The orbital cavity and the superior edge of the acoustic meatus are located in a flat direction due to the structural arrangement of the cranium; this is known as the cranium's anatomical position. The orbitomeatal plane is the most commonly used craniometric reference (Figure 9.1).

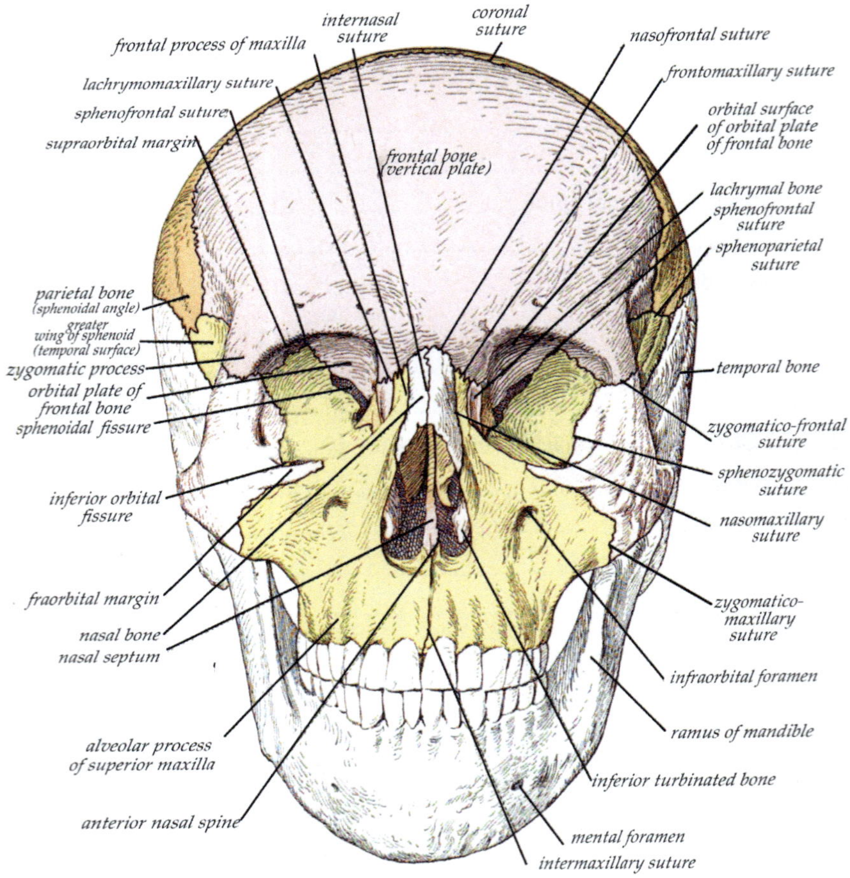

Figure 9.1. *Adult skull.*

Source: By Dr. Johannes Sobotta – Sobotta Atlas and Textbook of Human Anatomy 1909, Public Domain; https://commons.wikimedia.org/w/index.php?curid=29760948.

Orientation and Directional Terms

Term	Definition	Illustration
Orbital cavity	The orbital cavities are large bony sockets that house the eyeballs with associated muscles, nerves, blood vessels and fat. Each orbit is pear-shaped with the optic nerve representing the stem. The medial walls of the orbit are almost parallel and border the nasal cavity anteriorly.	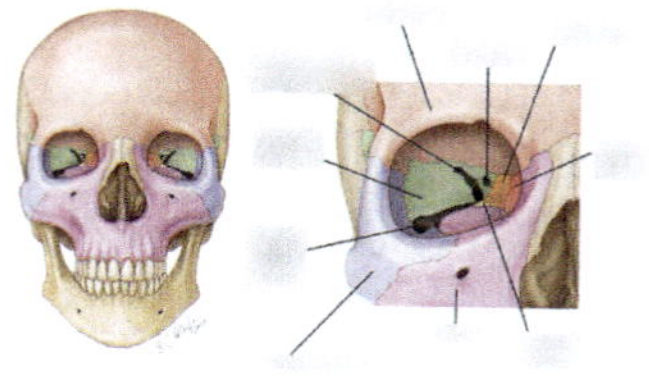
Neurocranium	The neurocranium, also known as the braincase, brainpan, or brain-pan, is the upper and back part of the skull, which forms a protective case around the brain. In the human skull, the neurocranium includes the calvaria or skullcap. The remainder of the skull is the facial skeleton.	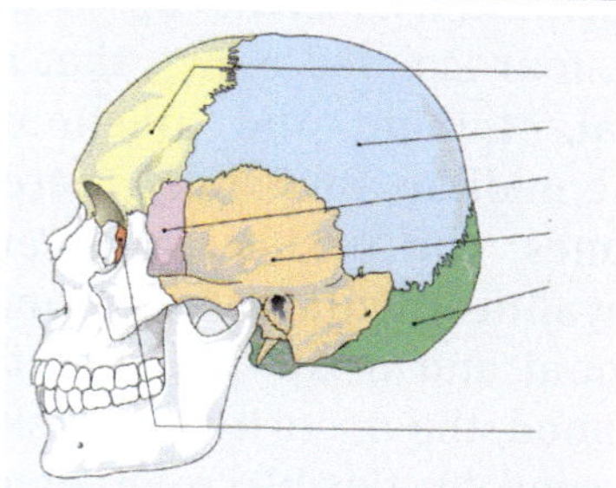
Zygomatic bones	One of a pair of bones on each upper side of the face that forms the cheek and part of the eye socket. The zygomatic bones help give shape and structure to the face and are connected to the jaw and bones near the ears, forehead, and skull.	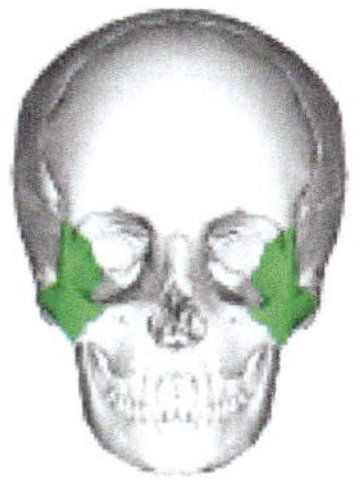
Cranial base	Cranial base is the most inferior part of the skull. It consists of the floor of the cranial cavity plus the inferior aspect of the viscerocranium, minus the mandible. Together with the cranial vault, which is the part of the skull that protects the brain, it contributes to the neurocranium.	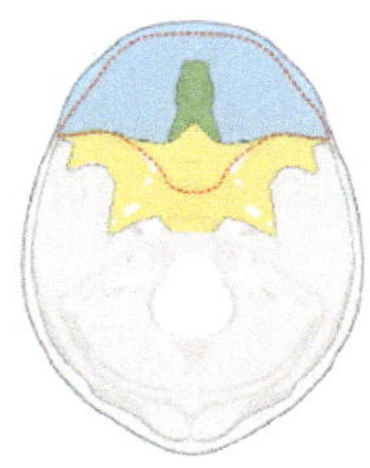
Deep cervical fascia	The deep cervical fascia lies, as its name suggests, 'deep' to the superficial fascia and platysma muscle. This fascia is organised into several layers. These layers act like a shirt collar, supporting the structures and vessels of the neck.	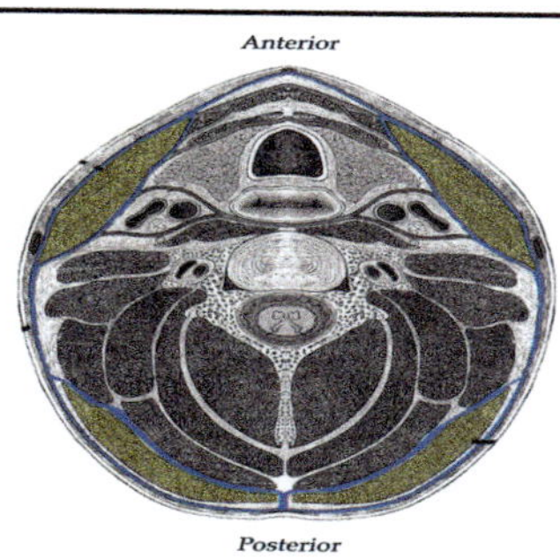

9.1. Cranium

The neurocranium and the viscerocranium are the two structural and functional components that make up the cranium. The brain and its membrane layers, known as the cranial meninges, are shielded from damage by the neurocranium, also known as the cranial vault. According to Caroline Berry & Berry (1967), the neurocranium has a ground (basicranium), a skullcap, and a roof shaped like a canopy. The neurocranium is made up of eight bones. Of these, four isolated bones, that is the occipital, frontal, ethmoid, and sphenoid are centered on the midline. Bilaterally, there are two pairs of bones: the parietal and temporal. While the hyaline cartilage (synchondroses) of the sphenoid and occipital bones develop during childhood, the majority of the skull's bones are connected by flexible interconnecting sutures (Sinclair & Scoffings, 2010). The mesenchyme of the embryonic pharyngeal arches is the principal site of development for the facial bones, which are in charge of creating the viscerocranium, or facial skeleton (Moore et al., 2012). The frontal area of the skull, or viscerocranium, is composed of the bones that encircle the orbits, lips, and nose. The 15 asymmetrical bones that make up the cranial base are divided into three central solo bones (the mandible, vomer, and ethmoid) and six bilaterally located coupled bones (Mitteroecker & Bookstein, 2008).

9.1.1. Facial Perspective of the Brain

The orbits, zygomatic bones, nasal region, mandible, and maxillae are among the anatomical features visible in the anterior view of the cranium (Nie, 2005). The frontal bone, which travels obliquely with the zygomatic and nasal bones, makes up the forehead skeleton. It also forms the floor of the cranial cavity and the upper area of the orbit by enclosing the lacrimal, ethmoid, and sphenoid bones. The nasal and frontal bones are joined by the nasion. The border between the orbital and plain sections of the frontal bone, known as the supra-orbital edge, has a supra-orbital notch. A rim that extends slightly above the supra-orbital boundary is known as the superciliary arch. In some adult crania, the metopic suture—a remnant of the developmental frontal suture—is visible in the flat area in the middle of the glabella, between the superciliary arches (Lieberman et al., 2000). The cheek prominences are caused by the zygomatic bones, which are situated inferolaterally on the orbits. A tiny zygomaticofacial foramen penetrates the lateral side of each bone.

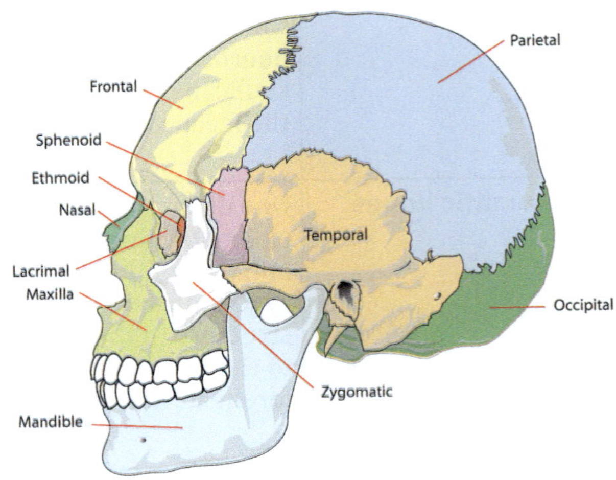

Figure 9.2. *Side view of the skull.*

Source: By LadyofHats Mariana Ruiz Villarreal – made it myself, Public Domain; https://commons.wikimedia.org/w/index.php?curid=1524860.

Located posterior to the nasal bones is the piriform orifice, which is the anterior side nasal orifice of the cranium. The nasal septum, which divides the nasal cavity into two equal sections, is clearly visible. Each nasal cavity contains elliptical bony plates called nasal conchae that are positioned laterally (Linnau et al., 2003). The upper jaw is composed of the maxillae. The transverse intermaxillary suture connects them. The alveolar processes that comprise the alveoli of maxillary teeth provide support for them. The majority of the piriform aperture is enclosed by the maxillae, which also form the infra-orbital borders. They have a foramen in the infra-orbital region, which is situated beneath each orbit, and a broad connection with the zygomatic bones. The mandible, the U-shaped bone that makes up the lower jaw, has an alveolar process that is in charge of keeping the mandibular teeth in place. It consists of a vertical area known as the ramus and a plane section called the body. The second premolar teeth are covered in mental foramina. The mental protuberance, a polygonal bone projection behind the mandibular symphysis, is what is known as the chin prominence. Within the orbits are apertures known as the optic canals and inferior and superior orbital fissures (Lieberman et al., 2000) (Figure 9.2).

9.1.2. Cranium's Lateral Aspect

The cranium's lateral side is produced by the combination of the neurocranium and viscerocranium. An approximate H-shaped structure is formed by the sutures that join the parietal, frontal, temporal, and sphenoid bones. Through the external acoustic meatus (ear canal) (eardrum), the external auditory aperture advances to the tympanic membrane. The mastoid process of the temporal bone is located posteroinferior to the external auditory meatus. The mastoid process and the narrow styloid process of the temporal bone are situated anteromedial to each other (Bout et al., 2001).

9.1.3. Cranium's Occipital View

The back of the skull, known as the occiput, contributes to the occipital aspect of the cranium. It consists of the occipital bone, portions of the parietal bones, and mastoid elements of the temporal bones. The occipital protuberance is usually a noticeable bump in the middle, with the upper nuchal line extending from it to define the upper boundary of the neck. In contrast, the lower nuchal line is less prominent. The lambda point, where the lambdoid and sagittal sutures intersect in the center of the occiput, may sometimes appear as a depression (Tuli et al., 1997) (Figure 9.3).

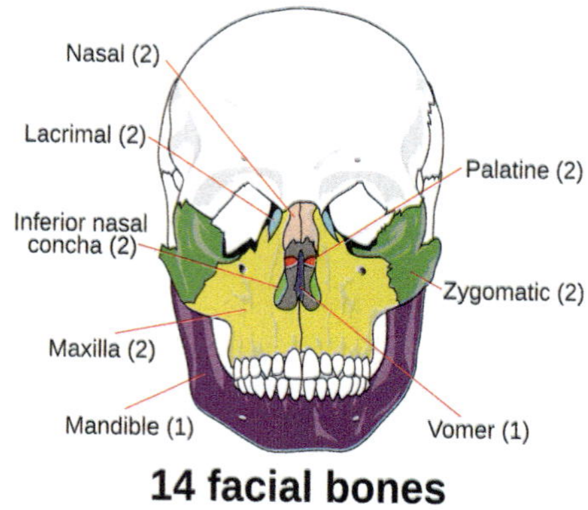

Figure 9.3. *The illustration of adult cranium.*

Source: By Own work – File:Es-Human skull front simplified (bones).svg, Public Domain; https://commons.wikimedia.org/w/index.php?curid=37631440.

9.1.4. Superior View of the Cranium

The superior view of the cranium, which is oval in shape, widens at the parietal edges. The four bones that comprise the calvaria of the neurocranium are visible from this angle: the frontal bone anteriorly, the right and left parietal bones laterally, and the occipital bone caudally. The frontoparietal bones are connected by the coronal suture, the sagittal suture is connected by the right and left parietal bones, and the lambdoid suture is connected by the occipital bone to the right and left parietal and temporal bones (Ucerler & Govsa, 2006).

9.1.5. Cranial Base Surface

The external aspect of the cranial base is composed of the palatine, sphenoid, vomer, temporal, and occipital bones, as well as the alveolar arch and palatine processes of the maxillae. The smooth plates of the palatine bones and the palatine processes of the maxillae combine to form the hard palate, also referred to as the bony palate. The central incisor teeth of the mouth are located behind the incisive fossa. The lower border of the choanae, or posterior nasal apertures, is formed by the palate's posterior margin. What distinguishes the choanae from one another is the vomer. A relatively flat and thin bone, the vomer is a part of the bony nasal septum (Stramrud, 1959).

The sphenoid bone is positioned in the space between the temporal, frontal, and occipital bones. It has a body and three sets of processes (Figure 9.4).

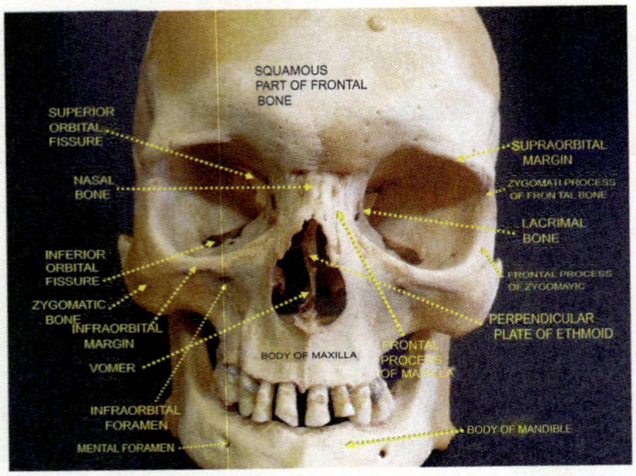

Figure 9.4. *Cranium.*

Source: By Anatomist90 – Own work, CC BY-SA 3.0; https://commons.wikimedia.org/w/index.php?curid=30039012.

Where the body and larger wings converge, the pterygoid processes extend obliquely onto the sphenoid. The pharyngotympanic tube's bony aperture and the cartilaginous part's sulcus are located inferior to the junction of the temporal bone's petrous portion and the sphenoid spine, respectively, and medial to the sphenoid spine. These are the midline structures of the sphenoid. The squamous part of the temporal bone has depressions called mandibular fossae that are formed when the mouth is closed. These fossae are big enough to hold the mandibular heads (Kreiborg et al., 1976).

The occipital bone articulates with the sphenoid bone in the anterior region and is responsible for the formation of the cranial base in the posterior region. The different parts of the occipital bone surround the large foramen magnum. Massive projections on either side of the foramen are known as the occipital condyles. These are the bones that enable the cranium and spinal column to articulate. The large fissure visible between the occipital bone and the petrous section of the temporal bone is called the jugular foramen. The internal carotid artery enters the carotid canal through the exterior aperture, which is located just in front of the deep foramen. Palpable mastoid processes serve as points of attachment for the surrounding muscles. The stylomastoid foramen is located between the mastoid and styloid processes (Jeffery, 2005).

9.2. Internal Surface of Cranial Base

The frontal, middle, and rear cranial fossae are located on the interior region of the cranial base and form the base of the cranial cavity. The posterior cranial fossa is located on the bottom, and the frontal cranial fossa is visible at the top (Rhoton, 2002).

The ethmoid bone forms the central cranial fossa, the frontal bone forms the anterior, the sphenoid body and wings form the posterior, and so on. The orbital plates of the frontal bone, which support the brain's frontal lobes and form the orbital roofs, contribute significantly to the formation of the frontal cranial fossa. The anterior bone's midline bony projection is known as the frontal crest. Arteries can pass through the foramen cecum, which is a hole in the base of the frontal bone, during the development of the embryo. The crista galli, a bone rim that extends medially from the ethmoid, is also referred to as the cock's comb in Latin. The cribriform plate, an ethmoid plate that resembles a sieve, is located on either side of the crista galli (Mori et al., 2010) (Figure 9.5).

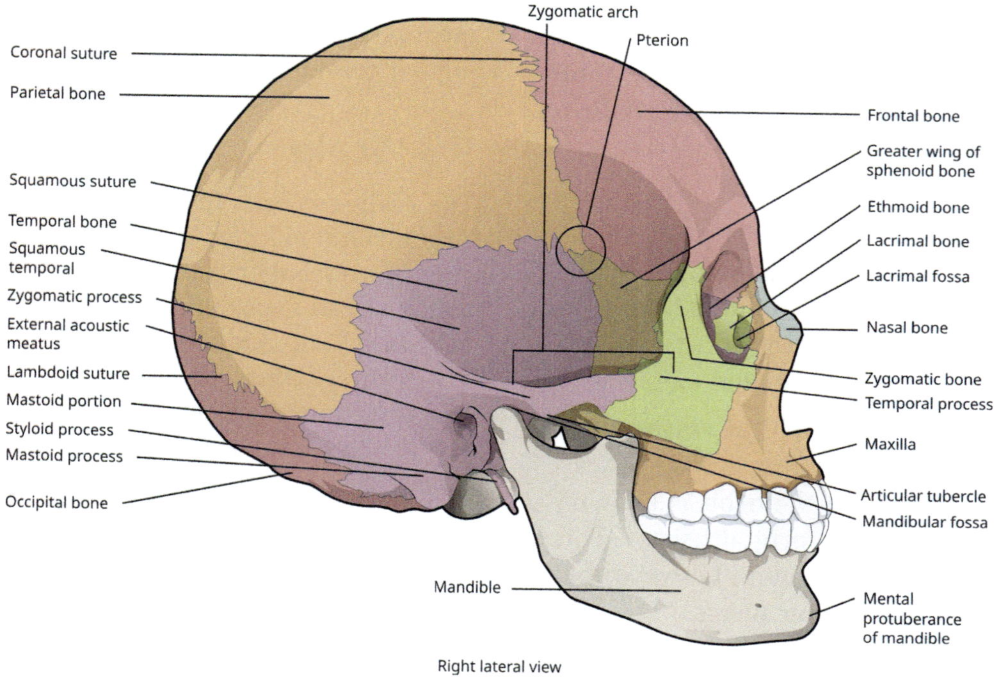

Figure 9.5. *Cranium.*

Source: By Original: OpenStax College Vector: Pixelsquid – This file was derived from: 705 Lateral View of Skull-01.jpg: CC BY 3.0; https://commons.wikimedia.org/w/index.php?curid=98006639.

The middle component of the butterfly-shaped middle cranial fossa is composed of the sella turcica on the sphenoid's body and lateral portions on either side. The sella turcica is encircled by the anterior and posterior clinoid processes (Besteiro et al., 1994).

The sella turcica is divided into two sections:

i. The *tuberculum sellae*, a slight elevation anteriorly on the sphenoid's body.

ii. The *hypophysial fossa*, a saddle-like pit in the center of the pituitary gland.

The dorsum sellae is created posteriorly by a bony plate on the sphenoid's body. The most obvious examples of superolateral angles are seen in the posterior clinoid processes (Labib et al., 2014).

The larger lateral portions of the central cranial fossa are made up of the sphenoid, squamous (flat) temporal bones, and petrous temporal bones. The temporal lobes are responsible for maintaining lateral areas of the central cerebral fossa. The partition between the posterior and middle cranial fossae is formed by the dorsum sellae of the sphenoid centrally and the upper boundary of the petrous section of the temporal bones laterally. The smaller wings of the sphenoid bones overhang the fossae anteriorly, and their sharp posterior borders are known as the sphenoidal crests.

The sphenoidal crests terminate medially at the two acute bony outcrops known as the anterior clinoid processes. The left and right optic canals are joined by the prechiasmatic sulcus. The foramen lacerum is located posterolaterally to the hypophysial fossa. Four foramina perforate the origins of the sphenoid's larger wings on either side of the sphenoid's body (Day et al., 1996):

1. **A Round Foramen:** The term "foramen rotundum" refers to the opening that can be found posterior to the superior orbital fissure's more developed medial end.
2. **The Superior Orbital Fissure:** An aperture resembling a drop of tear that links with the orbit is known as the superior orbital fissure. This opening can be found between the greater and lesser wings.
3. **Foramen Rotundum's Posterolateral Neighbor:** The foramen ovale, is an oval foramen.
4. **Foramen Spinosum:** Externally, it is situated posterolateral to the foramen ovale and extends anteriorly to the sphenoid's spine (Melsen & Melsen, 1980).

The posterior cranial fossa contains the cerebellum, medulla oblongata, and pons. This fossa is primarily composed of the occipital and temporal bones, with small contributions from the parietal and sphenoid bones. From the dorsum sellae, the clivus, a conspicuous elevation, reaches the foramen magnum. The landmark located posterior to this massive and deep foramen is the internal occipital crest, which divides the posterior portion of the fossae into two cerebellar fossae. The internal occipital protuberance is where the crest ends superiorly. This fossa has broad grooves made by the transverse and sigmoid sinuses. The temporal bones' petrous rims are the base where the jugular foramina are located. The hypoglossal canals pierce the occipital condyle roots above the foramen magnum, and the internal acoustic meatus is situated anteriorly superior to the jugular foramen (Kunz & Iliadis, 2007).

9.3. Scalp

The scalp encloses the neurocranium from the supraorbital margins of the frontal bone to the superior nuchal lines on the occipital bone. It is composed of skin, subcutaneous tissue, a layer of muscle, and aponeurotic tissue (Tolhurst et al., 1991). There are five layers in the scalp. The first three move forward as a unit and are closely connected to one another. The word "scalp" is made up of the letters that correspond to each of the five levels of the neurocranium (Miteva & Tosti, 2012) (Figure 9.6):

1. **Skin:** It is very thin, with the exception of the occipital area, and contains a large number of sweat glands, sebaceous glands, and hair follicles. The skin also benefits from an adequate artery supply as well as good venous and lymphatic circulation (Ilkit, 2010).
2. **Cutaneous Nerves:** These are abundant inside the connective tissue that contributes to the formation of the thick, dense, and highly vascularized subcutaneous layer.
3. **Aponeurosis:** A tendinous membrane that surrounds the calvaria, acts as the midway tendon of the occipitofrontalis muscle's frontal and occipital bellies, as well as the superior auricular muscle. These components comprise the musculo-aponeurotic epicranius (Mehrara et al., 2006).

4. **Loose Connective Tissues:** This provide for the unrestricted movement of the scalp. It is a layer that resembles a sponge and contains potential gaps that may become enlarged with fluid due to an injury or damage.
5. **Pericranium:** It is a compact sheath of connective tissue that forms the external periosteum of the neurocranium. It is strongly connected, but it can be removed easily from the calvaria of living people (Newman et al., 2004).

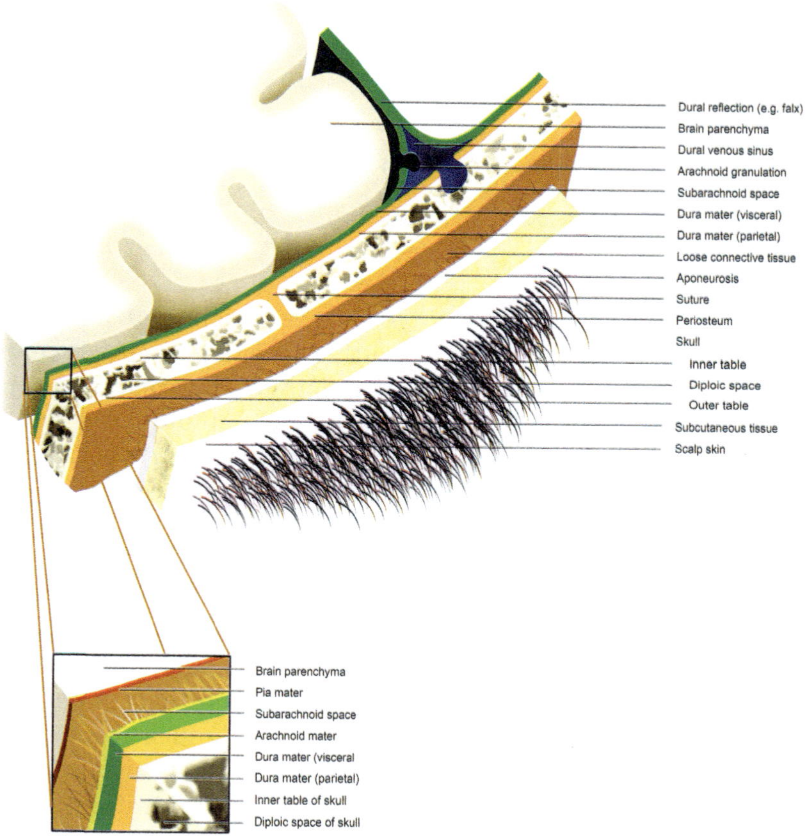

Figure 9.6. *Scalp.*

Source: By Frank Gaillard – Own work, CC BY-SA 3.0; https://commons.wikimedia.org/w/index.php?curid=8968406.

9.4. Cranial Meninges

The term "cranial meninges" refers to the brain membranes that are located directly inside the cranium. The brain is encased and shielded by a fluid-filled cavity called the subarachnoid space. The meninges are the name for this area. Additionally, they act as the framework for the body's venous sinuses, veins, and arteries. The cranial meninges are made up of three layers of membrane-like connective tissue, as seen in Figure 9.7 (Greenberg et al., 1994):

- **Dura Mater (Dura):** A dense and solid coating of external fibrous material.
- **Arachnoid Mater:** Also written as arachnoid refers to a thin middle layer.
- **Pia Matter:** Fragile interior vascular layer (Walsh et al., 2021).

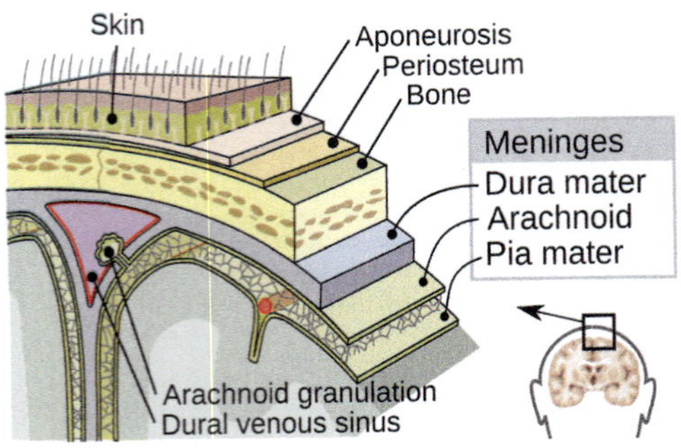

Figure 9.7. *Superior view of cranial meninges.*

Source: By SVG by Mysid, original by SEER Development Team, Jmarchn – Vectorized in Inkscape by Mysid, based on work by SEER Development Team, CC BY-SA 3.0; https://commons.wikimedia.org/w/index.php?curid=10485059.

The arachnoid and pia are the two continuous membranes that comprise the leptomeninges. The subarachnoid space, which contains the CSF, separates the arachnoid from the pia. Cerebrospinal fluid, or CSF, is a clear fluid with a composition quite similar to blood; however, it differs from blood in that it has a different ion concentration and fewer proteins. The brain's four ventricles contain choroid plexuses, which are primarily responsible for secreting CSF. CSF leaves the ventricular system of the brain and enters the subarachnoid space, where it pushes the arachnoid against the dura's inner surface while also supporting and nourishing the brain. This mechanism maintains the brain's structure (Sze et al., 1989).

9.4.1. Dura Mater

The dura mater (dura) is a double-layered membrane that adheres to the inner region of the cranium. It is composed of the following:

- *An outer periosteal layer* created by the periosteum covering the inner surface of the calvaria (Adeeb et al., 2012).
- A tough fibrous membrane called *the meninges* that covers and surrounds the spinal cord (Kerber & Newton, 1973).

9.4.2. Meningeal Spaces

In the absence of pathology, only one of the three meningeal spaces connected to the cranial meninges is present (Coureuil et al., 2012). The gap (epidural region) between the dura's outer periosteal layer and the cranium is not real because the dura is attached to the bones. It can only become a gap pathologically, for example, when blood from ruptured meningeal veins pushes the periosteum away from the skull and accumulates (Louveau et al., 2017). The dura-arachnoid junction is not a region that naturally occurs between the dura and the arachnoid, much like the subdural space. Any type of trauma, such as a blow to the head, can result in the dural border cell layer becoming perforated (Haines, 2006). The subarachnoid space, a separate area situated between the arachnoid and pia, contains bridging superior cerebral veins, cerebral arteries, CSF, and trabecular cells that empty into the upper sagittal sinus (Dietemann et al., 2005).

9.5. Brain

Given that neuroscience courses usually focus on the brain, the following provides a brief overview of the different parts of the brain, ventricular system, and blood vessels. Around 11 of the 12 cranial nerves originate in the brain, which is made up of the cerebrum, cerebellum, and brainstem (Raichle & Mintun, 2006) (Figure 9.8).

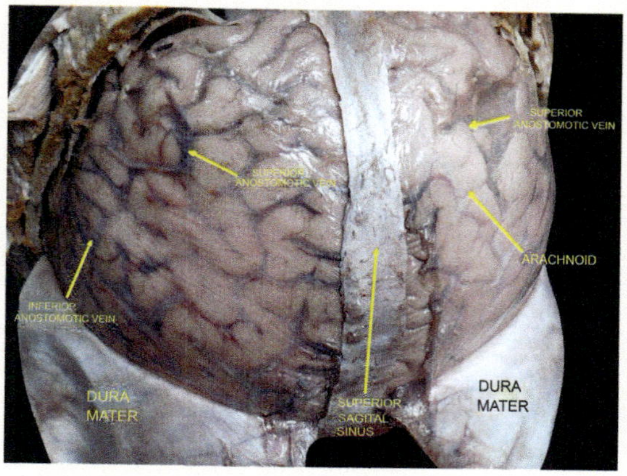

Figure 9.8. *Structure of brain.*

Source: By Anatomist90 – Own work, CC BY-SA 3.0; https://commons.wikimedia.org/w/index.php?curid=29606076.

These nerves carry out sensory, parasympathetic, or motor functions. Upon exiting the skull, they are usually surrounded by a protective dural sheath that connects with the connective tissue of the epineurium (Patel et al., 2009).

9.5.1. Parts of the Brain

When the calvaria and dura mater are removed, the gyri, sulci, and fissures of the cerebral cortex become visible through the delicate arachnoid-pia layer (Semenza, 1988):

1. The *cerebral hemispheres*, which make up most of the brain and are split by a sulcus, are included in the cerebrum. Four lobes – parietal, frontal, occipital, and temporal – make up each hemisphere. Frontal lobes reside in the anterior cranial fossa, temporal lobes in the lateral regions of the middle cranial fossa, and occipital lobes extend posteriorly across the tentorium cerebelli (Cowan, 1979).
2. *The thalamus, hypothalamus*, and *epithalamus* make up the central core of the brain. These parts are known as the *diencephalon.*
3. The *midbrain* is located at the intersection of the middle and posterior cranial fossae. The midbrain and CN III and IV are related (De Bellis et al., 1999).
4. *The pons*, related to CN V, is placed in the front region of the posterior cranial fossa. It is the portion of the brainstem that spans from the midbrain to the medulla oblongata caudally.
5. The tail-like portion of the brainstem (the *medulla oblongata*) is connected to the spinal cord and is located in the posterior cranial fossa. While CNs VI to VIII are situated at the medulla-pons intersection, CNs IX, X, and XII are connected to the medulla (Adam & Hye, 1966).

The cerebellum is the massive brain mass located posterior to the medulla and pons, as well as lower to the posterior region of the cerebrum. It is situated in the posterior cerebral fossa, beneath the tentorium cerebelli, and is composed of two hemispheres joined by a thin middle portion known as the vermis (Fornito et al., 2015).

9.5.2. Ventricular System of the Brain

The brain's ventricular structure consists of the midline third and fourth ventricles, two lateral ventricles, and the ventricular system. The lateral ventricles can enter the third ventricle (of Monro) through the interventricular foramina.

The cerebral aqueduct and the third ventricle, which separates the two diencephalon halves, are continuous. The posterior regions of the medulla and pons contain the fourth ventricle, which extends inferoposteriorly (Korzh, 2018) (Figure 9.9).

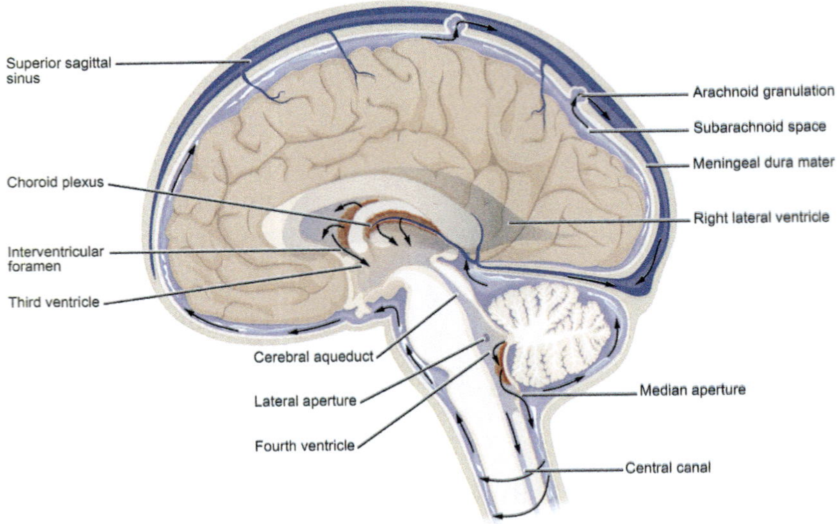

Figure 9.9. *Ventricular system.*

Source: By OpenStax – https://cnx.org/contents/FPtK1zmh@8.25:fEI3C8Ot@10/Preface, CC BY 4.0; https://commons.wikimedia.org/w/index.php?curid=30147960.

The central canal, which extends into the spinal cord, is formed when it tapers and narrows inferiorly. CSF exits the fourth ventricle through a single median opening and two lateral openings, allowing it to enter the subarachnoid space. These apertures are the only ways that CSF can get into the subarachnoid space. When they are blocked, the ventricles enlarge and compress the cerebral hemispheres. In certain regions, mainly near the base of the brain, the arachnoid and pia are divided by sizable cisterns (pools) of CSF (cerebrospinal fluid).

This creates a significant distance between the two layers (Stratchko et al., 2016):

1. The largest subarachnoid cistern, the cerebellomedullary cistern, is situated between the medulla and the cerebellum. It collects CSF via the fourth ventricle's openings and is separated into the posterior and lateral cerebellomedullary cisterns (*L. cisterna magna*).
2. The pontocerebellar cistern, also known as *the pontine cistern*, is a large space ventral to the pons.
3. The interpeduncular cistern, also known as the *basal cistern*, can be found in the interpeduncular fossa (Mortazavi et al., 2014).
4. The *quadrigeminal cistern* is a cistern of the cerebral vein that can be found in the brain between the superior surface of the cerebellum and the posterior region of the corpus callosum (Gonzalez et al., 2001).
5. CSF is secreted by the choroid plexuses' choroidal epithelial cells in the lateral,

third, and fourth ventricles. They are composed of vascular pia fringes (tela choroidea), which are surrounded by cuboidal epithelial cells. A portion of CSF exits the fourth ventricle and travels posterosuperiorly over the cerebellum and inferiorly into the subarachnoid space of the spinal cord (Bedussi et al., 2015).

The majority of CSF flow, however, is received by the quadrigeminal and interpeduncular cisterns. CSF can flow superiorly from the multiple cisterns thanks to the fissures and sulci on the superolateral and medial surfaces of the cerebral hemispheres. Furthermore, the subarachnoid space surrounding the cranial nerves is penetrated by CSF. As protuberances of arachnoid villi onto the walls of dural venous sinuses, particularly the superior sagittal sinus and its lateral venous lacunae, arachnoid granulations are the main site of CSF absorption into the venous system. CSF functions as a cushion with the meninges and calvaria to protect the brain from head trauma. By acting as a cushion, the CSF in the subarachnoid space keeps the weight of the brain from pressing against the blood vessels and cranial nerve roots (Yang et al., 2021).

9.6. The Neck

The neck, sometimes referred to as the collar or collum, serves as a vital conduit for organs and structures passing through it as well as a connecting point between the skull and the body's upper and lower limbs. Furthermore, several important organs with specific functions are located here, such as the trachea, parathyroid, and larynx (Lipan et al., 2006).

The bones that make up the neck are the cervical vertebrae (C1–C7), the hyoid bone (commonly called the hyoid), the manubrium of the sternum, and the clavicles. The movable hyoid is situated in the occipital region, at the mandibular bones, the position of the C3 vertebra, and the inclination created by the thyroid cartilage. Despite having no connections to other bones, the hyoid serves as a stabilizing element for the frontal neck and support for keeping the airways open (Bose et al., 2013) (Figure 9.10).

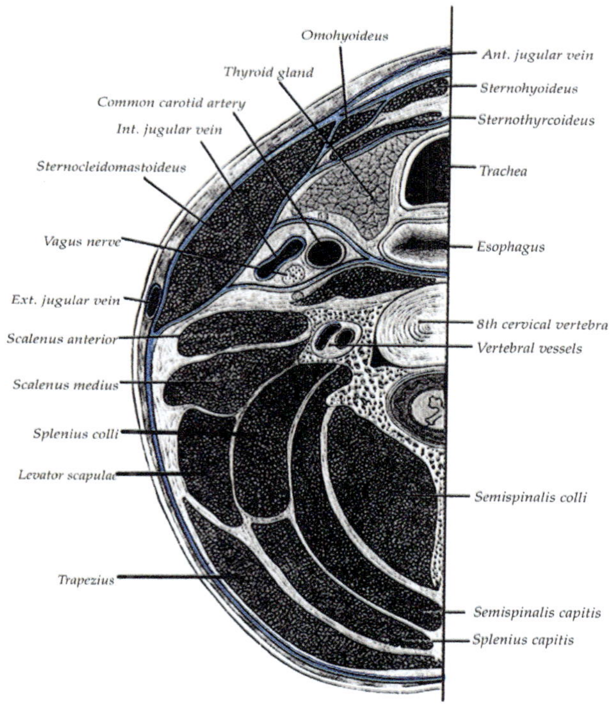

Figure 9.10. *Neck fascia.*

Source: By Henry Vandyke Carter – Henry Gray, (1918). Anatomy of the human body (see "Book" section below) Bartleby.com: Gray's Anatomy, Plate 384, Public Domain; https://commons.wikimedia.org/w/index.php?curid=561537.

9.7. Fascia of Neck

Parts of the neck that are covered in a layer of adipose subcutaneous tissue are categorized by sections of deeper cervical fascia. The fascial planes dictate the possible path of dissemination for the collar infection.

9.7.1. Cervical Subcutaneous Tissue and Platysma

The subcutaneous fat of the neck (superficial cervical fascia) is a layer of connective tissue that lies between the dermal layer of the skin and the investing surface of the deep cervical fascia. It has cutaneous neurons, lymphatic and circulatory systems, surface lymph nodes, and variable amounts of fat in addition to the platysma. The subcutaneous tissue covering the superior parts of the pectoralis major and deltoid muscles is the starting point of the platysma, a facial expression muscle that sweeps over the collarbone to the lower border of the jaw. It is a thin, thick layer of muscle (Nash et al., 2005).

9.7.2. Deep Cervical Fascia

The deep cervical fascia is composed of three layers of fascia: investing, pretracheal, and prevertebral. These layers provide support to the viscera, muscles, vessels, and deep lymph nodes in the neck. Their slippery nature allows for smooth movement of structures, such as swallowing and head movements. Additionally, the fascial layers form natural cleavage planes that aid in tissue separation during surgical procedures (Natale et al., 2015).

9.7.3. Investing Layer of Deep Cervical Fascia

The investing layer of the deep cervical fascia, which is the outermost superficial layer of deeper fascia, surrounds the entire neck. The investing layer encloses (includes) the left and right sternocleidomastoid (SCM) and trapezius musculature after dividing between the superficial and deep layers of the deep fascia at the four edges of the neck (Pandit et al., 2006). The hyoid and spinous processes of the neck spine, the mandibular lower border, the occipital bone's uppermost nuchal line, the mastoid processes of the temporal bones, the zygomatic arches, and the mandibular and temporal bone notable nuchal lines are all apically connected by this same investing layer of fascia.

Just below its attachment to the mandible, the submandibular gland is encased by the investing layer of deep fascia. It splits to form the parotid gland's entire fibrous capsule dorsal to the jaw (Guidera et al., 2012). The manubrium of the sternum, the collarbones, the acromions, and the scapular vertebrae are all connected to the fascia's lower border by the investing layer. The periosteum, contiguous with the investing layer posteriorly (ligamentum nuchae), covers the C7 spinous process and even the nuchal ligament. Just above the manubrium, the fascia is still divided into two levels, one of which is attached to the front and the other to the lower surface of the manubrium. These levels encircle the SCM. The jugular venous arch, fats, and a small number of deeper lymphatic nodes are located in the suprasternal region, which lies between levels (Guidera et al., 2014).

9.7.4. Pretracheal Layer of Deep Cervical Fascia

The deep delicate pretracheal membrane of the cervical fascia is found only in the front part of the neck. It extends inferiorly from the hyoid into the chest, where it blends in well with the fibrous pericardium encircling the ventricle. The pretracheal layer consists of a striated muscle portion covering the infrahyoid muscles and a visceral portion covering the thyroid, esophagus, and trachea completely. Similarly, the pretracheal membrane and the buccopharyngeal fascia merge horizontally and posterior-superiorly (Gavid et al., 2018) (Figure 9.11).

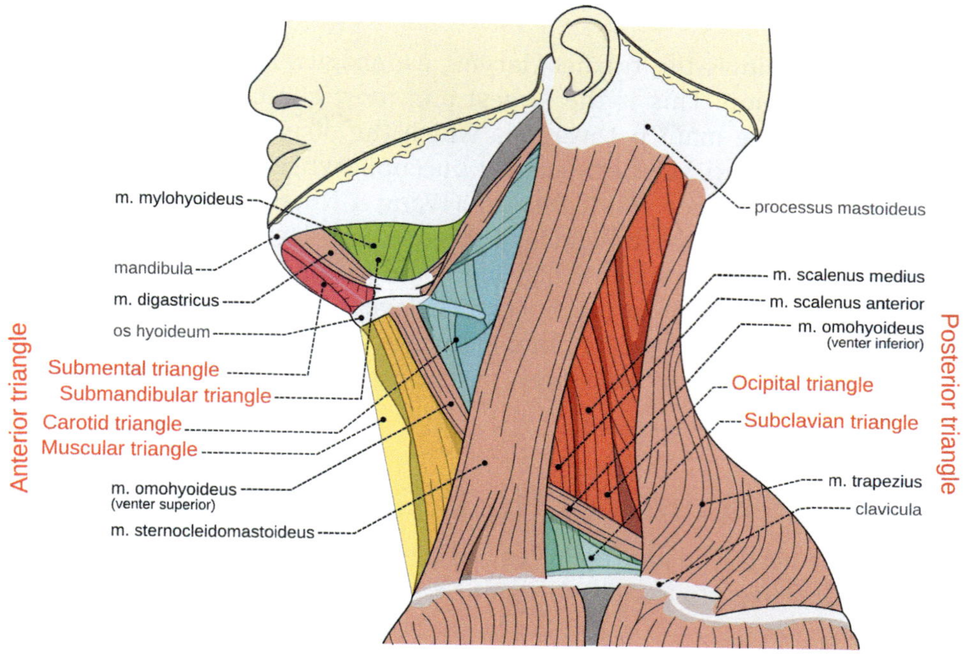

Figure 9.11. *Regions/triangles of the neck.*

Source: By Olek Remesz (wiki-pl: Orem, commons: Orem) Modified by user:madhero88 – original image File:Musculi coli base.svg, CC BY 3.0; https://commons.wikimedia.org/w/index.php?curid=6771884.

The carotid sheathing is a tubular fascial investment that extends from the base of the skull to the base of the neck. This sheathing fuses both the pretracheal and investing layers posteriorly, and apically with the prevertebral layer of the deeper cervical fascia. Located in the carotid sheathing are the following (Feigl et al., 2020):

- The internally shared carotid arteries;
- The greater inner jugular vein (IJV);
- The Vagus nerve (CN X);
- The deeper cervical lymphatic nodes;
- The carotid sinus nerve branching;
- The sympathetic nerve endings.

The cerebral chamber and the chest's mediastinum are connected apically by the pre-tracheal fascia and carotid sheathing, respectively. These interactions could act as conduits for the spread of illnesses and blood clots (Lindner, 1986).

9.7.5. Prevertebral Layer of Deep Cervical Fascia

The pre-vertebral layer of the deeper cervical fascia serves as a tubular covering for the vertebral column once more, as well as the surrounding muscles, such as the longus colli apically, the scalene laterally, and the longus capitis. Lastly, the deeper cervical muscles on the lower side. This layer of fascia is attached apically and on the lower border to the cranial base, where it unites squarely with the upper longitudinal ligament surrounding the T3 spine. The pre-vertebral membrane extends laterally to form the axillary sheathing, which encloses the brachial plexus and axillary arteries (Bilecenoglu et al., 2012).

9.7.6. Retropharyngeal Space

The retropharyngeal gap allows the trachea, larynx, esophagus, and pharynx to move relative to the vertebrae during ingestion. This is the largest and most clinically significant interfascial gap in the collar because it is the main pathway via which the disease spreads. There may be a gap composed of loose connective tissue between the buccopharyngeal fascia and the visceral part of the pre-vertebral layers of the deep cervical fascia (Wong & Novotny, 1978). The buccopharyngeal fascia is inferiorly connected to the pretracheal layer of the deep cervical fascia. The alar fascia runs through the retropharyngeal space. This thin coating extends from the skull to the position of the C7 vertebra. It is connected to the buccopharyngeal fascia along its entire length. It also has a carotid sheath. It does this by extending sideways to converge. The retropharyngeal space is superiorly sealed and covered on both sides by the carotid sheathing and the base of the skull (Davis et al., 1990).

9.8. Superficial Structures of Neck: Cervical Regions

There are regions on the neck. The four main regions are the anterior cervical region, lateral cervical region, posterior cervical region, and SCM region. Each zone can be divided more effectively by using simple triangles. .

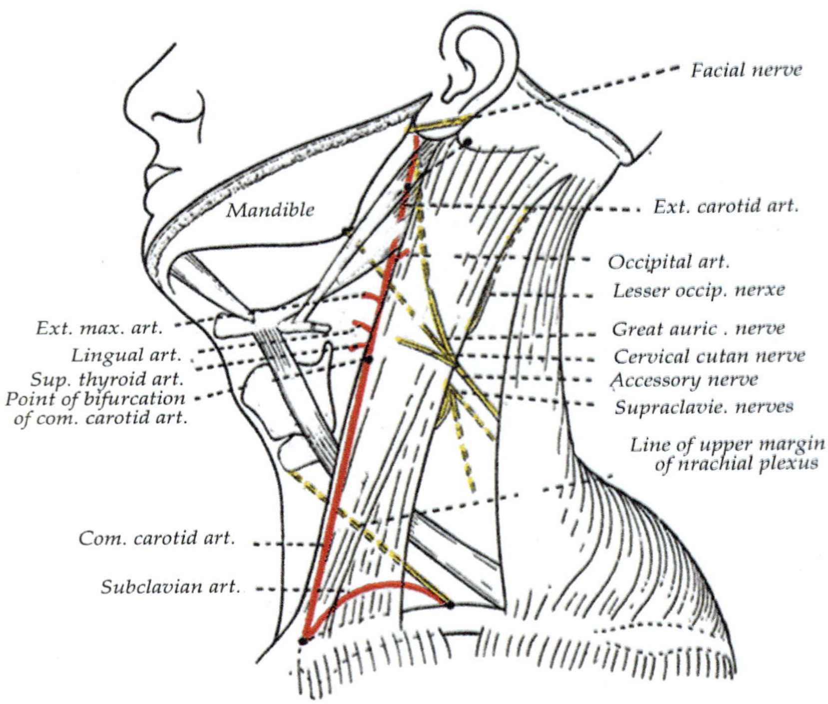

Figure 9.12. *Regions/triangles of the neck.*

Source: By Henry Vandyke Carter – Henry Gray, (1918). Anatomy of the human body (see "Book" section below) Bartleby.com: Gray's Anatomy, Plate 1210, Public Domain; https://commons.wikimedia.org/w/index.php?curid=564825.

The SCM muscle, which also defines the SCM region, clearly separates each half of the neck into a lateral and an anterior cervical region. The larger clavicular head and the rounder tendons of the sternal head are the two main branches that make up the SCM. The area beneath the two heads is called the lower supraclavicular fossa (Wilhelm et al., 2010) (Figure 9.12)

9.9. Lateral Cervical Region

9.9.1. Muscles in the Lateral Cervical Region

The flooring of the sidewise cervical region (L scalenus posterior) is made up of prevertebral fascia, which also covers the levator scapulae, splenius capitis, the middle scalene (the scalenus medius), and the rear scalene muscles. The scalenus anterior, which is part of the inferior border of the front scalene, is occasionally visible at the inferomedial inclination of the lateral cervical region (Kamibayashi & Richmond, 1998).

9.9.2. Nerves of Lateral Cervical Region

The junction of the superior and middle thirds of the posterior border of the SCM is where the spinal accessory nerve crosses before entering the lateral cervical area. It travels postero-inferiorly, inside or deeper to the investing membrane of deep cervical fascia, where a pre-vertebral membrane of fascia divides it from the levator scapulae. Before entering the muscle, CN XI disappears farther toward the anterior border of the muscle where the superior two-thirds and lower one-third of the trapezius meet (Bland & Boushey, 1990) (Figure 9.13).

The brachial plexus roots of the front rami of C5–C8 and T1 appear between the anterior and middle scalene muscles. Bogduk (2004) states that the brachial plexus trunks, which consist of five rami, descend inferior-laterally over the lateral cervical region.

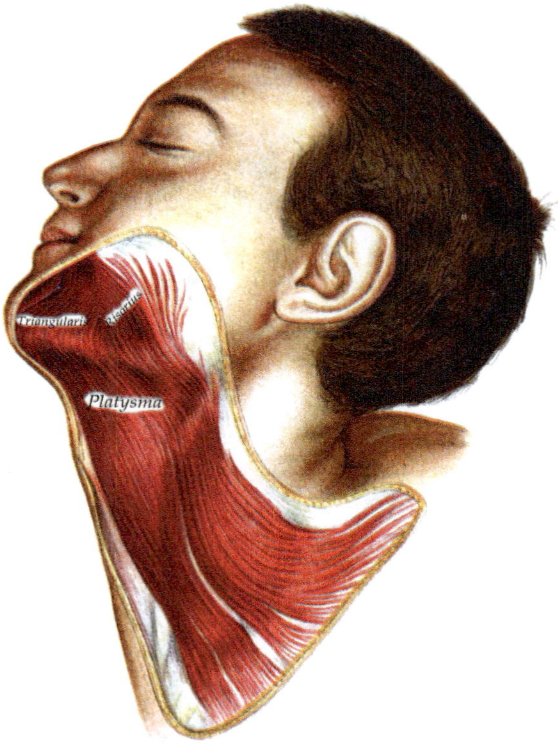

Figure 9.13. *Platysma.*

Source: By Dr. Johannes Sobotta - Sobotta's Atlas and Textbook of Human Anatomy, 1909, Public Domain; https://commons.wikimedia.org/w/index.php?curid=29817198.

The plexus then enters the axilla, innervating most of the upper limb extremities, passing through the cervico-axillary canal located between the clavicle, upper edge of the shoulder, and first rib. The suprascapular nerves originate from the upper part of the brachial plexus and travel through the lateral cervical region to provide nourishment to the infraspinatus and supraspinatus muscles located on the posterior aspect of the shoulder (Melamed et al., 2002).

Articular branching is also received by the glenohumeral joint from it. The network of neural loops that make up the cervical plexus's roots are known as the frontal rami of C1–C4. Deep to the SCM, the plexus extends anterior-medially to the levator scapulae and the middle scalene muscles. The shallow branches that mainly go posteriorly are the cutaneous branching of the plexus (Zhang et al., 2003). Among the deeper branches that travel anteromedially are the motor branches that comprise the phrenic nerves and the ansa cervicalis.

Called the neural points of the neck, cutaneous branching of the cervical plexus supplies the epidermis of the anterior-lateral collar, supero-lateral chest wall, and the forehead between the external occipital and the auricle protuberance. The cervical plexus bases receive the interconnecting branches, also known as L rami communicants, near their origin. Most of these branches originate from the uppermost cervical ganglion in the upper region of the neck (Bogduk, 2016).

The cervical plexus's branching that emerge out from the neural loop around C2 and C3 – the anterior rami of these possess the following features (Kochilas et al., 2008):

1. The lesser occipital nerve (C2) provides the epidermis on the back of the collar and forehead posterior-superior to the ear.
2. The great auricular nerve (C2 and C3) ascends straight across the SCM onto the parotid and separates there to supply the epidermis and sheathing covering the glands, the back of the ears, and the patch of skin covering the curve of the mandible to the mastoid bone.
3. The transverse cervical nerves (C2 and C3) supply the skin that covers the anterior cervical area. The nerves wrap around the posterior edge of the SCM and travel proximally and horizontally through it, deeper towards the EJV and platysma.

The supraclavicular nerve endings (C3 and C4) are branches of the cervical plexus that emerge from the loop here between the frontal rami of C3 and C4. They start as a common trunk under the SCM and send branches to the skin of the neck as well as crossing the clavicle to supply the skin over the shoulders (Johnson, 2004). Deeper motor branches that arise from the anterior rami of the cervical nerves supply the rhomboids (dorsal scapular nerve, C4 and C5), the serratus anterior (thoracic spinal nerve, C5–C7), and the surrounding prevertebral muscles.

9.9.3. Veins in Lateral Cervical Region

The external jugular venous system (EJV) is formed when the rear classification of the retromandibular vein connects with the rear auricular vein just below the outer ear auricle, near the mandibular curve. The EJV at the rear SCM boundary punctures the investment layer of the deeper cervical fascia, which acts as the region's roofing, after it diagonally crosses the SCM deeper to the platysma.

The EJV descends to the lower section of the sideways cervical area and ends at the subclavian vein. The primary vein supplying the upper limb extremity, the subclavian vein, passes in front of the anterior scalene muscles and phrenic nerve as it passes through the lower portion of the sideways cervical region. The union of the subclavian vein and IJV forms the brachiocephalic vein, which is located behind the midline tip of the clavicle. Just above the collarbone, the supra-scapular, cervicodorsal, and upper jugular veins all enter the EJV (Seoane & Rhoton Jr, 1999).

9.10. Anterior Cervical Region

9.10.1. Muscles in the Anterior Cervical Region

The hyoid in the anterior-lateral region of the neck (collar) is the attachment point for the infrahyoid and suprahyoid muscles. These hyoid muscles support or move the larynx and the hyoid (Vasavada et al., 1998) (Figure 9.14).

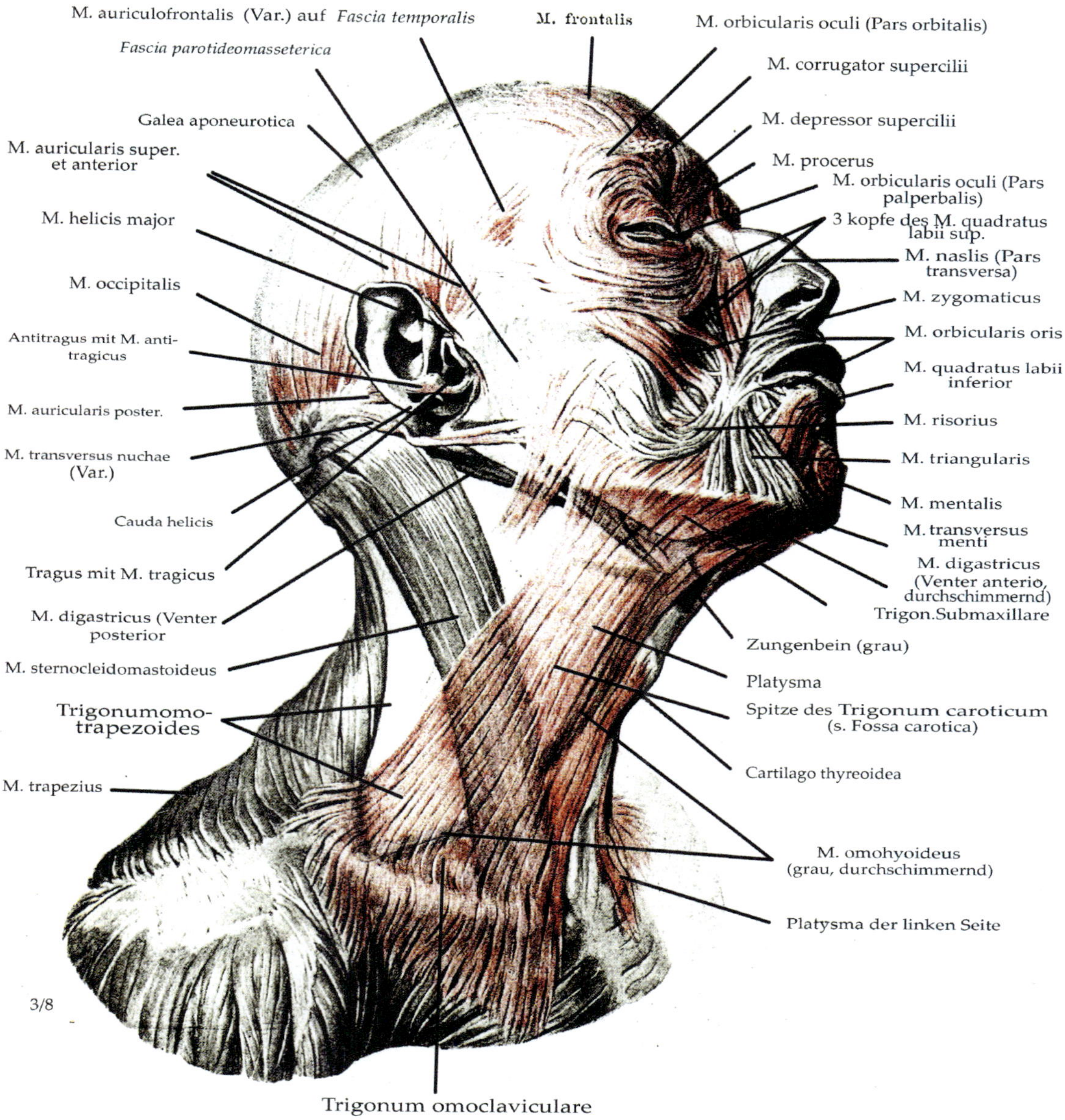

Figure 9.14. *The cervical region.*

Source: https://commons.wikimedia.org/wiki/File:Braus_1921_375.png.

The suprahyoid muscles, which are situated above the hyoid bone, connect it to the skull. This group includes the digastric, mylohyoid, geniohyoid, and stylohyoid muscles (Civelek et al., 2008). The group comprises most of the floor of the mouth; it raises the larynx and hyoid in relation to ingestion and sound production, while stabilizing the hyoid to create a base upon which the tongue can function. The middle tendon that runs between each digastric muscle's front and rear bellies descends towards the hyoid. A fibro loop that allows it to glide in both directions connects the intermediary tendons to the hyoid bone's greater horns and core (Ovsepyan et al., 2022).

The infrahyoid muscles, or strapped muscles, are inferior to the suprahyoid muscles. These four muscles attach to the sternum, clavicle, scapula, and compress the larynx and the hyoid. They are used for ingestion and speech. These work well with the suprahyoid muscles to stabilize the hyoid and provide a firm base for the tongue. The infrahyoid grouping of muscles is arranged in 2 planes: the shallow sternohyoid and omohyoid, and the deeper sternothyroid and thyrohyoid (Falla et al., 2006). An intermediary tendon connects the two omohyoid chambers, and it is affixed to the clavicle in this location by a ligamentous sling. It is situated beneath the sternothyroid, which is larger than the sternohyoid. In order to stop the upper development of a larger thyroid, the sternothyroid attaches to the slanted line of the thyroid bone sheet directly above the gland. It includes the thyroid's side lobe. Going apically out from the slanted line of the thyroid bone to the hyoid, the thyrohyoid appears to be an extension of the sternothyroid muscle (Panjabi et al., 2001) (Figure 9.15).

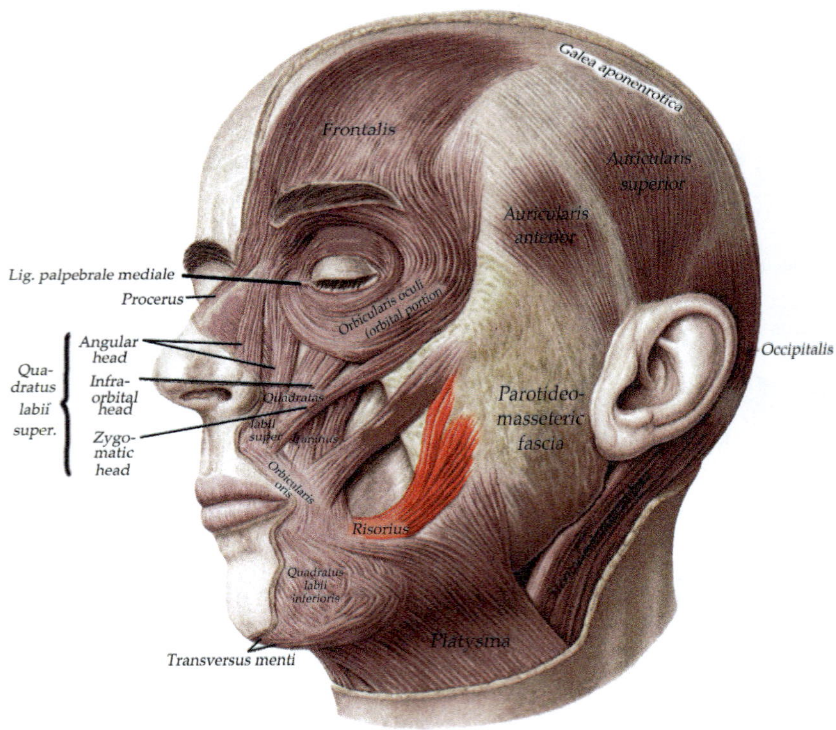

Figure 9.15. *Anterior cervical region and suprahyoid region.*

Source: By Sobotta, color changed by was_a_bee. – File:Sobo_1909_260.png, Public Domain; https://commons.wikimedia.org/w/index.php?curid=30471257.

9.10.2. Arteries in the Anterior Cervical Region

The anterior cervical region houses the carotid system, which is made up of the internal carotid artery and its terminal branches, the external and internal carotid arteries. This region is also home to the IJV and its branches, as well as the front jugular veins. The carotid artery and the external carotid artery, one of the terminal branches, are the main vascular arteries in the carotid triangle (Ackland et al., 2011). Every normal carotid artery ascends within the carotid sheathing to the location of the upper thyroid cartilage margin, together with the vagus nerve and the IJV. This is the point where each carotid artery ends, where the internal and external carotid arteries split. The common right carotid artery begins at the division of the brachiocephalic trunk. In contrast, the left common carotid artery ascends through the neck after emerging from the aortic arch. The standard carotid arteries lead to the carotid triangle. You can feel or palpate their pulses by gently pressing it against the lateral aspect of the neck spine (Peng et al., 2009).

9.11. Deep Structures of the Neck

The cervical side of the superior thoracic aperture, the root of the neck, contains structures on the cervical side as well as the prevertebral muscles, which are positioned posterior to the cervical viscera and anterolateral to the vertebral column (Zhu et al., 2019) (Figure 9.16).

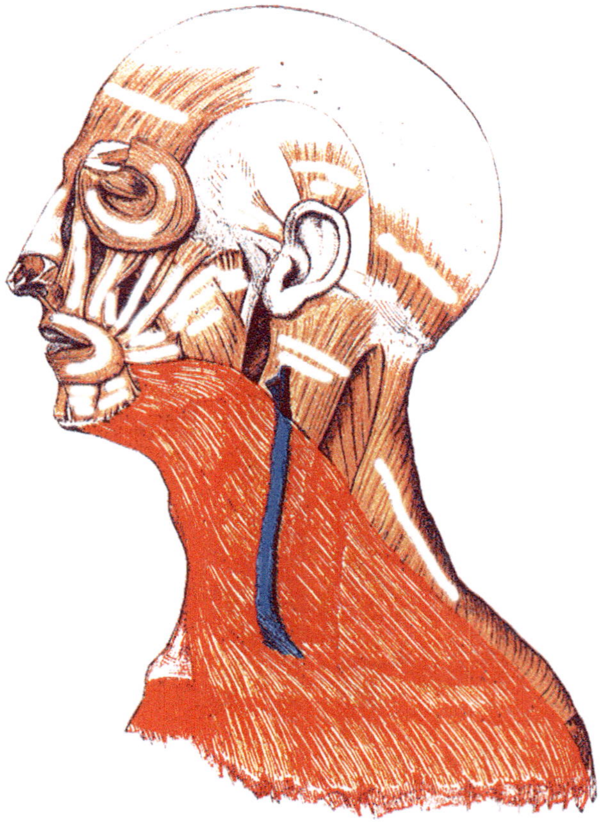

Figure 9.16. *The platysma muscle, located within the superficial cervical fascia.*

Source: https://commons.wikimedia.org/wiki/File:Gray_%E2%80%94_platysma.png.

9.11.1. Prevertebral Muscles

The lateral and anterior spinal muscles, also referred to as pre-vertebral muscles, are located directly behind the retropharyngeal region and are composed of the longus colli and the capitis, the anterior scalene muscle, and the rectus capitis anterior. The lateral vertebral muscles, which include the splenius capitis, the levator scapulae, the middle and posterior scalene muscles, and the subclavian artery and cervical plexuses, are situated on the back side of the neurovascular plane of the brachial. The rectus capitis lateralis is the only other muscle in the lateral cervical region (Offiah & Hall, 2009).

9.11.2. Root of Neck

The base of the neck is the area where the neck and thorax converge. The posterior and anterior limits of the lower root are formed by the manubrium of the chest, the first set of ribs and their corresponding costal cartilages, and the core of the T1 vertebra. This discussion is limited to the neurovascular aspects of the neck's root (Bogduk, 1981) (Figure 9.17).

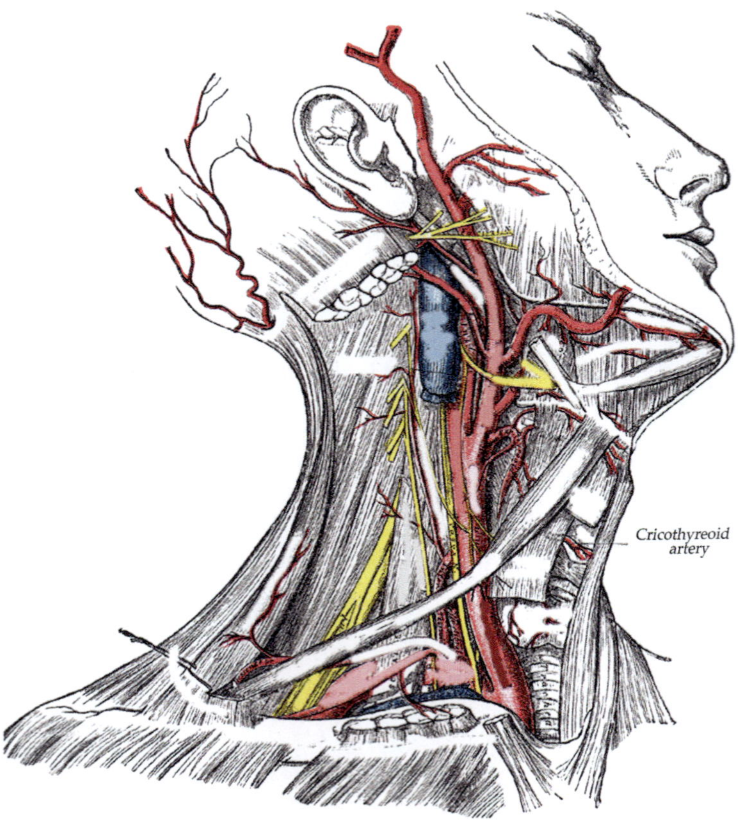

Figure 9.17. *Functional layers of the neck.*

Source: By Henry Vandyke Carter – Henry Gray, (1918). Anatomy of the human body (see "Book" section below) Bartleby.com: Gray's Anatomy, Plate 507, Public Domain; https://commons.wikimedia.org/w/index.php?curid=559526.

9.11.3. Arteries in Root of Neck

The brachiocephalic trunk, which is the largest branch of the aortic arch, is apically shielded by the sternohyoid and sternothyroid muscles. It begins development in the middle, behind the manubrium, and proceeds superior-laterally and rightward. It divides into the right subclavian and right common carotid arteries just behind the right sternoclavicular (SC) joint (Koizumi et al., 1994). Blood is supplied to the brain, neck, and upper limbs via the subclavian arteries. The right subclavian artery originates from the brachiocephalic trunk, whereas the left subclavian artery originates from the aortic arch. Their neck courses begin posterior to the corresponding SC joint as they rise through all of the upper thoracic openings. The arteries form a superolateral arch between their point of entry and the median edge of the front scalene muscle. As the clavicles begin to descend, the arteries pass the top edge of the first rib and continue deeper to the midpoint. At the outer edge of the first rib, their nomenclature changes to the underarm arteries (Chakravorty, 1971).

Every subclavian artery is split into 3 sections by the upper scalene muscle: the first section is medial to the musculature, the second is posterior to it, and the third is lateral to it. The autonomic trunk and cervical pleurae, which cover the apices of the lung, are located behind the arteries. The branches of the subclavian artery are (Siegmund et al., 2009):

1. The first segment of the subclavian artery, the spinal artery, the internal thoracic artery, and the thyrocervical trunk.
2. The second segment of the subclavian artery is the costo cervical trunk.
3. The lateral scapular artery, which often arises from the third part of the subclavian artery.

The cervical part of the spinal artery, which ascends in the pyramidal space formed by the longus and scalene muscles, is supported by the first segment of the subclavian artery. The vessel then passes through the transverse foramina of cervical vertebrae C1–C6. A foramen can be found above the C6 vertebra in the segment of the vertebral artery that courses through the spine. Prior to entering the cranial cavity and traversing the foramen magnum, the suboccipital part of the vertebral artery, which marks the beginning of the cranial part of the vertebral artery, runs in a groove on the posterior arches of the atlas (Lasjaunias et al., 1985).

The antero-inferior segment of the subclavian artery is where the internal thoracic artery emerges after entering the thorax inferomedially. The thyrocervical trunk begins near the medial aspect of the anterior scalene muscle, in the anterosuperior portion of the very first segment of the subclavian artery. The suprascapular artery, which supplies the musculature on the back of the shoulder, and the cervicodorsal trunks are its two lateral branches. The dorsal scapular and superficial cervical arteries emerge from the cervicodorsal trunk and provide branching to the muscles of the lateral cervical region, trapezius, and medial scapular musculature. The inferior thyroid artery, the main visceral artery of the neck, and the ascending cervical artery, which supplies the lateral neck muscles, are the final branches of the thyrocervical trunk (Mears, 1888).

The costocervical trunk lies posteriorly (behind the anterior scalene muscle on the right side and primarily just medial to the muscle on the left side) and is supported by the second part of the subclavian artery. As the trunk crosses posterior-superiorly, the superior intercostal and deep cervical arteries are formed. These arteries supply the first two intercostal spaces and the deep cervical muscles at the back, respectively. The transverse scapular artery often arises from the cervicodorsal trunk, although it may be a separate branch of the second or third part of the subclavian artery. It extends deeply to supply the rhomboid and levator scapulae muscles and also participates in the vascular anastomoses around the scapula (Ebraheim et al., 2003).

9.11.4. Veins in Root of Neck

Two major veins terminate at the base of the neck (AJV): the irregular anterior jugular vein (AJV) and the ejectory jugular vein (EJV), which drains fluid primarily from the head and face. The AJV is typically formed by the union of superficial submandibular veins near the hyoid bone (Kubo et al., 1994). The vein exits the body in the subclavian vein or ends in the EJV after bending sideways behind the SCM at the base of the neck. In the suprasternal region, the left and right AJVs normally unite above the manubrium to form the jugular vascular arch. The subclavian vein extends from the axillary vein at the lateral edge of the first rib to the point where it joins the IJV behind the clavicle's middle extremity to form the brachiocephalic vein. Here, the thoracic duct and the right lymph trunk converge to form the venous angle, which is the point at which lymph that has accumulated throughout the body is released into the venous circulation. The carotid sheathing surrounds the IJV throughout the entire way (Som & Laitman, 2017).

9.11.5. Nerves in Root of Neck

The three primary nerve groups that comprise the neck's roots are the sympathetic trunks, phrenic nerves, and vagus nerves. This chapter has already covered the cervical plexus and the phrenic nerves (Singh & Husain, 2011).

9.11.6. Vagus Nerves (CN X)

Once the vagus nerve ending leaves the jugular foramen, it travels inferiorly inside the neck, well within the posterior aspect of the carotid sheathing, at the inclination between the internal jugular vein and the carotid artery. The first segment of the subclavian artery is located anteriorly, while the right vagus nerve enters the thorax posterior to the SC and the brachiocephalic vein. According to Martinez et al. (2019), the left vagus nerve enters the thorax posterior to the SC joint, between the left subclavian and left main carotid arteries.

The recurrent laryngeal nerves are accessed through the vagus nerve, which is located in the lower neck. The nerves on the ends are arranged similarly in general, but they originate from different structures on opposing wings and recur (circle around) them at different times. While the other recurrent laryngeal nerve circles beneath the right subclavian artery, the left recurrent laryngeal nerve wraps beneath the aortic arch. All recurrent laryngeal nerves loop and then rise apically to the posteromedial aspect of the thyroid gland. There, they emerge in the tracheoesophageal trough and supply nourishment to all the innermost laryngeal muscles except the cricothyroid (George et al., 2003).

A Closer Look

Head and Neck Cancer

Head and neck cancer encompasses a diverse group of malignancies originating in the oral cavity, pharynx, larynx, nasal cavity, paranasal sinuses, and salivary glands. These cancers are predominantly squamous cell carcinomas, arising from the mucosal lining of these regions. Understanding the etiology, risk factors, diagnostic methods, and treatment options for head and neck cancer is essential for improving patient outcomes and advancing medical research.

The etiology of head and neck cancer is multifactorial, with tobacco and alcohol use being the primary risk factors. Smoking and excessive alcohol consumption have a synergistic effect, significantly increasing the risk of developing these cancers. Human papillomavirus (HPV) infection, particularly HPV-16, has emerged as a significant risk factor, especially for oropharyngeal cancers. Other risk factors include prolonged exposure to ultraviolet (UV) light, certain occupational hazards (such as exposure to wood dust and asbestos), poor oral hygiene, and genetic predisposition.

Symptoms of head and neck cancer vary depending on the specific site of the tumor but commonly include a persistent sore throat, difficulty swallowing, unexplained weight loss, a lump or sore that does not heal, changes in voice, and ear pain. Early detection is crucial for effective treatment, but symptoms are often nonspecific and may lead to delayed diagnosis.

Diagnostic evaluation begins with a thorough clinical examination and a detailed patient history. Imaging studies such as computed tomography (CT), magnetic resonance imaging (MRI), and positron emission tomography (PET) scans are utilized to assess the extent of the disease and guide biopsy procedures. Endoscopy allows direct visualization and biopsy of suspicious lesions. Histopathological examination of biopsy samples confirms the diagnosis, and molecular testing for HPV status is often performed in cases of oropharyngeal cancer due to its prognostic significance.

Treatment for head and neck cancer typically involves a multidisciplinary approach, including surgery, radiation therapy, and chemotherapy. The choice of treatment depends on the tumor's location, stage, and HPV status, as well as the patient's overall health and preferences. Early-stage cancers may be treated effectively with surgery or radiation alone, while advanced-stage cancers often require a combination of treatments. Chemoradiation, the concurrent use of chemotherapy and radiation, is a common approach for locally advanced cancers. Targeted therapies, such as cetuximab, and immunotherapies, like pembrolizumab, are emerging treatment options, particularly for recurrent or metastatic disease.

Surgical interventions can range from minimally invasive procedures to extensive resections, sometimes necessitating reconstructive surgery to restore form and function. Advances in surgical techniques, such as transoral robotic surgery (TORS) and microvascular free flap reconstruction, have improved outcomes and reduced morbidity. Radiation therapy techniques, including intensity-modulated radiation therapy (IMRT), allow for precise targeting of the tumor while sparing surrounding healthy tissue.

The prognosis for head and neck cancer varies based on factors such as the tumor's location, stage at diagnosis, HPV status, and response to treatment. HPV-positive oropharyngeal cancers generally have a better prognosis compared to HPV-negative counterparts. However, the overall survival rate for head and neck cancer has improved with advances in diagnostic and therapeutic techniques.

Supportive care and rehabilitation are essential components of the management plan, addressing issues such as speech and swallowing difficulties, nutritional support, pain management, and psychosocial support. Ongoing research aims to develop more effective treatments, improve early detection methods, and identify novel biomarkers for better prognosis and personalized therapy.

In conclusion, head and neck cancer is a complex and diverse group of diseases requiring a comprehensive and multidisciplinary approach to diagnosis and treatment. Continued advancements in medical research and clinical practice hold promise for improving patient outcomes and quality of life.

Summary

- The head and neck region of the human body is a complex and vital area that houses numerous structures essential for various functions such as sensory perception, communication, and basic physiological processes.
- The cranium is composed of two structural and functional elements: the neurocranium and the viscerocranium. The neurocranium *(cranial vault)* is a casing made of bones that protects the brain and its membrane layers, the *cranial meninges.*
- The forehead skeleton is composed of the frontal bone, which travels obliquely with the zygomatic and the nasal bones. It also encapsulates the lacrimal, ethmoid, and sphenoid bones, forming the orbit's upper area as well as the cranial cavity's floor.
- The viscerocranium and neurocranium combine to generate the cranium's lateral side. Sutures that connect the parietal, frontal, temporal, and sphenoid bones form an approximately H-shaped structure.
- The oval-shaped cranium widens at the parietal edges when viewed from above. The superior view reveals the four bones of the calvaria: the frontal bone in front, the parietal bones on the sides, and the occipital bone at the back.
- The alveolar arch of the maxillae, the palatine processes of the maxillae, and the palatine, sphenoid, vomer, temporal, and occipital bones make up the external aspect of the cranial base.
- The upper boundary of the petrous section of the temporal bones laterally and the dorsum sellae of the sphenoid centrally constitute the partition between the posterior and middle cranial fossae.
- Skin, subcutaneous tissue, and a layer of muscle and aponeurotic tissue make up the scalp, which encloses the neurocranium from the supraorbital margins of the frontal bone to the superior nuchal lines on the occipital bone.
- The membranes of the brain that are found directly inside the cranium are referred to as the *cranial meninges*. The subarachnoid space is a cavity that is filled with fluid and protects and encloses the brain.
- The neck (*collar*), also known as the cervix or collum, connects the skull to the body's upper and lower limbs and acts as a key passageway for structures/organs moving through them.
- The full neck is encircled by the investing layer of the deep cervical fascia, which comprises the most superficial deeper fascial layer.
- The deeper cervical fascia's pre-vertebral layer acts as a tubular coating for the vertebral column and also the muscles that surround it, including the scalene laterally, the longus capitis, and the longus colli apically, and finally, the *deeper cervical muscles* on the lower side.
- The hyoid serves as an attachment site for the infrahyoid muscles & suprahyoid muscles in the anterior-lateral region of the neck (collar).

- The carotid system, which consists of the internal carotid artery as well as its terminal extensions, the external and internal carotid arteries, is situated in the anterior cervical area.
- The greatest branching of the aortic arch is the brachiocephalic trunk, which is apically protected by the sternothyroid and the sternohyoid muscles.
- The EJV, which drains fluid primarily from the face and head, as well as the irregular anterior jugular vein, are two major veins that come to an end in the base of the neck (AJV).

References

1. Ackland, D. C., Merritt, J. S., & Pandy, M. G. (2011). Moment arms of the human neck muscles in flexion, bending and rotation. *Journal of Biomechanics, 44*(3), 475–486.
2. Adam, H. M., & Hye, H. K. (1966). Concentration of histamine in different parts of brain and hypophysis of cat and its modification by drugs. *British Journal of Pharmacology and Chemotherapy, 28*(1), 137.
3. Adeeb, N., Mortazavi, M. M., Tubbs, R. S., & Cohen-Gadol, A. A. (2012). The cranial dura mater: A review of its history, embryology, and anatomy. *Child's Nervous System, 28*(6), 827–837.
4. Bedussi, B., van Lier, M. G., Bartstra, J. W., de Vos, J., Siebes, M., VanBavel, E., & Bakker, E. N. (2015). Clearance from the mouse brain by convection of interstitial fluid towards the ventricular system. *Fluids and Barriers of the CNS, 12*(1), 1–13.
5. Besteiro, J. M., Aki, F. E., Ferreira, M. C., Medina, L. R., & Cernea, C. (1994). Free flap reconstruction of tumors involving the cranial base. *Microsurgery, 15*(1), 9–13.
6. Bilecenoglu, B., Onul, M., Altay, O. T., & Sakul, B. U. (2012). Cervicofacial emphysema after dental treatment with emphasis on the anatomy of the cervical fascia. *Journal of Craniofacial Surgery, 23*(6), e544–e548.
7. Bland, J. H., & Boushey, D. R. (1990, August). Anatomy and physiology of the cervical spine. *Seminars in Arthritis and Rheumatism, 20*(1), 1–20.
8. Bogduk, N. (2004). The neck and headaches. *Neurologic Clinics, 22*(1), 151–171.
9. Bogduk, N. (2016). Functional anatomy of the spine. *Handbook of Clinical Neurology, 136*, 675–688.
10. Bogduk, N. I. K. O. L. A. I. (1981). An anatomical basis for the neck-tongue syndrome. *Journal of Neurology, Neurosurgery & Psychiatry, 44*(3), 202–208.
11. Bose, P., Brockton, N. T., & Dort, J. C. (2013). Head and neck cancer: From anatomy to biology. *International Journal of Cancer, 133*(9), 2013–2023.
12. Bout, R. G., & Zweers, G. A. (2001). The role of cranial kinesis in birds. *Comparative Biochemistry and Physiology Part A: Molecular & Integrative Physiology, 131*(1), 197–205.
13. Brooks, D. N. (1991). The head-injured family. *Journal of Clinical and Experimental Neuropsychology, 13*(1), 155–188.
14. Carolineberry, A., & Berry, R. J. (1967). Epigenetic variation in the human cranium. *Journal of Anatomy, 101*(Pt 2), 361.

15. Chakravorty, B. G. (1971). Arterial supply of the cervical spinal cord (with special reference to the radicular arteries). *The Anatomical Record, 170*(3), 311–329.

16. Civelek, E., Karasu, A., Cansever, T., Hepgul, K., Kiris, T., Sabancı, A., & Canbolat, A. (2008). Surgical anatomy of the cervical sympathetic trunk during anterolateral approach to cervical spine. *European Spine Journal, 17*(8), 991–995.

17. Coureuil, M., Join-Lambert, O., Lécuyer, H., Bourdoulous, S., Marullo, S., & Nassif, X. (2012). Mechanism of meningeal invasion by Neisseria meningitidis. *Virulence, 3*(2), 164–172.

18. Cowan, W. M. (1979). The development of the brain. *Scientific American, 241*(3), 112–133.

19. Davis, W. L., Harnsberger, H. R., Smoker, W. R., & Watanabe, A. S. (1990). Retropharyngeal space: Evaluation of normal anatomy and diseases with CT and MR imaging. *Radiology, 174*(1), 59–64.

20. Day, J. D., Jordi, X. K., Manfred, T., & Takanori, F. (1996). Surface and superficial surgical anatomy of the posterolateral cranial base: Significance for surgical planning and approach. *Neurosurgery, 38*(6), 1079–1084.

21. De Bellis, M. D., Keshavan, M. S., Clark, D. B., Casey, B. J., Giedd, J. N., Boring, A. M., & Ryan, N. D. (1999). Developmental traumatology part II: Brain development. *Biological Psychiatry, 45*(10), 1271–1284.

22. Dietemann, J. L., Bogorin, A., Eid, A., Koob, M., Nogueira, T., Vargas, M. I., & Zöllner, G. (2005). Normal and abnormal meningeal enhancement: MRI features. *Journal de Radiologie, 86*(11), 1659–1683.

23. Ebraheim, N. A., An, H. S., Xu, R., Ahmad, M., & Yeasting, R. A. (1996). The quantitative anatomy of the cervical nerve root groove and the intervertebral foramen. *Spine, 21*(14), 1619–1623.

24. Falla, D., Jull, G., O'leary, S., & Dall'Alba, P. (2006). Further evaluation of an EMG technique for assessment of the deep cervical flexor muscles. *Journal of Electromyography and Kinesiology, 16*(6), 621–628.

25. Feigl, G., Hammer, G. P., Litz, R., & Kachlik, D. (2020). The intracarotid or alar fascia, other cervical fascias, and their adjacent spaces–A plea for clarification of cervical fascia and spaces terminology. *Journal of Anatomy, 237*(1), 197–207.

26. Fornito, A., Zalesky, A., & Breakspear, M. (2015). The connectomics of brain disorders. *Nature Reviews Neuroscience, 16*(3), 159–172.

27. Gavid, M., Dumollard, J. M., Habougit, C., Lelonge, Y., Bergandi, F., Peoc'h, M., & Prades, J. M. (2018). Anatomical and histological study of the deep neck fasciae: does the alar fascia exist? *Surgical and Radiologic Anatomy, 40*(8), 917–922.

28. George, M. S., Rush, A. J., Sackeim, H. A., & Marangell, L. B. (2003). Vagus nerve stimulation (VNS): utility in neuropsychiatric disorders. *International Journal of Neuropsychopharmacology, 6*(1), 73–83.

29. Gonzalez-Soriano, J., Garcia, P. M., Contreras-Rodriguez, J., Martinez-Sainz, P., & Rodríguez-Veiga, E. (2001). Age-related changes in the ventricular system of the dog brain. *Annals of Anatomy-Anatomischer Anzeiger, 183*(3), 283–291.

30. Greenberg, R. W., Lane, E. L., Cinnamon, J., Farmer, P., & Hyman, R. A. (1994, December). The cranial meninges: Anatomic considerations. *Seminars in Ultrasound, CT and MRI, 15*(6), 454–465.

31. Guidera, A. K., Dawes, P. J., & Stringer, M. D. (2012). Cervical fascia: A terminological pain in the neck. *ANZ Journal of Surgery, 82*(11), 786–791.

32. Guidera, A. K., Dawes, P. J., Fong, A., & Stringer, M. D. (2014). Head and neck fascia and compartments: No space for spaces. *Head & Neck, 36*(7), 1058–1068.

33. Haines, A., Kovats, R. S., Campbell-Lendrum, D., & Corvalán, C. (2006). Climate change and human health: Impacts, vulnerability and public health. *Public Health, 120*(7), 585–596.

34. Holland, J., Ramazanoglu, C., Sharpe, S., & Thomson, R. (1998). The male in the head. In J. Holland, C. Ramazanoglu, S. Sharpe, & R. Thomson (Eds.), *The Male in the Head: Young People, Heterosexuality and Power* (pp. 171–191). London: Tufnell Press.

35. Ilkit, M. (2010). Favus of the scalp: An overview and update. *Micropathological, 170*(3), 143–154.

36. Jeffery, N. (2005). Cranial base angulation and growth of the human fetal pharynx. *The Anatomical Record Part A: Discoveries in Molecular, Cellular, and Evolutionary Biology, 284*(1), 491–499.

37. Johnson, G. M. (2004). The sensory and sympathetic nerve supply within the cervical spine: Review of recent observations. *Manual Therapy, 9*(2), 71–76.

38. Kamibayashi, L. K., & Richmond, F. J. (1998). Morphometry of human neck muscles. *Spine, 23*(12), 1314–1323.

39. Kerber, C. W., & Newton, T. H. (1973). The macro and microvasculature of the dura mater. *Neuroradiology, 6*(4), 175–179.

40. Kochilas, X., Bibas, A., Xenellis, J., & Anagnostopoulou, S. (2008). Surgical anatomy of the external branch of the superior laryngeal nerve and its clinical significance in head and neck surgery. *Clinical Anatomy: The Official Journal of the American Association of Clinical Anatomists and the British Association of Clinical Anatomists, 21*(2), 99–105.

41. Koizumi, M., Sekiya, S. I., Horiguchi, M., & Harada, M. (1994). A study of the deep ascending cervical artery (new definition) and its relation to some other arteries in the human cervical region. *Annals of Anatomy-Anatomischer Anzeiger, 176*(3), 233–242.

42. Korzh, V. (2018). Development of brain ventricular system. *Cellular and Molecular Life Sciences, 75*(3), 375–383.

43. Kreiborg, S., Prydsoe, U., Dahl, E., & Fogh-Andersen, P. (1976). Clinical conference I. Calvarium and cranial base in Apert's syndrome: An autopsy report. *The Cleft Palate Journal, 13*(3), 296–303.

44. Kubo, Y., Waga, S., Kojima, T., Matsubara, T., Kuga, Y., & Nakagawa, Y. (1994). Microsurgical anatomy of the lower cervical spine and cord. *Neurosurgery, 34*(5), 895–902.

45. Kunz, A. R., & Iliadis, C. (2007). Hominid evolution of the arteriovenous system through the cranial base and its relevance for craniosynostosis. *Child's Nervous System, 23*(12), 1367–1377.

46. Labib, M. A., Prevedello, D. M., Carrau, R., Kerr, E. E., Naudy, C., Abou Al-Shaar, H., & Kassam, A. (2014). A road map to the internal carotid artery in expanded endoscopic endonasal approaches to the ventral cranial base. *Operative Neurosurgery, 10*(3), 448–471.

47. Lasjaunias, P., Vallee, B., Person, H., Ter Brugge, K., & Chiu, M. (1985). The lateral spinal artery of the upper cervical spinal cord: Anatomy, normal variations, and angiographic aspects. *Journal of Neurosurgery, 63*(2), 235–241.

48. Lieberman, D. E., Pearson, O. M., & Mowbray, K. M. (2000). Basicranial influence on overall cranial shape. *Journal of Human Evolution, 38*(2), 291–315.

49. Lieberman, D. E., Ross, C. F., & Ravosa, M. J. (2000). The primate cranial base: Ontogeny, function, and integration. *American Journal of Physical Anthropology: The Official Publication of the American Association of Physical Anthropologists, 113*(S31), 117–169.

50. Lindner, H. H. (1986). The anatomy of the fasciae of the face and neck with particular reference to the spread and treatment of intraoral infections (Ludwig's) that have progressed into adjacent fascial spaces. *Annals of Surgery, 204*(6), 705.

51. Linnau, K. F., Hallam, D. K., Lomoschitz, F. M., & Mann, F. A. (2003). Orbital apex injury: Trauma at the junction between the face and the cranium. *European Journal of Radiology, 48*(1), 5–16.

52. Lipan, M. J., Reidenberg, J. S., & Laitman, J. T. (2006). Anatomy of reflux: A growing health problem affecting structures of the head and neck. *The Anatomical Record Part B: The New Anatomist: An Official Publication of the American Association of Anatomists, 289*(6), 261–270.

53. Louveau, A., Plog, B. A., Antila, S., Alitalo, K., Nedergaard, M., & Kipnis, J. (2017). Understanding the functions and relationships of the glymphatic system and meningeal lymphatics. *The Journal of Clinical Investigation, 127*(9), 3210–3219.

54. Martin-Giménez, T., Cruz, A. M., Barragán, A., Montero, E., Sanchez, P. G., Caballero, G., & Corradini, I. (2019). Delayed onset vagus nerve paralysis after occipital condyle fracture in a horse. *Journal of Veterinary Internal Medicine, 33*(6), 2780–2785.

55. Mears, W. P. (1888). Abnormal distribution of arteries and veins in the neck. *Journal of Anatomy and Physiology, 22*(Pt 2), 304.

56. Mehrara, B. J., Disa, J. J., & Pusic, A. (2006). Scalp reconstruction. *Journal of Surgical Oncology, 94*(6), 504–508.

57. Melamed, H., Harris, M. B., & Awasthi, D. (2002). Anatomic considerations of superior laryngeal nerve during anterior cervical spine procedures. *Spine, 27*(4), E83–E86.

58. Melsen, B., & Melsen, F. (1980). The cranial base in anencephaly and microcephaly studied histologically. *Teratology, 22*(3), 271–277.

59. Miteva, M., & Tosti, A. (2012). Hair and scalp dermatoscopy. *Journal of the American Academy of Dermatology, 67*(5), 1040–1048.

60. Mitteroecker, P., & Bookstein, F. (2008). The evolutionary role of modularity and integration in the hominoid cranium. *Evolution: International Journal of Organic Evolution, 62*(4), 943–958.

61. Mori, K., Yamamoto, T., Nakao, Y., & Esaki, T. (2010). Development of artificial cranial base model with soft tissues for practical education. *Operative Neurosurgery, 66*(suppl_2), onsE339–onsE341.

62. Mortazavi, M. M., Adeeb, N., Griessenauer, C. J., Sheikh, H., Shahidi, S., Tubbs, R. I., & Tubbs, R. S. (2014). The ventricular system of the brain: A comprehensive review of its history, anatomy, histology, embryology, and surgical considerations. *Child's Nervous System, 30*(1), 19–35.

63. Nash, L., Nicholson, H. D., & Zhang, M. (2005). Does the investing layer of the deep cervical fascia exist? *The Journal of the American Society of Anesthesiologists, 103*(5), 962–968.

64. Natale, G., Condino, S., Stecco, A., Soldani, P., Belmonte, M. M., & Gesi, M. (2015). Is the cervical fascia an anatomical proteus? *Surgical and Radiologic Anatomy, 37*(9), 1119–1127.

65. Newman, M. I., Hanasono, M. M., Disa, J. J., Cordeiro, P. G., & Mehrara, B. J. (2004). Scalp reconstruction: A 15-year experience. *Annals of Plastic Surgery, 52*(5), 501–506.

66. Nie, X. (2005). Cranial base in craniofacial development: Developmental features, influence on facial growth, anomaly, and molecular basis. *Acta Odontologica Scandinavica, 63*(3), 127–135.

67. Offiah, C. E., & Hall, E. (2009). Acute calcific tendinitis of the longus colli muscle: Spectrum of CT appearances and anatomical correlation. *The British Journal of Radiology, 82*(978), e117–e121.

68. Ovsepyan, A. L., Smirnov, A. A., Pustozerov, E. A., Mokhov, D. E., Mokhova, E. S., Trunin, E. M., & Starchik, D. A. (2022). Biomechanical analysis of the cervical spine segment as a method for studying the functional and dynamic anatomy of the human neck. *Annals of Anatomy-Anatomischer Anzeiger, 240*, 151856.

69. Pandit, J. J., Dorje, P., & Satya-Krishna, R. (2006). Investing layer of the cervical fascia of the neck may not exist. *The Journal of the American Society of Anesthesiologists, 104*(6), 1344–1344.

70. Panjabi, M. M., Miura, T., Cripton, P. A., Wang, J. L., Nain, A. S., & DuBois, C. (2001). Development of a system for in vitro neck muscle force replication in whole cervical spine experiments. *Spine, 26*(20), 2214–2219.

71. Patel, M. M., Goyal, B. R., Bhadada, S. V., Bhatt, J. S., & Amin, A. F. (2009). Getting into the brain. *CNS Drugs, 23*(1), 35–58.

72. Peng, C. W., Chou, B. T., Bendo, J. A., & Spivak, J. M. (2009). Vertebral artery injury in cervical spine surgery: Anatomical considerations, management, and preventive measures. *The Spine Journal, 9*(1), 70–76.

73. Raichle, M. E., & Mintun, M. A. (2006). Brain work and brain imaging. *Annual Review of Neuroscience, 29*, 449–476.

74. Rhoton Jr, A. L. (2002). The anterior and middle cranial base. *Neurosurgery, 51*(suppl_4), S1–273.

75. Semenza, C. (1988). Impairment in localization of body parts following brain damage. *Cortex, 24*(3), 443–449.

76. Seoane, E., & Rhoton Jr, A. L. (1999). Compression of the internal jugular vein by the transverse process of the atlas as the cause of cerebellar hemorrhage after supratentorial craniotomy. *Surgical Neurology, 51*(5), 500–505.

77. Siegmund, G. P., Winkelstein, B. A., Ivancic, P. C., Svensson, M. Y., & Vasavada, A. (2009). The anatomy and biomechanics of acute and chronic whiplash injury. *Traffic Injury Prevention, 10*(2), 101–112.

78. Sinclair, A. G., & Scoffings, D. J. (2010). Imaging of the post-operative cranium. *Radiographics, 30*(2), 461–482.

79. Singh, R., & Husain, A. M. (2011). Neurophysiologic intraoperative monitoring of the glossopharyngeal and vagus nerves. *Journal of Clinical Neurophysiology, 28*(6), 582–586.

80. Som, P. M., & Laitman, J. T. (2017). Embryology, variations, and innervations of the human neck muscles. *Neurographics, 7*(3), 215–242.

81. Stramrud, L. (1959). External and internal cranial base a cross-sectional study of growth and of association in form. *Acta Odontologica Scandinavica, 17*(2), 239–266.

82. Stratchko, L., Filatova, I., Agarwal, A., & Kanekar, S. (2016, April). The ventricular system of the brain: Anatomy and normal variations. *Seminars in Ultrasound, CT and MRI, 37*(2), 72–83.

83. Sze, G., Soletsky, S., Bronen, R., & Krol, G. (1989). MR imaging of the cranial meninges with emphasis on contrast enhancement and meningeal carcinomatosis. *American Journal of Neuroradiology, 10*(5), 965–975.

84. Tolhurst, D. E., Carstens, M. H., Greco, R. J., & Hurwitz, D. J. (1991). The surgical anatomy of the scalp. *Plastic and Reconstructive Surgery, 87*(4), 603–612.

85. Tuli, S., Tator, C. H., Fehlings, M. G., & Mackay, M. (1997). Occipital condyle fractures. *Neurosurgery, 41*(2), 368–377.

86. Ucerler, H., & Govsa, F. (2006). Asterion as a surgical landmark for lateral cranial base approaches. *Journal of Cranio-Maxillofacial Surgery, 34*(7), 415–420.

87. Vasavada, A. N., Li, S., & Delp, S. L. (1998). Influence of muscle morphometry and moment arms on the moment-generating capacity of human neck muscles. *Spine, 23*(4), 412–422.

88. Walsh, D. R., Zhou, Z., Li, X., Kearns, J., Newport, D. T., & Mulvihill, J. J. (2021). Mechanical properties of the cranial meninges: A systematic review. *Journal of Neurotrauma, 38*(13), 1748–1761.

89. Wilhelm, T., Harlaar, J. J., Kerver, A., Kleinrensink, G. J., & Benhidjeb, T. (2010). Surgical anatomy of the floor of the oral cavity and the cervical spaces as a rationale for trans-oral, minimal-invasive endoscopic surgical procedures: Results of anatomical studies. *European Archives of Oto-Rhino-Laryngology, 267*(8), 1285–1290.

90. Wong, Y. K., & Novotny, G. M. (1978). Retropharyngeal space-a review of anatomy, pathology, and clinical presentation. *The Journal of Otolaryngology, 7*(6), 528–536.

91. Yang, S., Emelyanov, A., You, M. S., Sin, M., & Korzh, V. (2021). Camel regulates development of the brain ventricular system. *Cell and Tissue Research, 383*(2), 835–852.

92. Zhang, J., Tsuzuki, N., Hirabayashi, S., Saiki, K., & Fujita, K. (2003). Surgical anatomy of the nerves and muscles in the posterior cervical spine: A guide for avoiding inadvertent nerve injuries during the posterior approach. *Spine, 28*(13), 1379–1384.

93. Zhu, W., Huang, Y., Zeng, L., Chen, X., Liu, Y., Qian, Z., & Xie, X. (2019). AnatomyNet: Deep learning for fast and fully automated whole-volume segmentation of head and neck anatomy. *Medical Physics, 46*(2), 576–589.

Chapter

THE CENTRAL NERVOUS SYSTEM

10

Contents

Introduction

The human body's central nervous system (CNS), which includes the brain and spinal cord, is an essential component. It controls all physiological responses and processes and acts as the main hub for information processing and transmission. The CNS is investigated in clinical anatomy due to its intricate structure and vital function in preserving homeostasis, directing voluntary and involuntary movements, and promoting perception, cognition, and movement. The cerebrum, cerebellum, and brainstem are three areas of the brain that are contained inside the skull and are each in charge of particular functions. Higher order cognitive processes including memory, reasoning, and sensory processing are managed by the cerebrum. While the brainstem controls vital life-sustaining processes like breathing, heart rate, and sleep cycles, the cerebellum coordinates movement and balance. Signals between the brain and the body's other organs are transmitted via the spinal cord, which grows from the brainstem through the vertebral column. It transmits motor and sensory data and participates in reflex actions. For the purpose of diagnosing and treating neurological conditions like multiple sclerosis, epilepsy, stroke, and spinal cord injuries, a clinical understanding of the central nervous system is essential. Improvements in neurosurgery and neuroimaging have made it possible to see and treat CNS pathologies more effectively, which has improved patient outcomes.

Orientation and Directional Terms

Term	Definition	Illustration
Central nervous system (CNS)	The central nervous system (CNS) is made up of the brain and spinal cord. The CNS is the body's processing centre. The brain controls most of the functions of the body, including awareness, movement, thinking, speech, and the 5 senses.	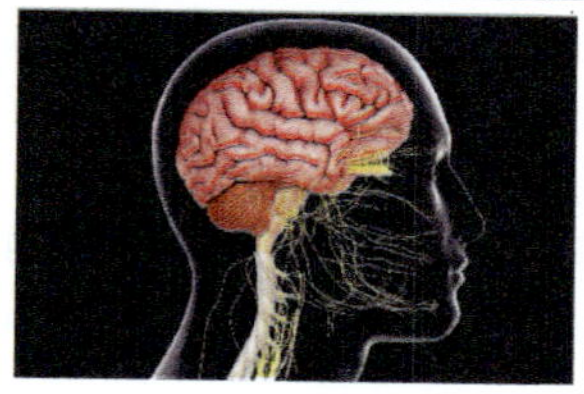
Pyramidal tract	The term pyramidal tracts refers to upper motor neurons that originate in the cerebral cortex and terminate in the spinal cord (corticospinal) or brainstem (corticobulbar).	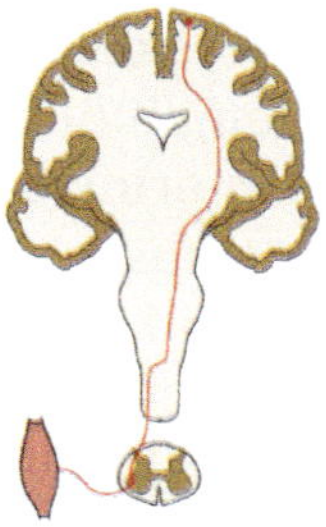
Cerebrospinal fluid (CSF)	Cerebrospinal fluid is a clear, colorless body fluid found within the tissue that surrounds the brain and spinal cord of all vertebrates. CSF is produced by specialized ependymal cells in the choroid plexus of the ventricles of the brain, and absorbed in the arachnoid granulations.	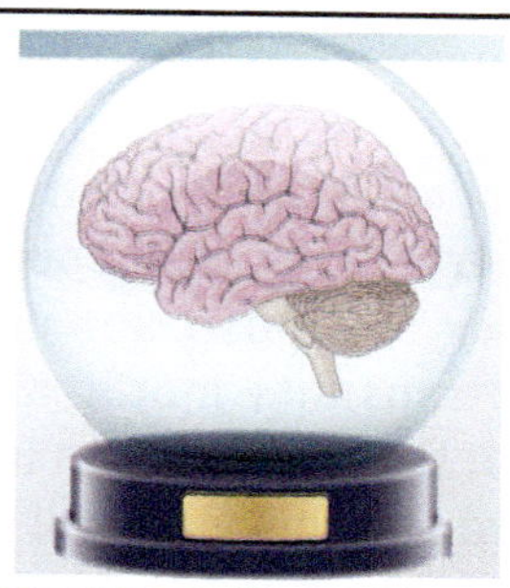
Hypothalamus	The hypothalamus is a structure deep within your brain. It's the main link between your endocrine system and your nervous system. Your hypothalamus keeps your body balanced in a stable state called homeostasis.	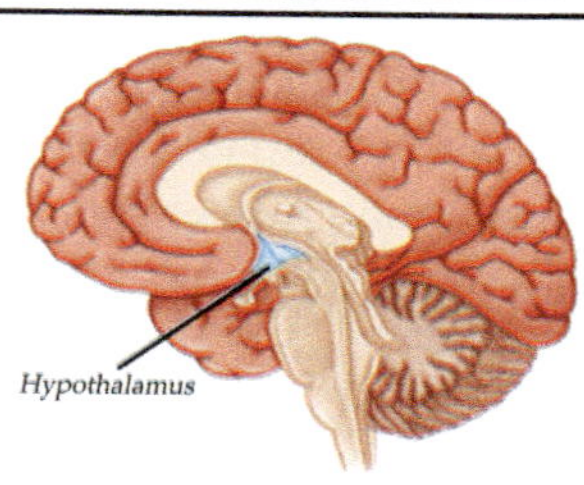
Basal ganglia	Basal ganglia are a group of subcortical nuclei found in the brains of vertebrates. In humans and other primates, differences exist, primarily in the division of the globus pallidus into external and internal regions, and in the division of the striatum.	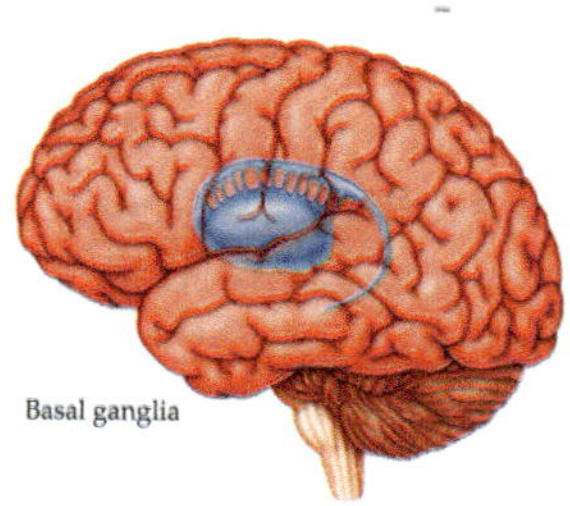

10.1. The Spinal Cord

The spinal cord has a length of 18 inches (45 cm). It ends at the lower level of the first lumbar vertebra or the upper level of the second. It is continuous above with the medulla oblongata at the level of the foramen magnum. It tapers inferiorly into the conus medullaris, from which the filum terminale, a prolongation of pia mater, descends to attach itself to the posterior aspect of the coccyx. The posterior (sensory) nerve roots are serially arranged along a posterolateral sulcus on either side of the cord, which also has a deeper longitudinal anterior fissure and a narrower posterior septum. Each of these posterior roots has a ganglion, which is the sensory nerves' initial cell station. On either side of the cord, the anterior (motor) nerve roots emerge sequentially along the anterolateral aspect. A number of rootlets emerge from the cord to give rise to the anterior and posterior nerves. The anterior and posterior nerve roots combine at each intervertebral foramen to form a spinal nerve. This spinal nerve then splits into its anterior and posterior primary rami, each of which transmits motor and sensory fibers. Because of the difference in length between the spinal cord and the vertebral column, the length of the roots grows gradually from top to bottom. The lumbar and sacral roots continue as a cauda equina, a leash of nerve roots, below the cord's termination at vertebral level L2 (Shipp, 2007; Stiles & Jernigan, 2010).

10.1.1. Age Differences

The spinal cord fills the entire vertebral canal up until the third month of fetal life. The cord only reaches the level of the 3rd lumbar vertebra at birth because the vertebrae continue to grow faster than the cord. The cord reaches its final position at the approximate level of the disc between the first and second lumbar vertebrae during additional differential growth until adolescence.

10.1.2. Structure

A transverse section of the cord reveals the central canal, which is encircled by the H-shaped gray matter and the long ascending and descending tracts that are contained in the white matter. Many of the sensory fibers that enter from the posterior nerve roots terminate within the posterior horns of the gray matter, which are capped by the substantia gelatinosa. The motor cells that give rise to the anterior root fibers are located in the large anterior horns.

The sympathetic system's origin cells are located in the lateral horns on either side of the thoracic and upper lumbar cords. The longer, more significant tracts in the white matter will now be addressed (Figures 10.1 and 10.2).

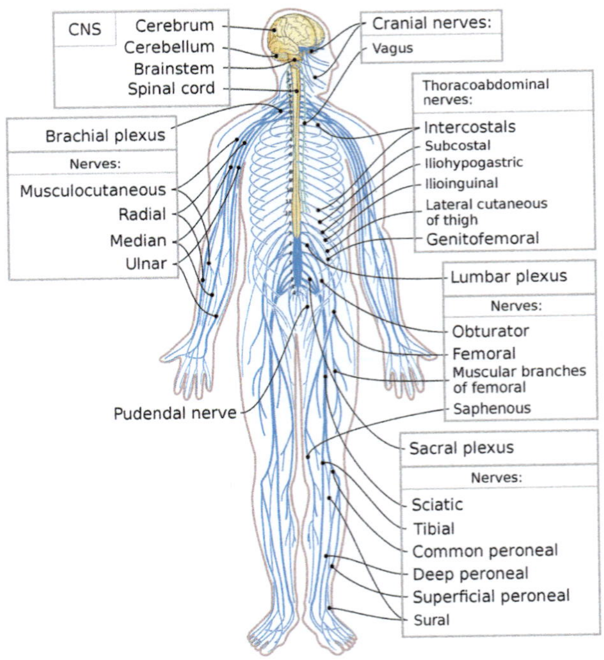

Figure 10.1. *The spinal cord.*

Source: By Medium69, Jmarchn – File:Nervous system diagram.png, CC BY-SA 4.0; https://commons.wikimedia.org/w/index.php?curid=36395693.

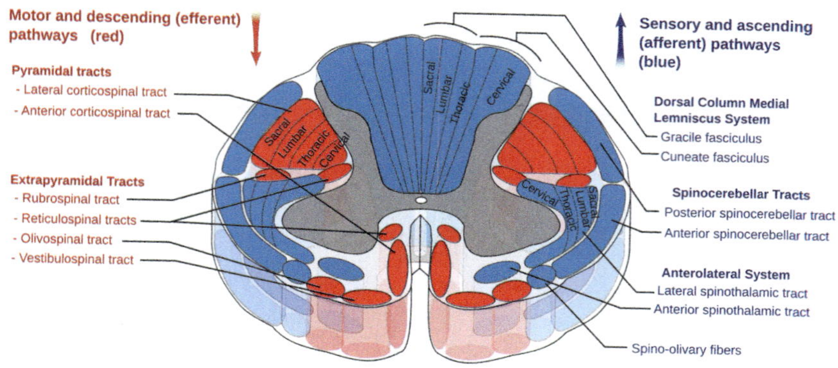

Figure 10.2. *The spinal cord.*

Source: By Polarlys and Mikael Häggström – File:Medulla spinalis – tracts – English.svg by Polarlys (translation by Selket), CC BY-SA 3.0; https://commons.wikimedia.org/w/index.php?curid=10909281.

10.1.3. Descending Tracts

The pyramidal tract, also known as crossed motor or lateral cerebrospinal. The motor pathway begins at the motor cortex's pyramidal cells, descends in the pyramidal tract on the opposite side of the cord, and then decusses in the medulla. Because fibers enter the anterior horn at each spinal segment and join up with the motor cells there, the tract gets smaller as it descends (Shipp, 2007; Stiles & Jernigan, 2010) (Figures 10.3 and 10.4).

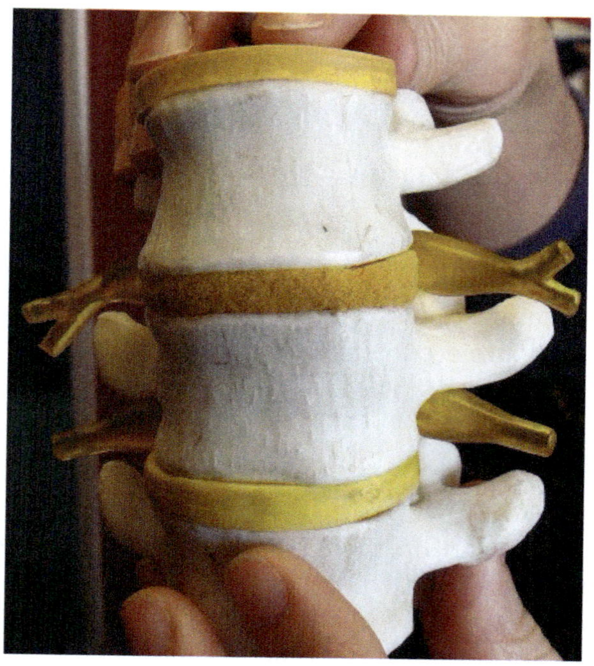

Figure 10.3. *The range of variation in the termination of the spinal cord in the adult.*

Source: By Tomwsulcer – Own work, CC0; https://commons.wikimedia.org/w/index.php?curid=15006027.

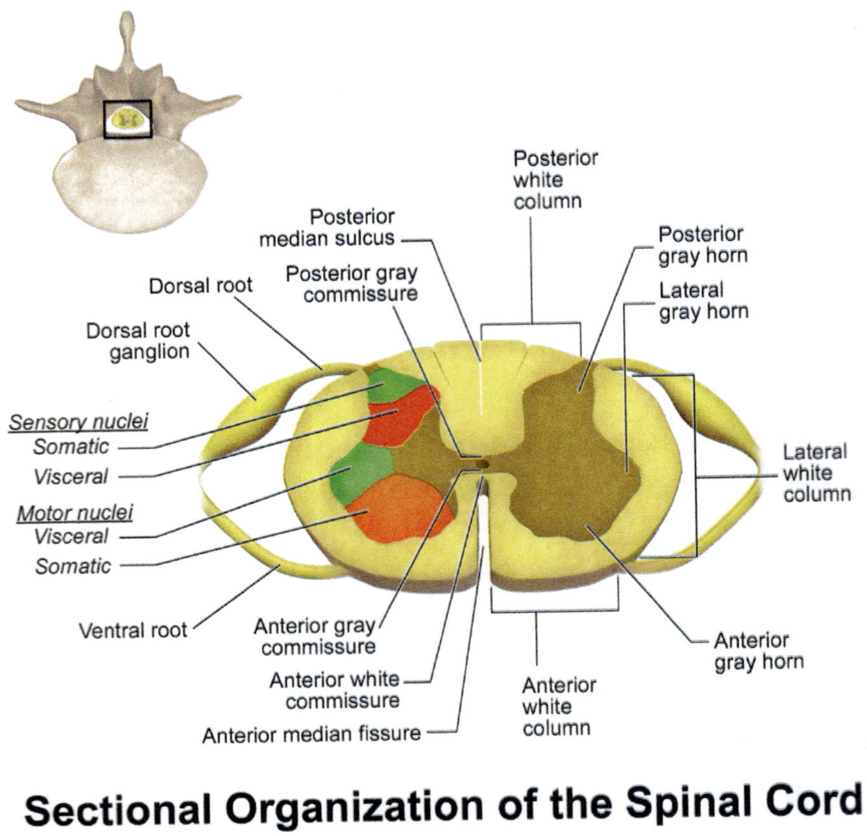

Figure 10.4. *The section of the spinal cord.*

Source: By BruceBlaus – Own work, CC BY-SA 4.0; https://commons.wikimedia.org/w/index.php?curid=46621399.

The direct pyramidal tract, also known as the anterior corticospinal or uncrossed motor tract, is a compact pathway that descends without crossing over in the medulla. However, at each segment, fibers from this tract project to the motor cells in the anterior (ventral) horn on the opposite side of the body.

10.1.4. Ascending Tracts

The inferior and superior cerebellar peduncles, respectively, are where the posterior and anterior spinocerebellar tracts, which ascend on the same side of the cord, enter the cerebellum. The spinothalamic tracts, anterior and lateral. Sensory cortex: Afferent nerve fibers responsible for pain and temperature travel through the posterior roots, climb a few segments, reroute in the substantia gelatinosa, and then traverse to the other side to ascend via these tracts to the thalamus. A medial and lateral tract, known as the fasciculus gracilis (of Goll) and fasciculus cuneatus (of Burdach), respectively, make up the posterior columns. They carry first-order sensory fibers, which are primarily uncrossed and serve fine touch and proprioception (position sense), to the medulla's gracile and cuneate nuclei. From there, second-order fibers decussate, travel to the thalamus, and then, following another synapse, third-order fibers are transmitted to the sensory cortex. Some fibers travel along the inferior cerebellar peduncle from the medulla to the cerebellum (Shipp, 2007; Stiles & Jernigan, 2010).

10.1.4.1. Blood Supply

The intracranial portion of the vertebral artery gives rise to the anterior and posterior spinal arteries, which descend in the pia. Branches from the lumbar arteries, intercostal, ascending cervical, and cervical portion of the vertebral column reinforce them sequentially.

10.1.4.2. Clinical Features

Complete cord transection is accompanied by flaccid muscle paralysis and complete loss of sensation in the areas supplied by the cord segments below the site of injury. After a period of spinal shock, the paralysis becomes spastic and the reflexes become exaggerated as the cord distal to the section heals. If the cord centers located in the sacral zone of the cord are not destroyed, voluntary sphincter control is lost but reflex bladder and rectum emptying then resumes. When the central nervous system is destroyed, as is the case with syringomyelia and certain intramedullary tumors, the decussating spinothalamic fibers are the first to be affected. This causes a bilateral loss of pain and temperature sense beneath the lesion at first, but proprioception and fine touch are retained until later in the uncrossed posterior columns. Brown-Sequard syndrome follows hemi section of the cord; the afflicted side experiences paralysis below the lesion (pyramidal tract), along with loss of proprioception and fine discrimination (dorsal columns). Since the affected spinothalamic tract contains fibers that have decussated below the level of cord hemi section, pain and temperature senses are lost on the opposite side below the lesion. Loss of proprioception is a characteristic of tabes dorsalis, a syphilitic degenerative lesion of the posterior columns and posterior nerve roots. The patient becomes ataxic, especially if he closes his eyes, as a result of losing his sense of position, which he can only partially compensate for with visual knowledge of his spatial relationship (Romberg's sign). In certain instances, intractable pain can be managed by dividing the spinothalamic tract on the side opposite the pain (cordotomy) or by excising the relevant posterior nerve roots (posterior rhizotomy). The pyramidal tract immediately posterior to the spinothalamic tract will remain intact if a knife is inserted 3 mm into the cord anterior to the denticulate ligament and then swept anteriorly from this point.

10.1.5. The Membranes of the Cord (The Meninges)

The pia mater envelops the spinal cord and the brain closely. The denticulate ligament is formed by this becoming thicker on either side in between the nerve roots and passing laterally to adhere to the dura. Below, the pia persists as the filum terminale, penetrating the dural sac's distal extremity and joining the coccyx.

Cerebrospinal fluid (CSF) is located in a large subarachnoid space that is left behind after the arachnoid mater lines the dura mater, in between the pia and it. The spinal nerve roots continue to carry both pia and arachnoid. The dura itself protects the cord with a strong sheath. At the level of the second sacral vertebra, it ends distally. Additionally, it persists along every nerve root and combines with the peripheral nerve sheaths (Figure 10.5).

The space between the spinal canal and the dural sheath is known as the extradural (or epidural) space. It reaches the sacral hiatus from the foramen magnum, below which the dura splits into two layers. It is filled with semiliquid fat, arteries, big, thin-walled veins, and lymphatics (though no lymphatics exist within the nervous system deep to the dura). These could be compared to the cerebral venous sinuses, which are located in the space between the cerebral dura's two layers. The extradural veins form a plexus that receives the basi vertebral veins, which emerge from each vertebral body on its posterior aspect, while the arteries of this space are rather insignificant. Furthermore, the veins connect to the cerebral veins above and the pelvic veins below, providing a channel for the spread of tumor cells and bacteria. This explains, for instance, why prostatic cancer can spread quickly to the sacrum and vertebrae (a condition known as "valveless vertebral venous plexus," described by Watson).

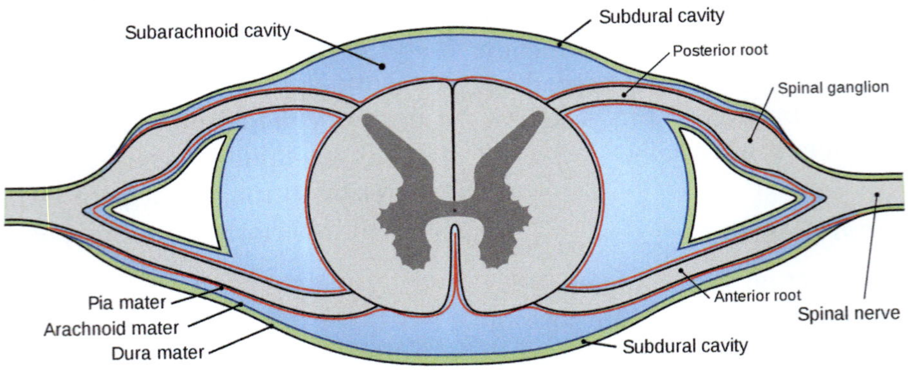

Figure 10.5. *The membranes of the spinal cord.*

Source: By Mysid – Made by Mysid Inkscape, based on plate 770 from Gray's Anatomy (1918, Public Domain), Public Domain; https://commons.wikimedia.org/w/index.php?curid=10496507.

10.1.5.1. Clinical Features

To remove CSF, a lumbar puncture must be carried out from the spinal subarachnoid space far away from the cord's termination. The intervertebral spaces directly above or below this landmark can be used safely because a line connecting the iliac crests passes through the fourth lumbar vertebra. To fully open the vertebral interspinous spaces, the patient's spine must be fully flexed, either while they are sitting or lying on their side. The dura, which has a noticeable "give," is punctured after the supraspinous and interspinous ligaments are crossed, and the needle is inserted inward, slightly cranially, in the midline, and at an angle to the spine. Occasionally, if a cauda equina root is impinged upon, root pain is felt; however, these typically float clear of the needle. CSF at spinal puncture is available for inspection; the CSF, radio-opaque contrast medium, or anesthetics can be injected into the subarachnoid space. Pressure can be approximated (normal, 80–180 mm CSF when lying on the side). A block in the spinal canal above the point of puncture, produced, for example, by a spinal tumor, can be revealed by Queckenstedt's test as follows.

The internal jugular veins are compressed by applying pressure to the neck, which decreases venous outflow from the cranium and increases intracranial pressure. As a result, CSF is transferred into both the spinal sac and the CSF. Pressure increases rapidly by at least 40 mm, as shown by lumbar puncture and manometry. If there is a spinal block, this pressure increase is not noticed. Blockage beyond the normal range. A needle can be inserted via the sacral hiatus or between the spinal laminae to reach the extradural space (Figure 10.6).

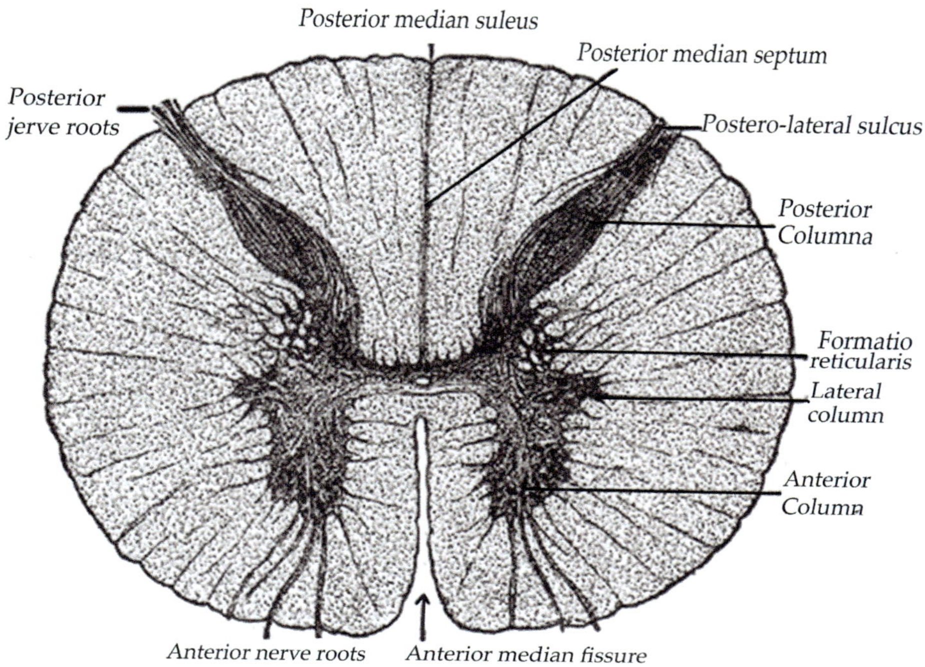

Figure 10.6. *Mid-thoracic level.*

Source: By Henry Vandyke Carter – Henry Gray, (1918). Anatomy of the human body (see "Book" section below) Bartleby.com: Gray's Anatomy, Plate 664, Public Domain; https://commons.wikimedia.org/w/index.php?curid=541456.

10.2. The Brain

10.2.1. The Medulla

The medulla has a length of 1 inch (25 mm) and a diameter of approximately 0.75 inch (18 mm). It is continuous with the spinal cord below via the foramen magnum and with the pons above; it is connected to the cerebellum posteriorly through the inferior cerebellar peduncles.

10.2.1.1. External Features

The pyramidal tract swellings are located on either side of an anteromedian fissure that grooves the anterior surface of the medulla. The anterolateral sulcus, where the rootlets of the XIIth cranial nerve emerge, divides these pyramids from the olivary eminences in turn (Figure 10.7).

The cranial nerves IX, X, and XI's rootlets emerge from a second groove that runs between the olive and the inferior cerebellar peduncle. This groove corresponds to the spinal cord's posterolateral sulcus. Halfway up the medulla, the posteromedian sulcus of the cord continues and widens to form the posterior region of the IVth ventricle. The gracile and cuneate nuclei are represented by the two distinct tubercles that are formed by the posterior columns of the spinal cord expanding on either side of the fissure.

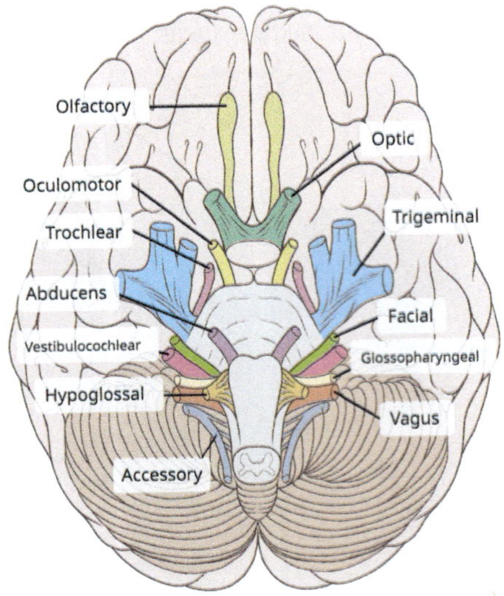

Figure 10.7. *The base of the brain showing the cranial nerve roots and their relationships to the circle of Willis.*

Source: By Brain_human_normal_inferior_view_with_labels_en.svg: *Brain_human_normal_inferior_view.svg: Patrick J. Lynch, medical illustrator derivative work: Beaoderivative work: Dwstultz (talk) – Brain_human_normal_inferior_view_with_labels_en.svg, CC BY 2.5, https://commons.wikimedia.org/w/index.php?curid=15108118.

10.2.1.2. Deep Structure

The best way to illustrate the deep structure of the medulla is to use diagrams that show how the medulla appears cross-sectionally at the level of the IVth ventricle and the sensory decussation (Figures 10.8 and 10.9).

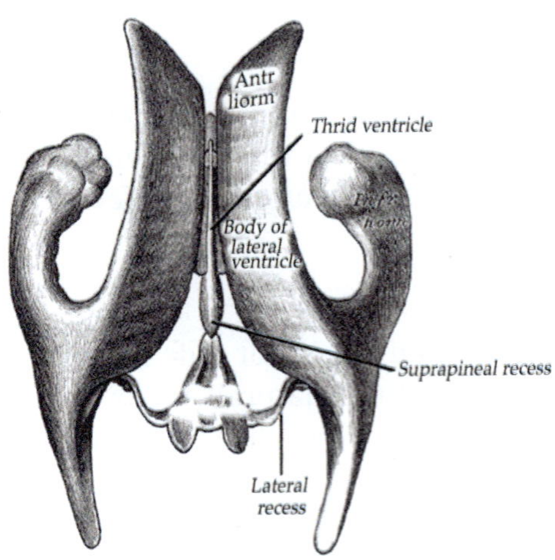

Figure 10.8. *The ventricles.*

Source: By Henry Vandyke Carter – Henry Gray, (1918). Anatomy of the human body (see "Book" section below) Bartleby.com: Gray's Anatomy, Plate 735, Public Domain; https://commons.wikimedia.org/w/index.php?curid=541555.

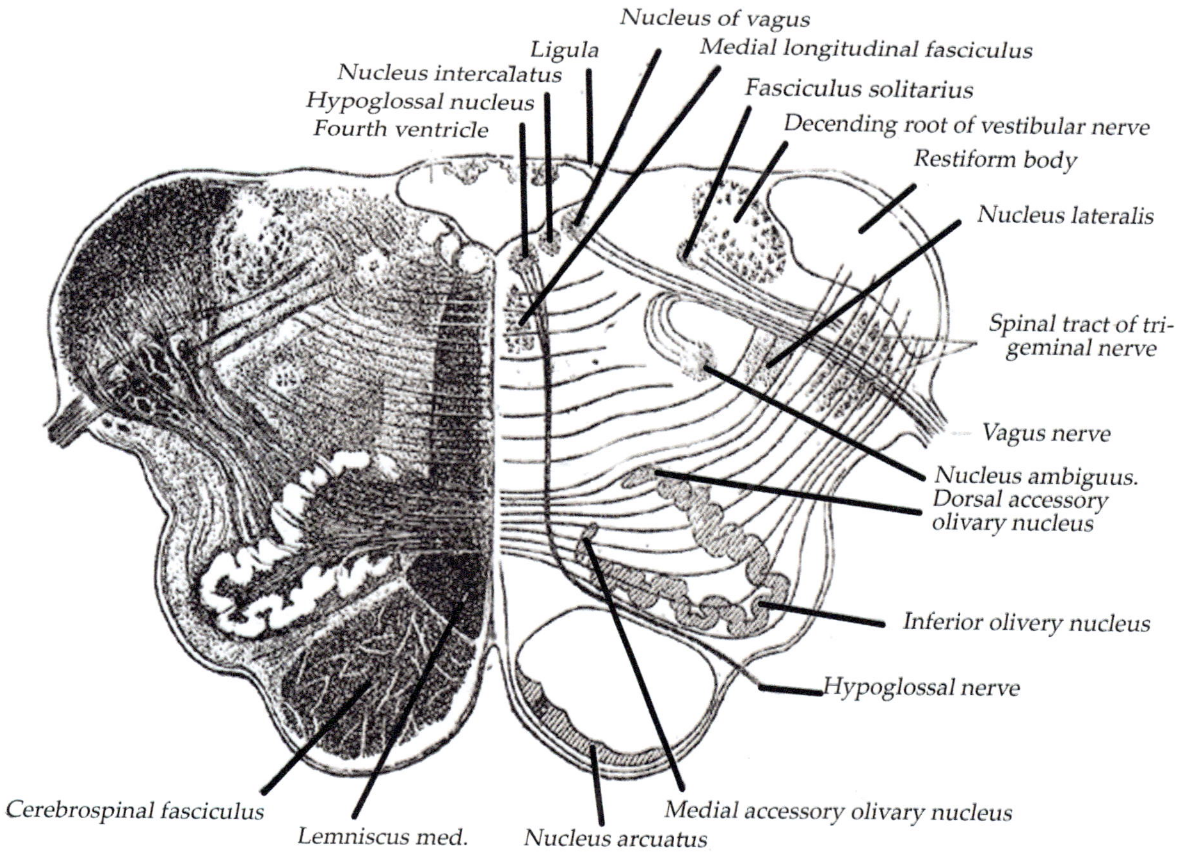

Figure 10.9. *Cross-section through the medulla at the level of the caudal part of the 4th ventricle.*

Source: By Henry Vandyke Carter – Henry Gray, (1918). Anatomy of the human body (see "Book" section below) Bartleby.com: Gray's Anatomy, Plate 695, Public Domain; https://commons.wikimedia.org/w/index.php?curid=541508.

The vertebral arteries directly supply the medulla with blood, as do their posterior inferior cerebellar branches.

10.2.1.3. Clinical Features

The "vital centers"—the respiratory, cardiac, and vasomotor—are found in the medulla. Respiratory failure resulting from compression, injury, or poliomyelitis is especially likely to affect the respiratory center.

10.2.2. The Pons

10.2.2.1. External Features

The middle cerebellar peduncles connect the pons, which is situated between the medulla and the midbrain, to the cerebellum. Its measurements are 1 in (25 mm) wide and 1.5 in (38 mm) long. Its ventral surface has multiple transverse ridges that run parallel to the middle cerebellar peduncle laterally, as well as a shallow median groove. The upper portion of the IVth ventricle's floor is formed by the pons' dorsal surface. The emergence of the VIth cranial nerves and the VIIth and VIIIth nerves in the angle formed by the pons and cerebellum indicate its junction with the medulla, which is located near the ventral midline. The lateral region of the pons, close to its upper border, is where the motor and sensory roots of V exit.

10.2.2.2. Internal Structure

The pons is primarily composed of several cell masses, known as the pontine nuclei, which are dispersed throughout the long pathways traveling up and down as well as the crossing pontocerebellar fibers. It also includes the pontine tegmentum, a part of the reticular formation, and the central connections of the Vth, VIth, and VIIth cranial nerves. The blood supply of the pons comes from the basilar artery, which is created by the merging of the two vertebral arteries, through various small pontine branches.

10.2.3. The Cerebellum

10.2.3.1. External Features

The posterior cranial fossa is mostly occupied by the cerebellum, which makes up the majority of the hindbrain. It consists of a median vermis and two lateral cerebellar hemispheres. On the inferior side, the vermis is easily distinguished from the two hemispheres and is situated at the base of the vallecula, a deep cleft; on the superior side, it is only identified as a low median elevation between the hemispheres. The portion of the hemisphere located on the middle cerebellar peduncle, known as the flocculus, is mostly isolated from the rest of the cerebellum. The cerebellum's surface is made up of multiple narrow folia and divided into lobules by deep fissures, creating the appearance of a branched tree in cross-section, known as the arbor vitae (Figure 10.10).

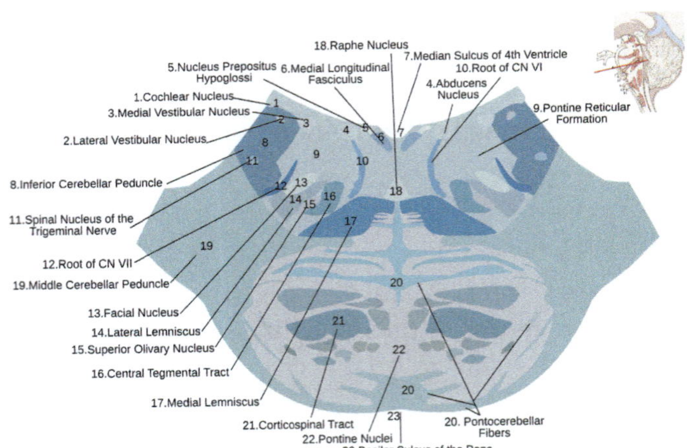

Figure 10.10. *The pons.*

Source: By Marshall Strother User:mcstrotherBrain_stem_sagittal_section.svg: Patrick J. Lynch, medical illustrator – Brain_stem_sagittal_section.svg, CC BY 3.0; https://commons.wikimedia.org/w/index.php?curid=15172679.

10.2.3.2. Internal Structure

The cerebellum has an exceptionally homogeneous structure. It is made up of a mass of white matter that contains the deep nuclei of gray matter buried beneath a cortex of gray matter, where all afferent fibers terminate. The dentate nucleus, which is located in the middle of each hemisphere, is by far the largest of these. Fastigii, globosus, and emboliformis are the other nuclei. Three pairs of cerebellar peduncles connect the cerebellum to the brainstem. It is connected to the dorsolateral aspect of the medulla by the inferior peduncles, to the pons by the middle cerebellar peduncles, and to the midbrain caudally by the superior peduncles. Dorsally, the tentorium cerebelli divides it from the cerebral hemispheres. Ventrally, the cerebellum is connected to the 4th ventricle, the medulla, and the pons; laterally, it is related to the sigmoid sinus, the mastoid antrum, and air cells.

The posterior inferior cerebellar branches of the vertebral arteries supply the posterior aspect of the vermis and hemispheres, while the anterior inferior and superior cerebellar branches of the basilar artery supply the anterolateral part of the under surface and the superior aspect of the cerebellum, respectively. These three pairs of arteries provide the blood supply for the cerebellum (Table 10.1).

Table 10.1. *Summary of Novel Treatment Strategies for Neurodegenerative Diseases*

Strategy	Model	Drugs	Dose	Results	References
Inhibiting protein aggregates	Rat	iAβ5 (Chaperon)	200 nmol	• Reduced size and number of cerebral amyloid plaques in AD.	[Sigurdsson E.M., et al. 2000]
Disaggregating misfolded proteins	Mouse	Hsp104	–	• Degradation of mutant HTT.	[Bauer P.O., et al. 2010]
Immunomodulation	Mouse	Geldanamycin	1 or 10 µg/kg	• Inhibition of HSP90. • Induction of HSP70. • Neuroprotection in MPTP induced PD.	[Shen H.Y., et al. 2005]
	Mouse	Amyloid-β-peptide	–	• Reduction of Aβ deposits in the frontal cortex and hippocampus in HD model. • Improved cognitive function. • Reduced astrogliosis and disease progression.	[Morgan D., et al. 2000, Janus C., et al. 2000, Schenk D., et al. 1999]

–	Mouse	Resveratrol	50 mg/kg	• Reduced glial activation in PD model. • Reduced ILs. • Improved TH expression.	[Lofrumento D.D., et al. 2014]
	Mouse	Tanshinone IIA	25 mg/kg	• Reduced degeneration of nigrostriatal DA neurons. • Increased striatal DA content.	[Ren B., et al. 2015]
	Mouse	Tanshinone I	10 mg/kg	• Reduced expression of pro-inflammatory factors. • Improved motor function and striatal neurotransmitters.	[Wang S., et al. 2015]
	Mouse	1H7, 5C1, 5D12	–	• Reduced α-synuclein accumulation. • Reduced synaptic and axonal pathology in PD model. • Improved cognitive function.	[Games D., et al. 2014]
	Mouse	mAb47	–	• Reduced α-synuclein accumulation in PD model. • Improved motor function.	[Lindström V., et al. 2014]
Induction of autophagy	Drosophila	Rapamycin	1 μM	• Enhanced clearance of pyroglutamine and polyalanine proteins. • Enhanced clearance of tau protein and decreased tau toxicity.	[Berger Z., et al. 2005]
	Verapamil	Mice	25 mg/kg	• Suppressed hepatosteatosis. • Reduced obesity-induced cytosolic calcium in liver. • Restored autophagic flux.	[Park H.-W., et al. 2014]

	Rapamycin ester (CCI-779)	Mice	20 mg/kg	• Enhanced clearance of mutant huntingtin. • Improved behavioral tasks.	[Ravikumar B., et al. 2004]
	Metformin	Mice	2 mg/mL of drinking water	• Prolonged survival time. • Decreased hindlimb clasping time.	[Ma T.C., et al. 2007]
	Nilotinib	Mice	10 mg/kg	• Reduced brain and peripheral α-synuclein and p-tau. • Improved immune profile.	[Hebron M.L., et al. 2014]
–	Nilotinib	Mice	–	• Increased β-amyloid clearance. • Reduced inflammation. • Improved immune profile.	[Lonskaya I., et al. 2015]

Source: Hussain, R., Zubair, H., Pursell, S., & Shahab, M., (2018). Neurodegenerative diseases: Regenerative mechanisms and novel therapeutic approaches. Brain Sciences, 8(9), 177. https://doi.org/10.3390/brainsci8090177.

10.2.3.3. Clinical Features

An unsteady gait, hypotonia, tremor, nystagmus, and dysarthria are among the symptoms of cerebellar lesions, which disrupt one or more of these motor functions. The cerebellum is primarily involved in balance, posture regulation, muscle tone, and muscular coordination. Symptoms and signs on the same side of the body are caused by lesions in the cerebellum. Ablation of the entire cerebellar hemisphere causes a disability almost as severe as destruction of the dentate nucleus or the superior cerebellar peduncle. Thrombosis of the posterior inferior cerebellar artery results in a distinctive syndrome characterized by signs of cranial nerve involvement (V to X), contralateral loss of pain and thermal sensibility (spinothalamic involvement), and ataxia and hypotonia of the homolateral limbs (Shipp, 2007; Stiles & Jernigan, 2010).

10.2.4. The Midbrain

The midbrain, which links the pons and cerebellum to the diencephalon, is the shortest segment of the brain stem. It is slightly less than 1 in (25 mm) long. It is mostly concealed by the surrounding structures and is located in the tentorium cerebelli gap.

10.2.4.1. External Features

The two cerebral peduncles, which emerge from the cerebral hemisphere's substance and travel downward and medially to connect the internal capsule to the pons, are the only parts of the midbrain that are visible from the ventral aspect of the brain. In the interpeduncular fossa, the third nerve fibers emerge between the two cerebral peduncles. The basis pedunculi ventrally, the midbrain tegmentum centrally, and the tectum dorsally are the three separate parts of the midbrain that are visible when viewed from the lateral aspect. This part of the midbrain is encircled by the optic tract, the trochlear nerve (IV), and the posterior cerebral artery. The superior medullary velum, situated between the two superior cerebellar peduncles, and the four colliculi, also known as the corpora quadrigemini, are visible on the dorsal surface of the midbrain. The pineal gland is connected to the posterior dorsal thalamus by a stalk and lies between the two superior colliculi. It plays a crucial part in establishing the circadian rhythm and secretes melatonin.

10.2.4.2. Internal Structure

Once more, cross-sectional diagrams at representative levels provide the best description of the interior structure of the midbrain: viz. in relation to the superior and inferior colliculi. It is noteworthy that these segments traverse the midbrain at the point where the superior cerebellar peduncle and the 4th nerve nucleus decussate, as well as the red nucleus and the III nucleus, respectively. These illustrations also make it easy to see the midbrain's three subdivisions. The gray matter of the tegmentum is situated between the cerebral aqueduct and the basis pedunculi, with the substantia nigra's deeply pigmented lamina standing between them. The tectum is located above the level of the cerebral aqueduct. The substantia nigra's neurons contain the pigment known as neuromelanin (Figures 10.11 and 10.12).

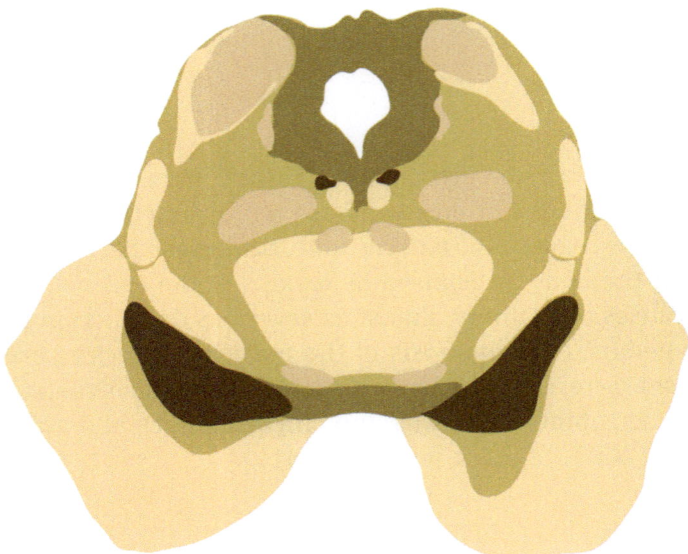

Figure 10.11. *The midbrain—level of the inferior colliculus and decussation of the superior cerebellar peduncle.*

Source: By Kevin Dufendach – Own work, CC BY-SA 3.0; https://commons.wikimedia.org/w/index.php?curid=28204164.

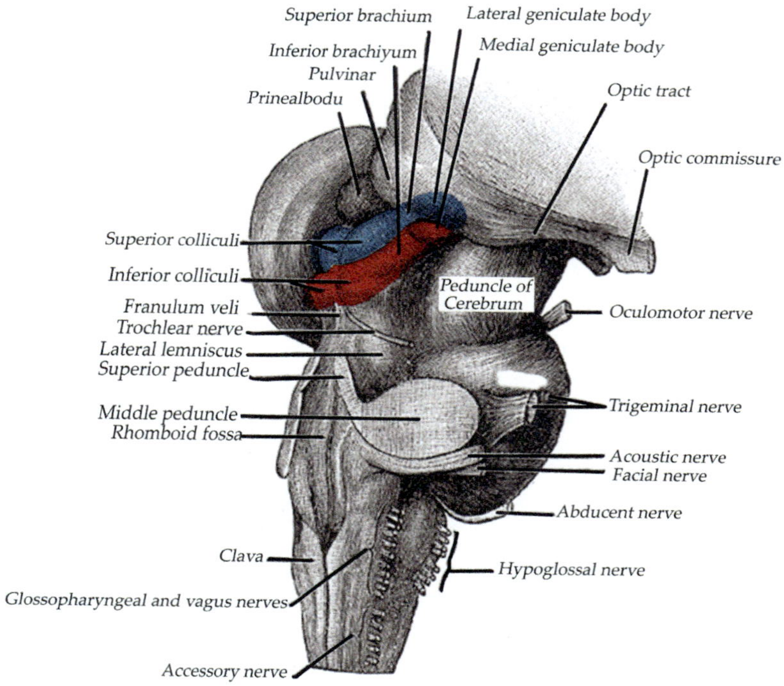

Figure 10.12. *The tectum.*

Source: By Henry Vandyke Carter – Henry Gray, (1918). Anatomy of the human body (see "Book" section below) Bartleby.com: Gray's Anatomy, Plate 719, Public Domain; https://commons.wikimedia.org/w/index.php?curid=526909.

10.2.4.3. Clinical Features

On skull radiographs, the pineal gland can be clearly seen when it has calcified. Then, it might show the crucial radiological signal of lateral displacement caused by a cerebral hemisphere space-occupying lesion.

10.2.5. The Diencephalon

The thalamus and hypothalamus make up the diencephalon. It is the region of the brain that encircles the ventricle.

10.2.6. The Hypothalamus

The third ventricle's floor is made up of the hypothalamus. It comprises the tuber cinereum, the mamillary bodies, the posterior perforated substance, the infundibular stalk (which descends to the pituitary's posterior lobe), and the optic chiasma, starting from the anterior direction. Each of these contains several cell masses or nuclei as well as the medial forebrain bundle, a fiber pathway that runs the entire length of the hypothalamus and connects it to the basal forebrain areas anteriorly and the midbrain posteriorly.

The hypothalamus is the head ganglion of the autonomic nervous system, according to Sherrington. It can be separated into an anterolateral area that deals with parasympathetic activity and a posteromedial sympathetic area that is primarily concerned with autonomic activity. Through the production of factors that either release or inhibit release, the hypothalamus plays a significant role in endocrine regulation. These chemicals affect the anterior pituitary cell synthesis of adrenocorticotrophin (ACTH), follicle-stimulating hormone, luteinizing hormone, prolactin, somatotrophin, thyrotrophin, and melanocyte-stimulating hormone after being secreted into the hypophyseal portal vessels (Figure 10.13).

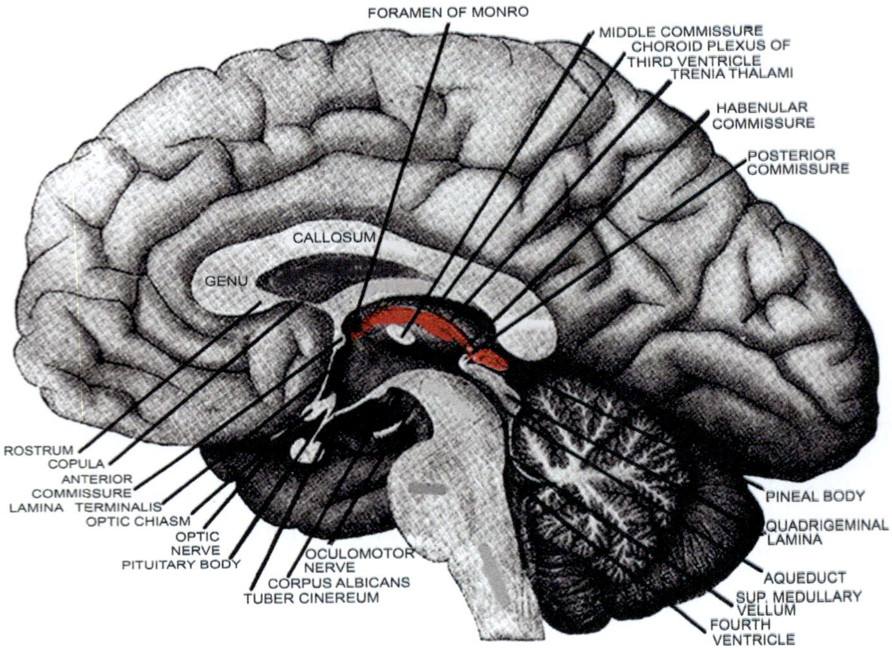

Figure 10.13. *The thalamus.*

Source: By Henry Gray (Lifetime: 1861) – Original publication: Anatomy: Descriptive and surgical immediate source: http://radiopaedia.org/images/23676, Public Domain; https://commons.wikimedia.org/w/index.php?curid=60000626.

Neurons in the hypothalamus produce the hormones oxytocin and vasopressin (also known as antidiuretic hormone, or ADH), which are then released at the axon terminals of these neurons in the posterior pituitary.

10.2.6.1. Clinical Features

- Lesions of the hypothalamus may result in a variety of autonomic disturbances, e.g., somnolence, disturbances of temperature regulation, and obesity, as well as a variety of endocrine abnormalities, e.g., hypogonadism and hypothyroidism.
- Damage to the supraoptic nuclei or the infundibular stalk leads to diabetes insipidus.

10.2.7. The Pituitary Gland (Hypophysis Cerebri)

Compare the two glandular components of the suprarenal cortex and medulla, as well as the exocrine and endocrine sections of the pancreas, testis, and ovary, to see an example of a "two in one" organ of which nature is so adept. The pituitary consists of two lobes: the larger anterior and the smaller posterior. The latter is joined to the tuber cinereum in the third ventricle's floor by the hollow infundibulum, also known as the pituitary stalk. The pars intermedia, a narrow zone, connects the two lobes. The diaphragma sellae, a dura mater fold, covers the pituitary, which is located in the pituitary fossa cavity. The infundibulum travels through the central aperture of this fold. The sphenoid body is located below, and intercavernous sinuses connect in front, behind, and below. Laterally, the cavernous sinus and its contents are divided by dura mater. Above and directly in front of the infundibulum is the optic chiasma.

10.2.7.1. Structure

The front lobe is highly cellular and is composed of chromophobe, eosinophilic, and basophilic cells. The middle part contains large colloid vesicles similar to those found in the thyroid. The back lobe is comprised of nerve fibers with cell bodies located in the hypothalamus.

10.2.7.2. Development

One type of cerebral diverticulum is the posterior lobe. From Rathke's pouch in the roof of the primitive buccal cavity, the anterior lobe and the pars intermedia develop. Occasionally, remnants of this pouch's epithelium give rise to a tumor (craniopharyngioma). These tumors are frequently calcified and cystic.

10.2.7.3. Clinical Features

In addition to developing intracranial space-occupying lesions, pituitary tumors can be distinguished by two unique characteristics: endocrine disruptions and a connection to the optic chiasma. The most prevalent pituitary tumor is chromophores adenoma. The pituitary fossa (sella turcica) expands as it grows, and radiological evidence of this can be provided. The very quick typical bitemporal hemianopia is caused by compression of the optic chiasma. The tumor slowly kills the normally functioning gland because it is not secretory in the first place. The patient experiences hypopituitarism, hypothyroidism, and hypoadrenalism along with a loss of sex characteristics. There is a growth arrest in childhood. Obesity and diabetes insipidus may be associated with hypothalamic involvement as the tumor grows.

The pituitary growth hormones are secreted by the eosinophil adenoma. It causes gigantism if it happens before puberty, which is unusual, and acromegaly if it happens after puberty. Small and without pressure effects, the basophil adenoma may be linked to Cushing's syndrome, though the condition is more frequently caused by hyperplasia or a tumor of the suprarenal cortex. Pituitary tumors can be accessed via a frontal bone flap or by passing a fiber-optic endoscope through the sphenoid sinus and nasal cavity. Fiber-optic instruments can be inserted into the pituitary gland using a trans nasal, transsphenoidal technique due to the pituitary's close relationship to the sphenoid sinus. Currently, this is the recommended method for operating on pituitary tumors.

10.2.8. The Thalamus

The third ventricle's lateral wall is formed by the oval mass of gray matter known as the thalamus, which stretches from the interventricular foramen caudally to the midbrain rostrally. It is connected dorsally to the floor of the lateral ventricle and laterally to the internal capsule (and via it, to the basal ganglia). It often shares a medial connection (the interthalamic connexus) with its counterpart on the other side. It has three distinct eminences on the posterior side: the pulvinar and the medial and lateral geniculate bodies, which are the thalamic relay nuclei for vision and hearing, respectively.

The primary sensory relay nucleus that relays impulses from the primary sensory pathways to the cerebral cortex is the thalamus. It accomplishes this through a variety of internal capsule thalamic radiations. The posterior cerebral artery provides the majority of the thalamus's blood supply through its thalamostriate branches, which pierce the posterior perforated substance and supply the posterior portion of the internal capsule as well. Loss of contralateral facial and body sensation is caused by thalamic damage due to blockage of this blood supply (Shipp, 2007; Stiles & Jernigan, 2010).

10.2.9. The Cerebral Hemispheres

The cerebral cortex, basal ganglia, and their afferent and efferent connections make up the cerebral hemispheres, which in humans have grown out of all proportion to the rest of the brain. At their center are the lateral ventricles, which hold the CSF.

10.2.10. The Cerebral Cortex

Topographically and functionally, the cerebral hemisphere cortex is separated into four lobes: frontal, parietal, temporal, and occipital (Figure 10.14).

- **The Motor Cortex:** A significant portion of the precentral gyrus is occupied by the primary motor area. It deals with voluntary movements and receives afferents from the cerebellum, thalamus, and premotor cortex. Distinct muscle contractions come from stimulation of this region.
- **The Premotor Cortex:** This is located in front of the lower portion of the frontal gyri that adjoins the precentral gyrus. It is also concerned with voluntary movement, but when it is stimulated, muscle groups that perform similar tasks move less deliberately.
- **Eye Motor Field:** This is located in front of the premotor cortex in the middle frontal area. When this region is injured, the gaze deviates to the side of the lesion, impairing eye movement.
- **Broca's Speech Area:** Broca demonstrated that the motor element in speech is impacted by lesions in the vicinity of the posterior portion of the inferior frontal gyrus of the dominant (typically left) hemisphere.
- **Frontal Association Cortex (Clinically Called the Prefrontal Cortex):** This is one of the amazing developments of the human brain and makes up a significant portion of the frontal lobe. Its efferents are most likely sent to the thalamus and hypothalamus,

while its afferents originate from the limbic region, thalamus, and other cortical areas. The lateral frontal lobe aspect appears to be associated with "intellectual activity" from a functional perspective, the management of autonomic activity, the medial and orbital surfaces to affective (or emotional) behavior, and cognitive processes such as analysis, judgment, and planning.

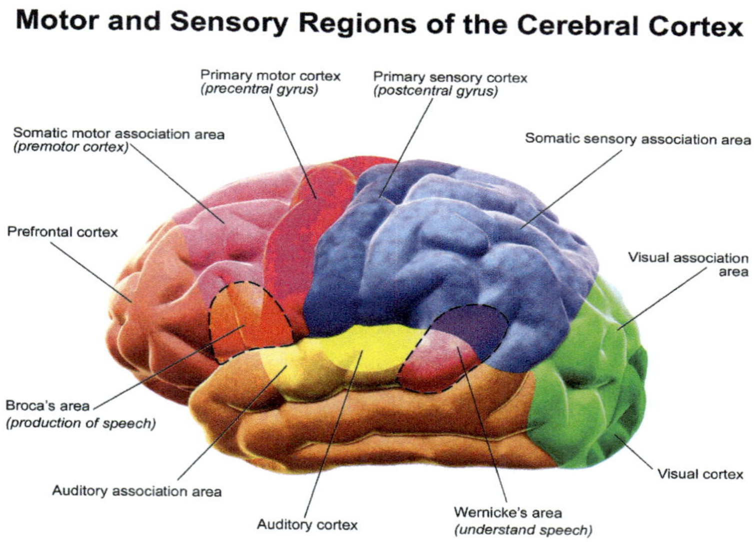

Figure 10.14. *Localization of function in the cerebral cortex.*

Source: By BruceBlaus. When using this image in external sources it can be cited as: Blausen.com staff (2014). "Medical gallery of Blausen Medical, 2014." Wiki Journal of Medicine, 1(2). doi: 10.15347/wjm/2014.010. ISSN: 2002-4436. Own work, CC BY 3.0; https://commons.wikimedia.org/w/index.php?curid=31574253.

10.2.10.1. Parietal Lobe

The parietal lobe is bounded anteriorly by the central sulcus and behind by a line drawn from the parieto-occipital sulcus to the posterior end of the lateral (Sylvian) sulcus. The important cortical areas of the parietal lobe are as follows:

1. The primary somatosensory cortex. The postcentral gyrus receives afferent fibers from the thalamus and is concerned with all forms of somatic sensation.
2. The remaining portion of the parietal lobe, known as the parietal association cortex, is primarily responsible for identifying somatic sensory stimulation and integrating it with other types of sensory data. Additionally, it receives afferents from the thalamus. Damage to it results in more complex defects than simple loss of sensation. One example is astereognosis, which is the inability to recognize somatic stimuli. If you place a coin or key in the patient's hand, for example, he will know what it is but will not be able to identify it. Language is largely controlled by the lower region

of the parietal lobe in the dominant hemisphere of the subject. It interacts with somatosensory visual and auditory associations.

10.2.10.2. The Temporal Lobe

A line drawn vertically downward from the upper end of the lateral sulcus arbitrarily divides this from the occipital lobe. The important cortical areas of the temporal lobe are the following:

1. **The Auditory Cortex:** This lies in the superior temporal gyrus on the lateral and superior surfaces of the hemisphere. Its afferent fibers are from the medial geniculate body and it is concerned with the perception of auditory stimuli.
2. **The Temporal Association Cortex:** The recognition of auditory stimuli and their integration with other sensory modalities are processes that take place in the region that surrounds the auditory cortex. Auditory agnosia is the result of lesions in this area and the incapacity to identify or comprehend the meaning of meaningful noises. The sensory components of language comprehension greatly depend on the cortical region (Wernicke's area) directly above and behind this area on the dominant hemisphere. The occipital lobe's visual region, which links to the temporal lobe, is involved in visual recognition. Behavior is the focus of the antero-inferior aspect of the frontal lobe, which is connected to the medial aspect of the temporal lobe.

10.2.11. The Para Hippocampal Gyrus

The para hippocampal gyrus, which makes up a large portion of the entorhinal cortex, is the most medial portion of the temporal lobe's undersurface cortex. It is one of the main sources of inputs to the hippocampal region and receives extensive association cortical afferent neural stimulation. It is connected to the uncus's olfactory cortex anteriorly. One of the most significant sources of afferents to this structure, the hippocampal layer of innervated cortex, is directly connected to it medially. The hippocampus extends to the amygdala and takes up the entire floor of the inferior horn of the lateral ventricle. It directs its efferents into the alveus, an underlying layer of white matter. The alveolar fibers assemble on the hippocampus's medial margin to form a compact bundle known as the fimbria. This bundle later becomes the fornix as it curves beneath the corpus callosum. The fornix travels in three directions: forward, downward, and backward through the interventricular foramen, ending in the mamillary body of the hypothalamus. It also supplies the thalamus and hypothalamus with fibers. The limbic system includes the projection of the hippocampus to the hypothalamus. This serves as a crucial foundation for memory, behavior, and emotions. Projections from the hypothalamus to the thalamus, the thalamus to the cingulate gyrus, and finally back to the hippocampus complete the circuit. Damage to both hippocampi impairs the ability to create new long-term memories (Shipp, 2007; Stiles & Jernigan, 2010).

10.2.12. The Amygdaloid Nuclear Complex

Located directly rostral to the hippocampus, the amygdaloid nuclear complex is another notable temporal lobe structure. It can be easily separated into three groups of nuclei: corticomedial, central, and basolateral. These groups, in turn, receive a significant amount of olfactory, gustatory, and association cortical afferents. The brainstem autonomic centers, ventral striatum, hypothalamus, and septum are all roughly separably connected to these divisions. The regulation of affective responses and learned behaviors is a function of the amygdala. Given that it can influence emotional reactions in the endocrine, autonomic, and motor domains, its neuroanatomical connections are obviously appropriate for such a role. While the extremely high density of benzodiazepine receptors here suggests amygdaloid involvement in anxiety and stress and their treatments, amygdaloid destruction is specifically linked to decreased aggressive behavior.

10.2.12.1. Occipital Lobe

The occipital lobe lies behind the parietal and temporal lobes. On its medial aspect, it presents the Y-shaped calcarine and post calcarine sulci. The following cortical areas are noteworthy:

- The visual cortex surrounds the calcarine and post calcarine sulci and receives its afferent fibers from the lateral geniculate body of the thalamus of the same side; it is concerned with the vision of the opposite half field of sight.
- The occipital association cortex lies anteriorly to the visual cortex. This area is particularly concerned with the recognition and integration of visual stimuli.

10.2.13. The Insula

There is a sizable portion of the cortex buried in the lateral sulcus floor when the lips of the sulcus are separated. The Reil Insula is the name given to this region. The middle cerebral artery crosses it and it is divided into several small gyri. The insula's function is unknown, with the exception of its upper portion, which borders the sensory cortex and likely represents the cerebral cortex's taste area. Visceral reactions like belching, increased salivation, stomach movements, and vomiting are triggered by its stimulation.

10.2.14. The Connections of the Cerebral Cortex

The thalamus is the primary source of afferent input for the majority of cerebral cortex regions, as previously mentioned. However, the corpus callosum facilitates established commissural connections between the corresponding areas of the opposite hemisphere. Long association pathways directly connect the frontal, occipital, and temporal lobes. Associational intracortical connections also connect neighboring cortical areas on the same side and, in certain situations, distant cortical areas.

10.2.14.1. Clinical Features

It is convenient to summarize here the clinical effects of lesions affecting the principal cortical areas:

1. **Frontal Cortex –** impairment of higher mental functions and emotions.
2. **Precentral (Motor) Cortex –** weakness of the opposite side of the body; lesions low down the cortex affecting the face and arm, high lesions affecting the leg. Midline lesions (meningioma, sagittal sinus thrombosis or a gunshot wound) may produce paraplegia by involving both leg areas.
3. **Sensory Cortex –** contralateral hemianesthesia (distributed in the same pattern as the motor cortex) affecting especially the higher sensory modalities such as stereognosis and two-point position sense. (For area localizations along the motor and sensory cortex).
4. **Occipital Cortex –** contralateral homonymous hemianopia.
5. Lesions adjacent to the lateral sulcus

in either the frontal, parietal or temporal lobes of the dominant hemisphere result in aphasia.

10.2.15. The Basal Ganglia

These compact masses of gray matter consist of the claustrum and the corpus striatum, which are located deep within the cerebral hemisphere and are made up of the caudate nucleus, putamen, and globus pallidus. They play a role in movement coordination and control alongside the cerebellum.

10.2.15.1. The Corpus Striatum

The caudate nucleus is a large, homogenous mass of gray matter made up of an elongated tail that forms the roof of the inferior (temporal) horn of the ventricle, a head that forms the lateral wall of the anterior horn of the lateral ventricle and is located anterior to the interventricular foramen. The internal capsule largely separates it from the putamen, although there is an anterior connection between the two structures. Together, they are referred to as the lentiform nucleus. The putamen is a roughly ovoid mass that is closely applied to the lateral aspect of the globus pallidus. From the cerebral cortex, the corpus striatum receives afferent connections and sends efferents to the globus pallidus. Fibers project from there to the thalamus and back to the premotor cortex. Efferent fibers also travel to the thalamus, hypothalamus, red nucleus, inferior olivary nucleus, and substantia nigra. Dopaminergic fibers originate in the substantia nigra and terminate in the corpus striatum (Figure 10.15).

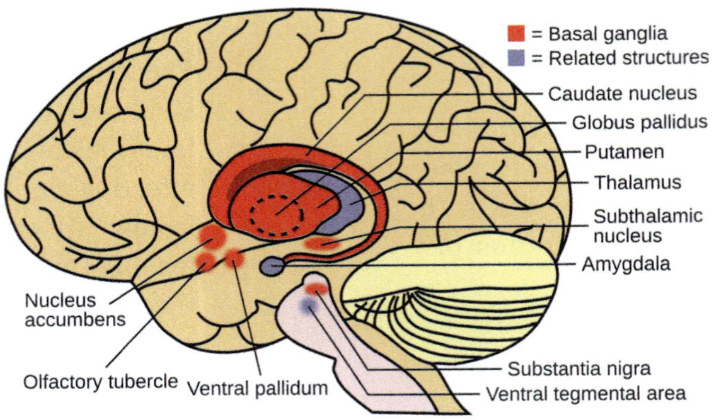

Figure 10.15. *The basal ganglia.*

Source: By File:BrainCaudatePutamen.svg: User: LeevanjacksonDerivative work: User:SUM1 – Derivative work based on File:BrainCaudatePutamen.svg, CC BY-SA 4.0; https://commons.wikimedia.org/w/index.php?curid=85845448.

10.2.16. The Long Ascending and Descending Pathways

10.2.16.1. The Somatic Afferent Pathways

The gracile and cuneate nuclei in the lower medulla receive proprioceptive and tactile impulses that travel through the ipsilateral posterior columns of the spinal cord and the posterior root ganglia without interruption. Afferent fibers are arranged fairly precisely in the posterior columns; fibers from the sacral and lumbar segments are positioned medially in the tracts, while fibers from the thoracic and cervical levels are added progressively to their lateral aspect. The arrangement based on body segments is upheld in the efferents that travel from the gracile and cuneate nuclei to the contralateral thalamus. In the medulla's sensory decussation, the fibers originating from the gracile and cuneate nuclei instantly switch to the opposing side and form a compact contralateral bundle known as the medial lemniscus that extends all the way to the thalamus.

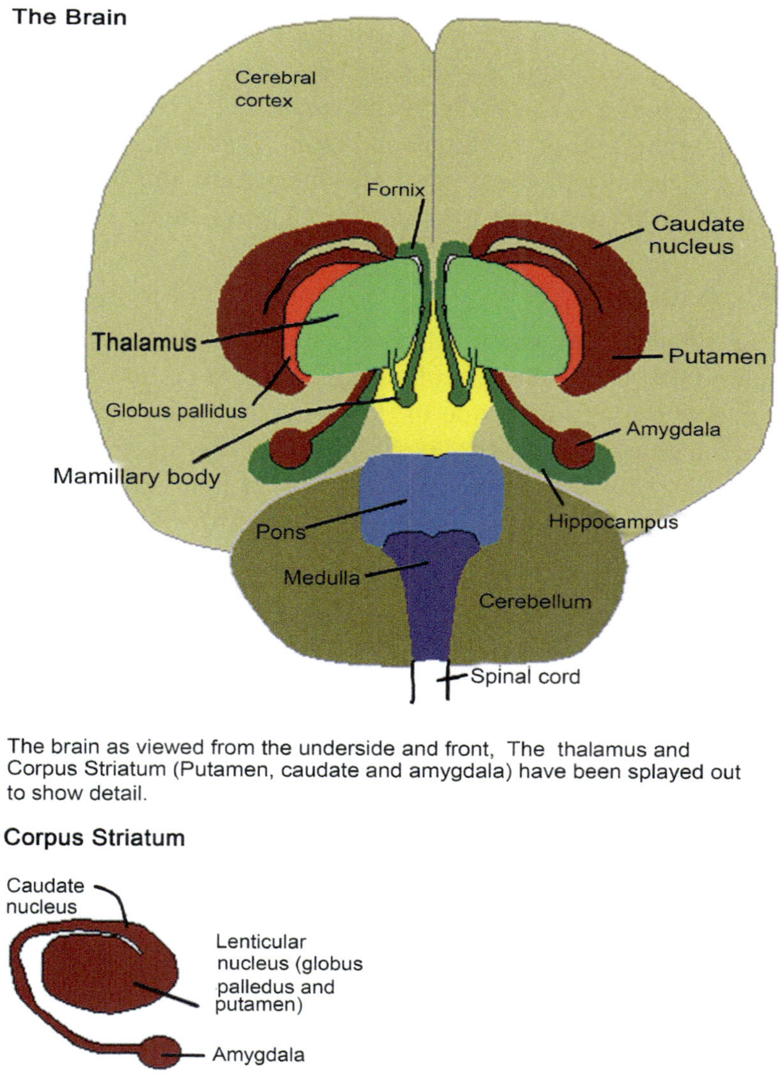

Figure 10.16. *The thalamus.*

Source: By The original uploader was RobinH at English Wiki books. Transferred from en.wikibooks to Commons, CC BY-SA 3.0; https://commons.wikimedia.org/w/index.php?curid=36970335.

The dorsal root fibers responsible for pain, temperature, and a few tactile afferents terminate ipsilaterally in the posterior horn's substantia gelatinosa. The contralateral thalamus receives them after they synapse, cross, and arrive at the contralateral anterior lateral columns of the cord. The anterior white commissure of the spinal cord is where the fiber crossing takes place. These fibers, which are sometimes referred to as the spinal lemniscus, emerge in the brainstem directly lateral to the medial lemniscus. In the thalamus, they come to an end (Figure 10.16).

The thalamus relays these somatic afferents to the somatic sensory cortex of the postcentral gyrus via the posterior limb of the internal capsule. The fibers in the internal capsule are arranged in the following order: face, arm, trunk, and leg. This pattern of arrangement is maintained in the sensory cortex, where the leg is positioned most inferiorly, the arm and trunk in the middle, and the face on the dorsal and medial portions of the cortex. There is a significant amount of distortion of the body image in the cortex, with the cortical representation of the face and hand being significantly greater than that of the limbs and trunk, because the size of the area of cortical representation reflects the density of the peripheral innervation and hence the complexity of the function being performed rather than the area of the receptive field.

10.2.16.2. Clinical Features

1. Lesions of the sensory pathway most commonly occur in the internal capsule following some form of cerebrovascular accident. If complete, these result in total hemianesthesia of the opposite side of the body. In partial lesions, the area of sensory loss will be determined by the site of the injury in the internal capsule, and from a knowledge of the sensory (and motor) loss, it is usually possible to determine with some degree of accuracy the site of a lesion in the capsule.
2. Since there is modality segregation below the decussation of the medial lemniscus, lesions of the sensory pathways at the cord level result in dissociation of sensation, with an area of analgesia contralaterally together with impairment of tactile sensibility ipsilaterally. The auditory, visual, and olfactory pathways are dealt with later under the appropriate cranial nerves.

10.2.16.3. The Motor Pathways

The brain and spinal cord's motor pathways are commonly classified as either extrapyramidal or pyramidal systems. Even though the latter is a vague idea, it offers a helpful collective term for the various motor structures in the medulla that are not restricted to the pyramidal tracts (Canedo, 1997).

A Closer Look

Central Nervous System PRN

The central nervous system (CNS), comprising the brain and spinal cord, is the primary control center of the body, coordinating sensory input, motor function, cognition, and emotion. This complex network of neurons and glial cells integrates information from the peripheral nervous system (PNS) and orchestrates appropriate responses to internal and external stimuli. Understanding the structure and function is crucial for diagnosing and treating neurological disorders.

The brain, protected by the skull, is divided into several key regions: the cerebrum, cerebellum, and brainstem. The cerebrum, the largest part, is responsible for higher cognitive functions such as thinking, memory, and voluntary movement. It is further divided into left and right hemispheres, each controlling the opposite side of the body and specialized for different functions. The cerebral cortex, the outermost layer, is involved in complex processes like language, problem-solving, and perception. The cerebellum, located under the cerebrum, coordinates voluntary movements, balance, and posture. The brainstem, connecting the brain to the spinal cord, controls vital involuntary functions such as heart rate, breathing, and sleep cycles.

The spinal cord, encased within the vertebral column, acts as a conduit for signals between the brain and the rest of the body. It is segmented into cervical, thoracic, lumbar, and sacral regions, each corresponding to different body parts. The spinal cord also houses reflex arcs, allowing for quick, involuntary responses to certain stimuli without involving the brain, such as the knee-jerk reflex.

Neurons, the functional units of the CNS, transmit information via electrical impulses and chemical signals. Each neuron consists of a cell body, dendrites, and an axon. Dendrites receive signals from other neurons, while the axon transmits impulses away from the cell body to other neurons or effector cells. Synapses, the junctions between neurons, facilitate the transmission of these signals using neurotransmitters, which are chemical messengers. Glial cells, including astrocytes, oligodendrocytes, and microglia, support and protect neurons, maintain homeostasis, and participate in signal transmission and immune responses.

The blood-brain barrier (BBB) is a selective permeability barrier that protects the CNS from harmful substances in the blood while allowing essential nutrients to pass through. It is formed by tightly packed endothelial cells lining the brain's capillaries, along with astrocytic end-feet. Disruption of the BBB can lead to neurological diseases such as multiple sclerosis, where the immune system attacks the myelin sheath, or in conditions like meningitis, where pathogens can infiltrate the CNS.

Neurological disorders affecting the CNS can be categorized into various types, including neurodegenerative diseases, traumatic injuries, infections, and congenital disorders. Alzheimer's disease, Parkinson's disease, and amyotrophic lateral sclerosis (ALS) are examples of neurodegenerative conditions characterized by the progressive loss of neuronal function and structure. Traumatic brain injury (TBI) and spinal cord injury (SCI) result from physical damage to the CNS, leading to long-term impairments. CNS infections such as encephalitis and meningitis, caused by bacteria, viruses, or fungi, can result in inflammation and significant neurological damage. Congenital disorders like spina bifida and cerebral palsy arise from developmental anomalies and can lead to lifelong disabilities.

Advances in neuroimaging techniques, such as MRI and CT scans, along with molecular biology and genetics, have enhanced our understanding of the CNS and improved diagnostic and therapeutic strategies for neurological disorders. Ongoing research aims to unravel the complexities of CNS function and pathology, to develop more effective treatments and potentially curative therapies for various neurological conditions (Shipp, 2007; Stiles & Jernigan, 2010).

Summary

- The central nervous system (CNS) is a pivotal part of the human body, encompassing the brain and spinal cord. It serves as the primary control center for processing and transmitting information, governing all bodily functions and responses.
- The brain, housed within the skull, comprises several regions including the cerebrum, cerebellum, and brainstem, each responsible for distinct functions. The cerebrum handles higher cognitive functions like reasoning, memory, and sensory processing.
- The spinal cord is 18 inches (45 cm) long. It is continuous above with the medulla oblongata at the level of the foramen magnum and ends below at the lower level of the 1st, or the upper level of the 2nd lumbar vertebra.
- The motor pathway commences at the pyramidal cells of the motor cortex, decussates in the medulla, then descends in the pyramidal tract on the contralateral side of the cord.
- Complete transection of the cord is followed by total loss of sensation in the regions supplied by the cord segments below the level of injury together with flaccid muscle paralysis. As the cord distal to the section recovers from a period of spinal shock, the paralysis becomes spastic, with exaggerated reflexes.
- The spinal cord, like the brain, is closely ensheathed by the pia mater. This is thickened on either side between the nerve roots to form the denticulate ligament, which passes laterally to adhere to the dura.
- Lumbar puncture to withdraw C.S.F. from the spinal subarachnoid space must be performed well clear of the termination of the cord.
- The blood supply of the medulla is derived from the vertebral arteries directly and from their posterior inferior cerebellar branches.
- The pons lies between the medulla and the midbrain and is connected to the cerebellum by the middle cerebellar peduncles. It is 1 in (25 mm) in length and 1.5 in (38 mm) in width. Its ventral surface presents a shallow median groove and numerous transverse ridges, which are continuous laterally with the middle cerebellar peduncle.
- The cerebellum is the largest part of the hindbrain and occupies most of the posterior cranial fossa. It is made up of two lateral cerebellar hemispheres and a median vermis.
- The hypothalamus forms the floor of the 3rd ventricle. It includes, from before backwards, the optic chiasma, the tuber cinereum, the infundibular stalk (leading down to the posterior lobe of the pituitary), the mamillary bodies, and the posterior perforated substance.

References

1. Canedo A. (1997). Primary motor cortex influences on the descending and ascending systems. *Progress in Neurobiology, 51*(3), 287–335. doi: 10.1016/S0301-0082(96)00061-1.
2. DeMaagd G, Philip A. (2015). Parkinson's disease and its management: Part 1: Disease entity, risk factors, pathophysiology, clinical presentation, and diagnosis. *P & T: A Peer-Reviewed Journal for Formulary Management, 40*(8), 504–532.

3. Flament-Durand J. (1980). The hypothalamus: Anatomy and functions. *Acta Psychiatrica Belgica, 80*(4), 364–375.
4. Fridriksson J, Fillmore P, Guo D, Rorden C. (2015). Chronic Broca's aphasia is caused by damage to Broca's and Wernicke's areas. *Cerebral Cortex, 25*(12), 4689–4696. doi: 10.1093/cercor/bhv114.
5. Gottschalk A, Van Aken H, Zenz M, Standl T. (2011). Is anesthesia dangerous? *Deutsches Ärzteblatt International, 108*(27), 469–474. doi: 10.3238/arztebl.2011.0469.
6. Lanciego JL, Luquin N, Obeso JA. (2012). Functional neuroanatomy of the basal ganglia. *Cold Spring Harbor Perspectives in Medicine, 2*(12), a009621. doi: 10.1101/cshperspect. a009621.
7. Mehndiratta MM, Mehndiratta P, Pande R. (2014). Poliomyelitis: Historical facts, epidemiology, and current challenges in eradication. *The Neurohospitalist, 4*(4), 223–229. doi: 10.1177/1941874414544978.
8. Nattie E, Li A. (2012). Central chemoreceptors: Locations and functions. *Comprehensive Physiology, 2*(1), 221–254. doi: 10.1002/cphy.c110027.
9. Raghavendra T. (2002). Neuromuscular blocking drugs: Discovery and development. *Journal of the Royal Society of Medicine, 95*(7), 363–367. doi: 10.1177/014107680209500714.
10. Rajmohan V, Mohandas E. (2007). The limbic system. *Indian Journal of Psychiatry, 49*(2), 132–139.
11. Schachter AS, Davis KL. (2000). Alzheimer's disease. *Dialogues in Clinical Neuroscience, 2*(2), 91–100.
12. Shipp S. (2007). Structure and function of the cerebral cortex. *Current Biology, 17*(12), R443–R449. doi: 10.1016/j.cub.2007.04.029.
13. Stiles J, Jernigan TL. (2010). The basics of brain development. *Neuropsychology Review, 20*(4), 327–348. doi: 10.1007/s11065-010-9148-4.
14. Vrselja Z, Brkic H, Mrdenovic S, Radic R, Curic G. (2014). Function of circle of Willis. *Journal of Cerebral Blood Flow & Metabolism, 34*(4), 578–584. doi: 10.1038/jcbfm.2013.248.
15. Gage F.H., Temple S. Neural stem cells: Generating and regenerating the brain. *Neuron.* 2013;80:588–601. doi: 10.1016/j.neuron.2013.10.037.
16. Malberg J.E., Eisch A.J., Nestler E.J., Duman R.S. Chronic antidepressant treatment increases neurogenesis in adult rat hippocampus. *J. Neurosci. Off. J. Soc. Neurosci.* 2000;20:9104–9110. doi: 10.1523/JNEUROSCI.20-24-09104.2000.
17. Kuhn H.G., Dickinson-Anson H., Gage F.H. Neurogenesis in the dentate gyrus of the adult rat: Age-related decrease of neuronal progenitor proliferation. *J. Neurosci. Off. J. Soc. Neurosci.* 1996;16:2027–2033. doi: 10.1523/JNEUROSCI.16-06-02027.1996.
18. Altman J. Are new neurons formed in the brains of adult mammals? *Science (New York)* 1962;135:1127–1128. doi: 10.1126/science.135.3509.1127.
19. Blokhuis A.M., Groen E.J.N., Koppers M., van den Berg L.H., Pasterkamp R.J. Protein aggregation in amyotrophic lateral sclerosis. *Acta Neuropathol.* 2013;125:777–794. doi: 10.1007/s00401-013-1125-6.
20. David M.A., Tayebi M. Detection of protein aggregates in brain and cerebrospinal fluid derived from multiple sclerosis patients. *Front. Neurol.* 2014;5:251. doi: 10.3389/fneur.2014.00251.

21. Lucke-Wold B.P., Turner R.C., Logsdon A.F., Bailes J.E., Huber J.D., Rosen C.L. Linking traumatic brain injury to chronic traumatic encephalopathy: Identification of potential mechanisms leading to neurofibrillary tangle development. *J. Neurotrauma.* 2014;31:1129–1138. doi: 10.1089/neu.2013.3303.

22. Hatters D.M. Protein misfolding inside cells: The case of huntingtin and Huntington's disease. *IUBMB Life.* 2008;60:724–728. doi: 10.1002/iub.111.

23. Martin J.B. Molecular basis of the neurodegenerative disorders. *N. Engl. J. Med.* 1999;340:1970–1980. doi: 10.1056/NEJM199906243402507.

24. Soto C., Estrada L.D. Protein misfolding and neurodegeneration. *Arch. Neurol.* 2008;65:184–189. doi: 10.1001/archneurol.2007.56.

25. Tuite M.F., Melki R. *Protein Misfolding and Aggregation in Ageing and Disease: Molecular Processes and Therapeutic Perspectives.* Taylor & Francis; Abingdon, UK: 2007.

26. Lepeta K., Lourenco M.V., Schweitzer B.C., Martino Adami P.V., Banerjee P., Catuara-Solarz S., de La Fuente Revenga M., Guillem A.M., Haidar M., Ijomone O.M., et al. Synaptopathies: Synaptic dysfunction in neurological disorders—A review from students to students. *J. Neurochem.* 2016;138:785–805. doi: 10.1111/jnc.13713.

27. Bae J.R., Kim S.H. Synapses in neurodegenerative diseases. *BMB Rep.* 2017;50:237–246. doi: 10.5483/BMBRep.2017.50.5.038.

28. Kiaei M. New hopes and challenges for treatment of neurodegenerative disorders: Great opportunities for young neuroscientists. *Basic Clin. Neurosci.* 2013;4:3–4.

29. Duraes F., Pinto M., Sousa E. Old drugs as new treatments for neurodegenerative diseases. *Pharmaceuticals (Basel, Switzerland)* 2018;11:44. doi: 10.3390/ph11020044.

30. Sehgal S.A., Hammad M.A., Tahir R.A., Akram H.N., Ahmad F. Current therapeutic molecules and targets in neurodegenerative diseases based on in silico drug design. *Curr. Neuropharmacol.* 2018;16:649–663. doi: 10.2174/1570159X16666180315142137.

31. Coppede F. The potential of epigenetic therapies in neurodegenerative diseases. *Front. Genet.* 2014;5:220. doi: 10.3389/fgene.2014.00220.

32. Amor S., Peferoen L.A., Vogel D.Y., Breur M., van der Valk P., Baker D., van Noort J.M. Inflammation in neurodegenerative diseases—An update. *Immunology.* 2014;142:151–166. doi: 10.1111/imm.12233.

33. Hussain R., Ghoumari A.M., Bielecki B., Steibel J., Boehm N., Liere P., Macklin W.B., Kumar N., Habert R., Mhaouty-Kodja S., et al. The neural androgen receptor: A therapeutic target for myelin repair in chronic demyelination. *Brain J. Neurol.* 2013;136:132–146. doi: 10.1093/brain/aws284.

34. Behl C. Oestrogen as a neuroprotective hormone. *Nat. Rev. Neurosci.* 2002;3:433–442. doi: 10.1038/nrn846.

35. Bondy C., Werner H., Roberts C.T., Jr., LeRoith D. Cellular pattern of type-I insulin-like growth factor receptor gene expression during maturation of the rat brain: Comparison with insulin-like growth factors I and II. *Neuroscience.* 1992;46:909–923. doi: 10.1016/0306-4522(92)90193-6.

36. Woolley J.D., Khan B.K., Murthy N.K., Miller B.L., Rankin K.P. The diagnostic challenge of psychiatric symptoms in neurodegenerative disease: Rates of and risk factors for

prior psychiatric diagnosis in patients with early neurodegenerative disease. *J. Clin. Psychiatry.* 2011;72:126–133. doi: 10.4088/JCP.10m06382oli.

37. Montero-Odasso M., Pieruccini-Faria F., Bartha R., Black S.E., Finger E., Freedman M., Greenberg B., Grimes D.A., Hegele R.A., Hudson C., et al. Motor phenotype in neurodegenerative disorders: Gait and balance platform study design protocol for the ontario neurodegenerative research initiative (ONDRI) *J. Alzheimer's Dis.* 2017;59:707–721. doi: 10.3233/JAD-170149.
38. Vadakkan K.I. Neurodegenerative disorders share common features of "loss of function" states of a proposed mechanism of nervous system functions. *Biomed. Pharmacother. Biomed. Pharmacother.* 2016;83:412–430. doi: 10.1016/j.biopha.2016.06.042.
39. Hervas R., Oroz J., Galera-Prat A., Goni O., Valbuena A., Vera A.M., Gomez-Sicilia A., Losada-Urzaiz F., Uversky V.N., Menendez M., et al. Common features at the start of the neurodegeneration cascade. *PLoS Boil.* 2012;10:e1001335. doi: 10.1371/journal.pbio.1001335.
40. Gitler A.D., Dhillon P., Shorter J. Neurodegenerative disease: Models, mechanisms, and a new hope. *Dis. Model Mech.* 2017;10:499–502. doi: 10.1242/dmm.030205.
41. Rubinsztein D.C. The roles of intracellular protein-degradation pathways in neurodegeneration. *Nature.* 2006;443:780–786. doi: 10.1038/nature05291.
42. Thompson L.M. Neurodegeneration: A question of balance. *Nature.* 2008;452:707–708. doi: 10.1038/452707a.
43. Alzheimer's Association 2012 Alzheimer's disease facts and figures. *Alzheimer's Dement. J. Alzheimer's Assoc.* 2012;8:131–168. doi: 10.1016/j.jalz.2012.02.001.
44. Bloom G.S. Amyloid-β and tau: The trigger and bullet in Alzheimer disease pathogenesis. *JAMA Neurol.* 2014;71:505–508. doi: 10.1001/jamaneurol.2013.5847.
45. Wenk G.L. Neuropathologic changes in Alzheimer's disease. *J. Clin. Psychiatry.* 2003;64:7–10.
46. Graham W.V., Bonito-Oliva A., Sakmar T.P. Update on Alzheimer's disease therapy and prevention strategies. *Annu. Rev Med.* 2017;68:413–430. doi: 10.1146/annurev-med-042915-103753.
47. Sanabria-Castro A., Alvarado-Echeverria I., Monge-Bonilla C. Molecular pathogenesis of Alzheimer's disease: An update. *Ann. Neurosci.* 2017;24:46–54. doi: 10.1159/000464422.
48. Schneider L. Alzheimer's disease and other dementias: Update on research. *Lancet Neurol.* 2017;16:4–5. doi: 10.1016/S1474-4422(16)30356-8.
49. Swerdlow R.H., Khan S.M. The Alzheimer's disease mitochondrial cascade hypothesis: An update. *Exp. Neurol.* 2009;218:308–315. doi: 10.1016/j.expneurol.2009.01.011.
50. Ottolini D., Cali T., Szabo I., Brini M. Alpha-synuclein at the intracellular and the extracellular side: Functional and dysfunctional implications. *Boil. Chem.* 2017;398:77–100. doi: 10.1515/hsz-2016-0201.
51. Davie C.A. A review of Parkinson's disease. *Br. Med. Bull.* 2008;86:109–127. doi: 10.1093/bmb/ldn013.
52. Alkhuja S. Parkinson disease: Research update and clinical management. *South Med. J.* 2013;106:334. doi: 10.1097/SMJ.0b013e318290f72a.
53. Frucht S.J. Parkinson disease: An update. *Neurologist.* 2004;10:185–194. doi: 10.1097/01.nrl.0000131146.08278.a5.

54. Rizek P., Kumar N., Jog M.S. An update on the diagnosis and treatment of Parkinson disease. *CMAJ.* 2016;188:1157–1165. doi: 10.1503/cmaj.151179.

55. Chung K.K., Zhang Y., Lim K.L., Tanaka Y., Huang H., Gao J., Ross C.A., Dawson V.L., Dawson T.M. Parkin ubiquitinates the alpha-synuclein-interacting protein, synphilin-1: Implications for Lewy-body formation in Parkinson disease. *Nat. Med.* 2001;7:1144–1150. doi: 10.1038/nm1001-1144.

56. Frigerio R., Fujishiro H., Maraganore D.M., Klos K.J., DelleDonne A., Heckman M.G., Crook J.E., Josephs K.A., Parisi J.E., Boeve B.F., et al. Comparison of risk factor profiles in incidental Lewy body disease and Parkinson disease. *Arch. Neurol.* 2009;66:1114–1119. doi: 10.1001/archneurol.2009.170.

57. Wood H. Parkinson disease: Antibodies reveal age of Lewy pathology in PD. *Nat. Rev. Neurol.* 2017;13:318–319. doi: 10.1038/nrneurol.2017.62.

58. Schneider J.S., Sendek S., Yang C. Relationship between motor symptoms, cognition, and demographic characteristics in treated mild/moderate Parkinson's disease. *PLoS ONE.* 2015;10:e0123231. doi: 10.1371/journal.pone.0123231.

59. Heinzel S., Bernhard F.P., Roeben B., Nussbaum S., Heger T., Martus P., Hobert M.A., Maetzler W., Berg D. Progression markers of motor deficits in Parkinson's disease: A biannual 4-year prospective study. *Mov. Disord. Off. J. Mov. Disord. Soc.* 2017;32:1254–1256. doi: 10.1002/mds.27062.

60. Walker F.O. Huntington's disease. *Lancet.* 2007;369:218–228. doi: 10.1016/S0140-6736(07)60111-1.

61. Kaplan A., Stockwell B.R. Therapeutic approaches to preventing cell death in Huntington disease. *Prog. Neurobiol.* 2012;99:262–280. doi: 10.1016/j.pneurobio.2012.08.004.

62. Messer A., McLear J. The therapeutic potential of intrabodies in neurologic disorders: Focus on Huntington and Parkinson diseases. *BioDrugs.* 2006;20:327–333. doi: 10.2165/00063030-200620060-00002.

63. Sciacca G., Cicchetti F. Mutant huntingtin protein expression and blood-spinal cord barrier dysfunction in Huntington disease. *Ann. Neurol.* 2017;82:981–994. doi: 10.1002/ana.25107.

64. Zhao T., Hong Y., Li X.J., Li S.H. Subcellular clearance and accumulation of Huntington disease protein: A mini-review. *Front. Mol. Neurosci.* 2016;9:27. doi: 10.3389/fnmol.2016.00027.

65. Zheng Z., Diamond M.I. Huntington disease and the huntingtin protein. *Prog. Mol. Biol. Transl. Sci.* 2012;107:189–214.

66. Frank S. Treatment of Huntington's disease. *Neurotherapeutics.* 2014;11:153–160. doi: 10.1007/s13311-013-0244-z.

67. Koutsis G., Panas M., Paraskevas G.P., Bougea A.M., Kladi A., Karadima G., Kapaki E. From mild ataxia to Huntington disease phenocopy: The multiple faces of spinocerebellar ataxia 17. *Case Rep. Neurol. Med.* 2014;2014:643289. doi: 10.1155/2014/643289.

68. Roxburgh R.H., Smith C.O., Lim J.G., Bachman D.F., Byrd E., Bird T.D. The unique co-occurrence of spinocerebellar ataxia type 10 (SCA10) and Huntington disease. *J. Neurol. Sci.* 2013;324:176–178. doi: 10.1016/j.jns.2012.09.030.

69. Hyman B.T., Van Hoesen G.W. Neuron numbers in Alzheimer's disease: Cell-specific pathology. *Neurobiol. Aging.* 1987;8:555–556. doi: 10.1016/0197-4580(87)90133-3.

70. Bendfeldt K., Kappos L., Radue E.W., Borgwardt S.J. Progression of gray matter atrophy and its association with white matter lesions in relapsing-remitting multiple sclerosis. *J. Neurol. Sci.* 2009;285:268–269. doi: 10.1016/j.jns.2009.05.020.

71. Datta G., Colasanti A., Rabiner E.A., Gunn R.N., Malik O., Ciccarelli O., Nicholas R., Van Vlierberghe E., Van Hecke W., Searle G., et al. Neuroinflammation and its relationship to changes in brain volume and white matter lesions in multiple sclerosis. *Brain J. Neurol.* 2017;140:2927–2938. doi: 10.1093/brain/awx228.

72. Hacohen Y., Ciccarelli O., Hemingway C. Abnormal white matter development in children with multiple sclerosis and monophasic acquired demyelination. *Brain J. Neurol.* 2017;140:1172–1174. doi: 10.1093/brain/awx075.

73. Lassmann H. Mechanisms of white matter damage in multiple sclerosis. *Glia.* 2014;62:1816–1830. doi: 10.1002/glia.22597.

74. Longoni G., Brown R.A., MomayyezSiahkal P., Elliott C., Narayanan S., Bar-Or A., Marrie R.A., Yeh E.A., Filippi M., Banwell B., et al. White matter changes in paediatric multiple sclerosis and monophasic demyelinating disorders. *Brain J. Neurol.* 2017;140:1300–1315. doi: 10.1093/brain/awx041.

75. Josephy-Hernandez S., Jmaeff S., Pirvulescu I., Aboulkassim T., Saragovi H.U. Neurotrophin receptor agonists and antagonists as therapeutic agents: An evolving paradigm. *Neurobiol. Dis.* 2017;97:139–155. doi: 10.1016/j.nbd.2016.08.004.

76. Moccia M., Quarantelli M., Lanzillo R., Cocozza S., Carotenuto A., Carotenuto B., Alfano B., Prinster A., Triassi M., Nardone A., et al. Grey:White matter ratio at diagnosis and the risk of 10-year multiple sclerosis progression. *Eur. J. Neurol.* 2017;24:195–204. doi: 10.1111/ene.13183.

77. Suzuki K., Kamoshita S., Eto Y., Tourtellotte W.W., Gonatas J.O. Myelin in multiple sclerosis. Composition of myelin from normal-appearing white matter. *Arch. Neurol.* 1973;28:293–297. doi: 10.1001/archneur.1973.00490230029002.

78. Chalah M.A., Ayache S.S. Psychiatric event in multiple sclerosis: Could it be the tip of the iceberg? *Rev. Bras. Psiquiatr.* 2017;39:365–368. doi: 10.1590/1516-4446-2016-2105.

79. de Cerqueira A.C., Semionato de Andrade P., Godoy Barreiros J.M., Teixeira A.L., Nardi A.E. Psychiatric disorders in patients with multiple sclerosis. *Compr. Psychiatry.* 2015;63:10–14. doi: 10.1016/j.comppsych.2015.08.001.

80. Honer W.G., Hurwitz T., Li D.K., Palmer M., Paty D.W. Temporal lobe involvement in multiple sclerosis patients with psychiatric disorders. *Arch. Neurol.* 1987;44:187–190. doi: 10.1001/archneur.1987.00520140053017.

81. Zambon A.A., Cecchetti G., Caso F., Santangelo R., Baldoli C., Natali Sora M.G., Comi G., Magnani G., Martinelli V. Primary progressive multiple sclerosis presenting with severe predominant cognitive impairment and psychiatric symptoms: A challenging case. *Mult. Scler.* 2017;23:1558–1561. doi: 10.1177/1352458517702550.

82. Desikan R.S., Fan C.C., Wang Y., Schork A.J., Cabral H.J., Cupples L.A., Thompson W.K., Besser L., Kukull W.A., Holland D., et al. Genetic assessment of age-associated Alzheimer disease risk: Development and validation of a polygenic hazard score. *PLoS Med.* 2017;14:e1002258. doi: 10.1371/journal.pmed.1002258.

83. Gaiteri C., Mostafavi S., Honey C.J., De Jager P.L., Bennett D.A. Genetic variants in Alzheimer disease-molecular and brain network approaches. *Nat. Rev. Neurol.* 2016;12:413–427. doi: 10.1038/nrneurol.2016.84.

84. Li Y., Hollingworth P., Moore P., Foy C., Archer N., Powell J., Nowotny P., Holmans P., O'Donovan M., Tacey K., et al. Genetic association of the app binding protein 2 gene (APBB2) with late onset Alzheimer disease. *Hum. Mutat.* 2005;25:270–277. doi: 10.1002/humu.20138.

85. Rosenberg R.N., Richter R.W., Risser R.C., Taubman K., Prado-Farmer I., Ebalo E., Posey J., Kingfisher D., Dean D., Weiner M.F., et al. Genetic factors for the development of Alzheimer disease in the Cherokee Indian. *Arch. Neurol.* 1996;53:997–1000. doi: 10.1001/archneur.1996.00550100071017.

86. Alcalay R.N., Caccappolo E., Mejia-Santana H., Tang M.X., Rosado L., Ross B.M., Verbitsky M., Kisselev S., Louis E.D., Comella C., et al. Frequency of known mutations in early-onset Parkinson disease: Implication for genetic counseling: The consortium on risk for early onset Parkinson disease study. *Arch. Neurol.* 2010;67:1116–1122. doi: 10.1001/archneurol.2010.194.

87. Scott W.K., Staijich J.M., Yamaoka L.H., Speer M.C., Vance J.M., Roses A.D., Pericak-Vance M.A. Genetic complexity and Parkinson's disease. Deane laboratory Parkinson disease research group. *Science (New York)* 1997;277:387–388. doi: 10.1126/science.277.5324.387.

88. Verstraeten A., Theuns J., Van Broeckhoven C. Progress in unraveling the genetic etiology of Parkinson disease in a genomic era. *Trends Genet.* 2015;31:140–149. doi: 10.1016/j.tig.2015.01.004.

89. Bates G.P. History of genetic disease: The molecular genetics of Huntington disease—A history. *Nat. Rev. Genet.* 2005;6:766–773. doi: 10.1038/nrg1686.

90. Pericak-Vance M.A., Conneally P.M., Merritt A.D., Roos R., Norton J.A., Jr., Vance J.M. Genetic linkage studies in Huntington disease. *Cytogenet. Cell Genet.* 1978;22:640–645. doi: 10.1159/000131042.

91. Pulst S.M. Neurodegenerative disease. Genetic discrimination in Huntington disease. *Nat. Rev. Neurol.* 2009;5:525–526. doi: 10.1038/nrneurol.2009.153.

92. Wilson R.S., Barral S., Lee J.H., Leurgans S.E., Foroud T.M., Sweet R.A., Graff-Radford N., Bird T.D., Mayeux R., Bennett D.A. Heritability of different forms of memory in the late onset Alzheimer's disease family study. *J. Alzheimer's Dis.* 2011;23:249–255. doi: 10.3233/JAD-2010-101515.

93. Lesage S., Brice A. Parkinson's disease: From monogenic forms to genetic susceptibility factors. *Hum. Mol. Genet.* 2009;18:R48–R59. doi: 10.1093/hmg/ddp012.

94. Dyment D.A., Ebers G.C., Sadovnick A.D. Genetics of multiple sclerosis. *Lancet Neurol.* 2004;3:104–110. doi: 10.1016/S1474-4422(03)00663-X.

95. Axisa P.P., Hafler D.A. Multiple sclerosis: Genetics, biomarkers, treatments. *Curr. Opin. Neurol.* 2016;29:345–353. doi: 10.1097/WCO.0000000000000319.

96. Baranzini S.E., Oksenberg J.R. The genetics of multiple sclerosis: From 0 to 200 in 50 years. *Trends Genet.* 2017;33:960–970. doi: 10.1016/j.tig.2017.09.004.

97. Cagliani R., Fumagalli M., Guerini F.R., Riva S., Galimberti D., Comi G.P., Agliardi C., Scarpini E., Pozzoli U., Forni D., et al. Identification of a new susceptibility variant for multiple sclerosis

in OAS1 by population genetics analysis. *Hum. Genet.* 2012;131:87–97. doi: 10.1007/s00439-011-1053-2.

98. Tizaoui K. Multiple sclerosis genetics: Results from meta-analyses of candidate-gene association studies. *Cytokine.* 2017 doi: 10.1016/j.cyto.2017.10.024.

99. Ryan J., Fransquet P., Wrigglesworth J., Lacaze P. Phenotypic heterogeneity in dementia: A challenge for epidemiology and biomarker studies. *Front. Public Health.* 2018;6:181. doi: 10.3389/fpubh.2018.00181.

100. Nelson P.T., Head E., Schmitt F.A., Davis P.R., Neltner J.H., Jicha G.A., Abner E.L., Smith C.D., Van Eldik L.J., Kryscio R.J. Alzheimer's disease is not "brain aging": Neuropathological, genetic, and epidemiological human studies. *Acta Neuropathol.* 2011;121:571–587. doi: 10.1007/s00401-011-0826-y.

101. Petrovitch H., White L., Ross G., Steinhorn S., Li C., Masaki K., Davis D., Nelson J., Hardman J., Curb J. Accuracy of clinical criteria for ad in the Honolulu–Asia aging study, a population-based study. *Neurology.* 2001;57:226–234. doi: 10.1212/WNL.57.2.226.

102. McKeith I.G., Dickson D., Lowe J., Emre M., O'brien J., Feldman H., Cummings J., Duda J., Lippa C., Perry E. Diagnosis and management of dementia with Lewy bodies third report of the DLB consortium. *Neurology.* 2005;65:1863–1872. doi: 10.1212/01.wnl.0000187889.17253.b1.

103. Delgado-Morales R., Esteller M. Opening up the DNA methylome of dementia. *Mol. Psychiatry.* 2017;22:485. doi: 10.1038/mp.2016.242.

104. Sperling R.A., Karlawish J., Johnson K.A. Preclinical Alzheimer disease—The challenges ahead. *Nat. Rev. Neurol.* 2013;9:54–58. doi: 10.1038/nrneurol.2012.241.

105. Citron M. Alzheimer's disease: Strategies for disease modification. *Nat. Rev. Drug Discov.* 2010;9:387–398. doi: 10.1038/nrd2896.

106. Levine A.J., Harris C.R., Puzio-Kuter A.M. The interfaces between signal transduction pathways: IGF-1/mTor, p53 and the Parkinson disease pathway. *Oncotarget.* 2012;3:1301–1307. doi: 10.18632/oncotarget.759.

107. Oddo S. The role of mTOR signaling in Alzheimer disease. *Front. Biosci.* 2012;4:941–952. doi: 10.2741/s310.

108. Tramutola A., Triplett J.C., Di Domenico F., Niedowicz D.M., Murphy M.P., Coccia R., Perluigi M., Butterfield D.A. Alteration of mTOR signaling occurs early in the progression of Alzheimer disease (AD): Analysis of brain from subjects with pre-clinical AD, amnestic mild cognitive impairment and late-stage AD. *J. Neurochem.* 2015;133:739–749. doi: 10.1111/jnc.13037.

109. Lan A.P., Chen J., Zhao Y., Chai Z., Hu Y. mTOR signaling in Parkinson's disease. *Neuromol. Med.* 2017;19:1–10. doi: 10.1007/s12017-016-8417-7.

110. Santini E., Heiman M., Greengard P., Valjent E., Fisone G. Inhibition of mtor signaling in Parkinson's disease prevents L-DOPA-induced dyskinesia. *Sci. Signal.* 2009;2:ra36. doi: 10.1126/scisignal.2000308.

111. Santini E., Valjent E., Fisone G. Mtorc1 signaling in Parkinson's disease and L-DOPA-induced dyskinesia: A sensitized matter. *Cell Cycle.* 2010;9:2713–2718. doi: 10.4161/cc.9.14.12180.

112. Cai Z., Chen G., He W., Xiao M., Yan L.J. Activation of mTOR: A culprit of Alzheimer's disease? *Neuropsychiatr. Dis. Treat.* 2015;11:1015–1030. doi: 10.2147/NDT.S75717.

113. Wang C., Yu J.T., Miao D., Wu Z.C., Tan M.S., Tan L. Targeting the mTOR signaling network for Alzheimer's disease therapy. *Mol. Neurobiol.* 2014;49:120–135. doi: 10.1007/s12035-013-8505-8.

114. Siman R., Cocca R., Dong Y. The mTOR inhibitor rapamycin mitigates perforant pathway neurodegeneration and synapse loss in a mouse model of early-stage Alzheimer-type tauopathy. *PLoS ONE.* 2015;10:e0142340. doi: 10.1371/journal.pone.0142340.

115. Pryor W.M., Biagioli M., Shahani N., Swarnkar S., Huang W.C., Page D.T., MacDonald M.E., Subramaniam S. Huntingtin promotes mTORc1 signaling in the pathogenesis of Huntington's disease. *Sci. Signal.* 2014;7:ra103. doi: 10.1126/scisignal.2005633.

116. Ravikumar B., Vacher C., Berger Z., Davies J.E., Luo S., Oroz L.G., Scaravilli F., Easton D.F., Duden R., O'Kane C.J., et al. Inhibition of mTOR induces autophagy and reduces toxicity of polyglutamine expansions in fly and mouse models of Huntington disease. *Nat. Genet.* 2004;36:585–595. doi: 10.1038/ng1362.

117. Hohlfeld R., Wekerle H. Autoimmune concepts of multiple sclerosis as a basis for selective immunotherapy: From pipe dreams to (therapeutic) pipelines. *Proc. Natl. Acad. Sci. USA.* 2004;101(Suppl. 2):14599–14606. doi: 10.1073/pnas.0404874101.

118. Frischer J.M., Bramow S., Dal-Bianco A., Lucchinetti C.F., Rauschka H., Schmidbauer M., Laursen H., Sorensen P.S., Lassmann H. The relation between inflammation and neurodegeneration in multiple sclerosis brains. *Brain J. Neurol.* 2009;132:1175–1189. doi: 10.1093/brain/awp070.

119. Perl A. Mtor activation is a biomarker and a central pathway to autoimmune disorders, cancer, obesity, and aging. *Ann. N. Y. Acad. Sci.* 2015;1346:33–44. doi: 10.1111/nyas.12756.

120. Carbone F., De Rosa V., Carrieri P.B., Montella S., Bruzzese D., Porcellini A., Procaccini C., La Cava A., Matarese G. Regulatory T cell proliferative potential is impaired in human autoimmune disease. *Nat. Med.* 2014;20:69–74. doi: 10.1038/nm.3411.

121. Pollizzi K.N., Patel C.H., Sun I.H., Oh M.H., Waickman A.T., Wen J., Delgoffe G.M., Powell J.D. Mtorc1 and mTORc2 selectively regulate CD8(+) T cell differentiation. *J. Clin. Investig.* 2015;125:2090–2108. doi: 10.1172/JCI77746.

122. Delgoffe G.M., Pollizzi K.N., Waickman A.T., Heikamp E., Meyers D.J., Horton M.R., Xiao B., Worley P.F., Powell J.D. The kinase mTOR regulates the differentiation of helper T cells through the selective activation of signaling by mTORc1 and mTORc2. *Nat. Immunol.* 2011;12:295–303. doi: 10.1038/ni.2005.

123. Tyler W.A., Gangoli N., Gokina P., Kim H.A., Covey M., Levison S.W., Wood T.L. Activation of the mammalian target of rapamycin (mTOR) is essential for oligodendrocyte differentiation. *J. Neurosci. Off. J. Soc. Neurosci.* 2009;29:6367–6378. doi: 10.1523/JNEUROSCI.0234-09.2009.

124. Bercury K.K., Dai J., Sachs H.H., Ahrendsen J.T., Wood T.L., Macklin W.B. Conditional ablation of raptor or rictor has differential impact on oligodendrocyte differentiation and cns myelination. *J. Neurosci. Off. J. Soc. Neurosci.* 2014;34:4466–4480. doi: 10.1523/JNEUROSCI.4314-13.2014.

125. Lebrun-Julien F., Bachmann L., Norrmen C., Trotzmuller M., Kofeler H., Ruegg M.A., Hall M.N., Suter U. Balanced mTORc1 activity in oligodendrocytes is required for accurate CNS myelination. *J. Neurosci. Off. J. Soc. Neurosci.* 2014;34:8432–8448. doi: 10.1523/JNEUROSCI.1105-14.2014.

126. Kim E.K., Choi E.-J. Pathological roles of MAPK signaling pathways in human diseases. *Biochim.*

Biophys. Acta (BBA) Mol. Basis Dis. 2010;1802:396–405. doi: 10.1016/j.bbadis.2009.12.009.

127. Lengfeld J.E., Lutz S.E., Smith J.R., Diaconu C., Scott C., Kofman S.B., Choi C., Walsh C.M., Raine C.S., Agalliu I., et al. Endothelial Wnt/β-catenin signaling reduces immune cell infiltration in multiple sclerosis. *Proc. Natl. Acad. Sci. USA.* 2017;114:E1168–E1177. doi: 10.1073/pnas.1609905114.
128. Bayat V., Jaiswal M., Bellen H.J. The bmp signaling pathway at the drosophila neuromuscular junction and its links to neurodegenerative diseases. *Curr. Opin. Neurobiol.* 2011;21:182–188. doi: 10.1016/j.conb.2010.08.014.
129. Holbert S., Dedeoglu A., Humbert S., Saudou F., Ferrante R.J., Neri C. Cdc42-interacting protein 4 binds to huntingtin: Neuropathologic and biological evidence for a role in Huntington's disease. *Proc. Natl. Acad. Sci. USA.* 2003;100:2712–2717. doi: 10.1073/pnas.0437967100.
130. Lione L.A., Carter R.J., Hunt M.J., Bates G.P., Morton A.J., Dunnett S.B. Selective discrimination learning impairments in mice expressing the human Huntington's disease mutation. *J. Neurosci. Off. J. Soc. Neurosci.* 1999;19:10428–10437. doi: 10.1523/JNEUROSCI.19-23-10428.1999.
131. Scheff S.W., Price D.A., Schmitt F.A., Scheff M.A., Mufson E.J. Synaptic loss in the inferior temporal gyrus in mild cognitive impairment and Alzheimer's disease. *J. Alzheimer's Dis. JAD.* 2011;24:547–557. doi: 10.3233/JAD-2011-101782.
132. Deininger M., Meyermann R., Schluesener H. Detection of two transforming growth factor-beta-related morphogens, bone morphogenetic proteins-4 and -5, in RNA of multiple sclerosis and Creutzfeldt-Jakob disease lesions. *Acta Neuropathol.* 1995;90:76–79. doi: 10.1007/BF00294462.
133. De Ferrari G.V., Avila M.E., Medina M.A., Perez-Palma E., Bustos B.I., Alarcon M.A. Wnt/beta-catenin signaling in Alzheimer's disease. *CNS Neurol. Disord. Drug Targets.* 2014;13:745–754. doi: 10.2174/1871527312666131223113900.
134. L'Episcopo F., Tirolo C., Testa N., Caniglia S., Morale M.C., Serapide M.F., Pluchino S., Marchetti B. Wnt/B-catenin signaling is required to rescue midbrain dopaminergic progenitors and promote neurorepair in ageing mouse model of Parkinson's disease. *Stem Cells (Dayton, Ohio)* 2014;32:2147–2163. doi: 10.1002/stem.1708.
135. Finkel S.I. Effects of rivastigmine on behavioral and psychological symptoms of dementia in Alzheimer's disease. *Clin. Ther.* 2004;26:980–990. doi: 10.1016/S0149-2918(04)90172-5.
136. Lee J.H., Jeong S.K., Kim B., Park K., Dash A. Donepezil across the spectrum of Alzheimer's disease: Dose optimization and clinical relevance. *Acta Neurol. Scand.* 2015;131:259–267. doi: 10.1111/ane.12386.
137. Quinn N. Drug treatment of Parkinson's disease. *BMJ Br. Med J.* 1995;310:575. doi: 10.1136/bmj.310.6979.575.
138. Bonuccelli U., Colzi A., Del Dotto P. Pergolide in the treatment of patients with early and advanced Parkinson's disease. *Clin. Neuropharmacol.* 2002;25:1–10. doi: 10.1097/00002826-200201000-00001.
139. Le W.-D., Jankovic J. Are dopamine receptor agonists neuroprotective in Parkinson's disease? *Drugs Aging.* 2001;18:389–396. doi: 10.2165/00002512-200118060-00001.
140. McMurray C.T. Huntington's disease: New hope for therapeutics. *Trends Neurosci.* 2001;24:S32–S38. doi: 10.1016/S0166-2236(00)01997-4.

141. Faissner S., Gold R. Oral therapies for multiple sclerosis. *Cold Spring Harb. Perspect. Med.* 2018 doi: 10.1101/cshperspect.a032011.

142. Stangel M., Kuhlmann T., Matthews P.M., Kilpatrick T.J. Achievements and obstacles of remyelinating therapies in multiple sclerosis. *Nat. Rev. Neurol.* 2017;13:742–754. doi: 10.1038/nrneurol.2017.139.

143. Zeydan B., Rodriguez M., Kantarci O.H. Timing of future remyelination therapies and their potential to stop multiple sclerosis progression. *Adv. Exp. Med. Biol.* 2017;958:161–170.

144. Plemel J.R., Liu W.Q., Yong V.W. Remyelination therapies: A new direction and challenge in multiple sclerosis. *Nat. Rev. Drug Discov.* 2017;16:617–634. doi: 10.1038/nrd.2017.115.

145. Kumar V., Sami N., Kashav T., Islam A., Ahmad F., Hassan M.I. Protein aggregation and neurodegenerative diseases: From theory to therapy. *Eur. J. Med. Chem.* 2016;124:1105–1120. doi: 10.1016/j.ejmech.2016.07.054.

146. Herczenik E., Gebbink M.F. Molecular and cellular aspects of protein misfolding and disease. *FASEB J.* 2008;22:2115–2133. doi: 10.1096/fj.07-099671.

147. Akiyama H., Barger S., Barnum S., Bradt B., Bauer J., Cole G.M., Cooper N.R., Eikelenboom P., Emmerling M., Fiebich B.L. Inflammation and Alzheimer's disease. *Neurobiol. Aging.* 2000;21:383–421. doi: 10.1016/S0197-4580(00)00124-X.

148. Smith M.A., Sayre L.M., Monnier V.M., Perry G. Radical ageing in Alzheimer's disease. *Trends Neurosci.* 1995;18:172–176. doi: 10.1016/0166-2236(95)93897-7.

149. Greenbaum E.A., Graves C.L., Mishizen-Eberz A.J., Lupoli M.A., Lynch D.R., Englander S.W., Axelsen P.H., Giasson B.I. The E46K mutation in α-synuclein increases amyloid fibril formation. *J. Boil. Chem.* 2005;280:7800–7807. doi: 10.1074/jbc.M411638200.

150. Azuaga A.I., Dobson C.M., Mateo P.L., Conejero-Lara F. Unfolding and aggregation during the thermal denaturation of streptokinase. *FEBS J.* 2002;269:4121–4133.

151. Iametti S., Gregori B., Vecchio G., Bonomi F. Modifications occur at different structural levels during the heat denaturation of β-lactoglobulin. *FEBS J.* 1996;237:106–112. doi: 10.1111/j.1432-1033.1996.0106n.x.

152. Giri K., Bhattacharyya N.P., Basak S. Ph-dependent self-assembly of polyalanine peptides. *Biophys. J.* 2007;92:293–302. doi: 10.1529/biophysj.106.091769.

153. Chaturvedi S.K., Alam P., Khan J.M., Siddiqui M.K., Kalaiarasan P., Subbarao N., Ahmad Z., Khan R.H. Biophysical insight into the anti-amyloidogenic behavior of taurine. *Int. J. Boil. Macromol.* 2015;80:375–384. doi: 10.1016/j.ijbiomac.2015.06.035.

154. Balch W.E., Morimoto R.I., Dillin A., Kelly J.W. Adapting proteostasis for disease intervention. *Science (New York)* 2008;319:916–919. doi: 10.1126/science.1141448.

155. Hartl F.U. Protein misfolding diseases. *Annu. Rev. Biochem.* 2017;86:21–26. doi: 10.1146/annurev-biochem-061516-044518.

156. Ross C.A., Poirier M.A. Protein aggregation and neurodegenerative disease. *Nat. Med.* 2004;10:S10–S17. doi: 10.1038/nm1066.

157. Sherman M.Y., Goldberg A.L. Cellular defenses against unfolded proteins: A cell biologist thinks about neurodegenerative diseases. *Neuron.* 2001;29:15–32. doi: 10.1016/S0896-6273(01)00177-5.

158. Chen S., Brown I.R. Neuronal expression of constitutive heat shock proteins: Implications for neurodegenerative diseases. *Cell Stress Chaperones.* 2007;12:51–58. doi: 10.1379/CSC-236R.1.

159. Jackrel M.E., Shorter J. Engineering enhanced protein disaggregases for neurodegenerative disease. *Prion.* 2015;9:90–109. doi: 10.1080/19336896.2015.1020277.

160. Hughes E., Burke R., Doig A. Inhibition of toxicity in the Alzheimer's disease peptide fragment β (25–35) using N-methylated derivatives. *Biochem. Soc. Trans.* 2000;28:A72. doi: 10.1042/bst028a072b.

161. Madine J., Doig A.J., Middleton D.A. Design of an N-methylated peptide inhibitor of α-synuclein aggregation guided by solid-state NMR. *J. Am. Chem. Soc.* 2008;130:7873–7881. doi: 10.1021/ja075356q.

162. Lu R.-C., Tan M.-S., Wang H., Xie A.-M., Yu J.-T., Tan L. Heat shock protein 70 in Alzheimer's disease. *BioMed Res. Int.* 2014;2014:435203. doi: 10.1155/2014/435203.

163. Hoshino T., Murao N., Namba T., Takehara M., Adachi H., Katsuno M., Sobue G., Matsushima T., Suzuki T., Mizushima T. Suppression of Alzheimer's disease-related phenotypes by expression of heat shock protein 70 in mice. *J. Neurosci.* 2011;31:5225–5234. doi: 10.1523/JNEUROSCI.5478-10.2011.

164. Patterson K.R., Ward S.M., Combs B., Voss K., Kanaan N.M., Morfini G., Brady S.T., Gamblin T.C., Binder L.I. Heat shock protein 70 prevents both tau aggregation and the inhibitory effects of preexisting tau aggregates on fast axonal transport. *Biochemistry.* 2011;50:10300–10310. doi: 10.1021/bi2009147.

165. Dou F., Netzer W.J., Tanemura K., Li F., Hartl F.U., Takashima A., Gouras G.K., Greengard P., Xu H. Chaperones increase association of tau protein with microtubules. *Proc. Natl. Acad. Sci. USA.* 2003;100:721–726. doi: 10.1073/pnas.242720499.

166. Hirakawa T., Rokutan K., Nikawa T., Kishi K. Geranylgeranylacetone induces heat shock proteins in cultured guinea pig gastric mucosal cells and rat gastric mucosa. *Gastroenterology.* 1996;111:345–357. doi: 10.1053/gast.1996.v111.pm8690199.

167. Chow A.M., Tang D.W., Hanif A., Brown I.R. Induction of heat shock proteins in cerebral cortical cultures by celastrol. *Cell Stress Chaperones.* 2013;18:155–160. doi: 10.1007/s12192-012-0364-0.

168. Bobkova N.V., Garbuz D.G., Nesterova I., Medvinskaya N., Samokhin A., Alexandrova I., Yashin V., Karpov V., Kukharsky M.S., Ninkina N.N. Therapeutic effect of exogenous hsp70 in mouse models of Alzheimer's disease. *J. Alzheimer's Dis.* 2014;38:425–435. doi: 10.3233/JAD-130779.

169. Vinokurov M., Ostrov V., Yurinskaya M., Garbuz D., Murashev A., Antonova O., Evgen'ev M. Recombinant human hsp70 protects against lipoteichoic acid-induced inflammation manifestations at the cellular and organismal levels. *Cell Stress Chaperones.* 2012;17:89–101. doi: 10.1007/s12192-011-0288-0.

170. Goldfarb S.B., Kashlan O.B., Watkins J.N., Suaud L., Yan W., Kleyman T.R., Rubenstein R.C. Differential effects of hsc70 and hsp70 on the intracellular trafficking and functional expression of epithelial sodium channels. *Proc. Natl. Acad. Sci. USA.* 2006;103:5817–5822. doi: 10.1073/pnas.0507903103.

171. Jinwal U.K., Akoury E., Abisambra J.F., O'Leary III J.C., Thompson A.D., Blair L.J., Jin Y., Bacon J., Nordhues B.A., Cockman M. Imbalance of hsp70 family variants fosters tau accumulation. *FASEB J.* 2013;27:1450–1459. doi: 10.1096/fj.12-220889.

172. Miyata Y., Li X., Lee H.-F., Jinwal U.K., Srinivasan S.R., Seguin S.P., Young Z.T., Brodsky J.L., Dickey C.A., Sun D. Synthesis and initial evaluation of YM-08, a blood-brain barrier permeable derivative of the heat shock protein 70 (Hsp70) inhibitor MKT-077, which reduces tau levels. *ACS Chem. Neurosci.* 2013;4:930–939. doi: 10.1021/cn300210g.

173. Morimoto R.I. Dynamic remodeling of transcription complexes by molecular chaperones. *Cell.* 2002;110:281–284. doi: 10.1016/S0092-8674(02)00860-7.

174. Kim S.A., Yoon J.H., Lee S.H., Ahn S.G. Polo-like kinase 1 phosphorylates heat shock transcription factor 1 and mediates its nuclear translocation during heat stress. *J. Boil. Chem.* 2005;280:12653–12657. doi: 10.1074/jbc.M411908200.

175. Hu Y., Mivechi N.F. Hsf-1 interacts with Ral-binding protein 1 in a stress-responsive, multiprotein complex with HSP90 in vivo. *J. Boil. Chem.* 2003;278:17299–17306. doi: 10.1074/jbc.M300788200.

176. Guo Y., Guettouche T., Fenna M., Boellmann F., Pratt W.B., Toft D.O., Smith D.F., Voellmy R. Evidence for a mechanism of repression of heat shock factor 1 transcriptional activity by a multichaperone complex. *J. Boil. Chem.* 2001;276:45791–45799. doi: 10.1074/jbc.M105931200.

177. Cushman M., Johnson B.S., King O.D., Gitler A.D., Shorter J. Prion-like disorders: Blurring the divide between transmissibility and infectivity. *J. Cell Sci.* 2010;123:1191–1201. doi: 10.1242/jcs.051672.

178. Lindberg I., Shorter J., Wiseman R.L., Chiti F., Dickey C.A., McLean P.J. Chaperones in neurodegeneration. *J. Neurosci.* 2015;35:13853–13859. doi: 10.1523/JNEUROSCI.2600-15.2015.

179. Takalo M., Salminen A., Soininen H., Hiltunen M., Haapasalo A. Protein aggregation and degradation mechanisms in neurodegenerative diseases. *Am. J. Neurodegener. Dis.* 2013;2:1–14.

180. Shorter J. Engineering therapeutic protein disaggregases. *Mol. Boil. Cell.* 2016;27:1556–1560. doi: 10.1091/mbc.e15-10-0693.

181. Shorter J. Hsp104: A weapon to combat diverse neurodegenerative disorders. *Neurosignals.* 2008;16:63–74. doi: 10.1159/000109760.

182. Jackrel M.E., Shorter J. Potentiated Hsp104 variants suppress toxicity of diverse neurodegenerative disease-linked proteins. *Dis. Model Mech.* 2014;7:1175–1184. doi: 10.1242/dmm.016113.

183. Lee S.J., Lim H.S., Masliah E., Lee H.J. Protein aggregate spreading in neurodegenerative diseases: Problems and perspectives. *Neurosci. Res.* 2011;70:339–348. doi: 10.1016/j.neures.2011.05.008.

184. Evans C.G., Wisén S., Gestwicki J.E. Heat shock proteins 70 and 90 inhibit early stages of amyloid beta (1-42) aggregation in vitro. *J. Boil. Chem.* 2006 doi: 10.1074/jbc.M606192200.

185. Bauer P.O., Goswami A., Wong H.K., Okuno M., Kurosawa M., Yamada M., Miyazaki H., Matsumoto G., Kino Y., Nagai Y., et al. Harnessing chaperone-mediated autophagy for the selective degradation of mutant huntingtin protein. *Nat. Biotechnol.* 2010;28:256–263. doi: 10.1038/nbt.1608.

186. Koyuncu S., Fatima A., Gutierrez-Garcia R., Vilchez D. Proteostasis of huntingtin in health and disease. *Int. J. Mol. Sci.* 2017;18:1568. doi: 10.3390/ijms18071568.

187. Maiti P., Manna J., Veleri S., Frautschy S. Molecular chaperone dysfunction in neurodegenerative

diseases and effects of curcumin. *BioMed Res. Int.* 2014;2014:495091. doi: 10.1155/2014/495091.

188. Dedmon M.M., Christodoulou J., Wilson M.R., Dobson C.M. Heat shock protein 70 inhibits alpha-synuclein fibril formation via preferential binding to prefibrillar species. *J. Boil. Chem.* 2005;280:14733–14740. doi: 10.1074/jbc.M413024200.

189. Ebrahimi-Fakhari D., Wahlster L., McLean P.J. Molecular chaperones in Parkinson's disease—Present and future. *J. Park. Dis.* 2011;1:299–320.

190. Schulte T.W., Neckers L.M. The benzoquinone ansamycin 17-allylamino-17-demethoxygeldanamycin binds to HSP90 and shares important biologic activities with geldanamycin. *Cancer Chemother. Pharmacol.* 1998;42:273–279. doi: 10.1007/s002800050817.

191. Shen H.Y., He J.C., Wang Y., Huang Q.Y., Chen J.F. Geldanamycin induces heat shock protein 70 and protects against MPTP-induced dopaminergic neurotoxicity in mice. *J. Boil. Chem.* 2005;280:39962–39969. doi: 10.1074/jbc.M505524200.

192. Ciechanover A., Kwon Y.T. Protein quality control by molecular chaperones in neurodegeneration. *Front. Neurosci.* 2017;11:185. doi: 10.3389/fnins.2017.00185.

193. Björkqvist M., Wild E.J., Thiele J., Silvestroni A., Andre R., Lahiri N., Raibon E., Lee R.V., Benn C.L., Soulet D., et al. A novel pathogenic pathway of immune activation detectable before clinical onset in Huntington's disease. *J. Exp. Med.* 2008;205:1869–1877. doi: 10.1084/jem.20080178.

194. Chen H., O'Reilly E.J., Schwarzschild M.A., Ascherio A. Peripheral inflammatory biomarkers and risk of Parkinson's disease. *Am. J. Epidemiol.* 2008;167:90–95. doi: 10.1093/aje/kwm260.

195. Mogi M., Harada M., Riederer P., Narabayashi H., Fujita K., Nagatsu T. Tumor necrosis factor-alpha (TNF-alpha) increases both in the brain and in the cerebrospinal fluid from parkinsonian patients. *Neurosci. Lett.* 1994;165:208–210. doi: 10.1016/0304-3940(94)90746-3.

196. Crotti A., Glass C.K. The choreography of neuroinflammation in Huntington's disease. *Trends Immunol.* 2015;36:364–373. doi: 10.1016/j.it.2015.04.007.

197. Tronel C., Largeau B., Santiago Ribeiro M.J., Guilloteau D., Dupont A.-C., Arlicot N. Molecular targets for pet imaging of activated microglia: The current situation and future expectations. *Int. J. Mol. Sci.* 2017;18:802. doi: 10.3390/ijms18040802.

198. Tai Y.F., Pavese N., Gerhard A., Tabrizi S.J., Barker R.A., Brooks D.J., Piccini P. Microglial activation in presymptomatic Huntington's disease gene carriers. *Brain J. Neurol.* 2007;130:1759–1766. doi: 10.1093/brain/awm044.

199. Rocha N.P., Ribeiro F.M., Furr-Stimming E., Teixeira A.L. Neuroimmunology of Huntington's disease: Revisiting evidence from human studies. *Mediat. Inflamm.* 2016;2016:8653132. doi: 10.1155/2016/8653132.

200. Sapp E., Kegel K.B., Aronin N., Hashikawa T., Uchiyama Y., Tohyama K., Bhide P.G., Vonsattel J.P., DiFiglia M. Early and progressive accumulation of reactive microglia in the Huntington disease brain. *J. Neuropathol. Exp. Neurol.* 2001;60:161–172. doi: 10.1093/jnen/60.2.161.

201. Miron V.E., Boyd A., Zhao J.W., Yuen T.J., Ruckh J.M., Shadrach J.L., van Wijngaarden P., Wagers A.J., Williams A., Franklin R.J.M., et al. M2 microglia and macrophages drive oligodendrocyte differentiation during CNS remyelination. *Nat. Neurosci.* 2013;16:1211–1218. doi: 10.1038/nn.3469.

202. Yang H.-M., Yang S., Huang S.-S., Tang B.-S., Guo J.-F. Microglial activation in the pathogenesis of Huntington's disease. *Front. Aging Neurosci.* 2017;9:193. doi: 10.3389/fnagi.2017.00193.

203. Chang K.H., Wu Y.R., Chen Y.C., Chen C.M. Plasma inflammatory biomarkers for Huntington's disease patients and mouse model. *Brain Behav. Immun.* 2015;44:121–127. doi: 10.1016/j.bbi.2014.09.011.

204. Politis M., Lahiri N., Niccolini F., Su P., Wu K., Giannetti P., Scahill R.I., Turkheimer F.E., Tabrizi S.J., Piccini P. Increased central microglial activation associated with peripheral cytokine levels in premanifest Huntington's disease gene carriers. *Neurobiol. Dis.* 2015;83:115–121. doi: 10.1016/j.nbd.2015.08.011.

205. Träger U., Andre R., Lahiri N., Magnusson-Lind A., Weiss A., Grueninger S., McKinnon C., Sirinathsinghji E., Kahlon S., Pfister E.L. HTT-lowering reverses Huntington's disease immune dysfunction caused by NFκB pathway dysregulation. *Brain J. Neurol.* 2014;137:819–833. doi: 10.1093/brain/awt355.

206. Brochard V., Combadiere B., Prigent A., Laouar Y., Perrin A., Beray-Berthat V., Bonduelle O., Alvarez-Fischer D., Callebert J., Launay J.M., et al. Infiltration of CD4+ lymphocytes into the brain contributes to neurodegeneration in a mouse model of Parkinson disease. *J. Clin. Investig.* 2009;119:182–192. doi: 10.1172/JCI36470.

207. Rees K., Stowe R., Patel S., Ives N., Breen K., Clarke C.E., Ben-Shlomo Y. Non-steroidal anti-inflammatory drugs as disease-modifying agents for Parkinson's disease: Evidence from observational studies. *Cochrane Database Syst. Rev.* 2011:Cd008454.

208. Du Y., Ma Z., Lin S., Dodel R.C., Gao F., Bales K.R., Triarhou L.C., Chernet E., Perry K.W., Nelson D.L., et al. Minocycline prevents nigrostriatal dopaminergic neurodegeneration in the MPTP model of Parkinson's disease. *Proc. Natl. Acad. Sci. USA.* 2001;98:14669–14674. doi: 10.1073/pnas.251341998.

209. Lofrumento D.D., Nicolardi G., Cianciulli A., Nuccio F.D., Pesa V.L., Carofiglio V., Dragone T., Calvello R., Panaro M.A. Neuroprotective effects of resveratrol in an MPTP mouse model of Parkinson's-like disease: Possible role of socs-1 in reducing pro-inflammatory responses. *Innate Immun.* 2014;20:249–260. doi: 10.1177/1753425913488429.

210. Zhang F., Shi J.-S., Zhou H., Wilson B.C., Hong J.-S., Gao H.-M. Resveratrol protects dopamine neurons against lipopolysaccharide-induced neurotoxicity through its anti-inflammatory actions. *Mol. Pharmacol.* 2010;94 doi: 10.1124/mol.110.064535.

211. Ren B., Zhang Y.-X., Zhou H.-X., Sun F.-W., Zhang Z.-F., Wei Z.-F., Zhang C.-Y., Si D.-W. Tanshinone IIA prevents the loss of nigrostriatal dopaminergic neurons by inhibiting NADPH oxidase and iNOS in the MPTP model of Parkinson's disease. *J. Neurol. Sci.* 2015;348:142–152. doi: 10.1016/j.jns.2014.11.026.

212. Wang S., Jing H., Yang H., Liu Z., Guo H., Chai L., Hu L. Tanshinone I selectively suppresses pro-inflammatory genes expression in activated microglia and prevents nigrostriatal dopaminergic neurodegeneration in a mouse model of Parkinson's disease. *J. Ethnopharmacol.* 2015;164:247–255. doi: 10.1016/j.jep.2015.01.042.

213. Borah A., Paul R., Choudhury S., Choudhury A., Bhuyan B., Das Talukdar A., Dutta Choudhury M., Mohanakumar K.P. Neuroprotective potential of silymarin against CNS disorders: Insight into the pathways and molecular mechanisms of action. *CNS Neurosci. Ther.* 2013;19:847–853. doi: 10.1111/cns.12175.

214. Gendelman H.E., Zhang Y., Santamaria P., Olson K.E., Schutt C.R., Bhatti D., Shetty B.L.D., Lu Y., Estes K.A., Standaert D.G. Evaluation of the safety and immunomodulatory effects of

sargramostim in a randomized, double-blind phase 1 clinical Parkinson's disease trial. *NPJ Park. Dis.* 2017;3:10. doi: 10.1038/s41531-017-0013-5.

215. Dobson L., Träger U., Farmer R., Hayardeny L., Loupe P., Hayden M.R., Tabrizi S.J. Laquinimod dampens hyperactive cytokine production in Huntington's disease patient myeloid cells. *J. Neurochem.* 2016;137:782–794. doi: 10.1111/jnc.13553.

216. Na S.Y., Mracsko E., Liesz A., Hunig T., Veltkamp R. Amplification of regulatory t cells using a CD28 superagonist reduces brain damage after ischemic stroke in mice. *Stroke.* 2015;46:212–220. doi: 10.1161/STROKEAHA.114.007756.

217. Chung E.S., Lee G., Lee C., Ye M., Chung H.S., Kim H., Bae S.J., Hwang D.S., Bae H. Bee venom phospholipase A2, a novel Foxp3+ regulatory t cell inducer, protects dopaminergic neurons by modulating neuroinflammatory responses in a mouse model of Parkinson's disease. *J. Immunol.* 2015;195:4853–4860. doi: 10.4049/jimmunol.1500386.

218. Games D., Valera E., Spencer B., Rockenstein E., Mante M., Adame A., Patrick C., Ubhi K., Nuber S., Sacayon P. Reducing C-terminal-truncated alpha-synuclein by immunotherapy attenuates neurodegeneration and propagation in Parkinson's disease-like models. *J. Neurosci.* 2014;34:9441–9454. doi: 10.1523/JNEUROSCI.5314-13.2014.

219. Lindström V., Fagerqvist T., Nordström E., Eriksson F., Lord A., Tucker S., Andersson J., Johannesson M., Schell H., Kahle P.J. Immunotherapy targeting α-synuclein protofibrils reduced pathology in (Thy-1)-h [A30P] α-synuclein mice. *Neurobiol. Dis.* 2014;69:134–143. doi: 10.1016/j.nbd.2014.05.009.

220. O'Nuallain B., Williams A.D., McWilliams-Koeppen H.P., Acero L., Weber A., Ehrlich H., Schwarz H.P., Solomon A. Anti-amyloidogenic activity of IgGs contained in normal plasma. *J. Clin. Immunol.* 2010;30:37–42. doi: 10.1007/s10875-010-9413-6.

221. Kayed R., Canto I., Breydo L., Rasool S., Lukacsovich T., Wu J., Albay R., Pensalfini A., Yeung S., Head E. Conformation dependent monoclonal antibodies distinguish different replicating strains or conformers of prefibrillar Aβ oligomers. *Mol. Neurodegener.* 2010;5:57. doi: 10.1186/1750-1326-5-57.

222. Lambert M.P., Velasco P.T., Chang L., Viola K.L., Fernandez S., Lacor P.N., Khuon D., Gong Y., Bigio E.H., Shaw P. Monoclonal antibodies that target pathological assemblies of Aβ *J. Neurochem.* 2007;100:23–35. doi: 10.1111/j.1471-4159.2006.04157.x.

223. Mizushima N., Levine B., Cuervo A.M., Klionsky D.J. Autophagy fights disease through cellular self-digestion. *Nature.* 2008;451:1069–1075. doi: 10.1038/nature06639.

224. Yen W.-L., Klionsky D.J. How to live long and prosper: Autophagy, mitochondria, and aging. *Physiology.* 2008;23:248–262. doi: 10.1152/physiol.00013.2008.

225. Boland B., Kumar A., Lee S., Platt F.M., Wegiel J., Yu W.H., Nixon R.A. Autophagy induction and autophagosome clearance in neurons: Relationship to autophagic pathology in Alzheimer's disease. *J. Neurosci.* 2008;28:6926–6937. doi: 10.1523/JNEUROSCI.0800-08.2008.

226. Nixon R.A. The role of autophagy in neurodegenerative disease. *Nat. Med.* 2013;19:983–997. doi: 10.1038/nm.3232.

227. Stoica L., Zhu P.J., Huang W., Zhou H., Kozma S.C., Costa-Mattioli M. Selective pharmacogenetic inhibition of mammalian target of rapamycin complex I (mTORc1) blocks long-term synaptic plasticity and memory storage. *Proc. Natl. Acad. Sci. USA.* 2011;108:3791–3796. doi: 10.1073/pnas.1014715108.

228. Pupyshev A.B., Korolenko T.A., Tikhonova M.A. A therapeutic target for inhibition of neurodegeneration: Autophagy. *Neurosci. Behav. Physiol.* 2017;47:1109–1127. doi: 10.1007/s11055-017-0519-7.

229. Nah J., Yuan J., Jung Y.-K. Autophagy in neurodegenerative diseases: From mechanism to therapeutic approach. *Mol. Cells.* 2015;38:381–389. doi: 10.14348/molcells.2015.0034.

230. Hara T., Nakamura K., Matsui M., Yamamoto A., Nakahara Y., Suzuki-Migishima R., Yokoyama M., Mishima K., Saito I., Okano H. Suppression of basal autophagy in neural cells causes neurodegenerative disease in mice. *Nature.* 2006;441:885–889. doi: 10.1038/nature04724.

231. Liang C.-C., Wang C., Peng X., Gan B., Guan J.-L. Neural-specific deletion of FIP200 leads to cerebellar degeneration caused by increased neuronal death and axon degeneration. *J. Boil. Chem.* 2010;285:3499–3509. doi: 10.1074/jbc.M109.072389.

232. Choi S.J., Panhelainen A., Schmitz Y., Larsen K.E., Kanter E., Wu M., Sulzer D., Mosharov E.V. Changes in neuronal dopamine homeostasis following 1-methyl-4-phenylpyridinium (MPP+) exposure. *J. Boil. Chem.* 2015;290:6799–6809. doi: 10.1074/jbc.M114.631556.

233. Javitch J.A., D'Amato R.J., Strittmatter S.M., Snyder S.H. Parkinsonism-inducing neurotoxin, N-methyl-4-phenyl-1,2,3,6-tetrahydropyridine: Uptake of the metabolite N-methyl-4-phenylpyridine by dopamine neurons explains selective toxicity. *Proc. Natl. Acad. Sci. USA.* 1985;82:2173–2177. doi: 10.1073/pnas.82.7.2173.

234. Steele J.W., Gandy S. Latrepirdine (Dimebon(R)), a potential alzheimer therapeutic, regulates autophagy and neuropathology in an Alzheimer mouse model. *Autophagy.* 2013;9:617–618. doi: 10.4161/auto.23487.

235. Chau S., Herrmann N., Ruthirakuhan M.T., Chen J.J., Lanctot K.L. *Latrepirdine for Alzheimer's Disease.* The Cochrane Library; London, UK: 2015.

236. Forlenza O.V., de Paula V.J., Machado-Vieira R., Diniz B.S., Gattaz W.F. Does lithium prevent Alzheimer's disease? *Drugs Aging.* 2012;29:335–342. doi: 10.2165/11599180-000000000-00000.

237. Berger Z., Ravikumar B., Menzies F.M., Oroz L.G., Underwood B.R., Pangalos M.N., Schmitt I., Wullner U., Evert B.O., O'kane C.J. Rapamycin alleviates toxicity of different aggregate-prone proteins. *Hum. Mol. Genet.* 2005;15:433–442. doi: 10.1093/hmg/ddi458.

238. Wang T., Lao U., Edgar B.A. Tor-mediated autophagy regulates cell death in drosophila neurodegenerative disease. *J. Cell Boil.* 2009;186:703–711. doi: 10.1083/jcb.200904090.

239. Park H.-W., Park H., Semple I.A., Jang I., Ro S.-H., Kim M., Cazares V.A., Stuenkel E.L., Kim J.-J., Kim J.S. Pharmacological correction of obesity-induced autophagy arrest using calcium channel blockers. *Nat. Commun.* 2014;5:4834. doi: 10.1038/ncomms5834.

240. Caccamo A., Majumder S., Richardson A., Strong R., Oddo S. Molecular interplay between mammalian target of rapamycin (mTOR), amyloid-beta, and tau: Effects on cognitive impairments. *J. Boil. Chem.* 2010;285:13107–13120. doi: 10.1074/jbc.M110.100420.

241. Sun Q., Wei L.-L., Zhang M., Li T.-X., Yang C., Deng S.-P., Zeng Q.-C. Rapamycin inhibits activation of ampk-mTOR signaling pathway-induced Alzheimer's disease lesion in hippocampus of rats with type 2 diabetes mellitus. *Int. J. Neurosci.* 2018;2018:1–22. doi: 10.1080/00207454.2018.1491571.

242. Wullschleger S., Loewith R., Hall M.N. Tor signaling in growth and metabolism. *Cell.* 2006;124:471–484. doi: 10.1016/j.cell.2006.01.016.

243. Ma T.C., Buescher J.L., Oatis B., Funk J.A., Nash A.J., Carrier R.L., Hoyt K.R. Metformin therapy in a transgenic mouse model of Huntington's disease. *Neurosci. Lett.* 2007;411:98–103.

244. Goedert M., Jakes R., Qi Z., Wang J.H., Cohen P. Protein phosphatase 2A is the major enzyme in brain that dephosphorylates tau protein phosphorylated by proline-directed protein kinases or cyclic amp-dependent protein kinase. *J Neurochem.* 1995;65:2804–2807. doi: 10.1046/j.1471-4159.1995.65062804.x.

245. Hebron M.L., Lonskaya I., Olopade P., Selby S.T., Pagan F., Moussa C.E. Tyrosine kinase inhibition regulates early systemic immune changes and modulates the neuroimmune response in α-synucleinopathy. *J. Clin. Cell. Immunol.* 2014;5:259. doi: 10.4172/2155-9899.1000259.

246. Lonskaya I., Hebron M., Selby S., Turner R., Moussa C.-H. Nilotinib and Bosutinib modulate pre-plaque alterations of blood immune markers and neuro-inflammation in Alzheimer's disease models. *Neuroscience.* 2015;304:316–327. doi: 10.1016/j.neuroscience.2015.07.070.

247. Iliff J.J., Nedergaard M. Is there a cerebral lymphatic system? *Stroke.* 2013;44:S93–S95. doi: 10.1161/STROKEAHA.112.678698.

248. Xie L., Kang H., Xu Q., Chen M.J., Liao Y., Thiyagarajan M., O'Donnell J., Christensen D.J., Nicholson C., Iliff J.J., et al. Sleep drives metabolite clearance from the adult brain. *Science (New York)* 2013;342:373–377. doi: 10.1126/science.1241224.

249. Nedergaard M. Neuroscience. Garbage truck of the brain. *Science (New York)* 2013;340:1529–1530. doi: 10.1126/science.1240514.

250. Iliff J.J., Lee H., Yu M., Feng T., Logan J., Nedergaard M., Benveniste H. Brain-wide pathway for waste clearance captured by contrast-enhanced MRI. *J. Clin. Investig.* 2013;123:1299–1309. doi: 10.1172/JCI67677.

251. Jessen N.A., Munk A.S., Lundgaard I., Nedergaard M. The glymphatic system: A beginner's guide. *Neurochem. Res.* 2015;40:2583–2599. doi: 10.1007/s11064-015-1581-6.

252. Kress B.T., Iliff J.J., Xia M., Wang M., Wei H.S., Zeppenfeld D., Xie L., Kang H., Xu Q., Liew J.A., et al. Impairment of paravascular clearance pathways in the aging brain. *Ann. Neurol.* 2014;76:845–861. doi: 10.1002/ana.24271.

253. Iliff J.J., Wang M., Liao Y., Plogg B.A., Peng W., Gundersen G.A., Benveniste H., Vates G.E., Deane R., Goldman S.A., et al. A paravascular pathway facilitates CSF flow through the brain parenchyma and the clearance of interstitial solutes, including amyloid beta. *Sci. Transl. Med.* 2012;4:147ra111. doi: 10.1126/scitranslmed.3003748.

254. Nedergaard M., Goldman S.A. Brain drain. *Sci. Am.* 2016;314:44–49. doi: 10.1038/scientificamerican0316-44.

255. de Leon M.J., Li Y., Okamura N., Tsui W.H., Saint Louis L.A., Glodzik L., Osorio R.S., Fortea J., Butler T., Pirraglia E., et al. CSF clearance in Alzheimer disease measured with dynamic pet. *J. Nucl. Med.* 2017;58:1471. doi: 10.2967/jnumed.116.187211.

256. Peng W., Achariyar T.M., Li B., Liao Y., Mestre H., Hitomi E., Regan S., Kasper T., Peng S., Ding F., et al. Suppression of glymphatic fluid transport in a mouse model of Alzheimer's disease. *Neurobiol. Dis.* 2016;93:215–225. doi: 10.1016/j.nbd.2016.05.015.

257. Oh H., Madison C., Baker S., Rabinovici G., Jagust W. Dynamic relationships between age,

amyloid-beta deposition, and glucose metabolism link to the regional vulnerability to Alzheimer's disease. *Brain J. Neurol.* 2016;139:2275–2289. doi: 10.1093/brain/aww108.

258. Gage F.H. Neurogenesis in the adult brain. *J. Neurosci.* 2002;22:612–613. doi: 10.1523/JNEUROSCI.22-03-00612.2002.
259. Reynolds B.A., Weiss S. Generation of neurons and astrocytes from isolated cells of the adult mammalian central nervous system. *Science (New York)* 1992;255:1707–1710. doi: 10.1126/science.1553558.
260. Shihabuddin L.S., Horner P.J., Ray J., Gage F.H. Adult spinal cord stem cells generate neurons after transplantation in the adult dentate gyrus. *J. Neurosci. Off. J. Soc. Neurosci.* 2000;20:8727–8735. doi: 10.1523/JNEUROSCI.20-23-08727.2000.
261. Pencea V., Bingaman K.D., Freedman L.J., Luskin M.B. Neurogenesis in the subventricular zone and rostral migratory stream of the neonatal and adult primate forebrain. *Exp. Neurol.* 2001;172:1–16. doi: 10.1006/exnr.2001.7768.
262. Allen S.J., Watson J.J., Dawbarn D. The neurotrophins and their role in Alzheimer's disease. *Curr. Neuropharmacol.* 2011;9:559–573. doi: 10.2174/157015911798376190.
263. Lindsay R.M., Altar C.A., Cedarbaum J.M., Hyman C., Wiegand S.J. The therapeutic potential of neurotrophic factors in the treatment of Parkinson's disease. *Exp. Neurol.* 1993;124:103–118. doi: 10.1006/exnr.1993.1181.
264. Grondin R., Gash D.M. Glial cell line-derived neurotrophic factor (GDNF): A drug candidate for the treatment of Parkinson's disease. *J. Neurol.* 1998;245:P35–P42. doi: 10.1007/PL00007744.
265. Bowenkamp K.E., Lapchak P.A., Hoffer B.J., Miller P.J., Bickford P.C. Intracerebroventricular glial cell line-derived neurotrophic factor improves motor function and supports nigrostriatal dopamine neurons in bilaterally 6-hydroxydopamine lesioned rats. *Exp. Neurol.* 1997;145:104–117. doi: 10.1006/exnr.1997.6436.
266. Duman R.S. Neuronal damage and protection in the pathophysiology and treatment of psychiatric illness: Stress and depression. *Dialogues Clin. Neurosci.* 2009;11:239–255.
267. Tsiperson V., Huang Y., Bagayogo I., Song Y., VonDran M.W., DiCicco-Bloom E., Dreyfus C.F. Brain-derived neurotrophic factor deficiency restricts proliferation of oligodendrocyte progenitors following cuprizone-induced demyelination. *ASN Neuro.* 2015;7 doi: 10.1177/1759091414566878.
268. Schindowski K., Belarbi K., Buée L. Neurotrophic factors in Alzheimer's disease: Role of axonal transport. *Genes Brain Behav.* 2008;7:43–56. doi: 10.1111/j.1601-183X.2007.00378.x.
269. Jiao S.S., Shen L.L., Zhu C., Bu X.L., Liu Y.H., Liu C.H., Yao X.Q., Zhang L.L., Zhou H.D., Walker D.G., et al. Brain-derived neurotrophic factor protects against tau-related neurodegeneration of Alzheimer's disease. *Transl. Psychiatry.* 2016;6:e907. doi: 10.1038/tp.2016.186.
270. Gold S.M., Chalifoux S., Giesser B.S., Voskuhl R.R. Immune modulation and increased neurotrophic factor production in multiple sclerosis patients treated with testosterone. *J. Neuroinflamm.* 2008;5:32. doi: 10.1186/1742-2094-5-32.
271. Cohen-Cory S., Kidane A.H., Shirkey N.J., Marshak S. Brain-derived neurotrophic factor and the development of structural neuronal connectivity. *Dev. Neurobiol.* 2010;70:271–288. doi: 10.1002/dneu.20774.

272. Henderson C.E. Role of neurotrophic factors in neuronal development. *Curr. Opin. Neurobiol.* 1996;6:64–70. doi: 10.1016/S0959-4388(96)80010-9.

273. Poo M.M. Neurotrophins as synaptic modulators. *Nat. Rev. Neurosci.* 2001;2:24–32. doi: 10.1038/35049004.

274. Huang E.J., Reichardt L.F. Neurotrophins: Roles in neuronal development and function. *Annu. Rev. Neurosci.* 2001;24:677–736. doi: 10.1146/annurev.neuro.24.1.677.

275. Nguyen T.L.X., Kim C.K., Cho J.-H., Lee K.-H., Ahn J.-Y. Neuroprotection signaling pathway of nerve growth factor and brain-derived neurotrophic factor against staurosporine induced apoptosis in hippocampal H19-7 cells. *Exp. Mol. Med.* 2010;42:583–595. doi: 10.3858/emm.2010.42.8.060.

276. Middlemas D.S., Kihl B.K., Zhou J., Zhu X. Brain-derived neurotrophic factor promotes survival and chemoprotection of human neuroblastoma cells. *J. Boil. Chem.* 1999;274:16451–16460. doi: 10.1074/jbc.274.23.16451.

277. Weissmiller A.M., Wu C. Current advances in using neurotrophic factors to treat neurodegenerative disorders. *Transl. Neurodegener.* 2012;1:14. doi: 10.1186/2047-9158-1-14.

278. Salehi A., Delcroix J.D., Swaab D.F. Alzheimer's disease and NGF signaling. *J. Neural Transm. (Vienna, Austria 1996)* 2004;111:323–345. doi: 10.1007/s00702-003-0091-x.

279. Higgins G.A., Mufson E.J. Ngf receptor gene expression is decreased in the nucleus basalis in Alzheimer's disease. *Exp. Neurol.* 1989;106:222–236. doi: 10.1016/0014-4886(89)90155-6.

280. Costa A., Peppe A., Carlesimo G.A., Zabberoni S., Scalici F., Caltagirone C., Angelucci F. Brain-derived neurotrophic factor serum levels correlate with cognitive performance in Parkinson's disease patients with mild cognitive impairment. *Front. Behav. Neurosci.* 2015;9:253. doi: 10.3389/fnbeh.2015.00253.

281. Howells D.W., Porritt M.J., Wong J.Y., Batchelor P.E., Kalnins R., Hughes A.J., Donnan G.A. Reduced bdnf mrna expression in the Parkinson's disease substantia nigra. *Exp. Neurol.* 2000;166:127–135. doi: 10.1006/exnr.2000.7483.

282. Pan W., Banks W.A., Kastin A.J. Permeability of the blood–brain barrier to neurotrophins. *Brain Res.* 1998;788:87–94. doi: 10.1016/S0006-8993(97)01525-4.

283. Pollack S.J., Harper S.J. Small molecule Trk receptor agonists and other neurotrophic factor mimetics. *Curr. Drug Targets CNS Neurol. Disord.* 2002;1:59–80. doi: 10.2174/1568007023339490.

284. Baulieu E.E., Robel P. Neurosteroids: A new brain function? *J. Steroid Biochem. Mol. Boil.* 1990;37:395–403. doi: 10.1016/0960-0760(90)90490-C.

285. Lv W., Du N., Liu Y., Fan X., Wang Y., Jia X., Hou X., Wang B. Low testosterone level and risk of Alzheimer's disease in the elderly men: A systematic review and meta-analysis. *Mol. Neurobiol.* 2016;53:2679–2684. doi: 10.1007/s12035-015-9315-y.

286. Paganini-Hill A., Henderson V.W. Estrogen deficiency and risk of Alzheimer's disease in women. *Am. J. Epidemiol.* 1994;140:256–261. doi: 10.1093/oxfordjournals.aje.a117244.

287. Carroll J.C., Rosario E.R., Villamagna A., Pike C.J. Continuous and cyclic progesterone differentially interact with estradiol in the regulation of Alzheimer-like pathology in female 3xtransgenic-Alzheimer's disease mice. *Endocrinology.* 2010;151:2713–2722. doi: 10.1210/en.2009-1487.

288. Rosario E.R., Chang L., Stanczyk F.Z., Pike C.J. Age-related testosterone depletion and

the development of Alzheimer disease. *JAMA.* 2004;292:1431–1432. doi: 10.1001/jama.292.12.1431-b.

289. Seidl J.N., Massman P.J. Relationships between testosterone levels and cognition in patients with Alzheimer disease and nondemented elderly men. *J. Geriatr. Psychiatry Neurol.* 2015;28:27–39. doi: 10.1177/0891988714541872.
290. Okun M.S., DeLong M.R., Hanfelt J., Gearing M., Levey A. Plasma testosterone levels in Alzheimer and Parkinson diseases. *Neurology.* 2004;62:411–413. doi: 10.1212/01.WNL.0000106840.72938.84.
291. Okun M.S., McDonald W.M., DeLong M.R. Refractory nonmotor symptoms in male patients with Parkinson disease due to testosterone deficiency: A common unrecognized comorbidity. *Arch. Neurol.* 2002;59:807–811. doi: 10.1001/archneur.59.5.807.
292. Markianos M., Panas M., Kalfakis N., Vassilopoulos D. Plasma testosterone in male patients with Huntington's disease: Relations to severity of illness and dementia. *Ann. Neurol.* 2005;57:520–525. doi: 10.1002/ana.20428.
293. Bove R., Musallam A., Healy B.C., Raghavan K., Glanz B.I., Bakshi R., Weiner H., De Jager P.L., Miller K.K., Chitnis T. Low testosterone is associated with disability in men with multiple sclerosis. *Mult. Scler.* 2014;20:1584–1592. doi: 10.1177/1352458514527864.
294. Trenova A.G., Slavov G.S., Manova M.G., Kostadinova, Vasileva T.V. Female sex hormones and cytokine secretion in women with multiple sclerosis. *Neurol. Res.* 2013;35:95–99. doi: 10.1179/1743132812Y.0000000120.
295. Zakrzewska-Pniewska B., Golebiowski M., Zajda M., Szeszkowski W., Podlecka-Pietowska A., Nojszewska M. Sex hormone patterns in women with multiple sclerosis as related to disease activity—A pilot study. *Neurol. I Neurochir. Polska.* 2011;45:536–542. doi: 10.1016/S0028-3843(14)60120-1.
296. Baker L.D., Sambamurti K., Craft S., Cherrier M., Raskind M.A., Stanczyk F.Z., Plymate S.R., Asthana S. 17beta-estradiol reduces plasma Abeta40 for HRT-naive postmenopausal women with Alzheimer disease: A preliminary study. *Am. J. Geriatr. Psychiatry.* 2003;11:239–244. doi: 10.1176/appi.ajgp.11.2.239.
297. Valen-Sendstad A., Engedal K., Stray-Pedersen B., Group A.S., Strobel C., Barnett L., Meyer N., Nurminemi M. Effects of hormone therapy on depressive symptoms and cognitive functions in women with Alzheimer disease: A 12 month randomized, double-blind, placebo-controlled study of low-dose estradiol and norethisterone. *Am. J. Geriatr. Psychiatry.* 2010;18:11–20. doi: 10.1097/JGP.0b013e3181beaaf4.
298. Cherrier M.M., Matsumoto A.M., Amory J.K., Asthana S., Bremner W., Peskind E.R., Raskind M.A., Craft S. Testosterone improves spatial memory in men with Alzheimer disease and mild cognitive impairment. *Neurology.* 2005;64:2063–2068. doi: 10.1212/01.WNL.0000165995.98986.F1.
299. Lu P.H., Masterman D.A., Mulnard R., Cotman C., Miller B., Yaffe K., Reback E., Porter V., Swerdloff R., Cummings J.L. Effects of testosterone on cognition and mood in male patients with mild Alzheimer disease and healthy elderly men. *Arch. Neurol.* 2006;63:177–185. doi: 10.1001/archneur.63.2.nct50002.
300. Moffat S.D., Zonderman A.B., Metter E.J., Kawas C., Blackman M.R., Harman S.M., Resnick S.M. Free testosterone and risk for Alzheimer disease in older men. *Neurology.* 2004;62:188–193. doi: 10.1212/WNL.62.2.188.

301. Martins R., Carruthers M. Testosterone as the missing link between pesticides, Alzheimer disease, and Parkinson disease. *JAMA Neurol.* 2014;71:1189–1190. doi: 10.1001/jamaneurol.2014.795.

302. Okun M.S., Fernandez H.H., Rodriguez R.L., Romrell J., Suelter M., Munson S., Louis E.D., Mulligan T., Foster P.S., Shenal B.V., et al. Testosterone therapy in men with Parkinson disease: Results of the test-PD study. *Arch. Neurol.* 2006;63:729–735. doi: 10.1001/archneur.63.5.729.

303. Okun M.S., Walter B.L., McDonald W.M., Tenover J.L., Green J., Juncos J.L., DeLong M.R. Beneficial effects of testosterone replacement for the nonmotor symptoms of Parkinson disease. *Arch. Neurol.* 2002;59:1750–1753. doi: 10.1001/archneur.59.11.1750.

304. Gold S.M., Voskuhl R.R. Estrogen and testosterone therapies in multiple sclerosis. *Prog. Brain Res.* 2009;175:239–251.

305. Kurth F., Luders E., Sicotte N.L., Gaser C., Giesser B.S., Swerdloff R.S., Montag M.J., Voskuhl R.R., Mackenzie-Graham A. Neuroprotective effects of testosterone treatment in men with multiple sclerosis. *Neuroimage Clin.* 2014;4:454–460. doi: 10.1016/j.nicl.2014.03.001.

306. Sicotte N.L., Giesser B.S., Tandon V., Klutch R., Steiner B., Drain A.E., Shattuck D.W., Hull L., Wang H.J., Elashoff R.M., et al. Testosterone treatment in multiple sclerosis: A pilot study. *Arch. Neurol.* 2007;64:683–688. doi: 10.1001/archneur.64.5.683.

307. Vukusic S., Ionescu I., El-Etr M., Schumacher M., Baulieu E.E., Cornu C., Confavreux C., Prevention of Post-Partum Relapses with Progestin. Estradiol in Multiple Sclerosis Study Group The prevention of post-partum relapses with progestin and estradiol in multiple sclerosis (POPART'MUS) trial: Rationale, objectives and state of advancement. *J. Neurol. Sci.* 2009;286:114–118. doi: 10.1016/j.jns.2009.08.056.

308. Palaszynski K.M., Loo K.K., Ashouri J.F., Liu H.B., Voskuhl R.R. Androgens are protective in experimental autoimmune encephalomyelitis: Implications for multiple sclerosis. *J. Neuroimmunol.* 2004;146:144–152. doi: 10.1016/j.jneuroim.2003.11.004.

309. Page S.T., Plymate S.R., Bremner W.J., Matsumoto A.M., Hess D.L., Lin D.W., Amory J.K., Nelson P.S., Wu J.D. Effect of medical castration on CD4+ CD25+ T cells, CD8+ T cell IFN-gamma expression, and NK cells: A physiological role for testosterone and/or its metabolites. *Am. J. Physiology. Endocrinol. Metab.* 2006;290:E856–E863. doi: 10.1152/ajpendo.00484.2005.

310. Malkin C.J., Pugh P.J., Jones R.D., Kapoor D., Channer K.S., Jones T.H. The effect of testosterone replacement on endogenous inflammatory cytokines and lipid profiles in hypogonadal men. *J. Clin. Endocrinol. Metab.* 2004;89:3313–3318. doi: 10.1210/jc.2003-031069.

311. Liva S.M., Voskuhl R.R. Testosterone acts directly on CD4+ T lymphocytes to increase IL-10 production. *J. Immunol. (Baltimore, Md. 1950)* 2001;167:2060–2067. doi: 10.4049/jimmunol.167.4.2060.

312. Simpkins J.W., Singh M., Brock C., Etgen A.M. Neuroprotection and estrogen receptors. *Neuroendocrinology.* 2012;96:119–130. doi: 10.1159/000338409.

313. Bryant D.N., Dorsa D.M. Roles of estrogen receptors alpha and beta in sexually dimorphic neuroprotection against glutamate toxicity. *Neuroscience.* 2010;170:1261–1269. doi: 10.1016/j.neuroscience.2010.08.019.

314. Deecher D.C., Daoud P., Bhat R.A., O'Connor L.T. Endogenously expressed estrogen receptors mediate neuroprotection in hippocampal cells (HT22) *J. Cell. Biochem.* 2005;95:302–312. doi: 10.1002/jcb.20413.

315. Labombarda F., Ghoumari A.M., Liere P., De Nicola A.F., Schumacher M., Guennoun R. Neuroprotection by steroids after neurotrauma in organotypic spinal cord cultures: A key role for progesterone receptors and steroidal modulators of Gaba(A) receptors. *Neuropharmacology.* 2013;71:46–55. doi: 10.1016/j.neuropharm.2013.03.010.

316. Liu A., Margaill I., Zhang S., Labombarda F., Coqueran B., Delespierre B., Liere P., Marchand-Leroux C., O'Malley B.W., Lydon J.P., et al. Progesterone receptors: A key for neuroprotection in experimental stroke. *Endocrinology.* 2012;153:3747–3757. doi: 10.1210/en.2012-1138.

317. Dubal D.B., Wise P.M. Neuroprotective effects of estradiol in middle-aged female rats. *Endocrinology.* 2001;142:43–48. doi: 10.1210/endo.142.1.7911.

318. Nuzzo M.T., Marino M. Estrogen/huntingtin: A novel pathway involved in neuroprotection. *Neural Regen. Res.* 2016;11:402–403.

319. Shen D., Tian X., Zhang B., Song R. Mechanistic evaluation of neuroprotective effect of estradiol on rotenone and 6-ohda induced Parkinson's disease. *Pharmacol. Rep. PR.* 2017;69:1178–1185. doi: 10.1016/j.pharep.2017.06.008.

320. Smith K., Dahodwala N. Neuroprotection by sex steroid hormones in Parkinson's disease (P3.068) *Neurology.* 2014;82 [Google Scholar]

321. Zárate S., Stevnsner T., Gredilla R. Role of estrogen and other sex hormones in brain aging. Neuroprotection and DNA repair. *Front. Aging Neurosci.* 2017;9:430. doi: 10.3389/fnagi.2017.00430.

322. Barker J.M., Galea L.A. Repeated estradiol administration alters different aspects of neurogenesis and cell death in the hippocampus of female, but not male, rats. *Neuroscience.* 2008;152:888–902. doi: 10.1016/j.neuroscience.2007.10.071.

323. Spencer J.L., Waters E.M., Romeo R.D., Wood G.E., Milner T.A., McEwen B.S. Uncovering the mechanisms of estrogen effects on hippocampal function. *Front. Neuroendocr.* 2008;29:219–237. doi: 10.1016/j.yfrne.2007.08.006.

324. Knoll J.G., Wolfe C.A., Tobet S.A. Estrogen modulates neuronal movements within the developing preoptic area/anterior hypothalamus. *Eur. J. Neurosci.* 2007;26:1091–1099. doi: 10.1111/j.1460-9568.2007.05751.x.

325. Tiwari-Woodruff S., Morales L.B.J., Lee R., Voskuhl R.R. Differential neuroprotective and antiinflammatory effects of estrogen receptor (ER)α and ERβ ligand treatment. *Proc. Natl. Acad. Sci. USA.* 2007;104:14813–14818. doi: 10.1073/pnas.0703783104.

326. Zhang Q.-G., Wang R., Tang H., Dong Y., Chan A., Sareddy G.R., Vadlamudi R.K., Brann D.W. Brain-derived estrogen exerts anti-inflammatory and neuroprotective actions in the rat hippocampus. *Mol. Cell. Endocrinol.* 2014;389:84–91. doi: 10.1016/j.mce.2013.12.019.

327. Shivers K.-Y., Amador N., Abrams L., Hunter D., Jenab S., Quiñones-Jenab V. Estrogen alters baseline and inflammatory-induced cytokine levels independent from hypothalamic–pituitary–adrenal axis activity. *Cytokine.* 2015;72:121–129. doi: 10.1016/j.cyto.2015.01.007.

328. Brown C.M., Mulcahey T.A., Filipek N.C., Wise P.M. Production of proinflammatory cytokines and chemokines during neuroinflammation: Novel roles for estrogen receptors α and β *Endocrinology.* 2010;151:4916–4925. doi: 10.1210/en.2010-0371.

329. Ahn J.-Y. Neuroprotection signaling of nuclear Akt in neuronal cells. *Exp. Neurobiol.* 2014;23:200–206. doi: 10.5607/en.2014.23.3.200.

330. Wang L., Zhou K., Fu Z., Yu D., Huang H., Zang X., Mo X. Brain development and Akt signaling: The crossroads of signaling pathway and neurodevelopmental diseases. *J. Mol. Neurosci.* 2017;61:379–384. doi: 10.1007/s12031-016-0872-y.

331. Itoh Y., Higuchi M., Oishi K., Kishi Y., Okazaki T., Sakai H., Miyata T., Nakajima K., Gotoh Y. PDK1–Akt pathway regulates radial neuronal migration and microtubules in the developing mouse neocortex. *Proc. Natl. Acad. Sci. USA.* 2016;113:E2955–E2964. doi: 10.1073/pnas.1516321113.

332. Liot G., Gabriel C., Cacquevel M., Ali C., MacKenzie E.T., Buisson A., Vivien D. Neurotrophin-3-induced PI-3 kinase/Akt signaling rescues cortical neurons from apoptosis. *Exp. Neurol.* 2004;187:38–46. doi: 10.1016/j.expneurol.2004.01.002.

333. Gross C., Bassell G.J. Neuron-specific regulation of class I PI3K catalytic subunits and their dysfunction in brain disorders. *Front. Mol. Neurosci.* 2014;7:12. doi: 10.3389/fnmol.2014.00012.

334. Guo W., Jiang H., Gray V., Dedhar S., Rao Y. Role of the integrin-linked kinase (ILK) in determining neuronal polarity. *Dev. Boil.* 2007;306:457–468. doi: 10.1016/j.ydbio.2007.03.019.

335. Hussain R., Macklin W.B. Integrin-linked kinase (ILK) deletion disrupts oligodendrocyte development by altering cell cycle. *J. Neurosci.* 2017;37:397–412. doi: 10.1523/JNEUROSCI.2113-16.2016.

336. Pereira J.A., Benninger Y., Baumann R., Gonçalves A.F., Özçelik M., Thurnherr T., Tricaud N., Meijer D., Fässler R., Suter U., et al. Integrin-linked kinase is required for radial sorting of axons and schwann cell remyelination in the peripheral nervous system. *J. Cell Boil.* 2009;185:147–161. doi: 10.1083/jcb.200809008.

337. Soltani M.H., Pichardo R., Song Z., Sangha N., Camacho F., Satyamoorthy K., Sangueza O.P., Setaluri V. Microtubule-associated protein 2, a marker of neuronal differentiation, induces mitotic defects, inhibits growth of melanoma cells, and predicts metastatic potential of cutaneous melanoma. *Am. J. Pathol.* 2005;166:1841–1850. doi: 10.1016/S0002-9440(10)62493-5.

338. Johnson G.V., Jope R.S. The role of microtubule-associated protein 2 (map-2) in neuronal growth, plasticity, and degeneration. *J. Neurosci. Res.* 1992;33:505–512. doi: 10.1002/jnr.490330402.

339. Chen W., Lu N., Ding Y., Wang Y., Chan L.T., Wang X., Gao X., Jiang S., Liu K. Rapamycin-resistant mTOR activity is required for sensory axon regeneration induced by a conditioning lesion. *eNeuro.* 2016;3 doi: 10.1523/ENEURO.0358-16.2016.

340. Maiese K. Driving neural regeneration through the mammalian target of rapamycin. *Neural Regen. Res.* 2014;9:1413. doi: 10.4103/1673-5374.139453.

341. Takei N., Nawa H. mTOR signaling and its roles in normal and abnormal brain development. *Front. Mol. Neurosci.* 2014;7:28. doi: 10.3389/fnmol.2014.00028.

342. Blázquez E., Velázquez E., Hurtado-Carneiro V., Ruiz-Albusac J.M. Insulin in the brain: Its pathophysiological implications for states related with central insulin resistance, type 2 diabetes and Alzheimer's disease. *Front. Endocrinol.* 2014;5:161. doi: 10.3389/fendo.2014.00161.

343. Hoyer S. Senile dementia and Alzheimer's disease. Brain blood flow and metabolism. *Prog. Neuro-Psychopharmacol. Boil. Psychiatry.* 1986;10:447–478. doi: 10.1016/0278-5846(86)90018-7.

344. Misiak B., Leszek J., Kiejna A. Metabolic syndrome, mild cognitive impairment and Alzheimer's disease—The emerging role of systemic low-grade inflammation and adiposity. *Brain Res. Bull.* 2012;89:144–149. doi: 10.1016/j.brainresbull.2012.08.003.

345. Gaspar J.M., Baptista F.I., Macedo M.P., Ambrósio A.N.F. Inside the diabetic brain: Role

of different players involved in cognitive decline. *ACS Chem. Neurosci.* 2015;7:131–142. doi: 10.1021/acschemneuro.5b00240.

346. de la Monte S.M., Wands J.R. Alzheimer's disease is type 3 diabetes—Evidence reviewed. *J. Diabetes Sci. Technol.* 2008;2:1101–1113. doi: 10.1177/193229680800200619.
347. de la Monte S.M., Tong M., Bowling N., Moskal P. si-RNA inhibition of brain insulin or insulin-like growth factor receptors causes developmental cerebellar abnormalities: Relevance to fetal alcohol spectrum disorder. *Mol. Brain.* 2011;4:13. doi: 10.1186/1756-6606-4-13.
348. Lee S., Tong M., Hang S., Deochand C., de la Monte S. CSF and brain indices of insulin resistance, oxidative stress and neuro-inflammation in early versus late Alzheimer's disease. *J. Alzheimer's Dis. Park.* 2013;3:128.
349. Shuvaev V.V., Laffont I., Serot J.-M., Fujii J., Taniguchi N., Siest G. Increased protein glycation in cerebrospinal fluid of Alzheimer's disease2. *Neurobiol. Aging.* 2001;22:397–402. doi: 10.1016/S0197-4580(00)00253-0.
350. Benedict C., Frey II W.H., Schiöth H.B., Schultes B., Born J., Hallschmid M. Intranasal insulin as a therapeutic option in the treatment of cognitive impairments. *Exp. Gerontol.* 2011;46:112–115. doi: 10.1016/j.exger.2010.08.026.
351. Reger M., Watson G., Frey Ii W., Baker L., Cholerton B., Keeling M., Belongia D., Fishel M., Plymate S., Schellenberg G. Effects of intranasal insulin on cognition in memory-impaired older adults: Modulation by APOE genotype. *Neurobiol. Aging.* 2006;27:451–458. doi: 10.1016/j.neurobiolaging.2005.03.016.
352. White M.F. Insulin signaling in health and disease. *Science (New York)* 2003;302:1710–1711. doi: 10.1126/science.1092952.
353. Boura-Halfon S., Zick Y. Phosphorylation of IRS proteins, insulin action, and insulin resistance. *Am. J. Physiol. Endocrinol. Metab.* 2009;296:E581–E591. doi: 10.1152/ajpendo.90437.2008.
354. Giordano G., Klintworth H., Kavanagh T., Costa L. Apoptosis induced by domoic acid in mouse cerebellar granule neurons involves activation of p38 and JNK MAP kinases. *Neurochem. Int.* 2008;52:1100–1105. doi: 10.1016/j.neuint.2007.11.004.
355. Andreozzi F., Laratta E., Procopio C., Hribal M.L., Sciacqua A., Perticone M., Miele C., Perticone F., Sesti G. Interleukin-6 impairs the insulin signaling pathway, promoting production of nitric oxide in human umbilical vein endothelial cells. *Mol. Cell. Boil.* 2007;27:2372–2383. doi: 10.1128/MCB.01340-06.
356. Bomfim T.R., Forny-Germano L., Sathler L.B., Brito-Moreira J., Houzel J.-C., Decker H., Silverman M.A., Kazi H., Melo H.M., McClean P.L. An anti-diabetes agent protects the mouse brain from defective insulin signaling caused by Alzheimer's disease–associated Aβ oligomers. *J. Clin. Investig.* 2012;122:1339–1353. doi: 10.1172/JCI57256.
357. Dineley K.T., Westerman M., Bui D., Bell K., Ashe K.H., Sweatt J.D. B-amyloid activates the mitogen-activated protein kinase cascade via hippocampal α7 nicotinic acetylcholine receptors: In vitro and in vivo mechanisms related to Alzheimer's disease. *J. Neurosci.* 2001;21:4125–4133. doi: 10.1523/JNEUROSCI.21-12-04125.2001.
358. Talbot K., Wang H.-Y., Kazi H., Han L.-Y., Bakshi K.P., Stucky A., Fuino R.L., Kawaguchi K.R., Samoyedny A.J., Wilson R.S. Demonstrated brain insulin resistance in Alzheimer's disease patients is associated with IGF-1 resistance, IRS-1 dysregulation, and cognitive decline. *J.*

Clin. Investig. 2012;122:1316–1338. doi: 10.1172/JCI59903.

359. Unger J.W., Livingston J.N., Moss A.M. Insulin receptors in the central nervous system: Localization, signalling mechanisms and functional aspects. *Prog. Neurobiol.* 1991;36:343–362. doi: 10.1016/0301-0082(91)90015-S.

360. Moroo I., Yamada T., Makino H., Tooyama I., McGeer P., McGeer E., Hirayama K. Loss of insulin receptor immunoreactivity from the substantia nigra pars compacta neurons in Parkinson's disease. *Acta Neuropathol.* 1994;87:343–348. doi: 10.1007/BF00313602.

361. Takahashi M., Yamada T., Tooyama I., Moroo I., Kimura H., Yamamoto T., Okada H. Insulin receptor mRNA in the substantia nigra in Parkinson's disease. *Neurosci. Lett.* 1996;204:201–204. doi: 10.1016/0304-3940(96)12357-0.

362. Bowen B.C., Block R.E., Sanchez-Ramos J., Pattany P.M., Lampman D.A., Murdoch J.B., Quencer R.M. Proton MR spectroscopy of the brain in 14 patients with Parkinson disease. *Am. J. Neuroradiol.* 1995;16:61–68.

363. Hu M., Taylor-Robinson S.D., Chaudhuri K.R., Bell J.D., Labbe C., Cunningham V., Koepp M., Hammers A., Morris R., Turjanski N. Cortical dysfunction in non-demented Parkinson's disease patients: A combined 31P-MRS and 18FDG-PET study. *Brain J. Neurol.* 2000;123:340–352. doi: 10.1093/brain/123.2.340.

364. Lalić N.M., Marić J., Svetel M., Jotić A., Stefanova E., Lalić K., Dragašević N., Miličić T., Lukić L., Kostić V.S. Glucose homeostasis in Huntington disease: Abnormalities in insulin sensitivity and early-phase insulin secretion. *Arch. Neurol.* 2008;65:476–480. doi: 10.1001/archneur.65.4.476.

365. Montojo M.T., Aganzo M., González N. Huntington's disease and diabetes: Chronological sequence of its association. *J. Huntington's Dis.* 2017;6:179–188. doi: 10.3233/JHD-170253.

366. Viollet B., Guigas B., Garcia N.S., Leclerc J., Foretz M., Andreelli F. Cellular and molecular mechanisms of metformin: An overview. *Clin. Sci.* 2012;122:253–270. doi: 10.1042/CS20110386.

367. Patrone C., Eriksson O., Lindholm D. Diabetes drugs and neurological disorders: New views and therapeutic possibilities. *Lancet Diabetes Endocrinol.* 2014;2:256–262. doi: 10.1016/S2213-8587(13)70125-6.

368. Bayliss J.A., Lemus M.B., Santos V.V., Deo M., Davies J.S., Kemp B.E., Elsworth J.D., Andrews Z.B. Metformin prevents nigrostriatal dopamine degeneration independent of AMPK activation in dopamine neurons. *PLoS ONE.* 2016;11:e0159381. doi: 10.1371/journal.pone.0159381.

369. Ismaiel A.A., Espinosa-Oliva A.M., Santiago M., García-Quintanilla A., Oliva-Martín M.J., Herrera A.J., Venero J.L., de Pablos R.M. Metformin, besides exhibiting strong in vivo anti-inflammatory properties, increases MPTP-induced damage to the nigrostriatal dopaminergic system. *Toxicol. Appl. Pharmacol.* 2016;298:19–30. doi: 10.1016/j.taap.2016.03.004.

370. Kang H., Khang R., Ham S., Jeong G.R., Kim H., Jo M., Lee B.D., Lee Y.I., Jo A., Park C. Activation of the ATF2/CREB-PGC-1α pathway by metformin leads to dopaminergic neuroprotection. *Oncotarget.* 2017;8:48603. doi: 10.18632/oncotarget.18122.

371. Chen F., Dong R.R., Zhong K.L., Ghosh A., Tang S.S., Long Y., Hu M., Miao M.X., Liao J.M., Sun H.B. Antidiabetic drugs restore abnormal transport of amyloid-β across the blood–brain barrier and memory impairment in db/db mice. *Neuropharmacology.* 2016;101:123–136. doi: 10.1016/j.neuropharm.2015.07.023.

372. Wahlqvist M.L., Lee M.-S., Hsu C.-C., Chuang S.-Y., Lee J.-T., Tsai H.-N. Metformin-inclusive

sulfonylurea therapy reduces the risk of Parkinson's disease occurring with type 2 diabetes in a Taiwanese population cohort. *Park. Relat. Disord.* 2012;18:753–758. doi: 10.1016/j.parkreldis.2012.03.010.

373. Ye F., Luo Y.-J., Xiao J., Yu N.-W., Yi G. Impact of insulin sensitizers on the incidence of dementia: A meta-analysis. *Dement. Geriatr. Cogn. Disord.* 2016;41:251–260. doi: 10.1159/000445941.
374. Koenig A.M., Mechanic-Hamilton D., Xie S.X., Combs M.F., Cappola A.R., Xie L., Detre J.A., Wolk D.A., Arnold S.E. Effects of the insulin sensitizer metformin in Alzheimer's disease: Pilot data from a randomized placebo-controlled crossover study. *Alzheimer Dis. Assoc. Disord.* 2017;31:107. doi: 10.1097/WAD.0000000000000202.
375. Hervás D., Fornés-Ferrer V., Gómez-Escribano A.P., Sequedo M.D., Peiró C., Millán J.M., Vázquez-Manrique R.P. Metformin intake associates with better cognitive function in patients with Huntington's disease. *PLoS ONE.* 2017;12:e0179283. doi: 10.1371/journal.pone.0179283.
376. Hampel H., Mesulam M.-M., Cuello A.C., Farlow M.R., Giacobini E., Grossberg G.T., Khachaturian A.S., Vergallo A., Cavedo E., Snyder P.J. The cholinergic system in the pathophysiology and treatment of Alzheimer's disease. *Brain J. Neurol.* 2018;141:1917–1933. doi: 10.1093/brain/awy132.
377. Mesulam M.M. Cholinergic circuitry of the human nucleus basalis and its fate in Alzheimer's disease. *J. Comp. Neurol.* 2013;521:4124–4144. doi: 10.1002/cne.23415.
378. Bowen D.M., Smith C.B., White P., Davison A.N. Neurotransmitter-related enzymes and indices of hypoxia in senile dementia and other abiotrophies. *Brain J. Neurol.* 1976;99:459–496. doi: 10.1093/brain/99.3.459.
379. Davies P., Maloney A. Selective loss of central cholinergic neurons in Alzheimer's disease. *Lancet.* 1976;308:1403. doi: 10.1016/S0140-6736(76)91936-X.
380. Mesulam M. A horseradish peroxidase method for the identification of the efferents of acetyl cholinesterase-containing neurons. *J. Histochem. Cytochem.* 1976;24:1281–1285. doi: 10.1177/24.12.826585.
381. Whitehouse P.J., Price D.L., Clark A.W., Coyle J.T., DeLong M.R. Alzheimer disease: Evidence for selective loss of cholinergic neurons in the nucleus basalis. *Ann. Neurol. Off. J. Am. Neurol. Assoc. Child Neurol. Soc.* 1981;10:122–126. doi: 10.1002/ana.410100203.
382. Drachman D.A., Leavitt J. Human memory and the cholinergic system: A relationship to aging? *Arch. Neurol.* 1974;30:113–121. doi: 10.1001/archneur.1974.00490320001001.
383. Summers W.K., Majovski L.V., Marsh G.M., Tachiki K., Kling A. Oral tetrahydroaminoacridine in long-term treatment of senile dementia, Alzheimer type. *N. Engl. J. Med.* 1986;315:1241–1245. doi: 10.1056/NEJM198611133152001.
384. Petersen R.C. Scopolamine induced learning failures in man. *Psychopharmacology.* 1977;52:283–289. doi: 10.1007/BF00426713.
385. Izquierdo I. Mechanism of action of scopolamine as an amnestic. *Trends Pharmacol. Sci.* 1989;10:175–177. doi: 10.1016/0165-6147(89)90231-9.
386. Lovestone S., Howard R. Alzheimer's disease: A treatment in sight? *J. Neurol. Neurosurgery, Psychiatry.* 1995;59:566. doi: 10.1136/jnnp.59.6.566.
387. Massoud F., Gauthier S. Update on the pharmacological treatment of Alzheimer's disease. *Curr. Neuropharmacol.* 2010;8:69–80. doi: 10.2174/157015910790909520.

388. Hansen R.A., Gartlehner G., Webb A.P., Morgan L.C., Moore C.G., Jonas D.E. Efficacy and safety of donepezil, galantamine, and rivastigmine for the treatment of Alzheimer's disease: A systematic review and meta-analysis. *Clin. Interv. Aging.* 2008;3:211.

389. Richter N., Beckers N., Onur O.A., Dietlein M., Tittgemeyer M., Kracht L., Neumaier B., Fink G.R., Kukolja J. Effect of cholinergic treatment depends on cholinergic integrity in early Alzheimer's disease. *Brain J. Neurol.* 2018;141:903–915. doi: 10.1093/brain/awx356.

390. Schmitz T.W., Spreng R.N., Weiner M.W., Aisen P., Petersen R., Jack C.R., Jagust W., Trojanowki J.Q., Toga A.W., Beckett L. Basal forebrain degeneration precedes and predicts the cortical spread of Alzheimer's pathology. *Nat. Commun.* 2016;7:13249. doi: 10.1038/ncomms13249.

391. Sigurdsson E.M., Permanne B., Soto C., Wisniewski T., Frangione B. In vivo reversal of amyloid-β lesions in rat brain. *J. Neuropathol. Exp. Neurol.* 2000;59:11–17. doi: 10.1093/jnen/59.1.11.

392. Morgan D., Diamond D.M., Gottschall P.E., Ugen K.E., Dickey C., Hardy J., Duff K., Jantzen P., DiCarlo G., Wilcock D. Aβ peptide vaccination prevents memory loss in an animal model of Alzheimer's disease. *Nature.* 2000;408:982–985. doi: 10.1038/35050116.

393. Janus C., Pearson J., McLaurin J., Mathews P.M., Jiang Y., Schmidt S.D., Chishti M.A., Horne P., Heslin D., French J. Aβ peptide immunization reduces behavioural impairment and plaques in a model of Alzheimer's disease. *Nature.* 2000;408:979–982. doi: 10.1038/35050110.

394. Schenk D., Barbour R., Dunn W., Gordon G., Grajeda H., Guido T., Hu K., Huang J., Johnson-Wood K., Khan K. Immunization with amyloid-β attenuates Alzheimer-disease-like pathology in the PDAPP mouse. *Nature.* 1999;400:173–177. doi: 10.1038/22124.

395. Vandenberghe R., Rinne J.O., Boada M., Katayama S., Scheltens P., Vellas B., Tuchman M., Gass A., Fiebach J.B., Hill D. Bapineuzumab for mild to moderate Alzheimer's disease in two global, randomized, phase 3 trials. *Alzheimer's Res. Ther.* 2016;8:18. doi: 10.1186/s13195-016-0189-7.

396. Lacey L., Bobula J., Rüdell K., Alvir J., Leibman C. Quality of life and utility measurement in a large clinical trial sample of patients with mild to moderate Alzheimer's disease: Determinants and level of changes observed. *Value Health.* 2015;18:638–645. doi: 10.1016/j.jval.2015.03.1787.

397. Honig L.S., Vellas B., Woodward M., Boada M., Bullock R., Borrie M., Hager K., Andreasen N., Scarpini E., Liu-Seifert H. Trial of solanezumab for mild dementia due to Alzheimer's disease. *N. Engl. J. Med.* 2018;378:321–330. doi: 10.1056/NEJMoa1705971.

398. Siemers E., Sundell K., Carlson C., Case M., Sethuraman G., Liu-Seifert H., Dowsett S., Pontecorvo M., Dean R., Demattos R. Phase 3 solanezumab trials: Secondary outcomes in mild Alzheimer's disease patients. *Alzheimer's Dement.* 1983;12:1–11. doi: 10.1016/j.jalz.2015.06.1893.

399. Bateman R.J., Benzinger T.L., Berry S., Clifford D.B., Duggan C., Fagan A.M., Fanning K., Farlow M.R., Hassenstab J., McDade E.M. The DIAN-TU next generation Alzheimer's prevention trial: Adaptive design and disease progression model. *Alzheimer's Dement. J. Alzheimer's Assoc.* 2017;13:8–19. doi: 10.1016/j.jalz.2016.07.005.

400. DeMattos R.B., Lu J., Tang Y., Racke M.M., DeLong C.A., Tzaferis J.A., Hole J.T., Forster B.M., McDonnell P.C., Liu F. A plaque-specific antibody clears existing β-amyloid plaques in Alzheimer's disease mice. *Neuron.* 2012;76:908–920. doi: 10.1016/j.neuron.2012.10.029.

401. Irizarry M.C., Sims J.R., Lowe S.L., Nakano M., Hawdon A., Willis B.A., Gonzales C., Liu P., Fujimoto S., Dean R.A. Safety, pharmacokinetics (PK), and florbetapir F-18 positron emission tomography

(PET) after multiple dose administration of LY3002813, a β-amyloid plaque-specific antibody, in Alzheimer's disease (AD) *Alzheimer's Dement. J. Alzheimer's Assoc.* 2016;12:P352–P353. doi: 10.1016/j.jalz.2016.06.665. [CrossRef] [Google Scholar]

402. Bohrmann B., Baumann K., Benz J., Gerber F., Huber W., Knoflach F., Messer J., Oroszlan K., Rauchenberger R., Richter W.F. Gantenerumab: A novel human anti-Aβ antibody demonstrates sustained cerebral amyloid-β binding and elicits cell-mediated removal of human amyloid-β *J. Alzheimer's Dis.* 2012;28:49–69. doi: 10.3233/JAD-2011-110977.

403. Blaettler T., Smith J., Smith J., Paul R., Asnaghi V., Fuji R., Quartino A., Honigberg L., Rabbia M.A., Yule S. Clinical trial design of cread: A randomized, double-blind, placebo-controlled, parallel-group phase 3 study to evaluate crenezumab treatment in patients with prodromal-to-mild Alzheimer's disease. *Alzheimer's Dement. J. Alzheimer's Assoc.* 2016;12:P609. doi: 10.1016/j.jalz.2016.06.1207. [CrossRef] [Google Scholar]

404. Adolfsson O., Pihlgren M., Toni N., Varisco Y., Buccarello A.L., Antoniello K., Lohmann S., Piorkowska K., Gafner V., Atwal J.K. An effector-reduced anti-β-amyloid (Aβ) antibody with unique Aβ binding properties promotes neuroprotection and glial engulfment of Aβ *J. Neurosci.* 2012;32:9677–9689. doi: 10.1523/JNEUROSCI.4742-11.2012.

405. Tucker S., Möller C., Tegerstedt K., Lord A., Laudon H., Sjödahl J., Söderberg L., Spens E., Sahlin C., Waara E.R. The murine version of BAN2401 (mAb158) selectively reduces amyloid-β protofibrils in brain and cerebrospinal fluid of tg-arcswe mice. *J. Alzheimer's Dis.* 2015;43:575–588. doi: 10.3233/JAD-140741.

406. Logovinsky V., Satlin A., Lai R., Swanson C., Kaplow J., Osswald G., Basun H., Lannfelt L. Safety and tolerability of BAN2401-a clinical study in Alzheimer's disease with a protofibril selective Aβ antibody. *Alzheimer's Res. Ther.* 2016;8:14. doi: 10.1186/s13195-016-0181-2.

407. Satlin A., Wang J., Logovinsky V., Berry S., Swanson C., Dhadda S., Berry D.A. Design of a bayesian adaptive phase 2 proof-of-concept trial for BAN2401, a putative disease-modifying monoclonal antibody for the treatment of Alzheimer's disease. *Alzheimer's Dement. Transl. Res. Clin. Interv.* 2016;2:1–12. doi: 10.1016/j.trci.2016.01.001.

408. Sevigny J., Chiao P., Bussière T., Weinreb P.H., Williams L., Maier M., Dunstan R., Salloway S., Chen T., Ling Y. The antibody aducanumab reduces Aβ plaques in Alzheimer's disease. *Nature.* 2016;537:50–56. doi: 10.1038/nature19323.

409. Kastanenka K.V., Bussiere T., Shakerdge N., Qian F., Weinreb P.H., Rhodes K., Bacskai B.J. Immunotherapy with aducanumab restores calcium homeostasis in Tg2576 mice. *J. Neurosci.* 2016;36:12549–12558. doi: 10.1523/JNEUROSCI.2080-16.2016.

INDEX

G

H

I

J

K

L

U

V

W

X

Z